Medical Response to Child Sexual Abuse

A Resource for Professionals Working With Children and Families

Second Edition

STM **Learning,** Inc.

Leading Publisher of Scientific, Technical, and Medical Educational Resources

Saint Louis

www.stmlearning.com

Dedication to the Second Edition

It seems appropriate that a physician who dedicated so much love and energy into caring for children, families, and other professionals was born on Valentine's Day. Rich Kaplan embodied our multidisciplinary approach throughout his career—political activist, social worker, pediatrician, and child abuse pediatrician. Rich established child advocacy centers in South Dakota and Minnesota; comprehensive child abuse programs, including the Center for Safe and Healthy Children in Minneapolis; and was a founding member of the Ray E. Helfer Society, a professional society designed to advance the clinical care, education, research, and advocacy of child maltreatment. Rich Kaplan was a medical leader in our profession serving as a mentor and educator to so many healthcare and child welfare professionals. It has been an honor to serve as authors of the 2nd edition of what we refer to as "the Kaplan textbook."

Randall Alexander, MD, PhD
Nancy S. Harper MD, FAAP

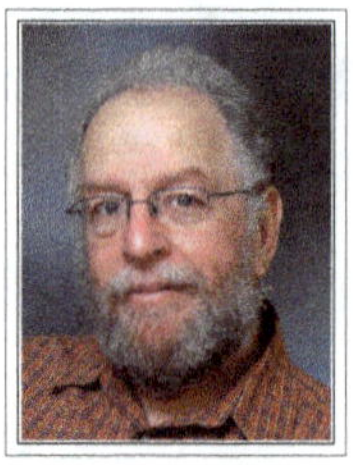

Rich Alan Kaplan
1950 – 2013

In Rich Kaplan's own words:

I know the work can be daunting
And I'm not helping with this rhyme
As everyone it seems is wanting
Pieces of your precious time

My very good friends
I trust you are doing well

Dedication to the First Edition

This book is dedicated to everyone who has been affected by child sexual abuse. It is our sincere hope that this will empower medical providers to give the most up-to-date and scientifically based care for victims. No one should undergo the trauma that these youngsters have undergone without high quality and responsive medical care in addition to other community interventions. It is our profound hope that this text makes a difference.

Rich Kaplan, MSW, MD, FAAP
Joyce A. Adams, MD
Suzanne P. Starling, MD, FAAP
Angelo P. Giardino, MD, PhD, MPH, FAAP

Medical Response to Child Sexual Abuse

A Resource for Professionals Working With Children and Families

Second Edition

Randell Alexander, MD, PhD
Professor and Chief
Division of Child Protection
and Forensic Pediatrics
University of Florida
Jacksonville, Florida

Nancy S. Harper, MD, FAAP
Director
Otto Bremer Trust Center for Safe
and Healthy Children
Child Abuse Pediatrics
Associate Professor
Department of Pediatrics
University of Minnesota

STM **Learning,** Inc.

Leading Publisher of Scientific, Technical, and Medical Educational Resources
Saint Louis
www.stmlearning.com

Publishers: Glenn E. Whaley and Marianne V. Whaley
Graphic Design Director: Glenn E. Whaley
Acquisitions Editor: Glenn E. Whaley
Associate Editor: Marika Betker
Book Design/Page Layout: Jennifer M. Jones and G.W. Graphics
Print/Production Coordinator: Jennifer M. Jones and G.W. Graphics
Cover Design: Jennifer M. Jones and G.W. Graphics
Color Repress Specialist: Kevin Tucker
Developmental Editor: Stavra Ketchmark
Copy Editor: Marika Betker
Proofreader: Marika Betker and Jessica Moore

Printed in the United States of America.

Publisher:
STM Learning, Inc.
Saint Louis, Missouri
Phone: (314) 434-2424
https://www.stmlearning.com orders@stmlearning.com

Library of Congress Cataloging-in-Publication Data

Names: Alexander, Randell, 1950- author. | Harper, Nancy S. (Nancy Sanders), 1969- author.
Title: Medical response to child sexual abuse : a resource for professionals working with children and families / Randell Alexander, Nancy S. Harper.
Description: Second edition. | Saint Louis : STM Learning, Inc., [2019] | Preceded by Medical response to child sexual abuse / Rich Kaplan ... [et al]. c2011. | Includes bibliographical references and index.
Identifiers: LCCN 2019008888 (print) | LCCN 2019009654 (ebook) | ISBN 9781936590759 (ebook) | ISBN 9781936590742 (pbk.)
Subjects: | MESH: Child Abuse, Sexual--diagnosis | Child Abuse, Sexual--therapy | Physical Examination--methods | Forensic Medicine--methods | Child | Adolescent
Classification: LCC RJ507.S49 (ebook) | LCC RJ507.S49 (print) | NLM WA 325 | DDC 618.92/85836--dc23
LC record available at https://lccn.loc.gov/2019008888

Contributors to the Second Edition

Joyce A. Adams, MD
Adams Pediatric Consulting
Retired Clinical Professor of Pediatrics
University of California, San Diego

Nora J. Baladerian, PhD
Counseling Center of West Los Angeles
Disability and Abuse Project of Spectrum Institute
Los Angeles, California

Craig L. Barlow, JD
Assistant Chief Criminal Deputy
Utah Attorney General's Office
Salt Lake City, Utah

Allan R. De Jong, MD
Co-Medical Director
Children at Risk Evaluation (CARE) Program
Nemours/Alfred I. duPont Hospital for Children
Wilmington, Delaware
Clinical Professor of Pediatrics
Sidney Kimmel Medical College
Thomas Jefferson University
Philadelphia, Pennsylvania

Stephanie A. Deutsch, MD, MS, FAAP
Department of General Pediatrics
Nemours/Alfred I. duPont Hospital for Children
Co-Medical Director
Children at Risk Evaluation (CARE) Program
Wilmington, Delaware

Karen J. Farst, MD, MPH
University of Arkansas for Medical Sciences
Section for Children at Risk
Arkansas Children's Hospital
Team for Children at Risk
Little Rock, Arkansas

Martin A. Finkel, DO, FACOP, FAAP
Professor of Pediatrics
Founder and Medical Director
Child Abuse Research Education & Service (CARES) Institute
Rowan University School of Osteopathic Medicine
Stratford, New Jersey

Jordan Greenbaum, MD
Staff physician
Stephanie V. Blank Center for Safe and Healthy Children
Children's Healthcare of Atlanta
Medical director
International Centre for Missing and Exploited Children

Jessica L. Griffin, PsyD
Associate Professor of Psychiatry and Pediatrics
Executive Director and Principal Investigator
Child Trauma Training Center
University of Massachusetts Medical School

Mark Hudson, MD
Midwest Children's Resource Center
Children's Hospitals and Clinics of Minnesota

Angela Kaufman, MA, CI/CT
ADA Consultant
Violence Against Persons with Disabilities
and Emergency Management
Los Angeles, California

Nancy D. Kellogg, MD
Division Chief and Professor of Pediatrics
Division of Child Abuse Pediatrics
University of Texas Health Science Center, San Antonio
San Antonio, Texas

Natalie Kissoon, MD, FAAP
Fellowship Program Director
Assistant Professor, Clinical
Department of Pediatrics
Division of Child Abuse
UT Health San Antonio
San Antonio, Texas

Kelly Liker, MD, FAAP
Chief, Division of Child Advocacy
Dayton Children's Hospital
Assistant Professor
Department of Pediatrics
Boonshoft School of Medicine
Wright State University
Dayton, Ohio

Marcellina Mian, MDCM, MHPE, FAAP, FRCPC
Professor Emerita of Pediatrics
Weill Cornell Medicine in Qatar
Doha, Qatar

Dena Nazer, MD, FAAP
Associate Professor of Pediatrics
Wayne State University
Chief, Child Protection Team
Child's Hospital of Michigan
Detroit, Michigan

Vincent J. Palusci, MD, MS, FAAP
Professor of Pediatrics
NYU School of Medicine
Chair, Hassenfeld Children's Hospital
Child Protection Committee
New York, New York

Carol A. Plummer, PhD
Retired Associate Professor
University of Hawai'i at Mānoa

Marcella F. Scott, MSPH
Crime Laboratory Analyst Supervisor
Florida Department of Law Enforcement
Jacksonville Regional Operations Center
Jacksonville, Florida

Lora Spiller, MD
Child Abuse Pediatrician
University of Texas Health San Antonio
San Antonio, Texas

Alice D. Swenson, MD, FAAP
Staff Physician
Midwest Children's Resource Center
Children's Hospitals and Clinics of Minnesota
Saint Paul, Minnesota

Jonathan D. Thackeray, MD
Vice-Chair and Professor of Pediatrics
Boonshoft School of Medicine
Wright State University
Chief Medical Community Health Officer
Dayton Children's Hospital
Dayton, Ohio

Supplemental Photo Contributions

Diana Faugno, MSN, RN, CPN, SANE-A, SANE-P, FAAFS, DF-IAFN, DF-AFN
Arne K. Myhre, MD
Tor Shwayder, MD, FAAP, FAAD
Mary J. Spencer, BA, MD, FAAP

Contributors to the First Edition

Michelle I. Amaya, MD, MPH
ABP Board Certified, Child Abuse Pediatrics
Associate Professor
Department of Pediatrics
Medical University of South Carolina
Charleston, South Carolina

Kathy Bell, MS, RN, SANE-A, SANE-P
Forensic Nursing Administrator
Tulsa Police Department
Tulsa, Oklahoma

Robert W. Block, MD, FAAP
Professor and Daniel C. Plunket Chair
Department of Pediatrics
School of Community Medicine
The University of Oklahoma-Tulsa

Daniel D. Broughton, MD
Professor of Pediatric and Adolescent Medicine
Mayo Clinic
Rochester, Minnesota

Michelle Clayton, MD, MPH, FAAP
Assistant Professor of Pediatrics
Eastern Virginia Medical School
Children's Hospital of the King's Daughter
Norfolk, Virginia

Judith A. Cohen, MD
Medical Director
Center for Traumatic Stress in Children & Adolescents
Allegheny General Hospital
Professor of Psychiatry
Drexel University College of Medicine
Pittsburgh, Pennsylvania

Sharon W. Cooper, MD, FAAP
Adjunct Professor of Pediatrics
University of North Carolina School of Medicine
Chapel Hill, North Carolina

Lori Frasier, MD
Professor of Pediatrics
Medical Director
Medical Assessment Team
Primary Children's Center for Safe and Healthy Families
Salt Lake City, Utah

Roberta A. Hibbard, MD
Professor of Pediatrics
Director
Section of Child Protection Programs
Indiana University School of Medicine
Indianapolis, Indiana

Jerry G. Jones, MD
Professor of Pediatrics
University of Arkansas for Medical Sciences
Director
Center for Children at Risk
University of Arkansas for Medical Sciences
Arkansas Children's Hospital
Little Rock, Arkansas

Anthony C. Leonard, PhD
Assistant Professor
Biostatistician
Department of Public Health Sciences
University of Cincinnati College of Medicine
Cincinnati, Ohio

Kathi L. Makoroff, MD
Assistant Professor of Pediatrics
University of Cincinnati College of Medicine
Mayerson Center for Safe and Healthy Children
Cincinnati Children's Hospital and Medical Center
Cincinnati, Ohio

Anthony P. Mannarino, PhD

Laura K. Murray, PhD
Assistant Professor of International Health
Boston University School of Public Health
Boston, Massachusetts

Robert A. Shapiro, MD
Professor of Clinical Pediatrics
University of Cincinnati College of Medicine
Medical Director
Mayerson Center for Safe and Healthy Children
Cincinnati Children's Hospital Medical Center
Cincinnati, Ohio

John Stirling, Jr., MD
Director
Center for Child Protection
Santa Clara Valley Medical Center
Medical Director
Santa Clara Country's Children Shelter
San Jose, California
Clinical Professor
Stanford University
Lucile Packard Children's Hospital
Palo Alto, California

Supplemental Photo Contributors

Michelle Ditton, RN, FNE, SANE-A, SANE-P
Margie Jessen, RN, FNP
Marilyn Kaufhold, MD
Carolyn Levitt, MD
Lynn Sheets, MD

Foreword to the Second Edition

In their landmark 1993 article, Olafson, Corwin, and Summit traced the history of the denial of child sexual abuse from the 17th Century to the 1970s (*Child Abuse Negl.* 1993;17(1):7-24). Re-reading this paper led me to realize how much has changed in our approach to this problem since then.

I am pleased to recommend this comprehensive reference, *Medical Response to Child Sexual Abuse, Second Edition.* It provides medical and nursing folks with everything they need to know about world-class sexual abuse evaluations. We have done more than *recognize* the importance of a robust response to children and adolescents who have experienced abuse. We have *embraced* this as an important component of health care.

So much has changed in the past forty plus years that doctors, nurses, physician assistants, and nurse practitioners have been taking care of children when sexual abuse is suspected. The amount of knowledge has expanded to an extent that keeping up with new developments is daunting. It's good to know there is one reference available to refine our practice in the 21st century.

The topics covered in this book are relevant to medical people, but other disciplines (perhaps law enforcement or prosecutors) might find the contents to be a valuable reference explaining everything medical. Particularly helpful are chapters on complex topics such as sexually transmitted diseases, DNA evidence, and mimics of physical findings of sexual abuse.

The list of contributors is impressive—all of them have added to the richness of the knowledge we now have available. This is a "who's who" of people who have advanced our understanding of this field.

One cannot approach the new edition of *Medical Response to Child Sexual Abuse* without remembering the originator of this book, Rich Kaplan. He was an inspiring figure in Child Abuse Pediatrics, and his humor and insight are still greatly missed.

Congratulations to Randy Alexander and Nancy Harper on this important book.

Carole Jenny, MD, MBA, FAAP
Professor of Pediatrics
University of Washington School of Medicine
Seattle Children's Hospital

Foreword to the Second Edition

By the time I began to see children and adolescents for alleged sexual abuse in the early 1990s, it was already becoming clear that diagnostic medical findings were uncommon. Over the subsequent 25 years, it has been established that in most cases the role of the health professional will not be to provide "proof" that the abuse took place, but to provide therapeutic healthcare as one part of a comprehensive multidisciplinary and multi-agency process. To see the child and family promptly; to approach them with empathy and respect; to give them time; to appreciate the child's developmental level and tailor an assessment accordingly; to recognize that sexual abuse may coexist with many other forms of abuse, violence, or neglect and with a wide variety of health, educational, and social needs; to conduct an examination with informed consent, in an appropriate physical environment, and with an appropriate support person; to know which examination findings are significant and which are not; to know when the collection of forensic evidence is appropriate and to collect it according to best practice standards; to document history and examination findings clearly in such a way that they can be subject to peer review; to provide medical treatment if needed; to debrief carefully with the child and family; to ensure appropriate follow-up (including for effects on mental health); to advocate for the child's safety and welfare; to communicate and collaborate effectively with child protective services and the police; and to be ready and able to assist the court as an expert witness within the parameters of current scientific knowledge.

This is demanding work. In the second edition of this authoritative textbook, a wide range of experts provide a superb resource for all who wish to do it well, and a challenge to consider new frontiers: recognition of sexual abuse in children with disabilities, commercial sexual exploitation (including online exploitation), and effective prevention. Of course, no book can replace the need for appropriate training, supervision, and peer review. It is crucial, for example, that healthcare providers learn practices for taking a history from sexually abused children that are endorsed by child protective services and the police in their own jurisdiction. Nonetheless, those who are already experts in the medical response to child sexual abuse will find both inspiration and new information in these pages; and for those who are not (both health professionals and our colleagues from other professions and other agencies), this book will provide an indispensable source of reference.

We have come a long way, but we still have a long way to go. May this book spur us all to advance our practice. In the words of a much-respected indigenous elder in my own country, Sir James Henare:

"Maha rawa wā tatou mahi te kore mahi tonu, tawhiti rawa to tatou haerenga, te kore haere tonu"—
"We have done too much to not do more, we have come too far to not go further."

Patrick Kelly, MBChB, FRACP
Service Clinical Director
Te Puaruruhau (Child Protection Team)
Starship Children's Health
Honorary Associate Professor
Department of Pediatrics: Child and Youth Health
Faculty of Medical and Health Sciences
University of Auckland
Auckland, New Zealand

Foreword to the First Edition

Substantiation of reports of sexual abuse of children has been declining since 1990, reduced by 51%, according to Jones (*Childhood Victimization: Violence, Crime, and Abuse in the Lives of Young People*). Researchers in this field expressed doubt that this steep decline could be real, and this prompted further investigation (*Child Abuse Negl.* 2001;25:1139-1158). The findings of this research suggested that the decline was real and did not reflect changed standards by agencies or other artifactual explanations (*Explanations for the Decline in Child Sexual Abuse Cases*). They found that this decline paralleled other social improvements: the fall in teen suicides, teenage births, numbers of children living in poverty, youth runaways, juvenile drug use, and improvements in child behavior problems and competence scores on the Child Behavior Checklist. While considering numerous factors to explain these trends, Finkelhor and Jones suggest that agents of social intervention "could well have curbed child victimization through a number of mechanisms" (*Childhood Victimization: Violence, Crime, and Abuse in the Lives of Young People*). These agents include police, victim advocates, legal advocates, teachers who educate about maltreatment and domestic violence, as well as the media, who have raised awareness of victimization by reporting on maltreatment and by portraying it in several films and television formats.

I believe another factor to be involved: more highly developed professional skills at all levels of the diagnostic process. Over the last 25 years, the evidence base in child sexual abuse has grown exponentially. Since 1994, over 300 peer-reviewed articles have been published in medical journals alone, and this figure doesn't include research published in the social sciences, mental health, legal, and law enforcement publications. In addition, the education and training of professionals for this field of practice has improved substantially. This ensures more accurate diagnosis in these cases and avoids confusing normal variants or other mimics of sexual abuse for true cases.

This is where this up-to-date, well-written book is so helpful. The authors of the various chapters in *Medical Response to Child Sexual Abuse* are truly experts in the field, with clinical experience and research to bolster their writing. There are chapters in this volume that are not available in other books on sexual abuse: the background and history of the field, special problems of adolescent patients, qualifications of medical examiners, child sexual abuse as a global issue, child sexual abuse as a symptom, an approach to the disabled child who may have been abused, and sexual abuse prevention strategies, to name just a few. These, in addition to the basics about anatomy and the medical approach to diagnosis, will equip the child abuse professional to be more proficient and precise in the performance and interpretation of a child sexual abuse evaluation.

Robert M. Reece, MD
Clinical Professor of Pediatrics
Tufts University School of Medicine
Director
Child Protection Program
The Floating Hospital for Children
Tufts New England Medical Center
Boston, Massachusetts
Editor
The Quarterly Update
North Falmouth, Massachusetts

Foreword to the First Edition

We may never truly know exactly how many children are sexually abused during their childhood years, but we do know that the numbers are enormous. Child sexual abuse is more common than childhood cancer, childhood diabetes, and congenital heart disease combined. Despite this, public discussion or even acknowledgement of this issue was not commonplace throughout most of history. This is no longer the case today. In fact, public awareness of the problem has never been higher. Internet predators, clergy abuse scandals, and cases involving child pornography regularly make local and national headlines alongside countless other stories of children being sexually abused by family members or other close contacts. Many of the television crime dramas watched by children and parents alike now routinely include stories about the sexual abuse of children. As our collective awareness of the problem of child sexual abuse has grown, so has the recognition that the response of the professional community must involve a collaborative, multidisciplinary approach in order to be successful. Law enforcement, social services, mental health, and medical providers now routinely work closely together to respond to cases of child sexual abuse, each providing their own specific services and expertise to respond to this problem. Of particular importance in this multidisciplinary approach to the care of sexually abused children is the medical component. There have been many changes over the past several decades with regard to what "having a medical evaluation" means for sexually abused children. Much has been learned about anatomy, interpretation of findings, evidence collection, medical management, therapy, and prevention. Consequently, the current standards of care for the medical management of sexually abused children are quite different today than in decades past. It is critical that all professionals who work with sexually abused children are familiar with what the medical response should involve.

It is in this context that Dr. Rich Kaplan has brought together many of the world's leading authorities regarding child sexual abuse to create *Medical Response to Child Sexual Abuse*. Dr. Kaplan brings his vast experience and his unique perspective to this text, having worked with abused children for over 30 years—first as a social worker and then as a pediatrician. His thoughtful, thorough, objective, meticulous, and hopeful approach to providing care to children is reflected throughout the book. Dr. Kaplan and his co-authors cover a vast amount of material in a clear and easily accessible manner. Although written from a medical perspective, *Medical Response to Child Sexual Abuse* is intended as a comprehensive resource for both medical as well as non-medical professionals. To know what the current, state-of-the-art standard of care approach to the medical evaluation of sexually abused children is, this text will serve as a primary resource.

The chapters that address basic anatomy of the genitalia and anus as well as the medical evaluation when sexual abuse is suspected should be mandatory reading not only for every clinician who provides medical care to children, but also to any other professional who works with sexually abused children. This book clarifies and demystifies the examination process, and most importantly, addresses what exams can and cannot "tell" us. We recognize that when children disclose sexual abuse, they do so in various timeframes, having experienced a wide variety of abuse. How does the care of a child who discloses an event that occurred yesterday differ from that of one who discloses an event from last summer? How does the care of an adolescent differ from that of a young child? What kind of medical management is required? We have learned that there is no "one exam fits all" response to child sexual abuse. This text addresses all these issues at length and allows the clinician to provide the best possible care to their patients. One of the most important issues in the medical evaluation of child sexual abuse is to ensure that physical findings are identified correctly for what they are. Dr. Kaplan's text addresses these issues at great length as well. *Medical Response to Child Sexual Abuse* also assists providers in working with children and families with the long term consequences of sexual abuse.

Quite simply, this text provides everything that professionals who work with sexually abused children and adolescents need to understand the medical response to child sexual abuse. Medical providers who are familiar with this information will provide even better care to the children they serve and will be more effective members of their community's multidisciplinary team. The non-medical professionals who use this book will better understand exactly what it is that medical providers can do for children and for them. We owe Dr. Kaplan and his co-authors a debt of gratitude for creating such a singularly useful text for all professionals who work with these children and their families.

James E. Crawford-Jakubiak, MD, FAAP
Medical Director
Center for Child Protection
Children's Hospital & Research Center Oakland
Oakland, California

Foreword to the First Edition

Medical Response to Child Sexual Abuse is a carefully crafted compendium of chapters taking the reader from an initial review of history to a glimpse of hope for the future. Along the way, we learn a great deal about what is known about child sexual abuse from basic anatomy to 5 chapters focused on medical evaluation issues, and other chapters presenting information on evidence-based literature review, the description and value of multidisciplinary teams, collaborative practice models, the importance of prevention, and expanding perspectives for the way we think about and react to the sexual maltreatment of children.

As the field of child abuse pediatrics has recently evolved into a pediatric subspecialty, we plan to increase the education of all health professionals in the many facets of violence and abuse involving children. The goal is to have informed health care providers at many levels, from those delivering primary care and those with increased knowledge and clinical competencies in child abuse to the pediatricians who are board certified in the subspecialty. We have learned a great deal over the last several years about the lifelong consequences of maltreatment. If we can properly discover, treat, and remedy the effects of sexual abuse, we can not only foster healthy lives, but we can also dramatically affect the huge economic costs of morbidity and mortality created by unrecognized abuse followed by health behaviors and physiologic responses to the stress created by the abuse.

An important outcome of having a uniformly informed cadre of clinicians evaluating children who may have been sexually abused will be consistency with the process of initial evaluation and treatment, follow-up care, documentation of important findings, and collaboration between physicians and other professionals. This text, complete with up-to-date information on interpretation of physical findings that include conditions that may mimic sexual abuse, sexually transmitted infections, and forensic interpretation, is a template for the consistency we desire. The reader will find well-referenced chapters, allowing easy access to the literature supporting authors' opinions and advice. Case scenarios and clear examples of clinical situations, as well as reports of successful approaches to child abuse prevention and intervention will assist readers in evaluating their own programs and/or developing new programs.

The contributors chosen by the authors are well known in the field and collectively have a great amount of experience, paving the way for the next generations of dedicated professionals that have a desire to work with children to both prevent their abuse and to intervene with an appropriate evaluation and diagnosis of sexual abuse when necessary.

We know now that most physical examinations of children alleging sexual abuse will be normal. Descriptions of these examinations are not only important medically, but legally as well. This is also true for descriptions of injuries when they are found. Appropriate treatment, whether for the emotional stability of the child, or for injuries or infections is an important facet of our work. *Medical Response to Child Sexual Abuse* clearly defines practical, evidence-informed advice for documenting and managing a variety of cases. When we are confronted with substantiating our findings and opinions in court, it is helpful to know that this text will be an accepted authority to support our work. For those future pediatricians who will bravely enter into fellowships in child abuse pediatrics, this book will pave the way to successful passage of certification examinations. For other health care providers, incorporating the information provided in the text will enable them to practice in an equivalent, evidence-based style consistent with the best practices all our children deserve. After all, it is our children for whom we seek the knowledge and skills necessary for their care.

Robert W. Block, MD, FAAP
Professor of Pediatrics
School of Community Medicine
The University of Oklahoma College of Medicine
Tulsa, Oklahoma

Preface to the Second Edition

Child sexual abuse has been increasingly appreciated as a broad subject, encompassing more than the core evaluation of a good forensic interview and medical examination. Building on the first edition of this book, there has been an increasing awareness of the importance of multidisciplinary collaboration in the approach to a case of suspected sexual abuse and the significance of history and physical findings.

This book has a particular focus on the medical evaluation of sexual abuse where the "evidence" is the history, not detectable damage to the genitalia. The importance of the medical history is usually key, but in those instances in which a physical finding is present, it is imperative that correct identification occur. Use of qualified medical examiners and working within a multidisciplinary team increases the sensitivity to sexual abuse and the need for a trauma-informed approach, but also decreases the risk for mistaken diagnoses and associated consequences for families.

Advances in DNA technology have changed some of the approaches to acute sexual assault. For example, a vaginal swab once thought to be useless for detection of specific male DNA has now been circumvented, in part by methods to detect the presence of male DNA amidst the plethora of female DNA. The epidemiology and pharmacological sensitivity of sexually transmitted infections has evolved. Methods to detect such infections have also improved with DNA based technology, and will continue to do so. Human trafficking and commercial sexual exploitation has been present throughout human history, but there is an increasing focus on detecting such cases, understanding the dynamics, and addressing the problem systemically.

There is also now a much deeper understanding of the harms of sexual abuse as a toxic stress or an adverse childhood experience and of the need for skilled trauma-focused therapists. Sexual abuse creates significant harms to the developing brain and results in long term health effects extending throughout adulthood. The brain has windows of sensitivity with age-dependent effects on brain structures. Sexual abuse is a neurobiological harm akin to a developmental disability—without the presence of an external injury—a point that is important for the legislative and legal communities to appreciate.

Ultimately, the goal is prevention. Not only tertiary identification of child victims, but primary prevention for those who would commit such acts. Understanding why children would be victimized is a frontier for the next decades. It should be approached with urgency—befitting the anguish and developmental harm this pandemic continues to cause.

We thank the authors of the previous edition: Rich Kaplan, Joyce Adams, Suzanne Starling, and Angelo Giardino for their impressive work. Our deep appreciation also goes to the wonderful contributors to this text. Collaboration with them was not only a pleasure, but educational for us as well.

Randell Alexander, MD, PhD
Nancy Harper, MD, FAAP

Preface to the First Edition

The concept of medical care for children who are possible victims of child sexual abuse is relatively new. In the last decade, we have seen the medical care for these children undergo a significant evolution in which we now see these children as patients who require medical attention and care. The focus of this book is to address the medical care for these children from a variety of perspectives.

Our central goal has been to demystify the medical care of these children, and it is emphasized that while there are special competencies involved, this is much more similar to medical care for other conditions than it is different. When caring for a child who is a possible victim of child sexual abuse, the same principles and standards of medical care exist, such as obtaining a complete and well-documented history and physical examination, performing an appropriate and scientifically driven laboratory evaluation, and forming a medical diagnosis to guide the ongoing care needs of the child. This is the definition of good pediatric medical care. It should be clear that the medical component is simply one part of the response to possible maltreatment, but we hope that this text will help crystallize the elements that make this component such an important part of the community response.

While the legal issues certainly are important for the safety and well-being of children, the focus of this text primarily will be on the medical and therapeutic care these children need to heal and, hopefully, to have a happy and productive life.

In *Medical Response to Child Sexual Abuse*, we have brought together national experts and scholars with a variety of expertise in the scientific fields that relate to the care of young victims. This group of contributors has created an impressive and helpful text that covers the entire range of the medical response to child sexual abuse. While the focus of this book is medical care, it is our hope that other members of the multidisciplinary team will find this to be a useful reference.

We would like to thank all the wonderful contributors for their hard work and their patience in the development of this text. Collaboration with them has been both gratifying and educational, and hopefully it will be the same for those who use this text as a reference.

Rich Kaplan, MSW, MD, FAAP
Joyce A. Adams, MD
Suzanne P. Starling, MD, FAAP
Angelo P. Giardino, MD, PhD, MPH, FAAP

Reviews to the Second Edition

Professionals working in the field of child sexual abuse have an important task. They should be dedicated to helping abused children and their families in the best possible way. This means that talking to children, performing the examination and tests, interpreting findings and results, and providing therapy should be based on best practice and scientific evidence. This text offers an excellent evidence based resource for the complete workup of sexually abused children in a multidisciplinary approach. This book also provides information about abused children with disabilities, child sexual exploitation, prevention, and the court process. Every professional working in this field should be familiar with this textbook.

Wouter A. Karst, MD
Forensic Physician
Netherlands Forensic Institute
The Hague, Netherlands

A valuable text for medical providers (physicians, forensic nurses, and advance practice providers) whether novice or expert, who provide care to children, adolescents, and their families when there is a suspicion of sexual abuse. Dr. Finkel provides meticulous detail describing elements of the medical history, components of the examination, screening for trauma symptoms, the value of anticipatory guidance on personal space and safety, and the mandate for precise and accurate medical documentation. An updated review is summarized regarding the collection and testing of items with potential evidentiary value with a forward focusing lens. Dr. Kellogg contributes a thorough blueprint on the testing, imaging, treatment, and reporting of STIs in addition to a valued approach to providing care to adolescents with concerns of sexual abuse. Dr. Nazer provides a detailed course on the structures of the genitalia and Dr. Adams provides the most recent information regarding the interpretation of medical findings in suspected child sexual abuse. This book is valuable to all members of the multidisciplinary team providing care, comfort, investigation, guidance, and resolution for children and adolescents affected by child sexual abuse.

Sonja Eddleman,
MSN, RN, SANE-A, SANE-P
Child Abuse Resource and
Evaluation (CARE) Team
Clinical Coordinator
Driscoll Children's Hospital
Corpus Christi, Texas

Readers across multiple disciplines—including healthcare providers, social workers, child protection teams, legal professionals, and law enforcement—will find this text highly relevant. The necessity of a multidisciplinary team to optimally care for children who have experienced sexual abuse and recommendations for the role of each team member are outlined. All disciplines will find practical applications for the information in Chapter 3: "The Medical Evaluation of a Suspected Child Abuse Victim." This chapter details key elements to approaching the child victim and family, the specifics of the history and physical exam, and highlights legal aspects of documentation with specific examples provided. Notably, this text ends with a review of the effects of sexual abuse on the genetic/epigenetic level of the brain and highlights the long term psychological and health consequences. For all who care for children and families affected by sexual abuse, I highly recommend this text as an engaging and thorough resource.

Kelly C. Dauk, MD
Professor of Pediatrics
University of Louisville
School of Medicine
Louisville, Kentucky

Dr. Alexander and Dr. Harper provide a bright and fast-moving discussion covering a wide expanse of multidisciplinary history, describing society's concept of the disease of child sexual abuse around the globe. The chapter maintains an optimistic tone even in the realistic criticism of past missteps and frames goals for the future of the field. Dr. Liker and Dr. Thackeray give an informative review addressing the application of evidence-based medicine criteria to the Child Abuse Pediatrics literature with a clever use of well-known publications for analysis of individual concepts. This chapter flows easily, reminiscent of participation in a journal club, and provides a grounded discussion that can (and no doubt will!) be referred to repeatedly by readers.

Marcella Donaruma, MD, FAAP
Associate Professor of Pediatrics
Baylor College of Medicine
Section of Public Health Pediatrics
Texas Children's Hospital
Houston, TX

This comprehensive digest offers a concise assimilation of chapters summarizing the latest research on child abuse practice for both advanced and beginner medical providers and multidisciplinary team members. Covering a broad range of topics with ample illustrations, this text will likely become the go-to resource on the shelves of child advocacy centers. In addition to a descriptive examination technique chapter, Dr. Harper provides useful explanations on the necessity of the non-acute examination beyond the forensics. The chapter on the importance of the post-examination conference offers lists and questions that are a must-read for practitioners and CAC family advocates. The chapter on therapy explains the unique effectiveness and application TF-CBT and the importance of parental engagement. Emphasizing how prevention efforts must move beyond child-based training, the prevention chapter describes new trends. Beyond child abuse pediatricians and medical providers, this book offers valuable information for all members of the multidisciplinary team.

Stacie LeBlanc, MEd, JD
Executive Director
New Orleans Children's
Advocacy Center
Department Head
Audrey Hepburn CARE Center
Children's Hospital of New Orleans
New Orleans, Louisiana

Reviews to the First Edition

This text is destined to be an excellent resource for novices as well as experienced providers of medical care to victims of sexual abuse. In addition, investigators and social workers without medical backgrounds will benefit from increased understanding of the nature, importance, and value of these medical assessments. Clinicians faced with the seemingly never-ending stream of victims will find the last chapter on prevention particularly helpful, providing hope that we can effect change.

Deborah Lowen, MD
Associate Professor of Pediatrics
Director
Child Abuse Pediatrics
Vanderbilt University School of Medicine
Nashville, Tennessee

This is a valuable, exhaustive resource combining anatomic, epidemiologic, therapeutic, and preventative strategies for children and young adults. Beginning with historical context and moving through basic anatomy, physiology, and pathology, the reader quickly learns best practices in health services for sexual abuse, assault, and exploitation. Team approaches, collaboration, telemedicine, training, treatment, and mental health services are reviewed in great detail, and there is a superlative discussion of research methods and the state of knowledge in the field topped off with legal and international issues and prevention. This book should be read by any professional who wants to responsibly provide services for children and families facing these difficult problems.

Vincent J. Palusci, MD, MS, FAAP
Professor of Pediatrics
New York University
School of Medicine
New York, New York

This comprehensive text ought to be available to each multidisciplinary team member tasked with treating and/or investigating child and adolescent sexual abuse and assault. Diverse topics are carefully addressed including interviewing children with impairments, commercial sexual exploitation, and efficacious mental health therapies. Dr. Allan De Jong's chapter on acute sexual abuse should be required reading for physicians and sexual assault nurse examiners tasked with forensic evidence collection and acute medical treatment. Dr. Martin Finkel details the highest standards to which clinicians should adhere as they elicit histories, conduct physical exams, and complete medicolegal documentation. This text is an excellent resource for both novice and established clinicians who serve child sexual abuse survivors and their families.

Tanya Hinds, MD, FAAP
Child Abuse Pediatrician
Children's National Medical Center
Washington DC

This comprehensive text will be an invaluable resource to any medical provider who has contact with children. With topics ranging from basic genital anatomy to court testimony and future directions for prevention, it is an excellent resource not only for those whose careers are primarily focused on child sexual abuse but also to those who simply desire a basic understanding. In recent decades, there have been tremendous advances in medicine related to child sexual abuse, and this book synthesizes all of this information.

Mark Hudson, MD
Midwest Children's Resource Center
Children's Hospitals and Clinics of Minnesota
St. Paul, Minnesota

Dr. Kaplan's new text is much more than a "how to do a sexual abuse exam" or "how to interpret the exam" handbook. The book includes chapters on how to talk with families after the examination, the history and future of child sexual abuse prevention, and child and youth prostitution and pornography. This is both a reference book and a thoughtful stimulus to broaden our thinking about the causes and effects of child sexual abuse and the role of the medical professional in caring for our patients and for the community.

Naomi F. Sugar MD
Clinical Professor of Pediatrics
University of Washington
Medical Director
Center for Sexual Assault and Traumatic Stress
Haborview Medical Center
Seattle, Washington

Contents in Brief

Contents in Detail

Medical Response to

Child Sexual Abuse

A Resource for Professionals Working With Children and Families

Second Edition

STM **Learning,** Inc.

Leading Publisher of Scientific, Technical, and Medical Educational Resources

Saint Louis

www.stmlearning.com

Chapter 1

The Medical Response to Child Sexual Abuse: An Historical Overview

Randell Alexander, MD, PhD
Nancy Sanders Harper, MD, FAAP
Rich A. Kaplan, MSW, MD, FAAP†

Introduction

Understanding the history of child sexual abuse (CSA) illuminates current attitudes toward and knowledge of CSA as well as what challenges remain in addressing it. Social, scientific, and clinical factors that have evolved over time are briefly reviewed in this chapter in order to provide an historical context through which to view current practice and perhaps a vantage point from which to view the future.

Not Just a Human Issue

Incest presents in a variety of species, often because an insufficient number of unrelated individuals exist in a small geographic area. Inbreeding diminishes genetic variability, which might yield a more adaptive organism, and potentially enhances the possibility for dysfunctional recessive genes. As genetic testing, such as chromosome microarray analysis, has advanced, ethical issues, such as the ability of the array to detect unsuspected consanguinity or relatedness, have arisen. In some cases, genetic testing may indicate parent-child incest.[1]

As a general principle, mammals usually do not engage in sex with prepubertal youth. Not only are pubertal olfactory and visual stimuli unlikely to be present in prepubertal individuals, sex with prepubertal youth is also effectively useless, if reproduction is understood to be the ultimate goal of sexual intercourse.

From the Dawn of Civilization

The sexual maltreatment of children is as old as civilization. Claude Lévi-Strauss[2] described the incest taboo as being present from the "dawn of culture." There are many descriptions of child sexual abuse from a variety of ancient cultures. The story of Lot being seduced by his daughters in Genesis suggests that both sexual contact with children and incest were social issues in ancient times. The Code of Hammurabi, a collection of laws developed during the reign of King Hammurabi of Babylon (1792-1750 BCE), includes several laws related to child sexual abuse, including the following[3]:

154. If a man be guilty of incest with his daughter, he shall be driven from the place (exiled).

157. If any one be guilty of incest with his mother after his father, both shall be burned.

In a survey of historic cases of child sexual abuse in the Byzantine Empire (324-1453 CE), the authors conclude that "child sexual abuse is an ancient social phenomenon" and that despite Byzantine political and religious prohibitions, "the problem seems to have remained endemic in all social classes."[4] Likewise, references to child sexual abuse among ancient Greeks, Romans, Egyptians, Hebrews, and others have been reported.[5]

Through the early modern and into the modern era, maltreatment, including sexual abuse, showed no evidence of abating. Accounts of sexual abuse from early 20th-century Scotland[6] and Canada[7] give disturbing insights into the response to child sexual abuse in the relatively recent past. Even as society articulates its abhorrence of child sexual abuse, such abuse persists and, with the advent of modern technology, manifests in new forms (eg, pornography, Internet pornography, digital abuses, human trafficking). Despite increased awareness and education, a variety of societally based myths and anxieties remain (eg, that hymens "break" and bleed with first intercourse, that a doctor can tell if a girl is a virgin) and perpetuate violent acts such as honor killings and genital mutilations.

The Early Medical Response

As pervasive as the sexual maltreatment of children has been, and as widespread as the religious, political, and cultural sanctions against such abuse have been, one might conclude that the medical community has, with equivalent consistency and vigor, responded to this abuse as it has to other major health concerns. However, for the better part of modern history, the medical response to child sexual abuse has been absent or, at best, sputtering and sporadic.

In the second half of the 19th century, a visionary French pathologist named Ambroise Tardieu wrote the remarkably accurate and, essentially, the first modern medical descriptions of both child physical and sexual abuse.[8,9] Tardieu described and analyzed more than 900 cases of sexual abuse of both boys and girls. His drawings of genital findings (**Figures 1-1** through **1-5**) are extremely accurate and hold up reasonably well, even today. Like so many

***Figures 1-1** and **1-2**. Tardieu's drawings of genital findings. Reprinted from Tardieu.[10]*

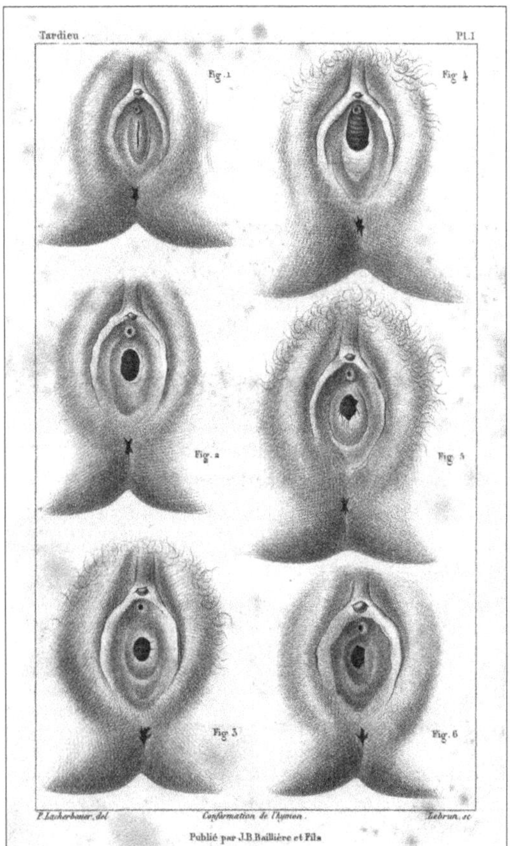

Figure 1-1

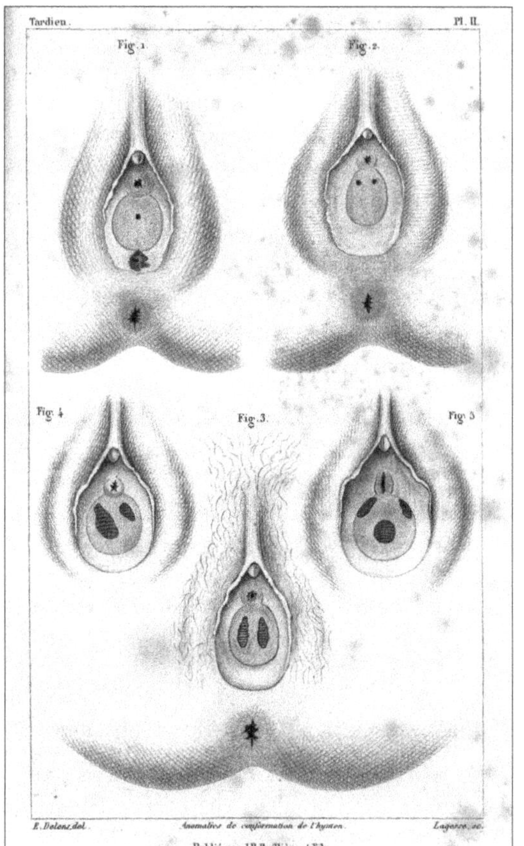

Figure 1-2

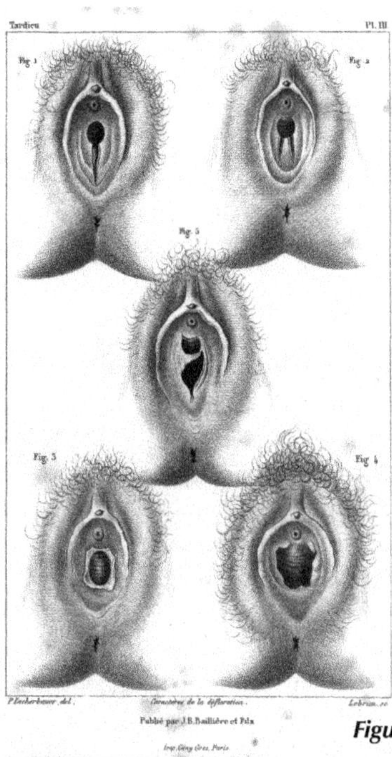

Figure 1-3

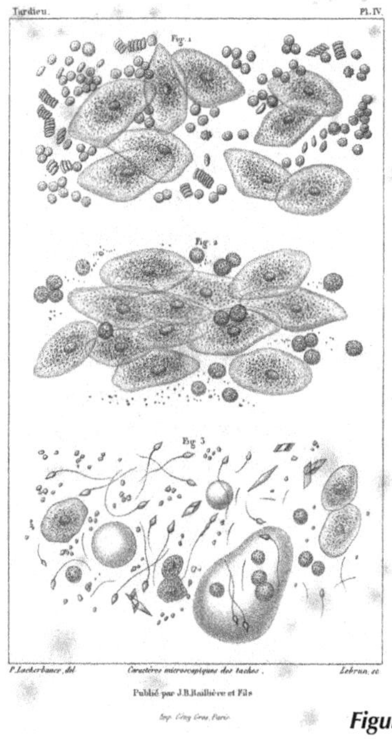

Figure 1-4

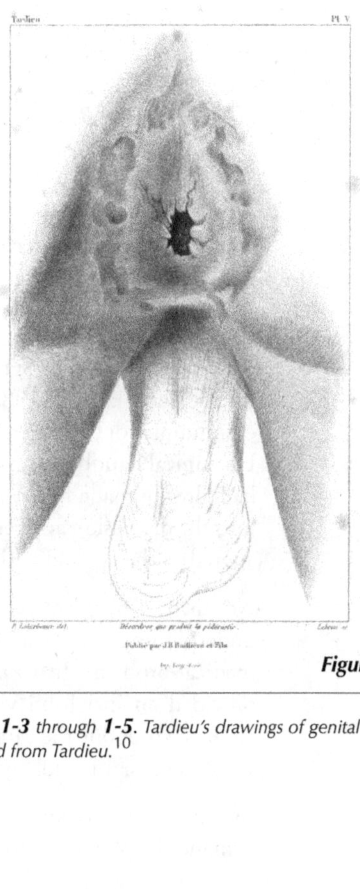

Figure 1-5

***Figures 1-3** through **1-5**. Tardieu's drawings of genital findings. Reprinted from Tardieu.*[10]

scientific innovators, Tardieu's work was underappreciated by his contemporaries. Rather than becoming the observational cornerstone for a burgeoning line of scientific inquiry and clinical practice, it faded into obscurity for well over a century.

However, Tardieu was not completely alone. Several other French physicians addressed the issue of child sexual abuse during this brief period of enlightenment. Masson[11] described works by Lacassagne, Garraud, and Bernard that supported Tardieu's work and elaborated on Lucas-Allen's work on the incidence and nature of the sexual abuse of children.[12] In fact, in *Des Attentats à la pudeur sur les petites filles (The Sexual Assault on Young Girls)*, Bernard noted 36 176 reported cases of "rape and assault on the morality of young children" between 1827 and 1870.[13] These works notwithstanding, considering the unsupportive and prevalent social and medical response to child sexual abuse, Tardieu was essentially a voice in the wilderness, quickly forgotten.

What stands as perhaps the best example of the 19th century's social and medical ambivalence toward the sexual abuse of children comes from a man who was certainly no stranger to ambivalence: Sigmund Freud. Long a source of great speculation and debate, it is clear that in less than 3 years, Freud abandoned (at least publicly) his revolutionary seduction theory, which identified sexual abuse as a cause of hysteria, in favor of the now-famous Oedipal complex, which contended that such patient accounts were fantasy. Whether Freud's reversal was the result of social and professional pressure[11,14] or a natural evolution of psychoanalytic theory[15] is well beyond the scope of this chapter to establish. Suffice it to say that at least on one level, the child victim became a seductress.[16] Postulating that children have sexual feelings toward a parent essentially made them co-conspirators in any incestuous abuse. As a consequence, sexual abuse remained relatively hidden and children were sometimes blamed when it was discovered.

If Tardieu's underappreciation and Freud's about-face exemplify 19th-century medicine's inability to respond scientifically to child sexual abuse, the issue of childhood gonorrhea suggests that a similar incapacity endured in the early 20th century. By that time, the science of medicine had clearly established a causal link between sexual contact and venereal diseases, including gonorrhea. However, it was not until the 1970s that the role of sexual abuse in the etiology of childhood gonococcal infections was generally accepted. Evans pointed out that, with respect to children, for the better part of the century, "physicians consistently downplayed and often denied the possibility of sexual transmission, providing other, less plausible explanations."[17] Arguments about differences in prepubertal anatomy and physiology that supported nonsexual transmission were proposed from multiple credible sources. Even when sexual transmission was acknowledged, it was not thought to occur in "good families." As late as 1973, physicians were not urged to consider child abuse in cases of gonococcal pharyngitis in prepubertal children.[18] In 1975 the sexual transmission of gonorrhea to children was described as a result of voluntary sex.[19]

In the 20th century, there was an awakening to the notion of child abuse in general. Although it is true that the seminal American child abuse case, that of Mary Ellen Wilson, occurred in 1874, the medical community only truly took notice with the publication of Kempe's *The Battered-Child Syndrome*.[20] Child physical abuse was acknowledged as a legitimate diagnosis, and additional medical research and other scholarly work began to appear in the medical literature. Sixteen years later, while delivering the 1977 C. Anderson Aldrich lecture, Kempe described another hidden form of abuse,[21] saying he "hoped to stimulate broader awareness among pediatricians about the problem of sexual abuse."

The Modern Response

A groundswell of interest in child sexual abuse had developed by the time Kempe gave his lecture. In 1979, Sgroi would publish a landmark article on childhood venereal disease[22] and later, in 1982, a second article on the same subject, rebuking the medical community for burying its head in the sand.[23] In that same period, she published the first US clinical handbook on child sexual abuse.[24] Shortly thereafter, Vincent Fontana, who had already made his mark as a medical pioneer in the area of physical abuse, entered into the discussion and reenergized the effort.[25] As a result, the medical community was alerted to the age-old affliction of child sexual abuse.

Nonmedical pioneers were at work as well, providing key psychological and epidemiologic underpinnings to the scientific understanding of this complex and troublesome "new" medical problem. In *Child Sexual Abuse Accommodation Syndrome*,[26] Roland Summit provided an insightful view into the sometimes counterintuitive behavior of young victims. At about the same time, David Finkelhor began his remarkable and ongoing work in the epidemiology of sexual abuse and exploitation.[27]

As authorities received reports of suspected child sexual abuse, there was an increased demand for physicians to evaluate children for medical signs of maltreatment. In 1986,

Woodling and Heger[28] reported on the utility of the colposcope to provide magnified views of the genital and anal tissues in children. The colposcope, equipped with a camera to document examination findings, was purported to detect minute injuries not easily visible to the naked eye. The hymen in the prepubertal girl, a previously obscure tissue, was now being seen, literally, in an entirely new light. With magnification, a new lexicon of mounds, bumps, notches (both U- and V-shaped), folds, ridges, clefts, and innumerable other variations were photographically documented. Given these new observations, the concept of an "intact" hymen was deemed too vague and became archaic.

Physicians who evaluated children and used a colposcope for magnification and documentation of their findings began to publish in the pediatric and gynecologic literature. The first papers were descriptive studies, usually of children who were referred for suspected sexual abuse to specialty centers. This led to additional scientific research on the examination findings of children without concern for sexual abuse, such as the seminal paper by Jenny and associates establishing the presence of a hymen in all normal newborns.[29] Shortly thereafter, McCann and associates published the results of the first studies of perianal[30] and genital[31] findings in children selected for nonabuse.

These new clinical data raised a question: Could the newfound understanding of hymenal morphology provide clear evidence to prove or disprove sexual abuse? With that, the medical role in sexual abuse cases took on a new dimension. Medical evaluators were now often called on to identify and document genital and perianal evidence to confirm or disprove sexual abuse. In many cases the medical caregiver's role had less to do with provision of care and much more to do with legal proceedings. In certain jurisdictions, this trend has persisted, at times compromising children's access to much-needed medical and mental health care.

The Role of Law Enforcement

As the role of the physician was emerging, the legal, law enforcement, and child protection communities were gearing up as well. From the beginning, sexual abuse cases were legally difficult. It was difficult for the community at large and for the juror in particular to accept that such horrendous things actually happened. At about the same time, famous and scandalous sexual abuse cases, such as the McMartin childcare center case in California and the debacle in Jordan, Minnesota, contributed to public skepticism. These early attempts at interviewing possible child victims were sometimes so leading it was not possible to garner the truth. Prosecutors and detectives looked to the medical examination as probative in breaking through the denial. This was only occasionally helpful. The daycare cases of the 1980s created a common supposition that professionals had overreached, but this was not necessarily true.[32] As terminology and science improved, Alexander,[33] in a review of such cases, later found that some medical findings were present that would be considered abusive even today. At the time, however, community professionals were forced to look in another direction, and the medical role was often limited to performing forensic examinations. In some communities, that is still the case.

In 1978, Jay Whitworth began in Florida what became the first statewide system to assess child abuse as a medical issue. Coupling forensic interviewing and other interviewing techniques with trained physicians and advanced nurse examiners, Florida enacted a series of laws that defined child protection teams (CPTs) as "medically led" and provided coverage to every child in the state. With a statewide database, continuous quality improvement, medical review of every child abuse report made via hotline (more than 200 000 per year), and access to every hospital, the Florida CPT system helps to ensure that every child with a significant abuse concern can at any time receive a health-oriented intervention conducted by trained medical providers. Similar systems have been developed in Kuwait and Mississippi, and portions of this approach have been instituted in New Jersey. Some areas in Texas provide online medical consultation for child protection and law enforcement, and several other states, including Missouri, provide training to general medical providers. Missouri's Sexual Assault Forensic Examination–Child Abuse Resource and Education Program, or SAFE-CARE, is a statewide network of medical providers who receive initial and annual training on medical forensic evaluations for cases of alleged child maltreatment. SAFE-CARE providers who meet annual training standards are eligible for increased reimbursement by the state for medical forensic evaluations of children. Additionally, all reports in Missouri of alleged maltreatment in children younger than age of 4 years are reviewed by a SAFE-CARE provider to determine if a medical forensic evaluation is needed. If in a given case a SAFE-CARE provider makes a medical diagnosis of abuse, that case must by law be sent by child protective services (CPS) to family court for consideration of intervention.

In 1984, Huntsville prosecutor and later Alabama Congressman Robert E. "Bud" Kramer, noting the difficulty of prosecuting child sexual abuse cases, founded what was called the first "child advocacy center" in Madison County, Alabama. Not long afterward, with collaboration from national child abuse experts, including medical child abuse pioneer Dr. Carolyn Levitt, the National Network of Child Advocacy Centers was born. This organization has evolved into the National Children's Alliance (NCA). The NCA has become the accrediting body for approximately 800 child advocacy centers across the country. These centers use medical services in a variety of ways. Some centers are hospital based and thus focus on medical care for victims of all types of maltreatment. Some centers are based in the community and focus on medical care largely for victims of sexual abuse. Others are associated with prosecutors' offices, and decisions regarding medical care are often made by individuals with no medical training. There are a host of models in between. Unlike the Florida and Mississippi models, such centers are usually not medically led, do not have systematic state funding, and are often prosecution based rather than health based. In practice, however, children often receive excellent services regardless of model.

Scientific Advances

Building on the pioneering work of Heger and McCann and associates, researchers such as Berenson,[34-38] Adams, and Kellogg[39] provided strong evidence-based support for the notion that the vast majority of child sexual abuse victims will have no diagnostic genital findings, even on magnified examination. This raises a new and more difficult question: Why examine these children at all? The answer, which must be given in the context of appropriate medical care, follows.

Medical Care of the Child Abuse Victim: Now and Beyond

Even at the beginning of the 21st century, the role of the child sexual abuse medical provider is still being defined. This special practice swelled with potential in 19th-century France only to disappear for the next 100 years in the face of denial, ambivalence, and deception. A medical reawakening of sorts has occurred, but many questions still need to be answered. For example, should victims of child sexual abuse be seen as patients or rather as potential witnesses who simply need a genital check?

There is an ongoing and concerted effort to answer such questions. In 2002 a group of pediatric child abuse consultants began meeting in an effort to develop a consensus on the medical care of possible sexual abuse victims. Blending current evidence-based research on physical findings with consensus on best practice, their work led to the development of an article titled "Guidelines for Medical Care of Children Who May Have Been Sexually Abused"[40] and a revised version issued in 2016.[41] In 2005, the American Academy of Pediatrics' Committee on Child Abuse and Neglect (COCAN) issued an updated edition of *The Evaluation of Sexual Abuse in Children*,[42] later supplemented with a clinical report intended to guide pediatricians through cases of suspected sexual abuse.[43] By 2006 the American Board of Pediatrics and the American Board of Medical Specialties approved ***child abuse pediatrics*** as a pediatric subspecialty,[44] with the first child abuse pediatricians' certified in 2009. As of August 2017, there were around 350 subspecialty-certified child abuse pediatricians in the United States.

What does all this mean for the future of the medical response to child sexual abuse? It means several steps forward and one critical step back. The new subspecialty is certainly a major step forward. It will allow for the further development of the child abuse research infrastructure and increased support of child abuse pediatrics fellowship programs. It should also serve to enhance efforts at professional peer review and continuous quality improvement among child abuse centers and medical providers. The work by the guidelines consensus group and COCAN also represents a step forward as they summarize the current state of the science of child sexual abuse and provide structure to the medical evaluation. Significant advances in DNA testing have also improved documentation in instances where that might prove useful. A much deeper understanding of the neurobiological harms of sexual abuse (ie, recognizing sexual abuse as an adverse childhood experience affecting a lifetime of health) and what might be its genetic and epigenetic consequences are the new frontiers that health research may illuminate.

The step back is the return to the notion that the child sexual abuse evaluation is, first and foremost, a provision of medical detection. For the sexually abused child, comprehensive care requires much more than looking for evidence in a magnified hymen, swabbing for body fluids, conducting a forensic interview, and providing court testimony. In such cases, comprehensive care requires a good history, a thorough physical examination, appropriate testing, and referrals to and collaboration with other health care professionals (eg, psychotherapists), as well as appropriate follow-up. Medical care providers must also be prepared to offer patient and family education; anticipatory guidance; and when indicated, much-needed reassurance for the child and family regarding the child's health, safety, and well-being.[45] Most critically, there must be a revolution in understanding what drives a perpetrator to sexually abuse a child and how abuse can be prevented.

Conclusion

There is great potential for the evolution of medical care for the young sexual abuse victim. Bolstered by a legal climate that grants increased credibility to providers of medical diagnoses and treatment, there can be a return to the professional practice that launched this specialized care: the practice of medicine.

References

1. Miller DT, Adam MP, Aradhya S, et al. Consensus statement: chromosomal microarray is a first-tier clinical diagnostic test for individuals with developmental disabilities or congenital anomalies. *Am J Hum Genet.* 2010;86(5):749-764.

2. Lévi-Strauss C. *The Elementary Structure of Kinship*. London, United Kingdom: Eyre & Spotterswoode; 1969.

3. Hammurabi. *The Code of Hammurabi*. King LW, trans. New Haven, CT: Lillian Goldman Law Library; 2008. The Avalon Project Web site. http://avalon.law.yale.edu/ancient/hamframe.asp. Accessed December 13, 2017.

4. Lascaratos J, Poulakou-Rebelakou E. Child sexual abuse: historical cases in the Byzantine Empire (324-1453 AD). *Child Abuse Negl.* 2000;24(8):1085-1090.
5. Kahr B. The sexual molestation of children: historical perspectives. *J Psychohist.* 1991;19(2):191-214.
6. Davidson R. "This pernicious delusion": law, medicine, and child sexual abuse in early-twentieth-century Scotland. *J Hist Sex.* 2001;10(1):62-77.
7. Sangster J. Masking and unmasking the sexual abuse of children: perceptions of violence against children in "the Badlands" of Ontario, 1916-1930. *J Fam Hist.* 2000;25(4):504-526.
8. Labbé J. Ambroise Tardieu: the man and his work on child maltreatment a century before Kempe. *Child Abuse Negl.* 2005;29(4):311-324.
9. Roche AJ, Fortin G, Labbé J, Brown J, Chadwick D. The work of Ambroise Tardieu: the first definitive description of child abuse. *Child Abuse Negl.* 2005;29(4):325-334.
10. Tardieu A. *Étude médico-légale sur les attentats aux moeurs.* 7th ed. Paris, France: Librairie JB Baillière et Fils; 1878.
11. Masson J. *The Assault on Truth: Freud's Suppression of the Seduction Theory.* New York, NY: Penguin; 1984.
12. Olafson E, Corwin DL, Summit RC. Modern history of child sexual abuse awareness: cycles of discovery and suppression. *Child Abuse Negl.* 1993;17(1):7-24.
13. Bernard P. *Des Attentats à la pudeur sur les petites filles.* Octave Dion, ed. Lyon, France: Laboratoire de Médecine Légale de Lyon; 1886.
14. Powell RA, Boer DP. Did Freud mislead patients to confabulate memories of abuse? a reply to Gleaves and Hernandez (1999). *Psychol Rep.* 2004;95(3 pt 1):863-877.
15. Gleaves DH, Hernandez E. Wethinks the author doth protest too much: a reply to Esterson. *Hist Psychol.* 2002;5(1):92-98.
16. Birken L. From seduction theory to Oedipus complex: a historical analysis. *New Ger Crit.* 1988;43:83-96.
17. Evans H. Physician denial and child sexual abuse in America. In: Warsh CK, Strong-Boag V, eds. *Children's Health Issues in Historical Perspective.* Waterloo, Ontario: Wilfrid Laurier University Press; 2005:327-352.
18. Abbott SL. Gonococcal tonsillitis-pharyngitis in a 5-year-old girl. *Pediatrics.* 1973;52(2):287-289.
19. Israel KS, Rissing KB, Brooks GF. Neonatal and childhood gonococcal infections. *Clin Obstet Gynecol.* 1975;18(1):143-151.
20. Kempe CH, Silverman FN, Steele BF, Droegemueller W, Silver HK. The battered-child syndrome. *JAMA.* 1962;181:17-24.
21. Kempe CH. Sexual abuse, another hidden pediatric problem: the 1977 C. Anderson Aldrich lecture. *Pediatrics.* 1978;62(3):382-389.
22. Sgroi SM. Pediatric gonorrhea beyond infancy. *Pediatr Ann.* 1979;8(5):326-336.
23. Sgroi SM. Pediatric gonorrhea and child sexual abuse: the venereal disease connection. *Sex Transm Dis.* 1982;9(3):154-156.
24. Sgroi SM. *Handbook of Clinical Intervention in Child Sexual Abuse.* Lexington, MA: Lexington Books; 1981.

25. Fontana VJ. When systems fail: protecting the victim of child sexual abuse. *Child Today*. 1984;13(4):14-18.
26. Summit RC. The child sexual abuse accommodation syndrome. *Child Abuse Negl.* 1983;7(2):177-93.
27. Finkelhor, D. How widespread is child sexual abuse? *Child Today*. 1984;13(4):18-20.
28. Woodling BA, Heger A. The use of the colposcope in the diagnosis of sexual abuse in the pediatric age group. *Child Abuse Negl.* 1986;10(1):111-114.
29. Jenny C, Kuhns ML, Arakawa F. Hymens in newborn female infants. *Pediatrics.* 1987;80(3):399-400.
30. McCann J, Voris J, Simon M, Wells R. Perianal findings in prepubertal children selected for nonabuse: a descriptive study. *Child Abuse Negl.* 1989;13(2):179-193.
31. McCann J, Wells R, Simon M, Voris J. Genital findings in prepubertal girls selected for nonabuse: a descriptive study. *Pediatrics.* 1990;86(3):428-439.
32. Cheit R. *The Witch-Hunt Narrative: Politics, Psychology, and the Sexual Abuse of Children.* New York, NY: Oxford University Press; 2014.
33. Alexander R. Medical evaluations then and now. *J Interpers Violence.* 2017;32(6):826-852.
34. Berenson AB. Appearance of the hymen at birth and one year of age: a longitudinal study. *Pediatrics.* 1993;91(4):820-825.
35. Berenson AB. The prepubertal genital exam: what is normal and abnormal. *Curr Opin Obstet Gynecol.* 1994;6(6):526-530.
36. Berenson AB. A longitudinal study of hymenal morphology in the first 3 years of life. *Pediatrics.* 1995;95(4):490-96.
37. Berenson AB, Chacko MR, Wiemann CM, Mishaw CO, Friedrich WN, Grady JJ. Use of hymenal measurements in the diagnosis of previous penetration. *Pediatrics.* 2002;109(2):228-235.
38. Berenson AB, Grady JJ. A longitudinal study of hymenal development from 3 to 9 years of age. *J Pediatr.* 2002;140(5):600-607.
39. Kellogg ND, Menard SW, Santos A. Genital anatomy in pregnant adolescents: "normal" does not mean "nothing happened". *Pediatrics.* 2004;113(1 pt 1):e67-e69.
40. Adams JA, Kaplan RA, Starling SP, et al. Guidelines for medical care of children who may have been sexually abused. *J Pediatr Adolesc Gynecol.* 2007;20(3):163-172.
41. Adams JA, Kellogg ND, Farst KJ, et al. Updated guidelines for the medical assessment and care of children who may have been sexually abused. *J Pediatr Adolesc Gynecol.* 2016;29(2):81-87.
42. Kellogg ND; American Academy of Pediatrics Committee on Child Abuse and Neglect. The evaluation of sexual abuse in children. *Pediatrics.* 2005;116(2):506-512.
43. Jenny C, Crawford-Jakubiak JE; Committee on Child Abuse and Neglect, American Academy of Pediatrics. The evaluation of children in the primary care setting when sexual abuse is suspected. *Pediatrics.* 2013;132(2):e558-e567.
44. Block RW, Palusci VJ. Child abuse pediatrics: a new pediatric subspecialty. *J Pediatr.* 2006;148(6):711-712.
45. National Children's Alliance. *Standards for Accredited Members.* Washington, DC: National Children's Alliance; 2017.

Chapter 2

Basic Anatomy of the Genitalia and Anus

Dena Nazer, MD, FAAP
Joyce A. Adams, MD

Introduction

To recognize signs of child sexual abuse, it is necessary to first be familiar with normal genital anatomy, its variations, and its development. Although this may seem obvious, the lack of understanding and knowledge of the many variations in normal appearance of the genital and anal tissues in children has led to misunderstandings among medical and nonmedical professionals alike. Even after the publication of the first detailed descriptions of anal and genital anatomy in nonabused prepubertal children,[1-3] some physicians and nurses who perform child sexual abuse medical evaluations are not familiar with the findings from those and subsequent studies.[4-9]

In 2009, Starling et al[10] surveyed 462 third-year residents on their training in and knowledge of child abuse. The residents were presented with an image of female genitalia and asked to identify 3 anatomical structures: the labia minora, urethral meatus, and hymen. Overall, only 19% of the residents correctly labeled all 3 structures, with the highest rate of correct identification among pediatric residents, followed by family medicine and emergency department residents. In this study, many residents, including 67% of all family medicine residents, incorrectly diagnosed a normal genital examination. This lack of knowledge may translate into misdiagnoses and a lack of comfort when performing the medical evaluations for children. In another study there was poor agreement in the results of the genital examinations performed by pediatric emergency department physicians when reviewed by physicians with training in child sexual abuse.[11] When reexamined by physicians with training in child sexual abuse, 70% of the examination results identified as abnormal by the emergency department physicians were found to be normal.[11]

When a child's examination is thought to show signs of injury or abuse but actually represents normal findings or evidence of another medical condition, the medical provider may contact child protection or law enforcement officials to report the suspicions. The child and family would then be unnecessarily traumatized by a referral and investigation of those suspicions. Misdiagnosis may also lead to delayed recognition and treatment of medical conditions, with persistence of symptoms and development of complications.

It is important for medical and nursing professionals, as well as nonmedical professionals, to be able to speak the same language when describing features of genital and anal anatomy in children and adolescents. Anatomy courses in medical and nursing schools rarely provide the necessary details about the features of genital anatomy in children, usually focusing on adults and on pathological conditions common to adult patients rather than children.

In the early 1990s a group of physicians met at conferences to agree on proper terminology for describing features of genital and anal anatomy, and the results of a 4-year consensus development process were published by the American Professional Society on the Abuse of Children in 1995.[12] Some of the definitions were taken from standard medical dictionaries and anatomy textbooks, but out of necessity, other definitions were created by specialists working in the field of sexual abuse medical evaluation. **Table 2-1** is a list of terms and definitions adapted from that publication.[12]

Table 2-1. Basic Genital Anatomy and Related Terminology

FEMALE ANATOMICAL STRUCTURES

— ***Mons pubis:*** The rounded, fleshy prominence, created by the underlying fat pad that lies over the symphysis pubis (pubic bone).

— ***Vulva:*** The external genitalia or pudendum of the female. Includes the anterior commisure, clitoris, labia majora, labia minora, vaginal vestibule, urethral orifice, vaginal orifice, hymen, and posterior commisure.

— ***Anterior commisure:*** The union of the two labia minora anteriorly/superiorly.

— ***Clitoris:*** A small, cylindrical, erectile body, situated at the anterior (superior) portion of the vulva, covered by a sheath of skin called the clitoral hood; homologous with the penis in the male.

— ***Labia majora (singular: labium majus):*** Rounded folds of skin forming the lateral boundaries of the vulva.

— ***Labia minora (singular: labium minus):*** Longitudinal thin folds of tissue enclosed within the labia majora. In the prepubertal child, these folds extend from the clitoral hood to approximately the midpoint on the lateral walls of the vestibule. In the adult, they enclose the structures of the vestibule.

— ***Vaginal vestibule:*** An anatomic cavity containing the opening of the vagina, the urethra, and the ducts of Bartholin's glands. Bordered by the clitoris superiorly, the labia minora laterally, and the posterior commisure inferiorly.

— ***Urethral orifice:*** External opening of the canal (urethra) from the bladder.

— ***Vestibular bands:*** Small bands of tissue lateral to the urethral orifice that connect the periurethral tissues to the anterior lateral walls of the vestibule (urethral support ligaments), or bands of tissue lateral to the hymen connecting to the vestibular wall.

— ***Vaginal orifice:*** The opening to the uterovaginal canal.

— ***Vagina:*** The internal structure extending from the uterine cervix to the inner edge of the hymen.

— ***Hymen:*** A membrane that partially, or rarely completely, covers the vaginal orifice.

— ***Fossa navicularis/posterior fossa:*** Concavity on the lower part of the vestibule situated inferiorly to the vaginal orifice and extending to the posterior commisure or posterior fourchette.

— ***Posterior commisure:*** The union of the two labia majora inferiorly (toward the anus).

(continued)

Table 2-1. Basic Genital Anatomy and Related Terminology ***(continued)***

MALE ANATOMICAL STRUCTURES

— ***Penis:*** Male sex organ composed of erectile tissue through which the urethra passes. Homologous with the clitoris in the female.

— ***Shaft:*** The part of the penis between the glans and the body.

— ***Glans (or "glans penis," "balanus"):*** The cap-shaped expansion of the spongiosum at the end of the penis. It is covered by mucous membrane and sheathed by the prepuce (foreskin) in uncircumcised males.

— ***Corona of the glans penis:*** The rounded, prominent border of the glans on the distal portion of the penile shaft.

— ***Scrotum:*** The pouch that contains the testicles and their accessory organs located inferiorly to the penis.

— ***Median raphe:*** A ridge or furrow that marks the line of union of the two halves of the perineum. This visible line extends from the anus to the perineum (between the scrotum and anus in males and vestibule and anus in females). (See **Appendix Figure 2-1-a** and **b**.)

DESCRIPTIVE TERMS RELATED TO THE PERINEUM AND ANUS

— ***Perineum:*** The external surface or base of the perineal body, lying between the vulva and the anus in the female and the scrotum and the anus in the male. Underlying the external surface of the perineum is the pelvic floor and its associated structures occupying the pelvic outlet, which is bounded anteriorly by the pubic symphysis (pubic bone), laterally by the ischial tuberosity (pelvic bone), and posteriorly by the coccyx (tail bone).

— ***Perineal body:*** The central tendon of the perineum located between the vulva and the anus in the female and between the scrotum and anus in the male.

— ***Anus:*** The anal orifice, which is the lower opening of the digestive tract, lying in the fold between the buttocks through which feces is extruded.

— ***Anal skin tag:*** A protrusion of anal verge tissue that interrupts the symmetry of the perianal skin folds.

— ***Anal verge:*** The tissue overlying the subcutaneous division of the external anal sphincter at the most distal portion of the anal canal (anoderm) and extending exteriorly to the margin of the anal skin.

— ***Pectinate/dentate line:*** The saw-toothed line of demarcation between the distal (lower) portion of the anal valves and the pectin, the smooth zone of stratified epithelium that extends to the anal verge. This line may be apparent when the external and internal anal sphincters relax and the anus dilates.

Adapted with permission from American Professional Society on the Abuse of Children.[12]

EMBRYOLOGY

An appreciation of the wide variation in the appearance of the genital and anal tissues in children requires an understanding of embryology and how the external genital tissues develop. For the first 6 weeks of development, the genital structures of the human embryo are in an undifferentiated state. In males, a transcription factor encoded on the sex-determining region of the Y chromosome (SRY) is produced during the seventh week, which triggers male development. In the absence of a Y chromosome and SRY production, female development progresses.

Figures 2-1 and **2-2** show the development of the male and female external genital structures from the indifferent stage (4 to 7 weeks) through the 12th week. The genital tubercle differentiates into the glans and shaft of the penis in the male and into the glans and shaft of the clitoris in the female. The definitive urogenital sinus develops into the penile urethra in the male and the vestibule of the vagina in the female. The urethral fold becomes the penis surrounding the penile urethra in the male or the labia minora in the female. The labioscrotal fold develops into either the scrotum in the male or the labia majora in the female.[13]

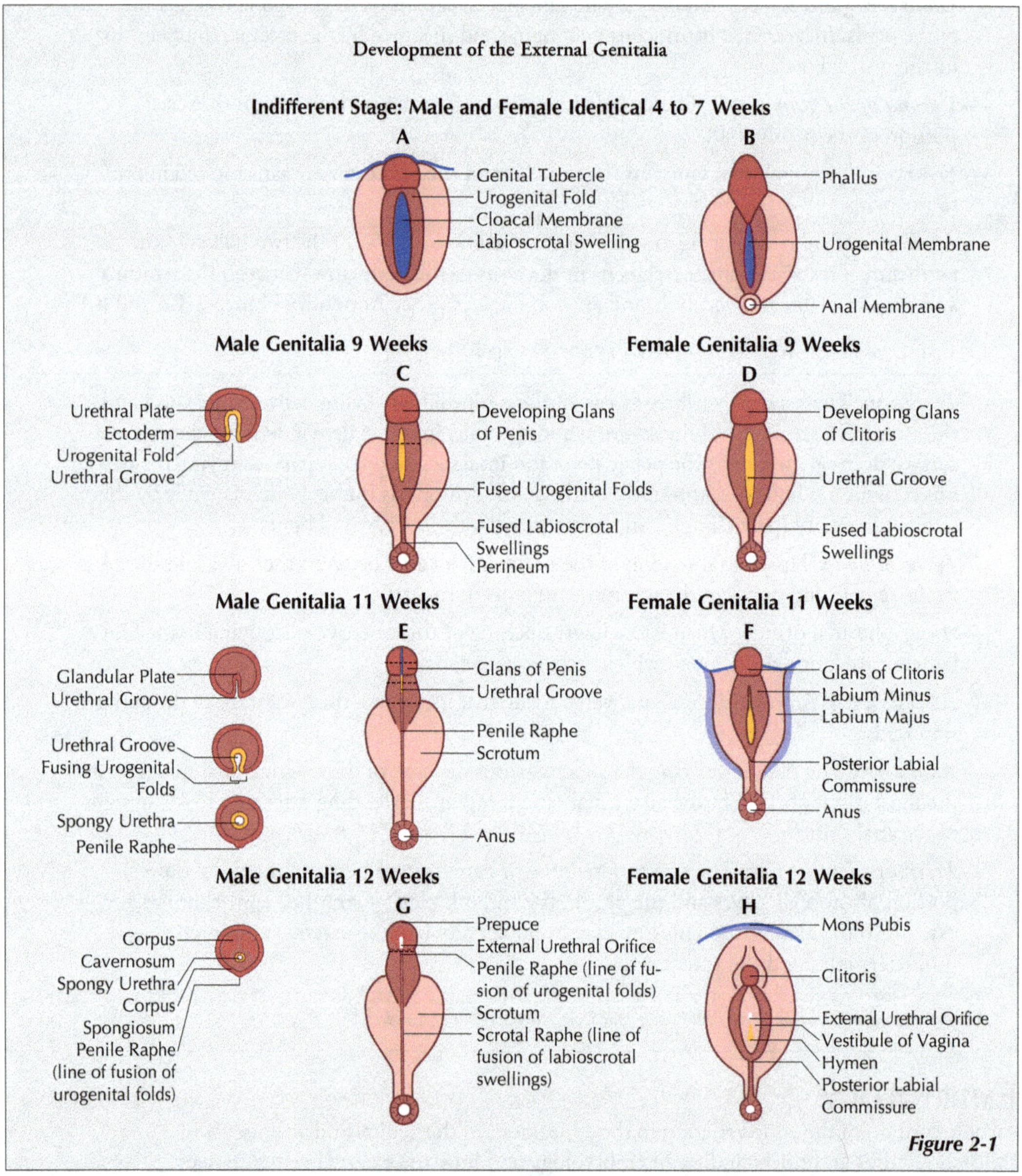

Figure 2-1. *Development of the external genitalia. Diagrams A and B illustrate the appearance of the genitalia during the indifferent stage (fourth to seventh week). Diagrams C, E, and G illustrate stages in the development of the male external genitalia at 9, 11, and 12 weeks, respectively. To the left are schematic transverse sections of the developing penis, illustrating the formation of the spongy urethra. Diagrams D, F, and H illustrate stages in the development of the female external genitalia at 9, 11, and 12 weeks, respectively. Figures and legend reprinted with permission from: Moore KL, Persaud TVN.* The Developing Human, Clinically Oriented Embryology, *6th ed. Philadelphia, PA: WB Saunders;1998, p332.*

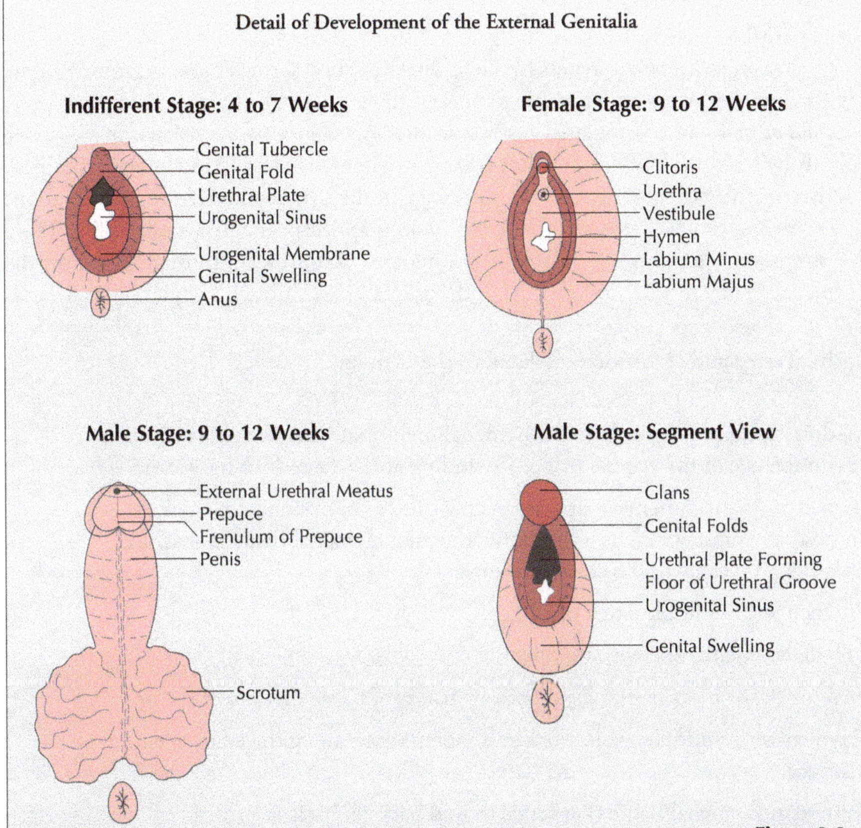

Figure 2-2

Figure 2-2. *Detail of development of the external genitalia in the female and the male. Reprinted with permission of Lippincott Williams & Wilkins, from: Snell RS.* Clinical Anatomy for Medical Students. *Baltimore, MD: Lippincott Williams & Wilkins; 2004.*

A detailed study of the development of the perineum was published in 2005, which provided a new understanding of the formation of the vagina and hymen.[14] In the undifferentiated state, the distal ends of the fused paramesonephric ducts are separated from the urogenital sinus by the dense stroma of the Müllerian tubercle. In females, the mesonephric ducts regress and the fused paramesonephric ducts form the uterus and vagina. The mesonephric orifices are incorporated into the orifice of the developing vagina, and the epithelium is replaced by the epithelium from the Müllerian tubercle.

The vagina expands and extends downward to bulge into the vestibulum, and the paramesonephric epithelium is transformed into vaginal epithelium. The glycogen-filled cells begin to disintegrate, forming the lumen of the vagina.

The lengthening of the vagina into the vestibulum, where it meets the dense stromal tissue of the Müllerian tubercle, forms the hymen.[15] Folds in the urogenital sinus contribute to the lateral folds of the hymen. The deepening of the dorsal vestibular groove accentuates the dorsal segment of the hymen, which in clinical terms is referred to as the posterior or inferior rim. Both the inner side and the outer side of the hymen are made up of sinus epithelium.

The opening in the hymen develops as the stromal tissue between the descending vagina and the urogenital sinus regresses. It is postulated that the denser the column of stromal tissue, the more likely it is that the tissue will not completely regress, which leads to a microperforate or imperforate hymen. If the tissue is denser in some areas than others, the uneven regression could also produce a septate or cribriform hymen.

Normal Variations

The Hymen

The increasing societal awareness of the problem of child sexual abuse, beginning in the 1980s, and the involvement of physicians in the evaluation of children with suspected child sexual abuse stimulated interest in the appearance of the hymen in neonates. A study by Jenny et al[16] identified the presence of a hymen in all 1131 neonates examined, and Berenson et al[17] described the morphology of the hymen and anatomical variations in 449 neonates who were examined and photographed in the first week of life. **Table 2-2** summarizes terminology related to the hymen.[12] **Figures 2-3** through **2-4** show the normal anatomy in a 5 year old child and **Figures 2-5-a** through **f** depict normal varia-

Table 2-2. Descriptive Terms and Definitions Related to the Hymen*

— ***Annular:*** Variation in morphology where the hymenal membrane tissue extends completely around the circumference of the vaginal orifice (including at the 12 o'clock location).

— ***Crescentic:*** Hymen with attachments at approximately the 11 o'clock and 1 o'clock positions with no tissue present between the 2 attachments. Hymenal tissue is absent at some point above the 3 o'clock to 9 o'clock locations.

— ***Cribriform:*** Hymen with multiple small openings.

— ***Imperforate:*** Hymenal membrane with no opening.

— ***Septate:*** Hymen with 2 or more openings, caused by bands of tissue that bisect the opening.

— ***Fimbriated:*** Hymen with multiple projections and indentations along the edge, creating a ruffled appearance.

— ***Redundant:*** Abundant hymenal tissue that tends to fold back on itself or protrude.

— ***Hymenal mound or bump:*** A solid elevation of hymenal tissue that is wider than or as wide as it is long, located on the edge of the hymenal membrane. This structure may be seen at the site where an intravaginal column attaches to the hymen.

— ***Hymenal tag:*** An elongated projection of tissue arising from any location on the hymenal rim.

— ***Hymenal cyst:*** A fluid-filled elevation of tissue, confined within the hymenal tissue.

— ***Hymenal cleft:*** An angular or v-shaped indentation on the edge of the hymenal membrane.

— ***External hymenal ridge:*** A midline longitudinal ridge of tissue on the external surface of the hymen. May be either anterior or posterior and usually extends to the edge of the hymen.

**According to the 2016 and the updated 2018 guidelines on interpretation of medical findings in children suspected of sexual abuse, normal variants that are unrelated to the child's disclosure of sexual abuse include the normal variations in the appearance of the hymen (annular, crescentic, imperforate, microperforate, septate, redundant, tags, mounds, and a narrow rim of the hymen).*[18,19]

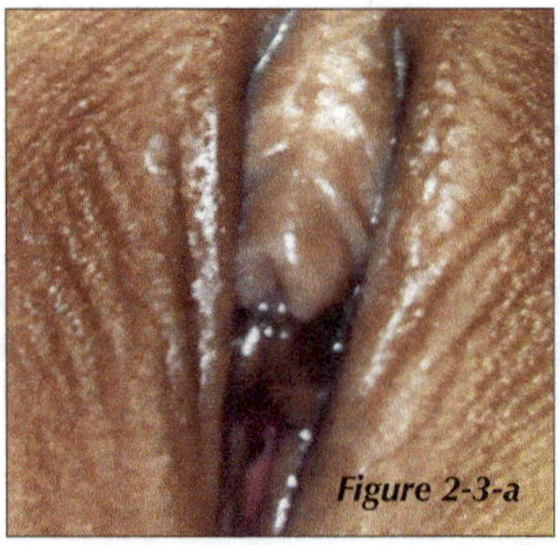

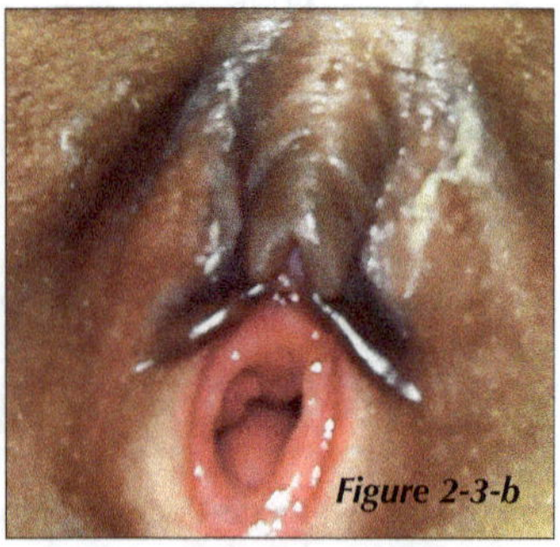

Figure 2-3-a *and* ***b.*** *A 5-year-old examined in the supine frog leg position. Figure 2-3-a shows the anatomy as visualized prior to labial separation. Notice the clitoral hood, glans of the clitoris, labia minora, and a slight view of the hymen. Figure 2-3-b shows the genital anatomy with labial separation.*

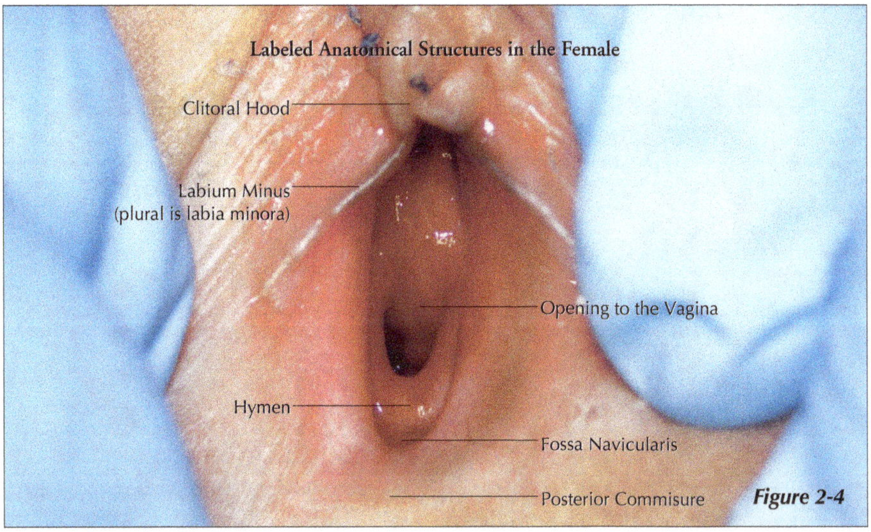

Figure 2-4. *Labeled anatomical structures in a 5-year-old girl examined in the supine position using labial separation. See Table 2-1 for definitions.*

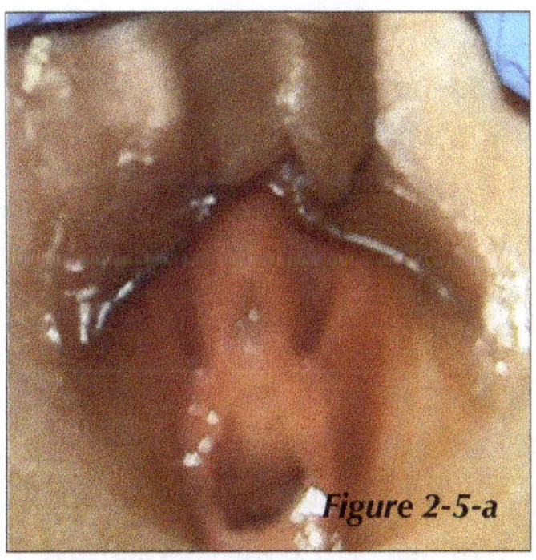

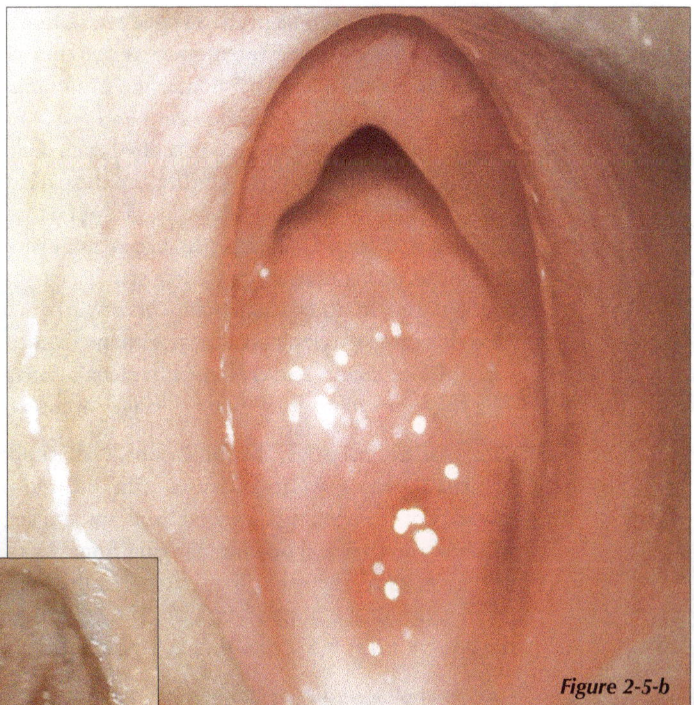

Figure 2-5-a. *Crescentic hymen examined in the supine frog leg position. Notice the periurethral support ligaments.*

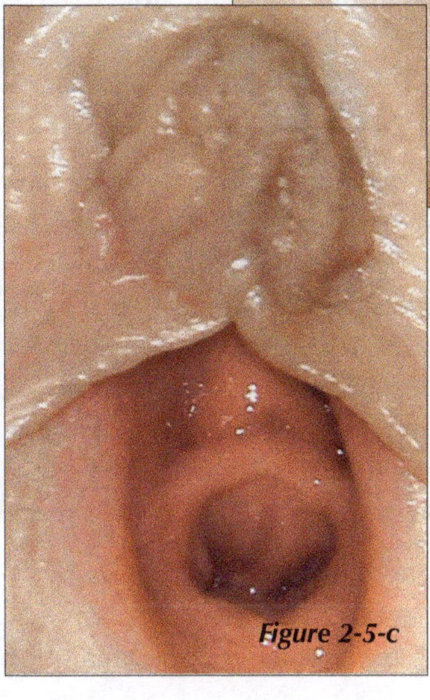

Figure 2-5-b. *Crescentic hymen. Child was examined in the prone knee-chest position.*

Figure 2-5-c. *Annular hymen extending completely around the circumference of the vaginal orifice.*

Figure 2-5-d. *Cribriform hymen.*

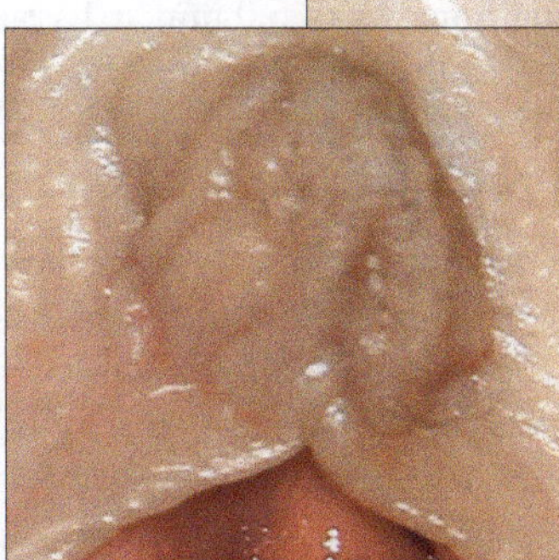

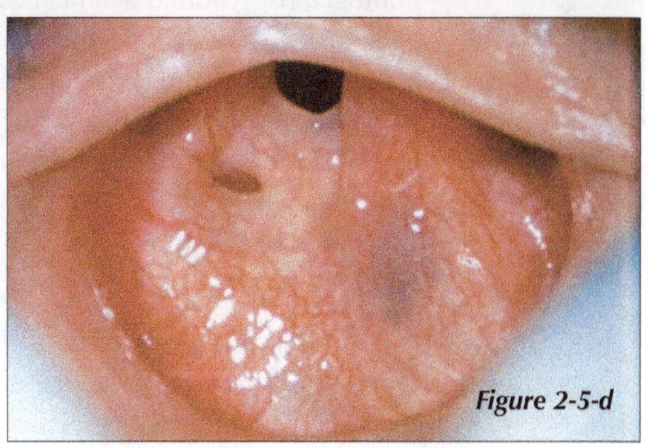

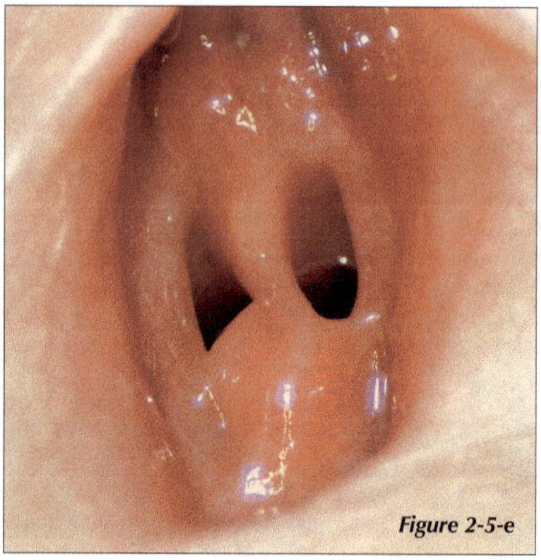

Figure 2-5-e

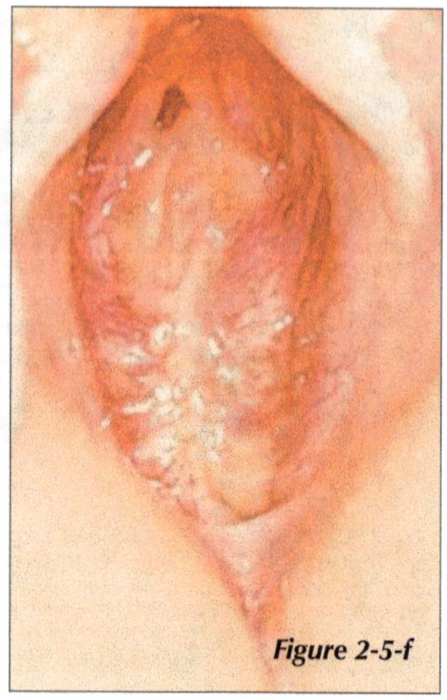

Figure 2-5-f

Figure 2-5-e. *Septate hymen. Note the band of tissue that bisects the opening.*

Figure 2-5-f. *Imperforate hymen. Note the absence of a hymenal opening.*

tions in the hymen. The neonates were found to have primarily annular hymens (ie, the hymenal tissue extended 360 degrees around the opening to the vagina). Hymenal clefts, cysts, tags, mounds, external ridges, and intravaginal ridges were noted. (See **Appendix Figures 2-2** through **2-28** for examples of anatomical variations of the hymen.) The location of various features was described using a clock face, with the 12 o'clock position defined as directly below the urethra and the 6 o'clock position in the midline above the posterior commissure. In a follow-up study of 62 infants examined at 1 year, Berenson et al[4] noted that 10 of 13 infants who had an annular hymen with a notch in the 12 o'clock position as neonates had a crescentic hymen at 1 year. A crescentic hymen is defined as a configuration in which the attachments of the hymen are at the 1 o'clock to 2 o'clock and 10 o'clock to 11 o'clock positions, with an absence of hymenal tissue in between. At 1 year, 28% of infants had crescentic hymens compared with none in the neonate period. The frequency of external hymenal ridges decreased from 82% to 14% at 1 year.

The longitudinal study by Berenson et al[4] supported the clinical observation that hymenal opening width increases with the age of the child. The mean horizontal diameter of the opening increased from 3.8 mm at 1 year to 6.1 mm at 9 years, with the width of the hymenal opening ranging from 2.5 to 6.0 mm at 1 year to 1.75 to 12.25 mm at 9 years. The other trend noted in the follow-up study was the decrease in the mean width of the posterior/inferior rim of the hymen. The range of measurements of the posterior rim was 2 to 4 mm at 1 year but changed to 0.75 to 5.5 mm at 7 years.

Cross-sectional studies of children selected for nonabuse, examined using colposcopy and photographs, reported a similar range of measurements of the diameter of the hymenal opening and the width of the posterior rim of the hymen. McCann et al[3] reported measurements of the horizontal diameter of the hymenal opening using labial traction of 2 to 8 mm in girls aged 2 to 5 years, 1 to 9 mm in girls aged 5 to 7 years, and 2.5 to 10.5 mm in girls 8 years through Tanner stage 2 development. Although there were not enough girls in each age group to compare width of the posterior hymenal rim by age, researchers reported that among girls who were examined in the prone knee-chest position, the range of posterior rim width was 1 to 8 mm, with a mean width of 2.8 mm.

A cross-sectional study of 211 girls aged 1 month to 7 years by Berenson et al[1] also found that the mean horizontal diameter of the hymenal opening varied significantly by age (2.5 ± 0.8 mm to 3.6 ± 1.2 mm) and that the measurement of the posterior rim of the hymen was as small as 0.9 to 1.0 mm in girls between 1 and 7 years of age who were considered to be nonabused. A study of 195 nonabused girls between 5 and 7 years by Myhre et al[9] also found that the range of measurement of the posterior hymenal rim, using labial traction, was 1.1 to 7.9 mm wide.

The Clitoris

Physical examination of the female genitalia entails examination of the clitoris and clitoral hood. The clitoris consists of the following components: hood, glans, suspensory ligament, body or corpora, crura, root, and bulbs.[20] The clitoris has not been very well described in anatomical textbooks; however, in recent years detailed descriptions and measurements are being published to further understand reconstructive surgery when indicated for sex development disorders.[21,22] The glans is the only external portion of the clitoris and is a short cylindrical erectile organ in the superior portion of the vestibule. **Figures 2-6**, **2-7**, and **2-8** show the clitoral hood and the glans of the clitoris visible upon gentle retraction of the hood.

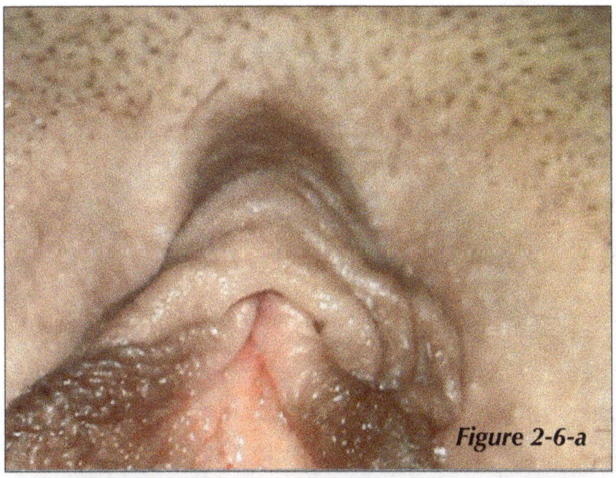
Figure 2-6-a

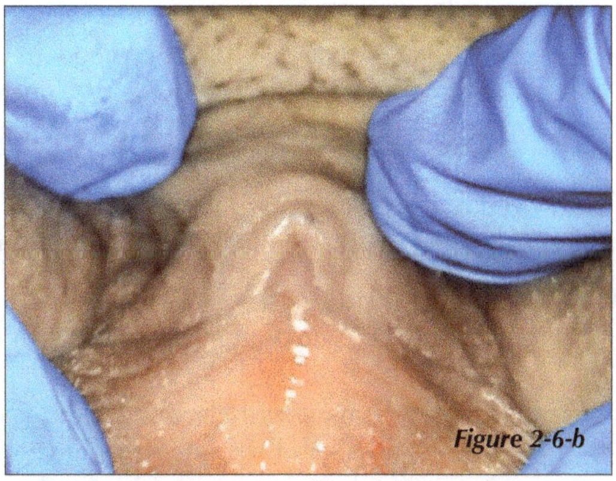
Figure 2-6-b

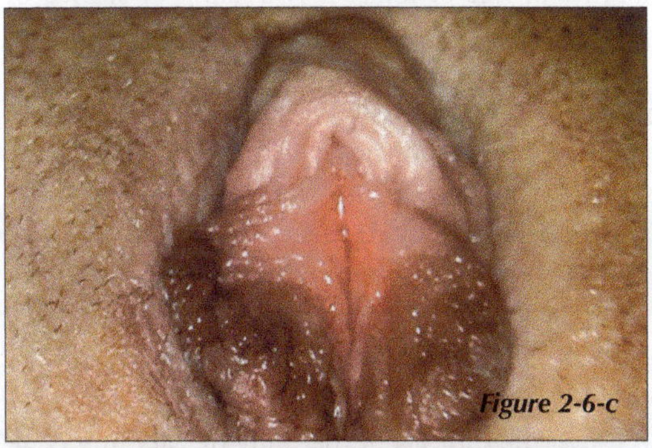
Figure 2-6-c

***Figure 2-6-a** through **c.** A 16-year-old child's examination showing the clitoral hood. Figure 2-6-b shows gentle retraction of the clitoral hood during the examination in order to visualize the glans of the clitoris. Figure 2-6-c shows the glans of the clitoris visible and the relationship between the clitoral hood and labia. The bleeding is due to the child's menstrual cycle.*

***Figure 2-7-a** and **b.** An 18-year-old examined in the supine lithotomy position. Figure 2-7-a shows the clitoral hood. Figure 2-7-b shows the gentle retraction of the clitoral hood to examine the glans of the clitoris.*

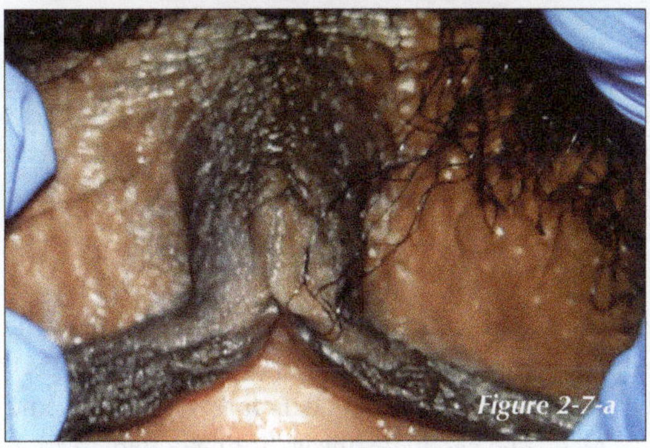
Figure 2-7-a

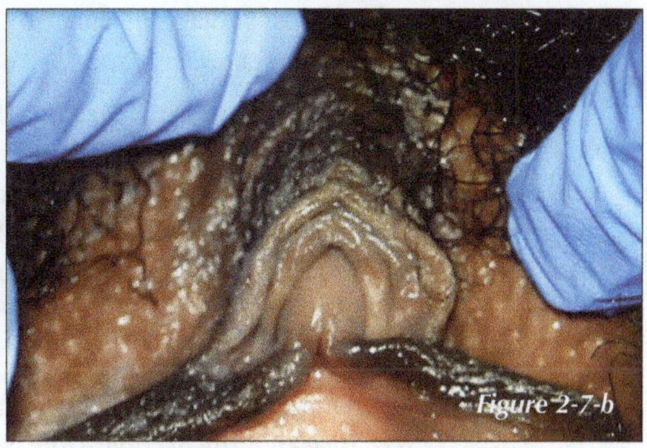
Figure 2-7-b

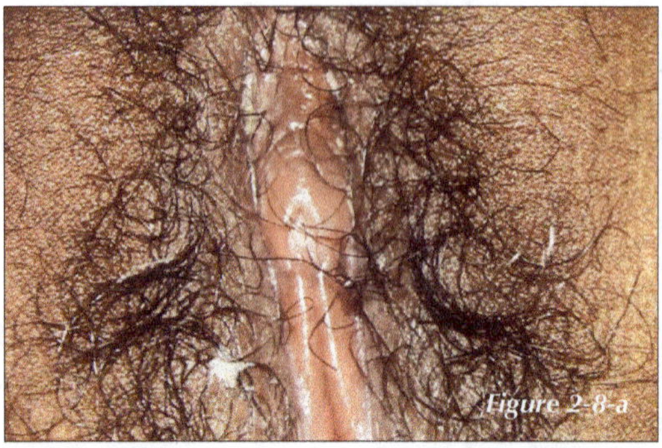

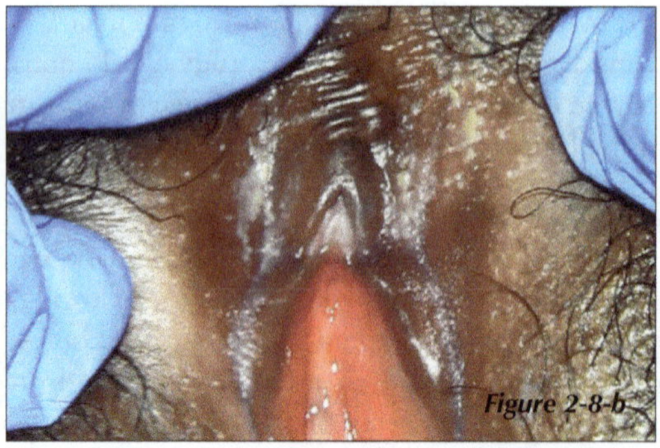

***Figure 2-8-a** and **b.** An 11-year-old examined in the supine frog leg position. Figure 2-8-a shows the clitoral hood, the glans of the clitoris and the labia minora. Figure 2-8-b shows the glans of the clitoris becoming more visible with the gentle retraction of the clitoral hood.*

In a 2016 study on 58 girls, Brodie et al[23] documented measurements and qualitative descriptions of the clitoral hood, clitoris, and labia minora. The authors found great variations in the morphology and size of female genitalia. The clitoral hood, which was observed to be a distinct structure separated from the labia minora, was noted to have 4 different shapes: coffee bean, horseshoe, tent, and trumpet. The most common was the tent-shaped clitoral hood, in which the hood forms a peak and then divides into left and right leaflets alongside a linear opening where the glans is located. The coffee bean shaped hood, with the left and right sides fused over the glans, was the most commonly observed shape in infants.[23] In addition to the variation in measurements in the same age category, the clitoral hood to urethral orifice distance and labia minora length and depth exhibited steep growth during puberty.

The Anus

The skin around the anus, when the external anal sphincter is contracted and the anus is closed, takes on a wrinkled appearance. The tighter the contraction of the sphincter, the more wrinkles or folds are seen. In some children there is a gap in the subcutaneous division of the external sphincter muscle, which causes an area in the midline, usually at the 6 o'clock position, to be smooth and free of folds. It is usually a v-shaped or a wedge-shaped area. This condition was named "diastasis ani" by Dr. John McCann[2] who observed this finding in 26% of the children in his study of perianal findings in nonabused children (**Appendix Figure 2-29**). Berenson et al,[5] in a study of 89 female infants younger than 18 months, also noted this smooth area in 26% of subjects. Myhre et al[8] studied children 5 to 7 years with no history or suspicion of sexual abuse and noted that more boys than girls were found to have diastasis ani and that it was more commonly observed in the prone knee-chest position than in the left lateral position. In the knee-chest position, 12% of subjects had the finding. Diastasis ani is considered a normal variant and unrelated to a child's disclosure of sexual abuse.[18,19]

Anal tags and thickened midline skin folds are common findings in children who have not been abused. Tags were seen in 11% of the subjects in the study by McCann et al[2] and in 6% of subjects in the study by Myhre et al.[8] **Appendix Figure 2-30** is an example of a midline tag.

The skin in the perianal area may have darker pigmentation than elsewhere on the body. This was first described in the study by McCann et al,[2] where the prevalence varied by race and ethnicity. Among white children, 22% had hyperpigmentation of the perianal skin, compared with 53% of the African American children and 58% of the Hispanic children studied (**Appendix Figures 2-31** through **2-33-a**).

When the external anal sphincter relaxes but the internal sphincter remains closed, the anal opening may have an irregular appearance (**Appendix Figures 2-33-b** and **2-34**). When both the internal and external anal sphincters relax, the anal canal is visualized, and in some views, the pectinate line can be seen. The pectinate line is the line of demarcation between the skin of the anal canal (pectin) and the anal mucosa and can have a jagged appearance because of the anal columns and crypts (**Appendix Figure 2-35**).

Anal dilation, with both internal and external sphincters relaxed, was found in 49% of 267 children selected for nonabuse in the study by McCann et al,[2] in which all children were examined in the prone knee-chest position, some for as long as 4 minutes. A smaller number of children had complete anal dilation within 30 seconds (14.6%). Myhre et al[8] reported the frequency of complete anal dilation seen in 100 boys and 167 girls between the ages of 4 and 6 years who were examined in the prone knee-chest position for 30 seconds as part of a study of findings in nonabused children. Complete anal dilation was seen in 3% of the boys and 5.6% of the girls, for a rate of 4.7% overall. In the Myhre study,[8] complete anal dilation was very rare (0.7%) when the child was examined in the left lateral position.

Another feature described in the studies by McCann et al[2] and Myhre et al[8] is that of venous pooling or venous congestion of the blood vessels in the perianal area. McCann et al[2] reported that at the midpoint of the examination in the knee-chest position, 52% of the subjects had venous pooling. In the Myhre et al[8] study, children were not kept in the knee-chest position as long as in the McCann et al[2] study (average time 30 seconds compared with up to 4 minutes), and venous congestion was documented in 20% of subjects. The perianal area has a rich blood supply, and the veins become engorged when the child is positioned so that venous return from the plexus is impaired. This can lead to a rather alarming purple-blue coloration of the surrounding skin, which should not be mistaken for trauma. See **Appendix Figures 2-36** through **2-38** for examples of venous pooling.

The congenital defect known as failure of midline fusion, or perineal groove, is another finding on anogenital examination that may cause concern of trauma and sexual abuse if it is not recognized (see **Appendix Figures 2-39-a** and **b**). In 1984, Dr. Anthony Shaw published photos of 6 children with this defect in the "Picture of the Month" section of the *American Journal of Diseases of Childhood*.[24] His report stated that the condition required no treatment and that the defect would eventually fill in. The groove results from the failure of midline fusion of the genital folds during embryonic development with the genital folds forming the sides and the floor of the groove in the perineal mound.[25]

A 2006 report described the results of a surgical correction of a perineal groove in a 6-month-old girl.[26] Clinically the sulcus has a wet mucus membrane and hypertrophic tails of the labia minora surround the sulcus.[26] Histological analysis of the excised tissue revealed squamous epithelial tissue at both ends, with rectal mucosa in between. There was also edema, patchy hemorrhage, and scattered inflammatory cell infiltrate in the lamina propria surrounding normal rectal crypts. The authors postulate that the anomaly represents an embryological remnant of the urorectal septum rather than a failure of midline fusion.

According to the 2018 updated guidelines on medical evaluation of children suspected of sexual abuse, normal variations of the anus that are unrelated to a child's disclosure of sexual abuse include diastasis ani, perianal skin tag, and hyperpigmentation of the perianal tissues in children of color. Conditions involving the anus that may be mistaken for sexual abuse include failure of midline fusion, also called perineal groove; visualization of the pectinate/dentate line at the juncture of the anoderm and rectal mucosa; and partial dilation of the external anal sphincter with the internal sphincter closed, causing the appearance of deep creases in the perianal skin.

Effects of Puberty

Puberty is the time children develop secondary sexual characteristics and reproductive function as a result of a complex sequence of biological events.[27,28] During this critical time, multiple physical changes occur, including changes in the external genitalia in boys and girls. The pubertal genitalia varies from the prepubertal genitalia, and recognition of these differences is essential to recognizing the normal variations and any genital disorders or signs of trauma.[28]

The Hymen

From infancy to age 2 years, the hymen is thick, pale, and redundant under the influence of the maternal hormone.[28] Later, as a result of lack of estrogen, the prepubertal hymen is usually pink-red and thin.[28] With the onset of puberty, the hymen and other genital tissues show the effects of hormonal influence, especially estrogen. The hymen becomes thicker, more elastic, paler, less sensitive to touch, and more likely to fold on itself (**Figures 2-9** through **2-11**). In a follow-up study of girls examined at 5 to 7 years, Myhre et al[9] reexamined a subset of subjects at 10 to 13 years. They found that the hymen, vagina, and labia show the effects of development, as seen in **Appendix Figures 2-40** through **2-43**.

Adolescent girls from 13 to 19 years with and without a history of penile-vaginal intercourse were examined in a study to compare the appearance of the hymen.[31] **Appendix Figures 2-44** through **2-47** show some of these variations, from a very thick, tulip-shape hymen with an anterior opening (see **Appendix Figure 2-44-a** and **b**) to a relatively narrow rim of the hymen (see **Appendix Figure 2-46**).

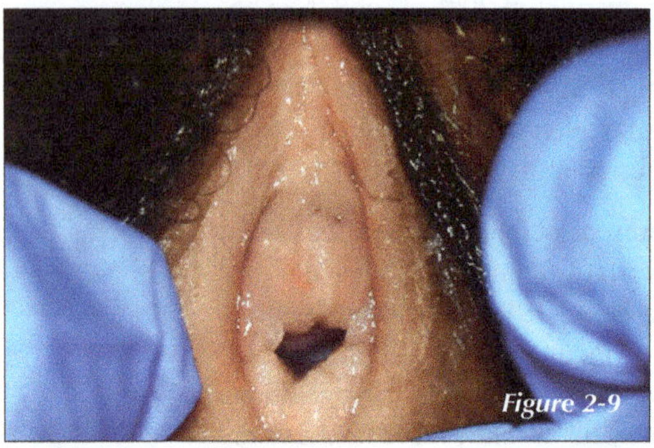

Figure 2-9. *A 15-year-old child with an estrogenized hymen. Notice the thick hymen and also notice the hyperpigmentation and elongation of the labia minora (all changes caused by puberty in this child).*

Figure 2-10-a. *A 15-year-old child who was sexually assaulted by multiple men a month before the examination. Notice the thickened and darkened labia minora and the clitoral hood and the glans appearing under the hood.*

Figure 2-10-b. *Same child examined with labial traction. Notice her annular estrogenized hymen.*

Figure 2-11-a. *A 10-year-old child who disclosed penile genital penetration by her 18-year-old cousin. Notice the clitoral hood and the thickened, hyperpigmented labia minora.*

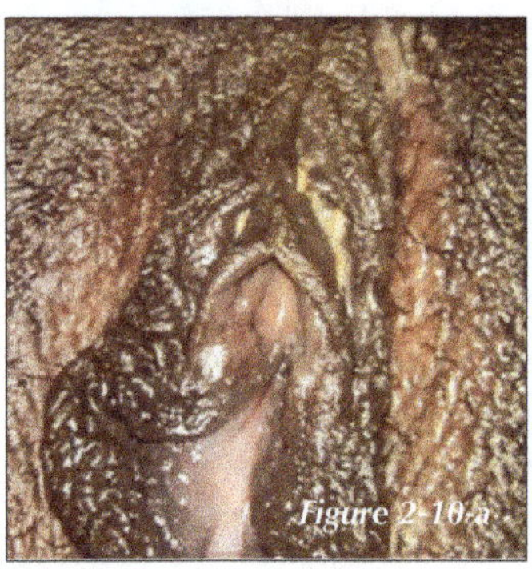

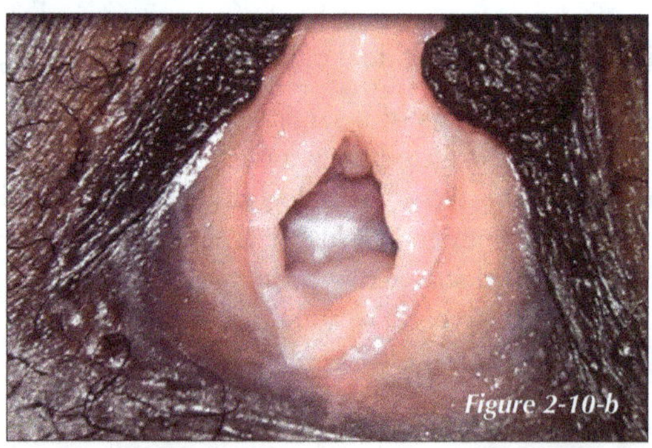

Figure 2-11-b. *Same child with gentle labial separation and retraction of the hood. Notice the glans of the clitoris.*

Figure 2-11-c. *Notice the estrogenized crescentic hymen.*

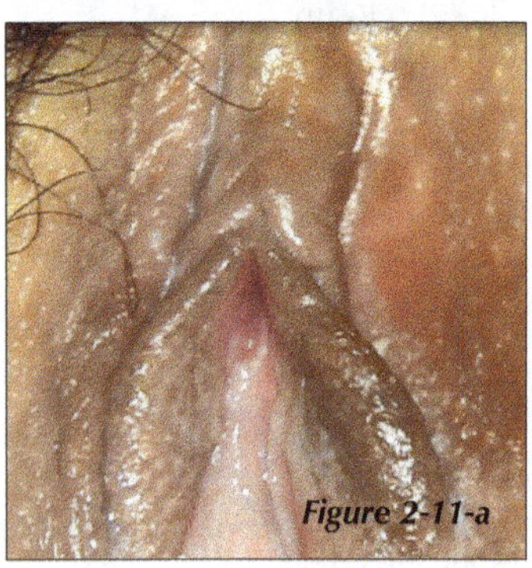

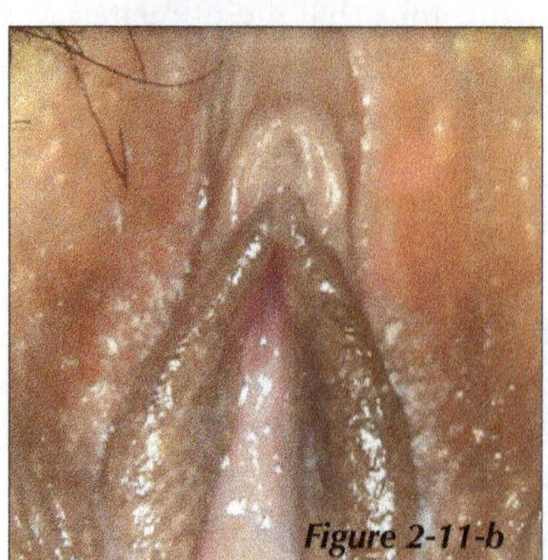

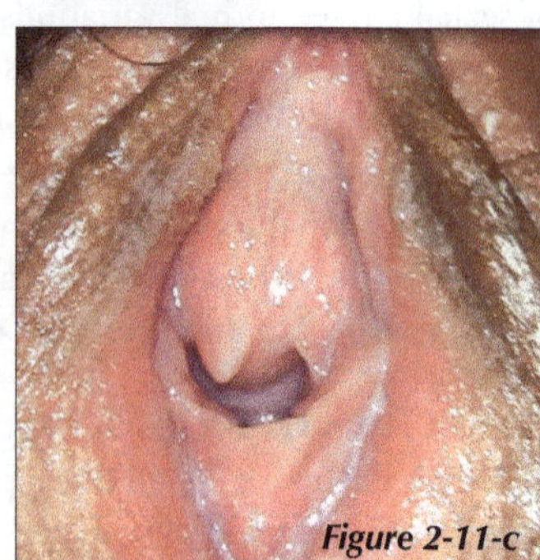

Because estrogen causes the tissues of both the hymen and vagina to thicken and become pale, it is sometimes difficult to identify the edge of the hymen. The use of a large swab covered by a balloon for color contrast (see **Appendix Figure 2-45**) or a regular cotton-tipped applicator to stretch out the edge of the hymen (see **Appendix Figures 2-46** and **2-47**) can assist the examiner in determining the integrity of the hymenal rim.

The Vagina

As pubertal development progresses, all the tissues and structures of the vaginal vestibule show the effects of estrogen. **Appendix Figures 2-48** and **2-49** are examples of the fossa groove that develops in some patients during early puberty as a result of the effect of estrogen on the inner aspect of the labia minora. The external surface of the labia minora is also affected by androgenic hormones in the same way the scrotal skin changes in boys. The skin becomes darker, thicker, and develops folds or rugae. For reasons not fully understood, the labia minora can be affected on one side more than another, which causes an asymmetry that can be quite pronounced (**Appendix Figures 2-50** and **2-51**).

The Cervix

The cervix may also take on a different appearance as puberty progresses (**Appendix Figure 2-52**). In the younger adolescent the columnar epithelium of the endocervix is visible on the outer surface, which gives it a darker red, sometimes pebbled appearance (**Appendix Figure 2-53**). This pattern changes as the neck of the cervix lengthens and the endocervical tissues regress inward.

Conclusion

It should not be surprising that there is considerable variation in the appearance of the structures of the external genitalia and anal tissues in children. Every child is a unique individual, and although there may be common patterns in how tissues develop, there is much not understood about anatomic variations. For example, it is not clear exactly why the hymen changes from primarily annular to primarily crescentic as a child grows and estrogen effects regress, or what factors are involved in the development of the septate, microperforate, or imperforate hymen.

Additional studies of children with no history or concern for abuse are needed, especially studies of the appearance of the genital tissues in girls between 9 and 13 years. Further studies are also needed of the appearance of the anal tissues in children of different ages and of the prevalence of dilation in children with and without a history of constipation. Further research will help to answer some of the remaining questions regarding what is normal when it comes to the appearance of the genital and anal tissues in children.

Appendix 2-1: Features of Genital and Anal Anatomy

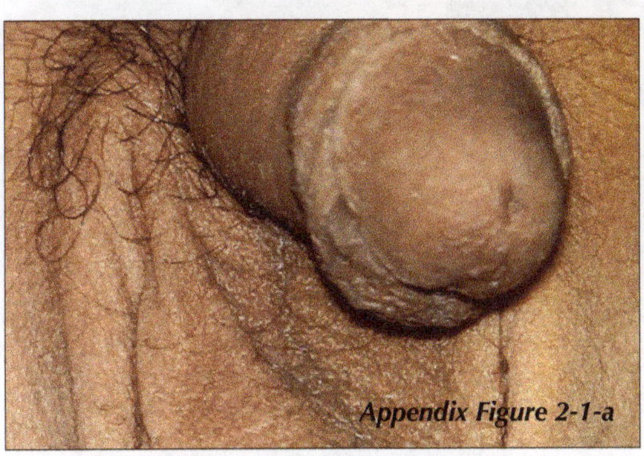

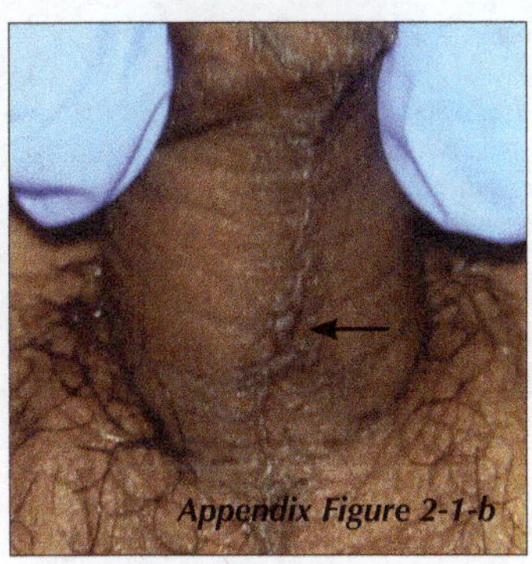

Appendix Figure 2-1-a** and **b. *An examination of a 12-year-old boy. Notice the median raphe in Appendix Figure 2-1-b.*

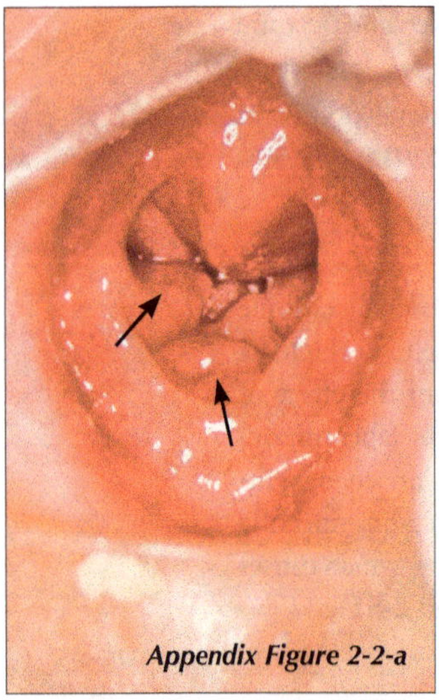

Appendix Figure 2-2-a

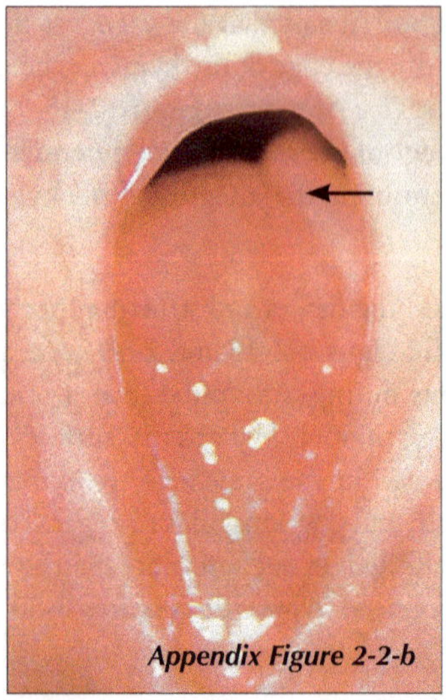

Appendix Figure 2-2-b

Appendix Figure 2-2-a. *An 8-year-old girl examined in the supine position, using labial traction. Arrows point to intravaginal ridges at 6 and 9 o'clock, which are normal structures. (See Table 2-2).*

Appendix Figure 2-2-b. *Same patient examined in the prone, knee-chest position. Arrow points to an intravaginal ridge. The hymen is smooth and without interruption. This is a normal examination.*

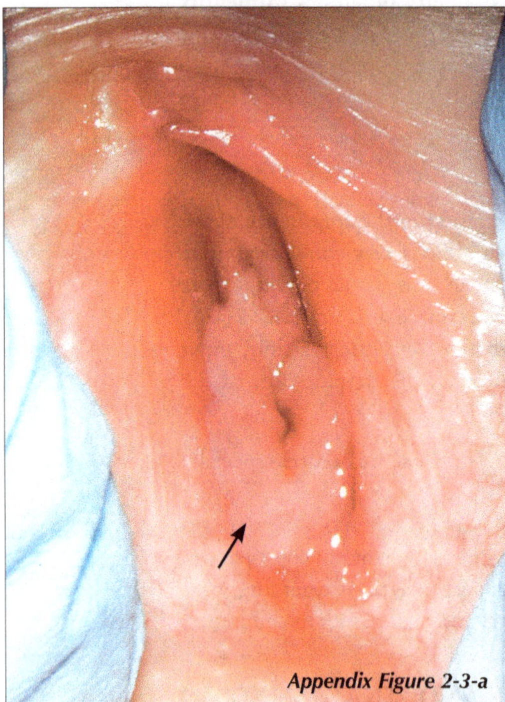

Appendix Figure 2-3-a

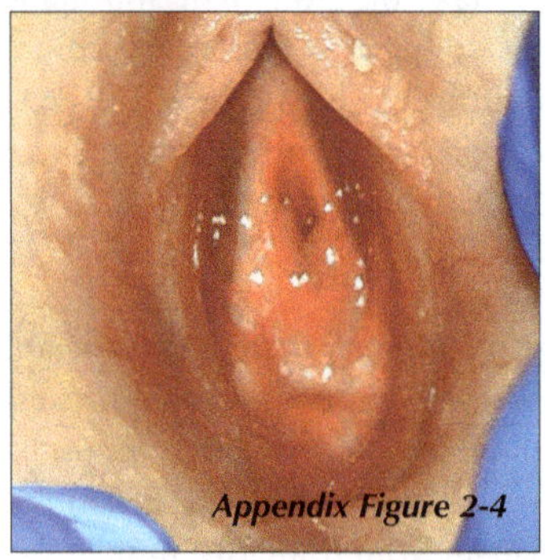

Appendix Figure 2-4

Appendix Figure 2-4. *A prepubertal child examined in the supine frog leg positon. Notice her prominent urethral opening (a normal finding) and normal annular hymen.*

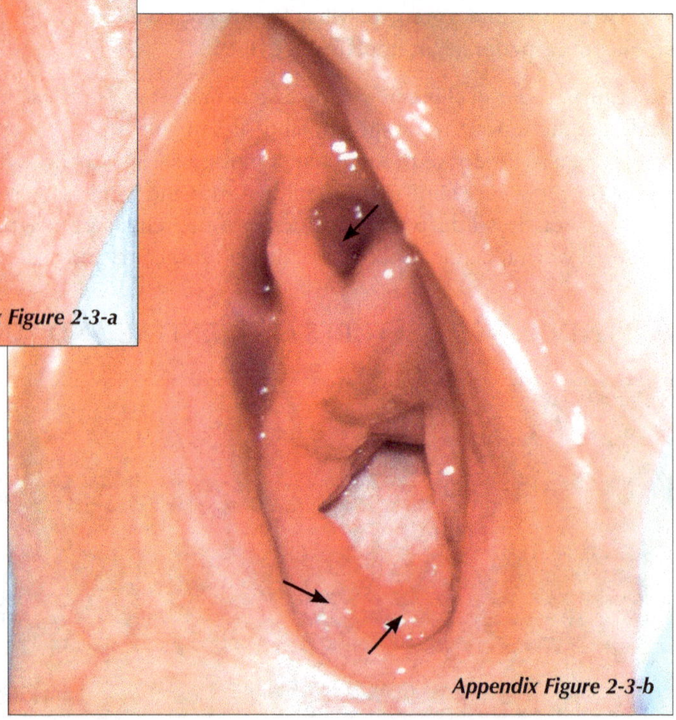

Appendix Figure 2-3-b

Appendix Figure 2-3-a. *A 2-year-old girl examined using labial separation. The hymen at 7 o'clock location is thick and shows the effects of estrogen. The hymen is redundant and folded, and in this view neither the hymenal edge nor the hymenal opening can be seen.*

Appendix Figure 2-3-b. *Using labial traction, with the examiner grasping the labia majora and gently pulling forward, the hymen at 7 o'clock opens, as does the urethral orifice shown at 12 o'clock, and an intravaginal ridge at 5 o'clock can be visualized extending into the vagina at the 8 o'clock location.*

Appendix Figure 2-5. *A 6-year-old female with a normal annular hymen. Photo contributed by Diana Faugno, MSN, RN, CPN, SANE-A, SANE-P, FAAFS, DF-IAFN, DF-AFN.*

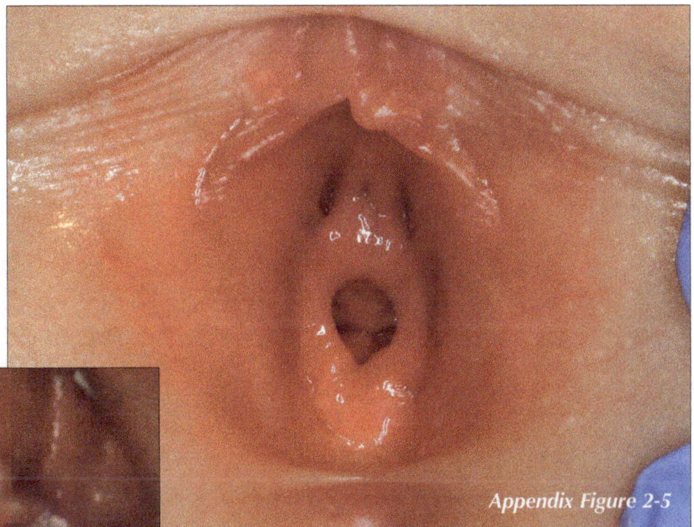

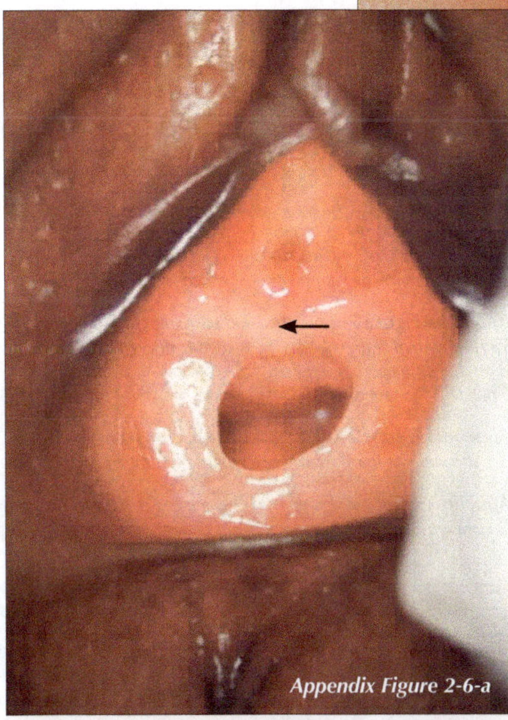

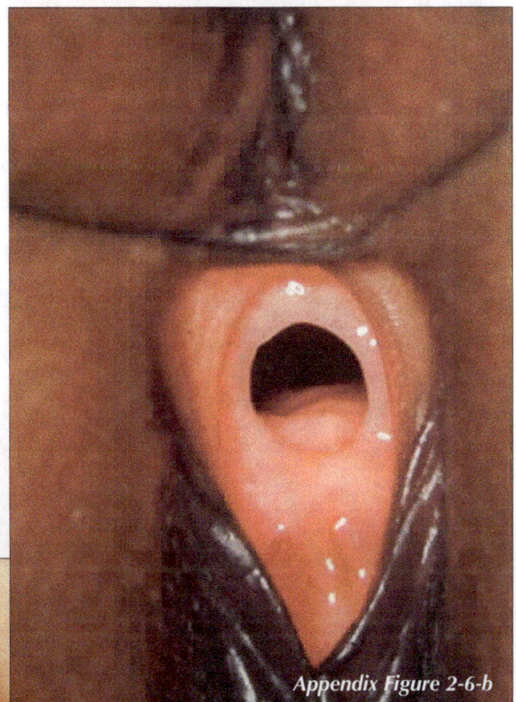

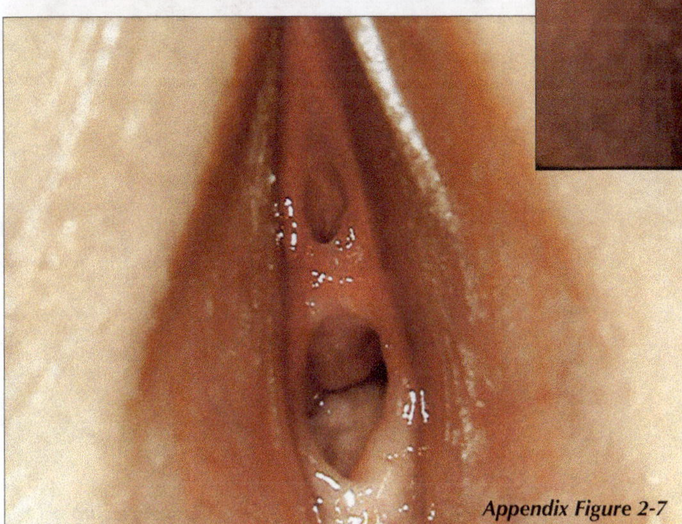

Appendix Figure 2-6-a. *A 6-year-old girl with no suspicion of sexual abuse. The photograph shows an annular hymen with tissue all the way around the hymenal opening, including at the 12 o'clock position.*

Appendix Figure 2-6-b. *In the prone knee-chest position, the smooth, noninterrupted edge of the hymen is clearly demonstrated.*

Appendix Figure 2-7. *An 11-year-old child evaluated in the supine frog-leg position. Notice the intravaginal ridge at the 6 o'clock position (a normal finding).*

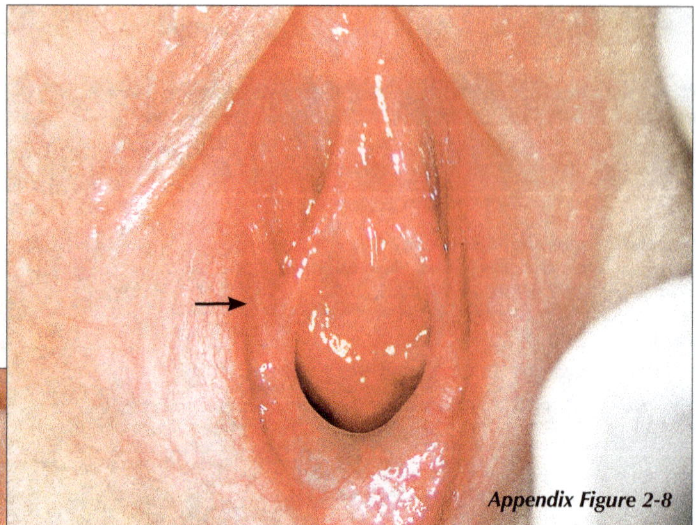

Appendix Figure 2-8

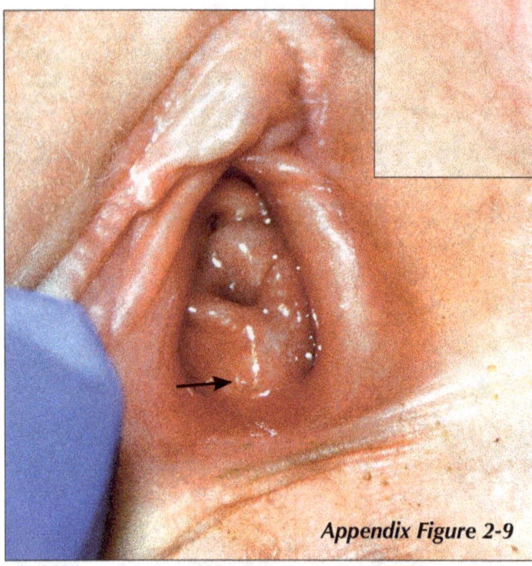

Appendix Figure 2-9

Appendix Figure 2-8. *An 11-year-old girl with no history of sexual abuse. This photo shows a normal, crescentic hymen, with attachments at the 2 o'clock and 10 o'clock position. The arrow points to periurethral support bands, which are normal structures.*

Appendix Figure 2-9. *A 2-year-old Hispanic girl brought for suspicion of sexual abuse. The hymen is sleeve-like, with a ventral opening and an external hymenal ridge in the midline at 6 o'clock. The redness in the fossa is not specific for sexual abuse.*

Appendix Figure 2-10. *Annular hymen in a 6-month-old white girl, showing the thick appearance typical of estrogen effect.*

Appendix Figure 2-11. *Annular hymen in a 16-month-old girl, shown using labial separation.*

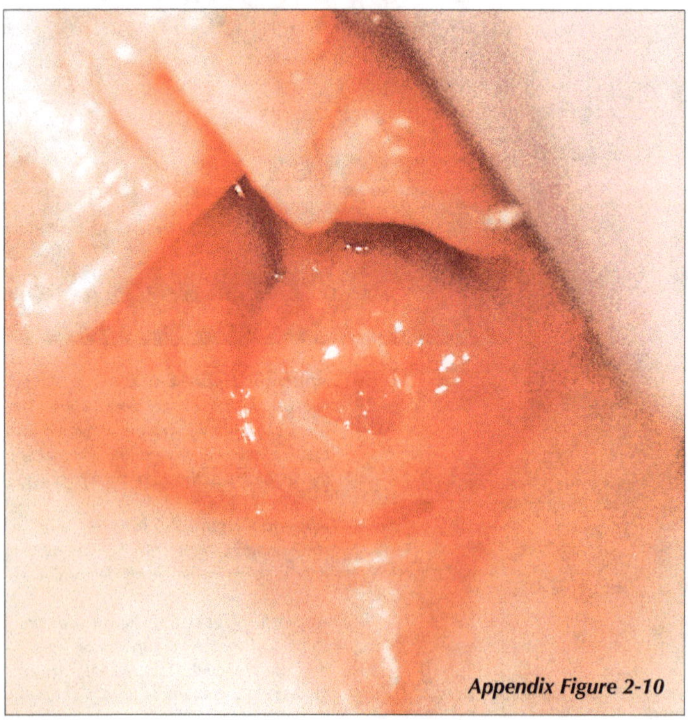

Appendix Figure 2-10

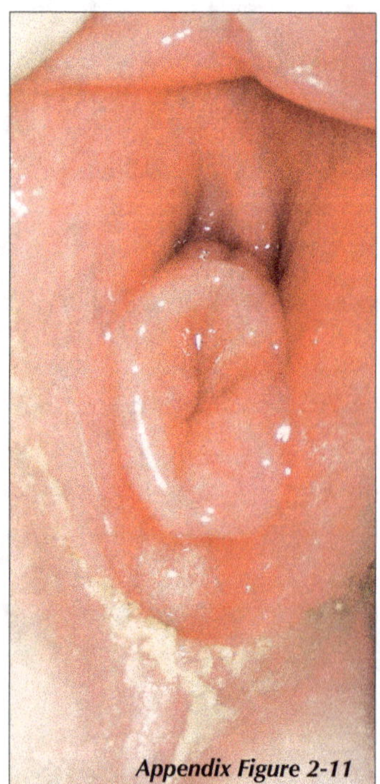

Appendix Figure 2-11

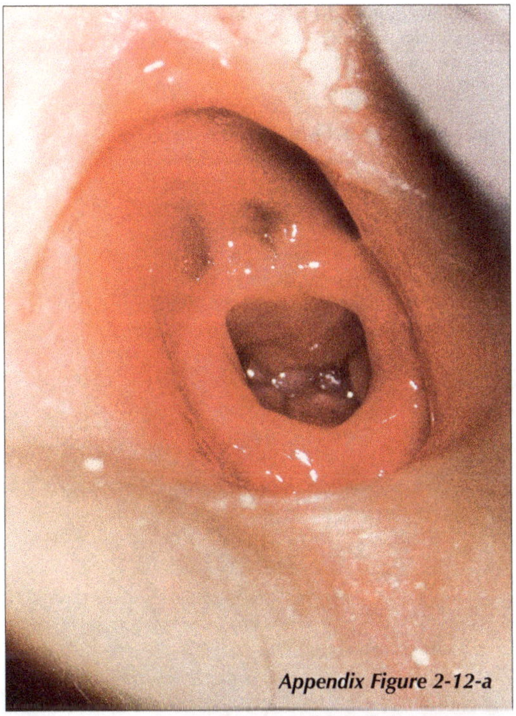

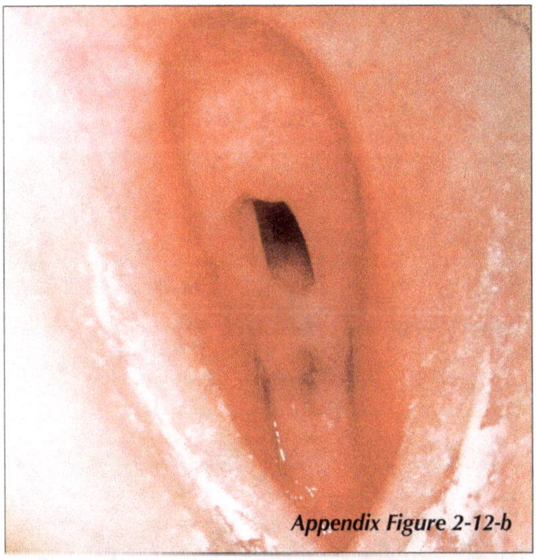

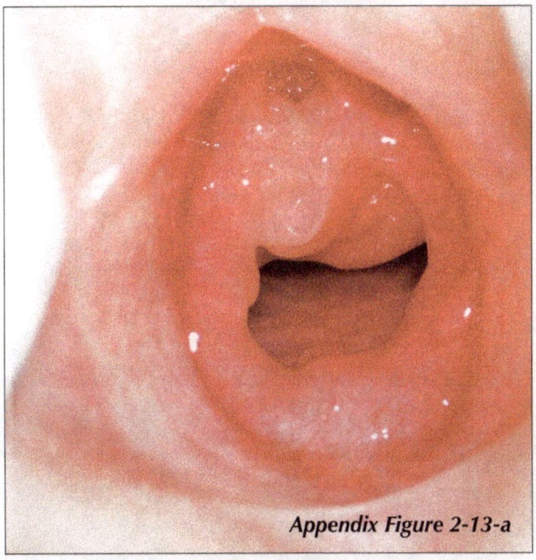

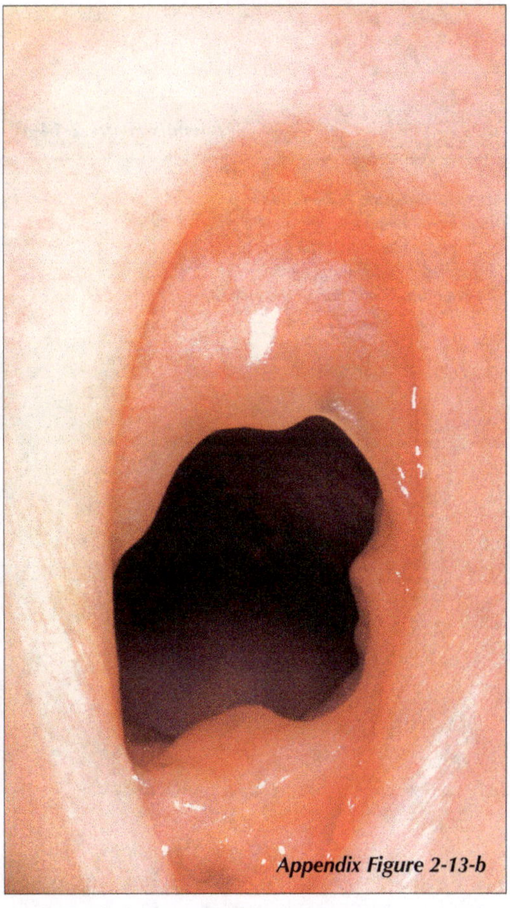

Appendix Figure 2-12-a. *A 3-year-old girl examined using labial traction. The hymen is thick, suggesting estrogen effect, and the inner edge of the hymen is smooth.*

Appendix Figure 2-12-b. *In the knee-chest position, the hymen edge looks sharper, but the rim is smooth and without interruption.*

Appendix Figure 2-13-a. *A 2-year-old white girl examined using labial traction. The crescentic hymen has attachments at 11 o'clock and 2 o'clock. There is a small mound or bump on the hymen at 6 o'clock and at 9 o'clock.*

Appendix Figure 2-13-b. *In the prone knee-chest position, the mound at 6 o'clock is now seen at 12 o'clock, and the mound at 9 o'clock is seen at 3 o'clock.*

Appendix Figure 2-14-a. *This 4-year-old girl, examined using labial traction, has a thick, redundant hymen. The edge is not well defined. She has no history or suspicion of sexual abuse.*

Appendix Figure 2-14-b. *Using labial traction, the hymenal opening is easily seen. The inner edge of the hymen is smooth except for a mound or tag at 6 o'clock. Although the opening may appear "large" to a caregiver or inexperienced medical provider, it is normal for the labial traction technique to produce the largest measurements of the horizontal diameter of the hymenal opening.*

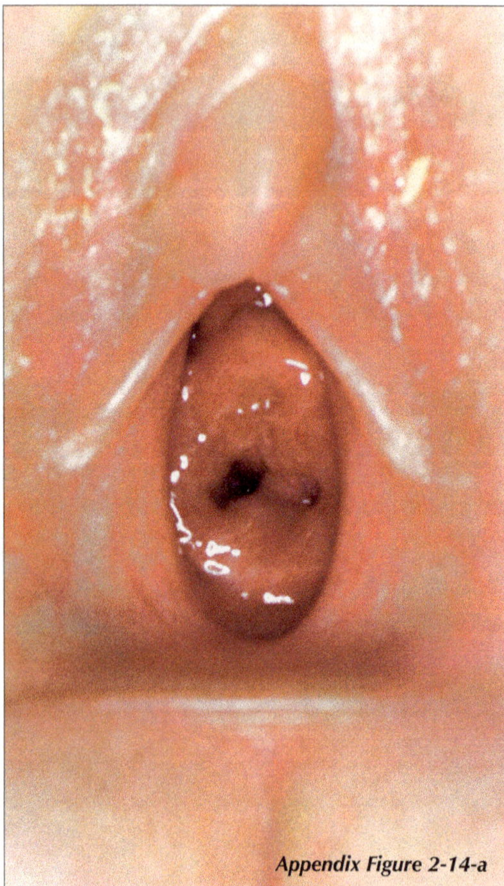

Appendix Figure 2-14-a

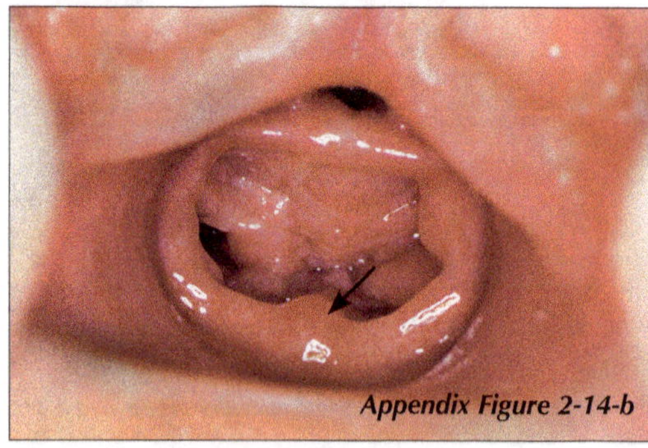

Appendix Figure 2-14-b

Appendix Figure 2-14-c. *In the prone knee-chest view, the mound on the hymen appears as a thickening, possibly a resolving hymenal tag from birth. This is a normal variation in the hymen.*

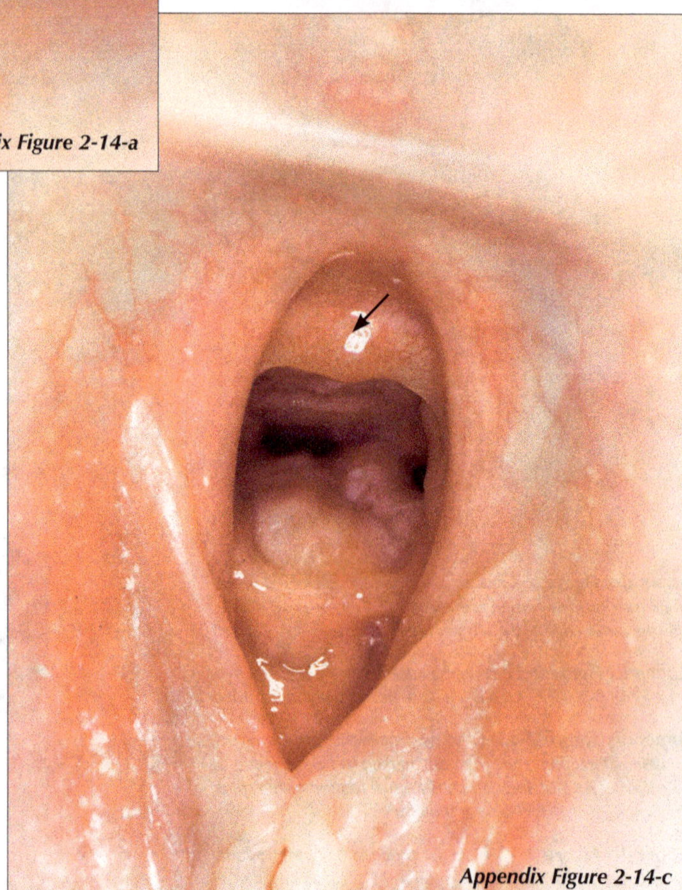

Appendix Figure 2-14-c

Appendix Figure 2-15-a. *This 8-year-old African American girl gave a history of penile-vaginal contact by an uncle. Using supine labial traction, the hymen appears to have a superficial cleft at 3 o'clock.*

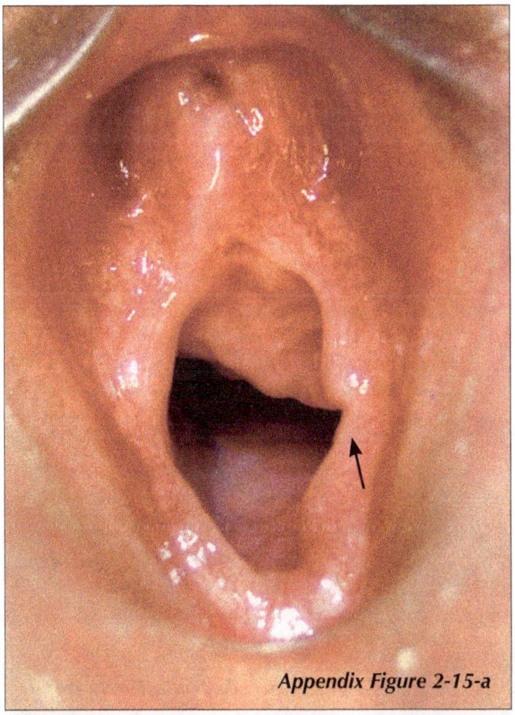

Appendix Figure 2-15-a

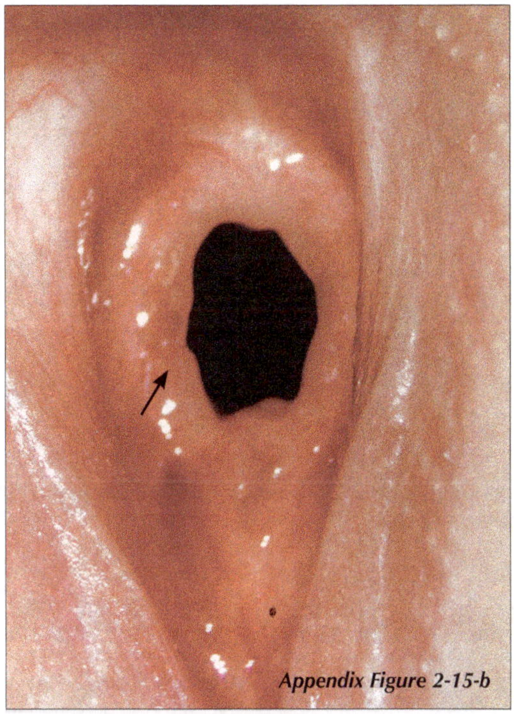

Appendix Figure 2-15-b

Appendix Figure 2-15-b. *In this prone knee-chest view, there is now a notch in the hymen at 9 o'clock, which would correlate with the 3 o'clock location when she was examined supine. A mound caused by an intravaginal ridge can give the impression of a notch adjacent to the mound, so additional techniques are needed to stretch out the edge of the hymen for a better view.*

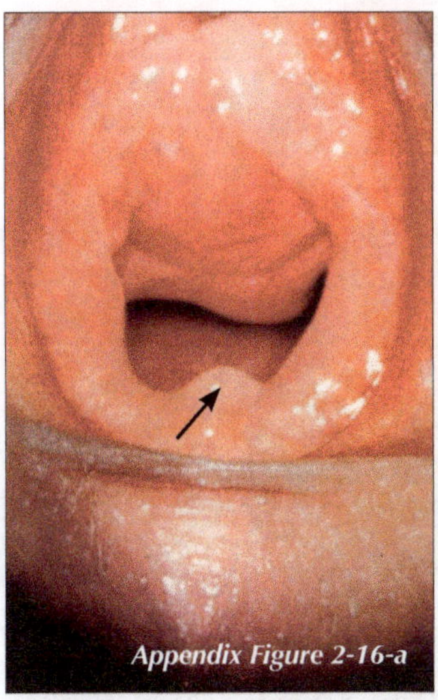

Appendix Figure 2-16-a

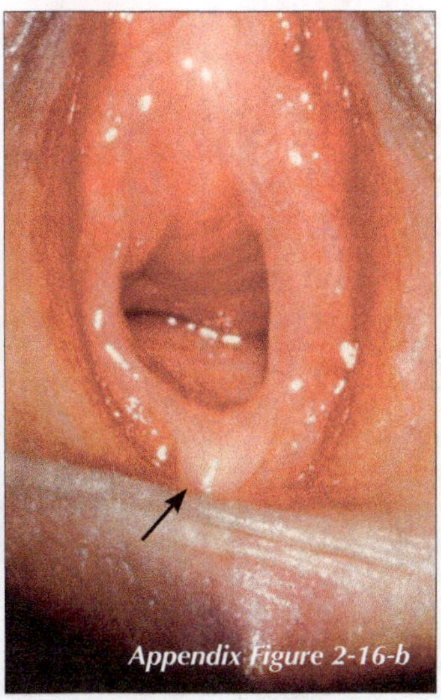

Appendix Figure 2-16-b

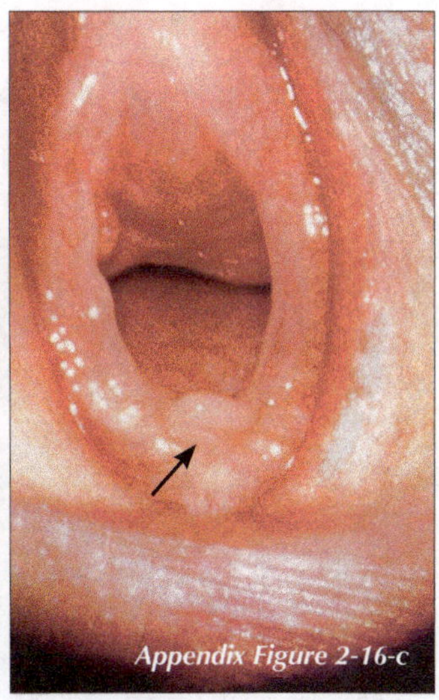

Appendix Figure 2-16-c

Appendix Figure 2-16-a. *A 3-year-old girl with no complaint of abuse, examined using labial traction. There is a small mound on the hymen at the 6 o'clock location, but otherwise the hymen appears smooth and normal.*

Appendix Figure 2-16-b. *In this view the mound appears to be a tag on the hymen, which is now folded outward.*

Appendix Figure 2-16-c. *The midline tag has again folded inward, causing the appearance of a mound.*

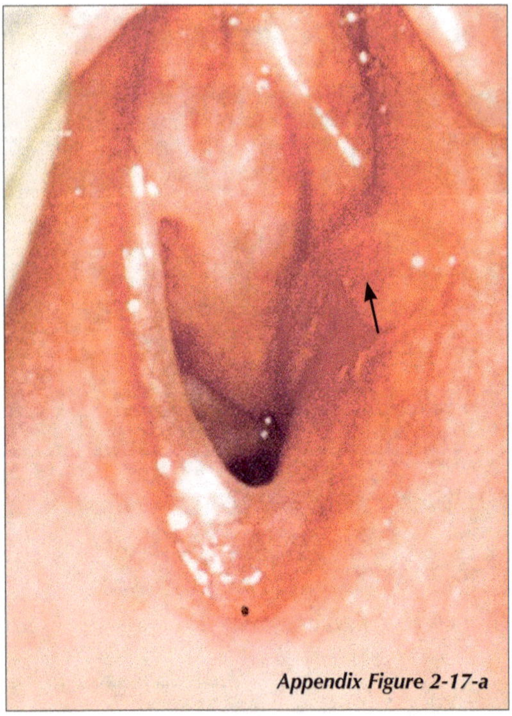

Appendix Figure 2-17-a

Appendix Figure 2-17-a. *This 3-year-old girl also has a tag on the hymen, at 3 o'clock, which is folded outward against the vestibular wall on the patient's left side.*

Appendix Figure 2-17-b. *By using labial traction to separate and then oppose the labia majora, the tag has been released and is now folded across the hymenal opening, touching the vestibular wall at 9 o'clock.*

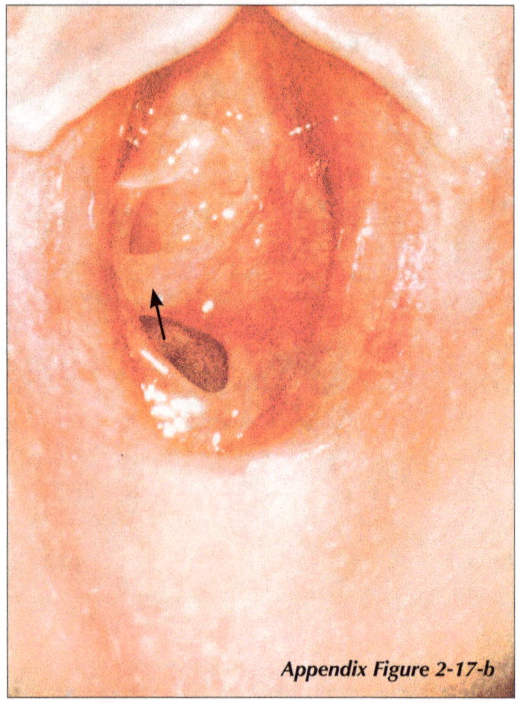

Appendix Figure 2-17-b

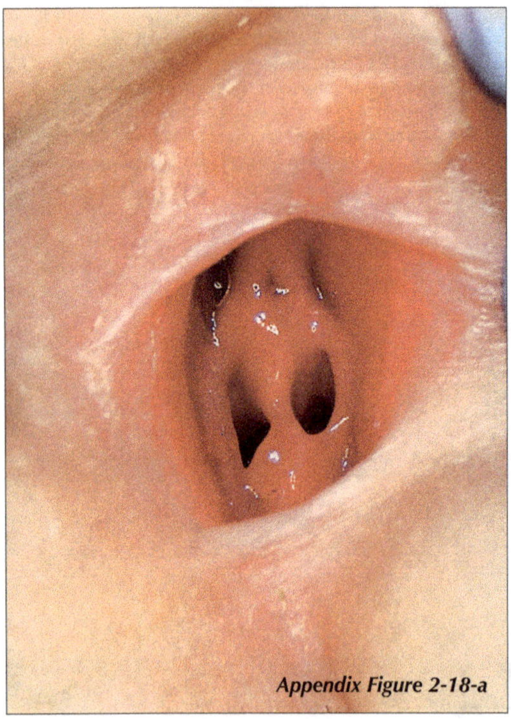

Appendix Figure 2-18-a

Appendix Figure 2-18-a. *A 3-year-old girl with a septate hymen.*

Appendix Figure 2-18-b. *Showing the septum extending from 12 o'clock to 6 o'clock across the vaginal opening. To be sure this is only a hymenal septum and not a vaginal septum, a small swab or probe should be passed behind the septum.*

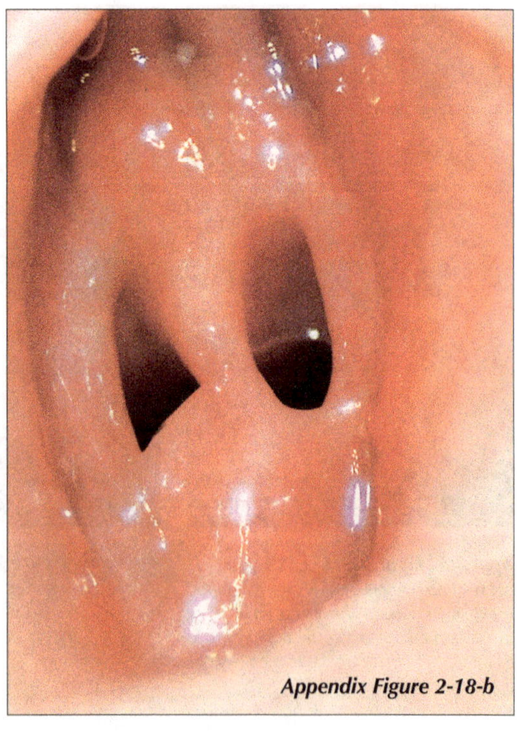

Appendix Figure 2-18-b

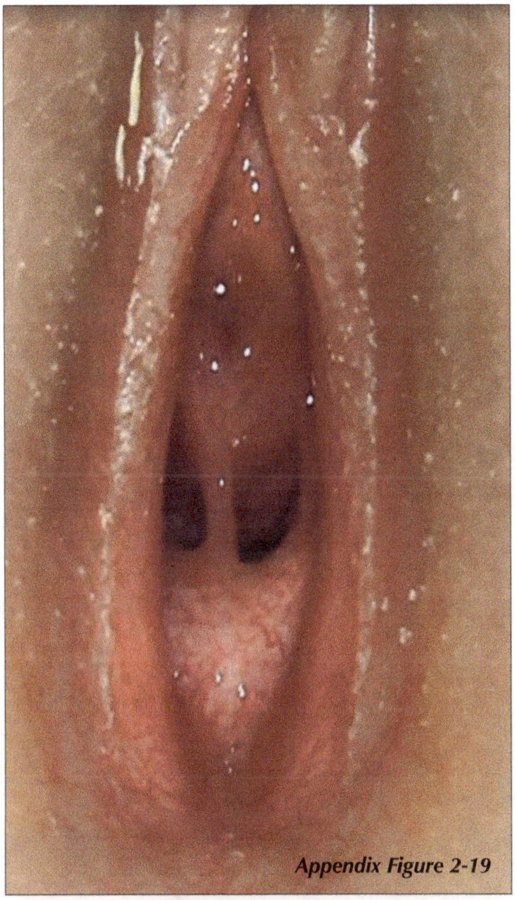

Appendix Figure 2-19

Appendix Figure 2-19. *This 9-year-old girl presented for a medical evaluation after she disclosed being sexually abused. She has a septate hymen.*

Appendix Figure 2-20. *This 6-year-old girl has a vertical septum, which is clearly seen to involve only the hymen. Image reprinted with permission from eMedicine.com, 2010. Available at: https://emedicine.medscape.com/article/954024-overview.*

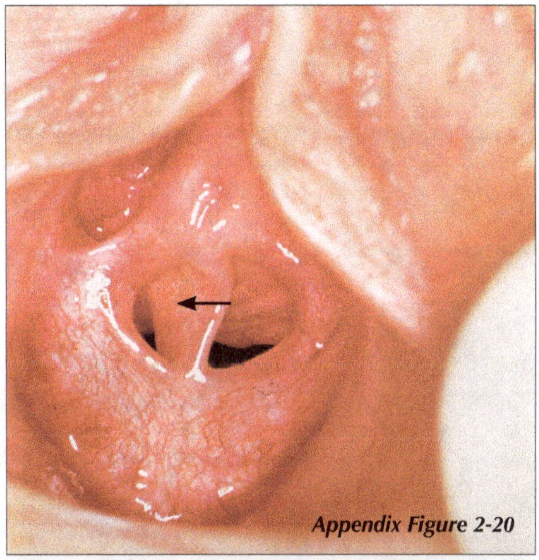

Appendix Figure 2-20

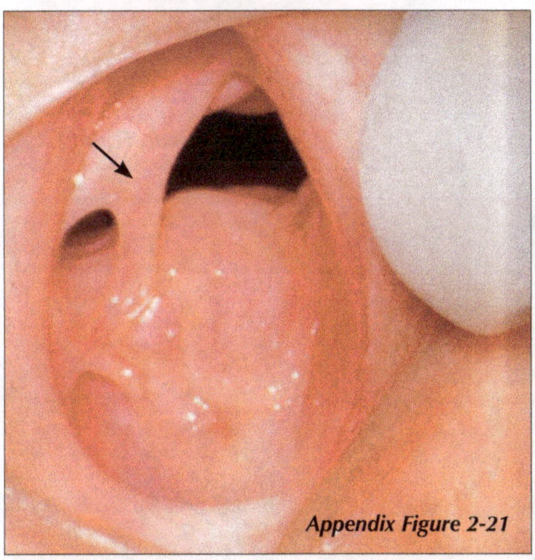

Appendix Figure 2-21

Appendix Figure 2-21. *This 3-year-old girl had an unusual appearance to the hymen. In the prone knee-chest position, a vertical septum is seen extending across the introitus, resulting in 2 asymmetrical hymenal openings.*

Appendix Figure 2-22. *Normal periurethral support bands in a 16-year-old girl with a redundant, closed hymen.*

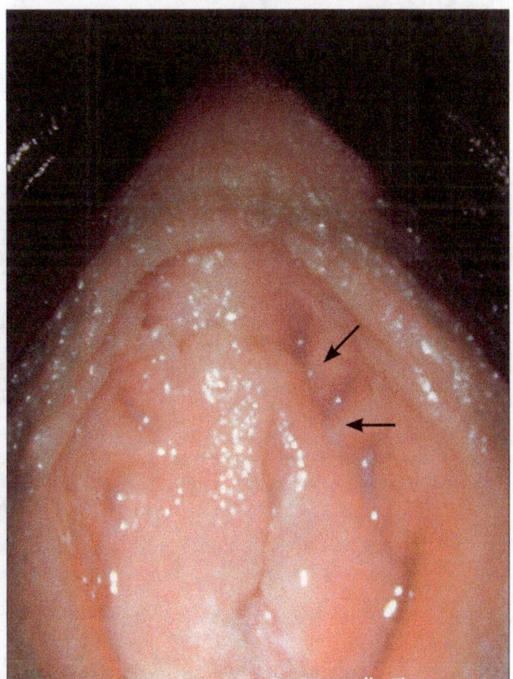

Appendix Figure 2-22

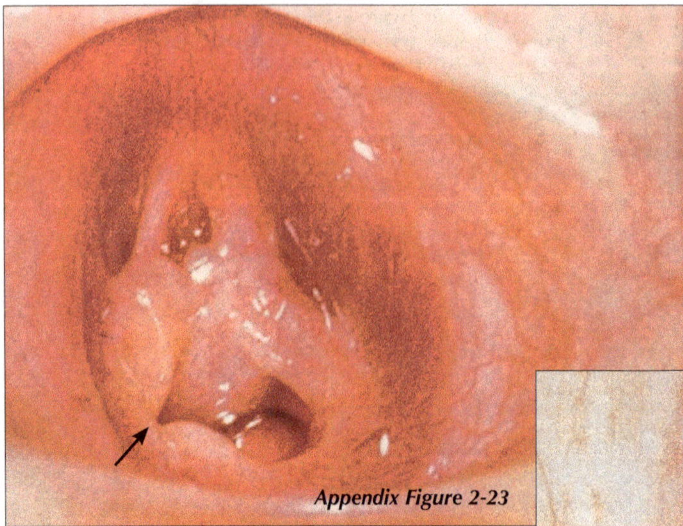
Appendix Figure 2-23

Appendix Figure 2-23. *A 3-year-old girl with a notch in the hymen at 9 o'clock and no history of penetration.*

Appendix Figure 2-24. *A 5-year-old African American girl with asymmetry in the thickness and pigmentation of the labia minora at 2 o'clock and 10 o'clock and a midline pale area in the fossa, likely linea vestibularis 6 o'clock, a normal finding.*

Appendix Figure 2-25. *Microperforate hymen in an 8-year-old girl.*

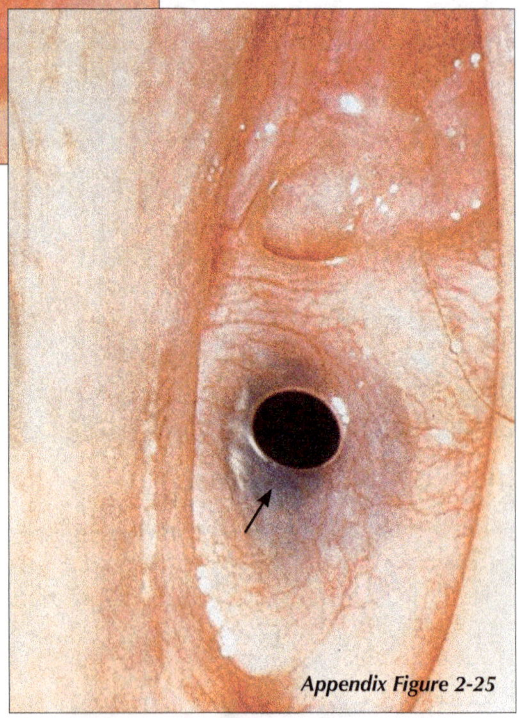
Appendix Figure 2-25

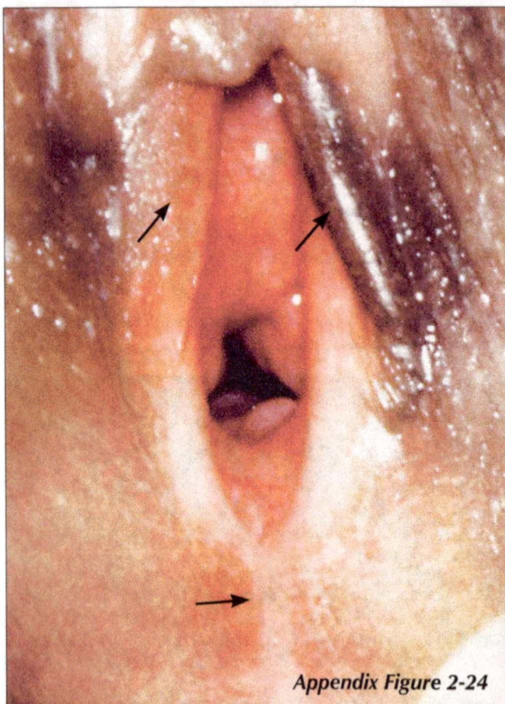
Appendix Figure 2-24

Appendix Figure 2-26. *Superficial notches at 3 o'clock and 6 o'clock in the hymen of a 6-year-old girl. Alternatively, one could describe this as representing 2 mounds on the hymen at 5 o'clock and 7 o'clock.*

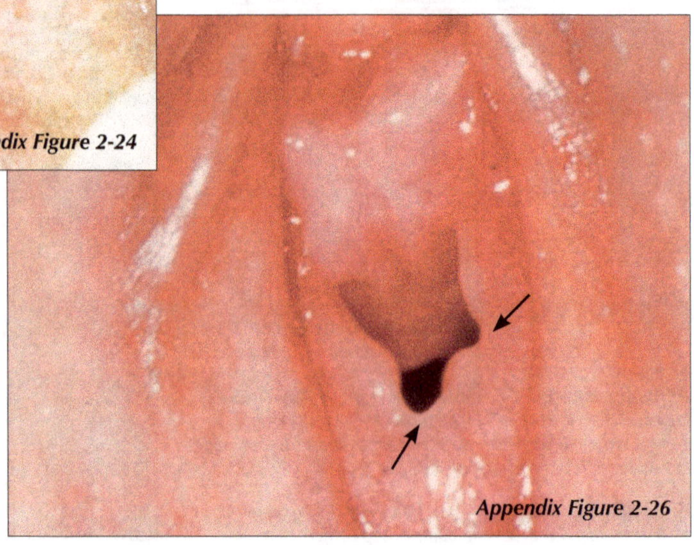
Appendix Figure 2-26

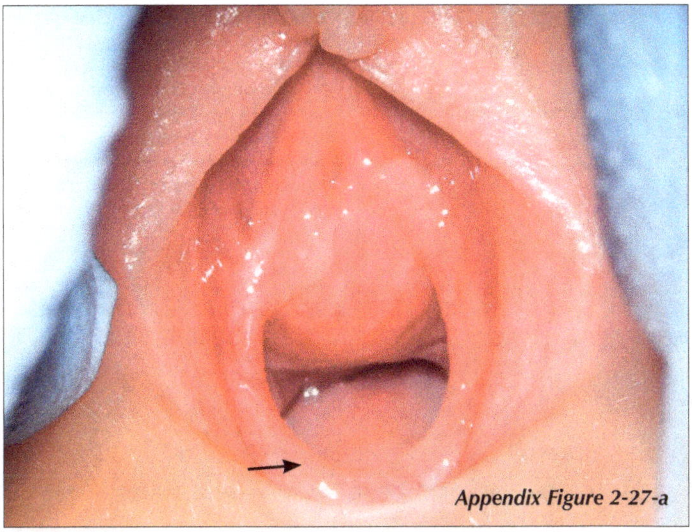

Appendix Figure 2-27-a

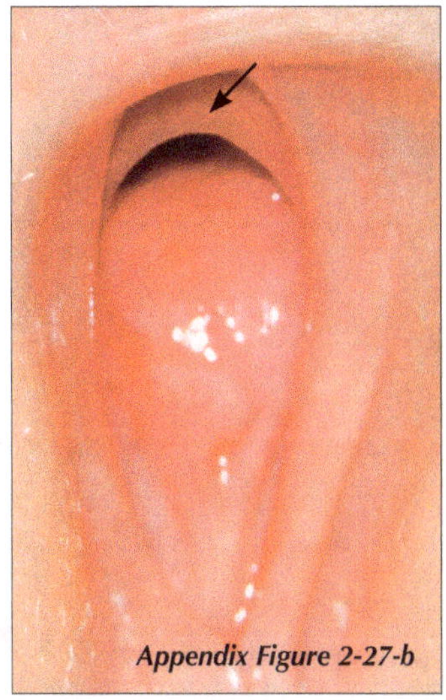

Appendix Figure 2-27-b

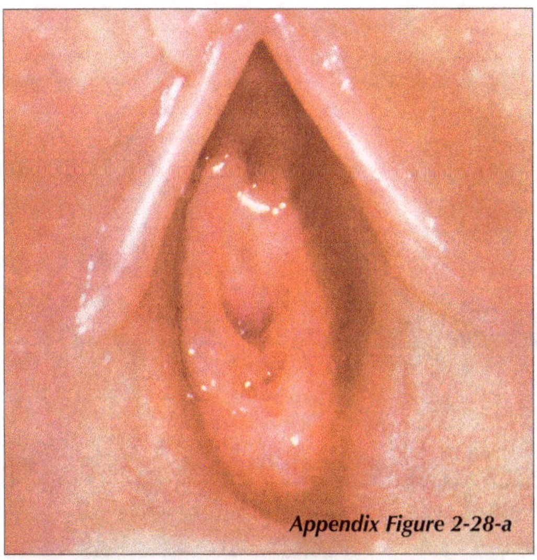

Appendix Figure 2-28-a

Appendix Figure 2-27-a. *An 8-year-old girl who described "sex" with an 11-year-old boy. In the supine position, using labial traction, the hymen is crescentic, with a smooth edge.*

Appendix Figure 2-27-b. *In the prone knee-chest position, the posterior rim of the hymen is smooth and without interruption.*

Appendix Figure 2-28-a. *This 2-year-old girl was referred because of sexual acting out behaviors. Using labial separation, the hymen is closed.*

Appendix Figure 2-28-b. *Using labial traction, both the urethral opening at 12 o'clock and the hymenal opening at 7 o'clock are revealed. It is difficult to assess the integrity of the posterior hymenal rim.*

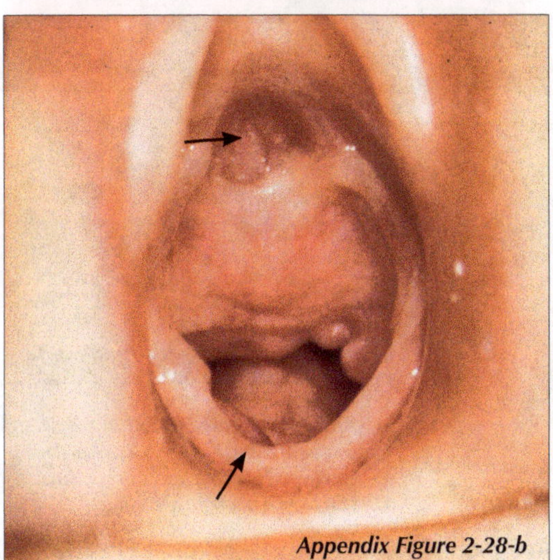

Appendix Figure 2-28-b

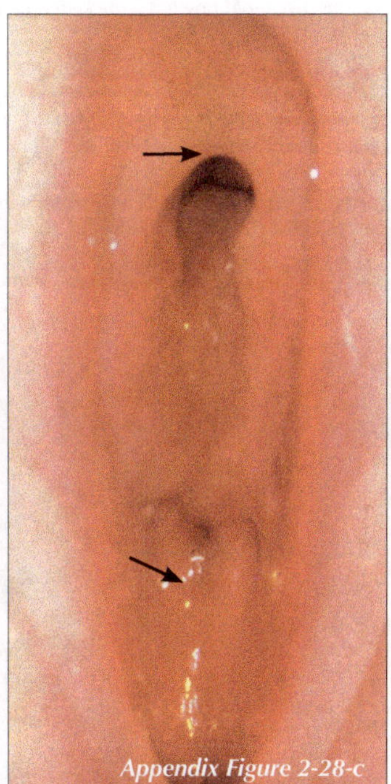

Appendix Figure 2-28-c

Appendix Figure 2-28-c. *In the prone knee-chest position, the posterior rim, although relatively narrow for a child of this age, is smooth and without signs of injury.*

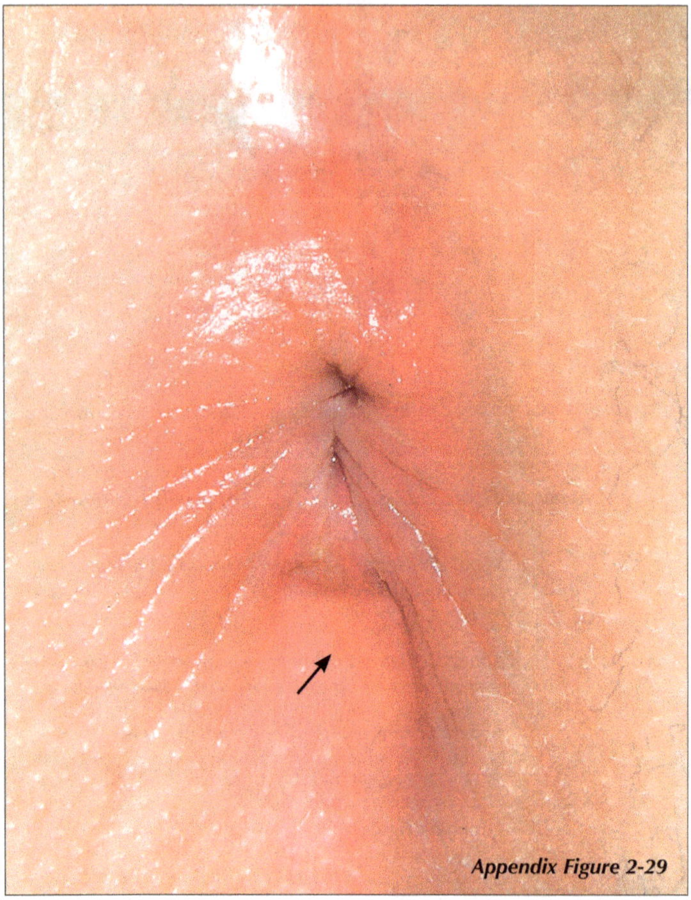

Appendix Figure 2-29

Appendix Figure 2-29. *Normal pattern of anal folds in a 5-year-old girl, showing a smooth area at 6 o'clock, called diastasis ani. This appearance is thought to be caused by a break in the fibers of the subcutaneous division of the external anal sphincter muscle. It is the contraction of the external sphincter that caused the circular pattern of folds in the perianal skin.*

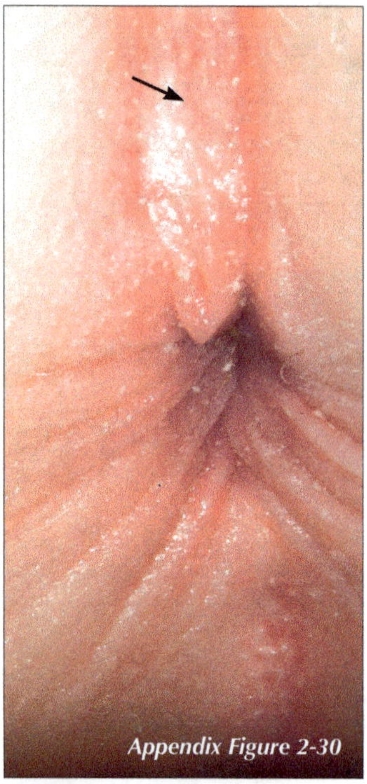

Appendix Figure 2-30

Appendix Figure 2-30. *This 3-year-old boy has a thickened perianal fold in the midline, which can appear as a tag.*

Appendix Figure 2-31. *This 3-year-old African American girl has normal anal folds and normal increased pigmentation of the perianal skin. Hyperpigmented skin in the perianal area and vulva is common in children of color.*

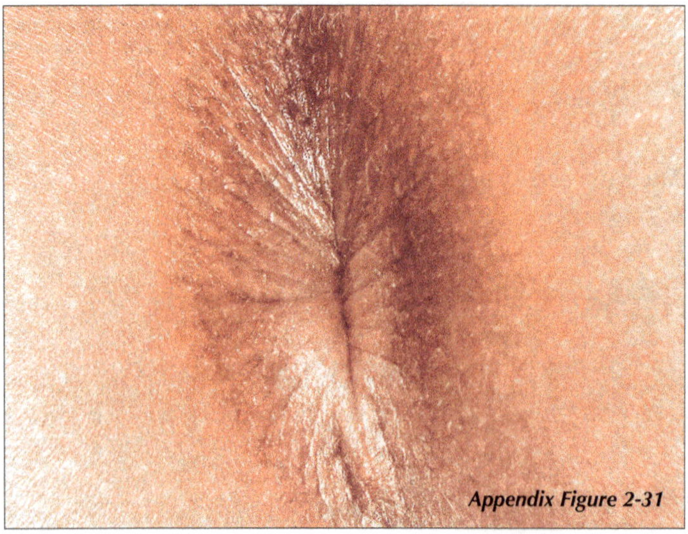

Appendix Figure 2-31

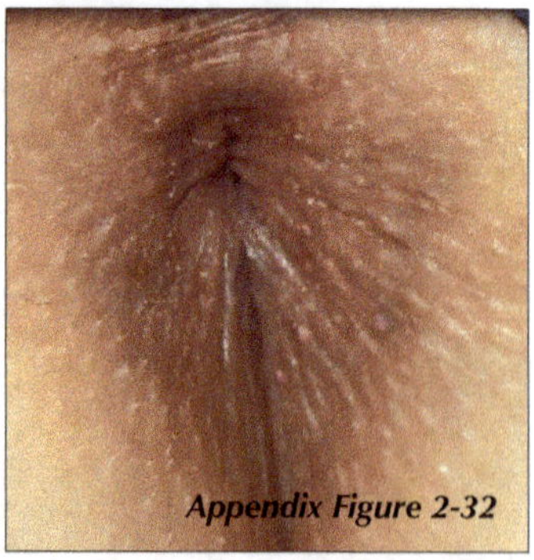

Appendix Figure 2-32

Appendix Figure 2-32. *This 8-year-old white child also has normal perianal folds and hyperpigmentation of the perianal skin, which is a normal finding.*

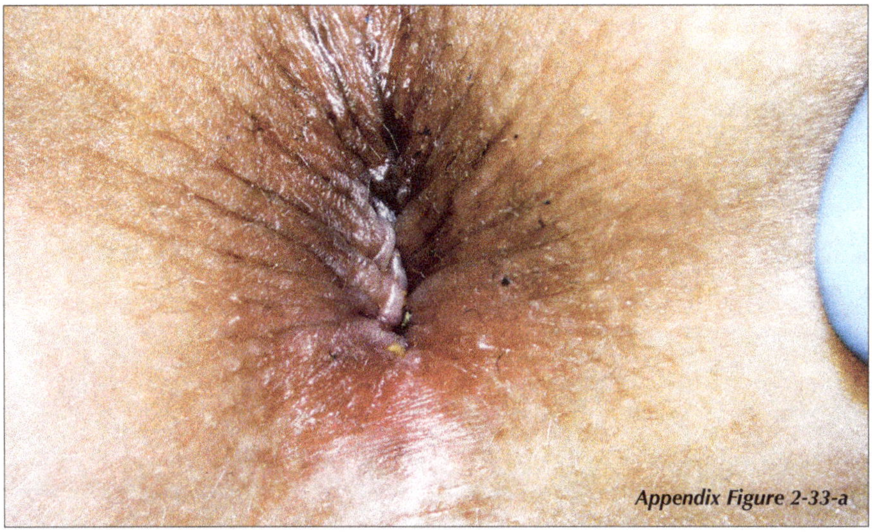

Appendix Figure 2-33-a

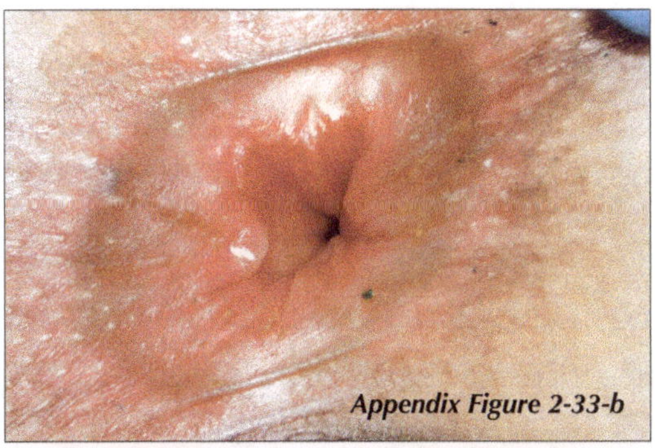

Appendix Figure 2-33-b

Appendix Figure 2-33-a. *This 5-year-old Mexican American girl gave a history of being fondled. The perianal folds are normal.*

Appendix Figure 2-33-b. *With separation of the buttocks, the external anal sphincter relaxes and the internal sphincter remains closed. This causes an irregular appearance that should not be mistaken for trauma.*

Appendix Figure 2-34. *A 9-year-old girl who reported fondling. The anus shows the appearance when the external sphincter is relaxed, but the internal sphincter is closed. This is normal.*

Appendix Figure 2-35. *Photograph of the anus of a 4-year-old child in the prone knee-chest position who is relaxed enough for the anus to dilate. Both external and internal anal sphincters are relaxed. The arrows show the anal verge at 12 o'clock, the pectin at 6 o'clock upper, the pectinate line at 6 o'clock lower, and an anal column at 9 o'clock.*

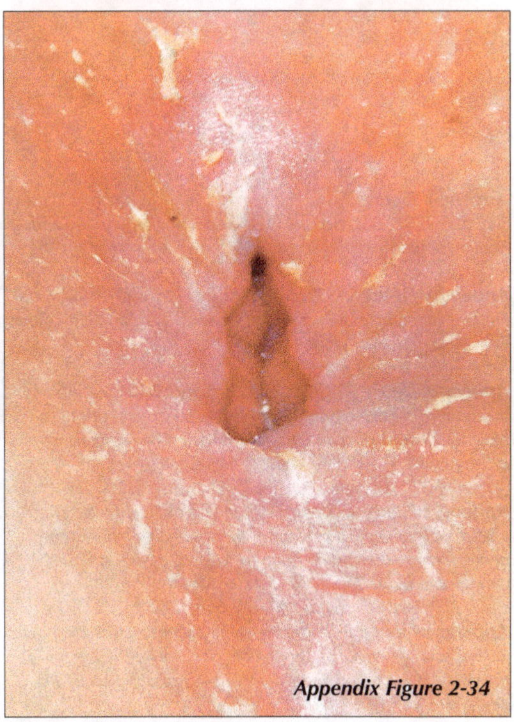

Appendix Figure 2-34

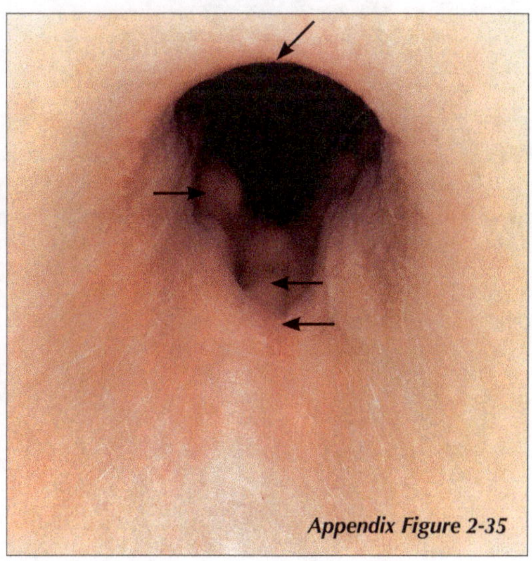

Appendix Figure 2-35

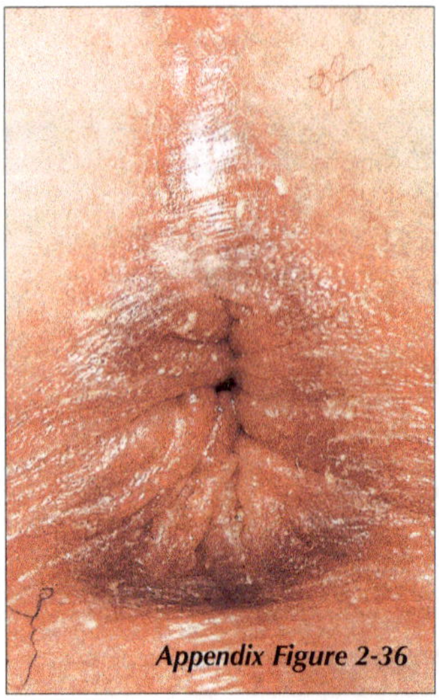
Appendix Figure 2-36

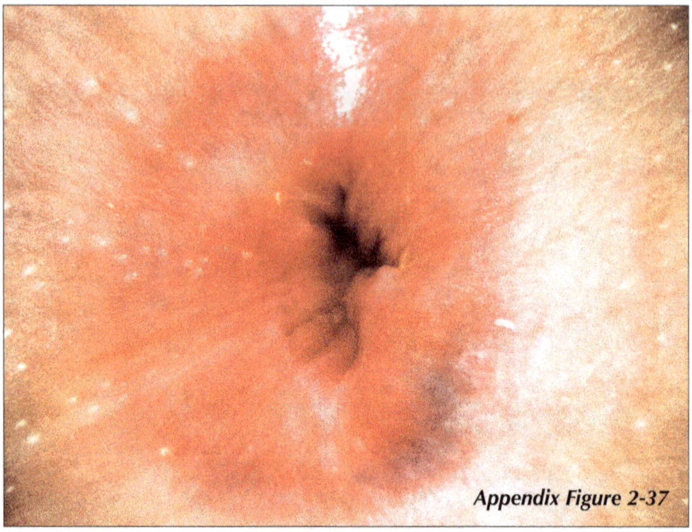
Appendix Figure 2-37

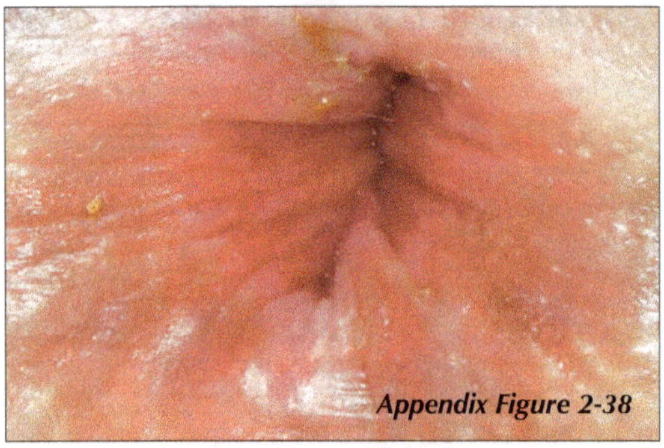
Appendix Figure 2-38

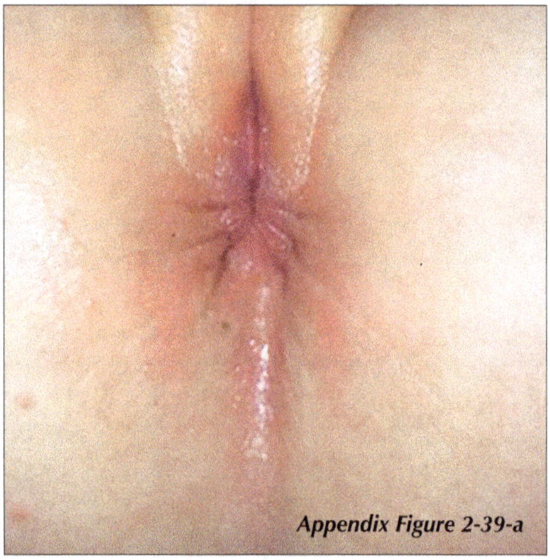
Appendix Figure 2-39-a

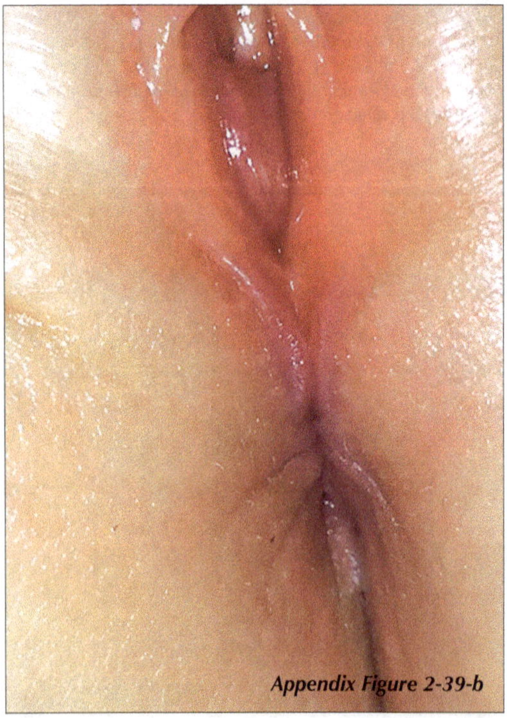
Appendix Figure 2-39-b

Appendix Figure 2-36. *A 2-year-old girl with no complaints of anal discomfort or constipation. The dark ring around the anus is pooling of blood in the plexus of veins and is a normal finding.*

Appendix Figure 2-37. *An 11-year-old boy with venous pooling and flattening of the anal folds as a result of partial relaxation of the external anal sphincter.*

Appendix Figure 2-38. *8-year-old patient who presented for acute touching of the anus, examined in the supine position. Note the venous pooling. Photo contributed by Diana Faugno, MSN, RN, CPN, SANE-A, SANE-P, FAAFS, DF-IAFN, DF-AFN.*

Appendix Figure 2-39-a. *A 20 month old child referred for a suspected perianal tear since 5 months of age. Notice the perineal groove extending from the fossa to the anus. Photo contributed by Tor Shwayder, MD, FAAP, FAAD.*

Appendix Figure 2-39-b. *The same patient pictured in Figure 2-39-a, with gentle labial separation. The skin at the border of the defect has a rolled appearance. Photo contributed by Tor Shwayder, MD, FAAP, FAAD.*

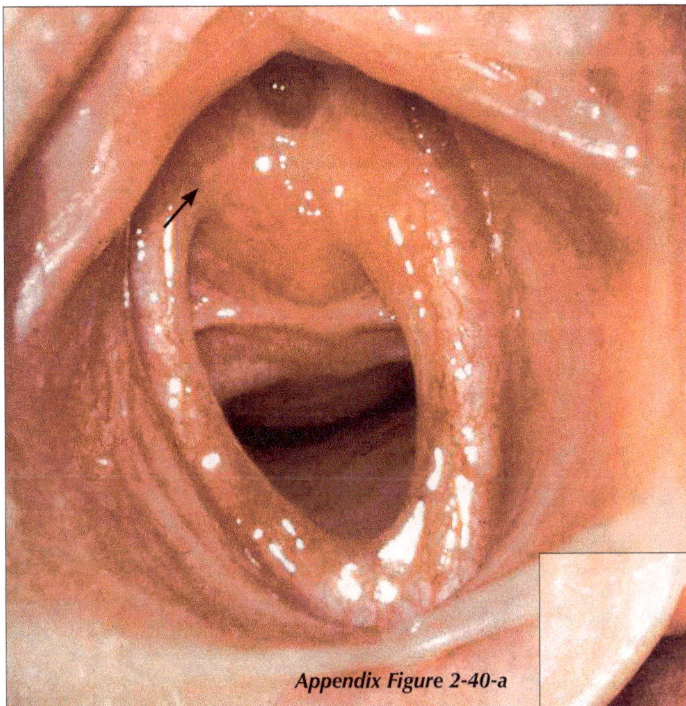

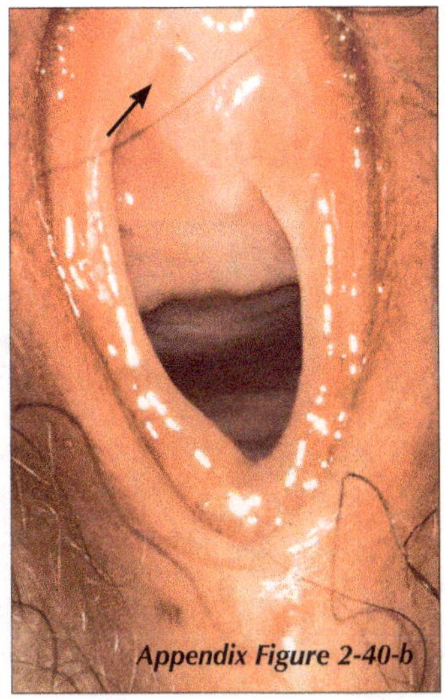

Appendix Figure 2-40-a. *A 7-year-old girl examined as part of a study of normal anatomy in nonabused children, done in Trondheim, Norway. This is a crescentic hymen with the attachment at 11 o'clock and 2 o'clock. Photo contributed by Arne K. Myhre, MD.*

Appendix Figure 2-40-b. *Same child pictured in Figure 2-40-a, reexamined as part of a follow-up study, now aged 12 years and 9 months. The hymen has a very similar appearance but now is thicker and paler in color. Photo contributed by Arne K. Myhre, MD.*

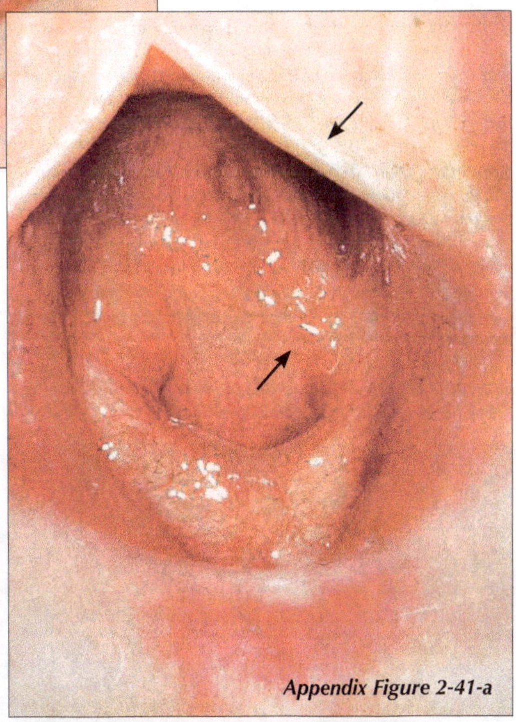

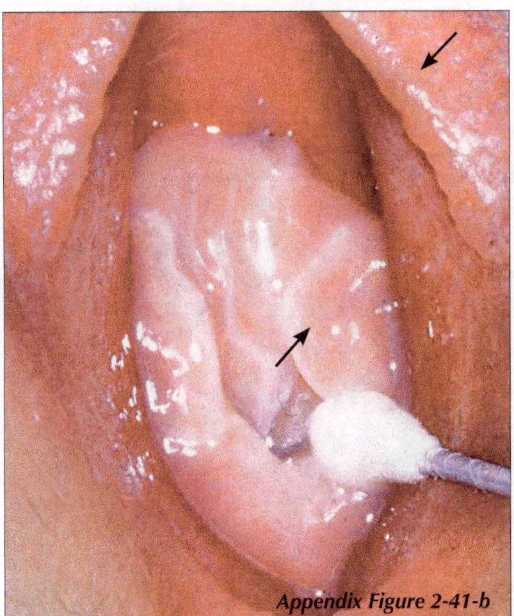

Appendix Figure 2-41-a. *A girl aged 6 years, 9 months, examined as part of the study by Myhre et al.[8] Note the appearance of the labia minora at 1 o'clock. There is a flap of hymen noted at 2 o'clock to 3 o'clock. Photo contributed by Arne K. Myhre, MD.*

Appendix Figure 2-41-b. *Same child, seen at follow-up at age 12 years and 7 months. The labia minora at 1 o'clock are thicker, longer, and more pigmented. The flap of hymen is more prominent, with the effect of endogenous estrogen shown at 3 o'clock. Photo contributed by Arne K. Myhre, MD.*

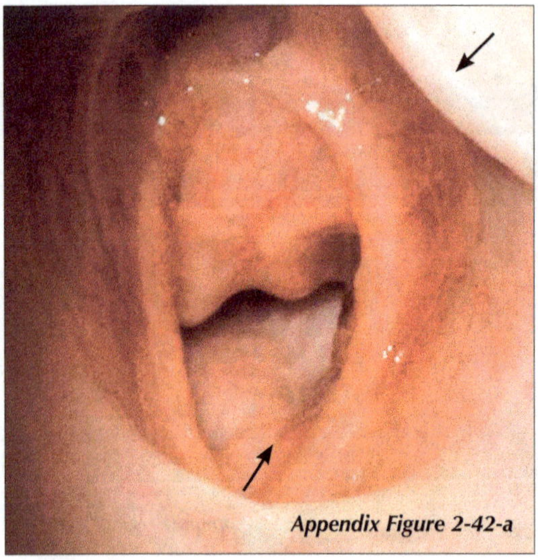

Appendix Figure 2-42-a

Appendix Figure 2-42-a. *This child was 5 years and 11 months old at the time of her first examination. The labium minus, seen here, is thin and smooth at the 1 o'clock position. The hymenal edge at 7 o'clock is not seen clearly, but there is an intravaginal ridge at that location.*

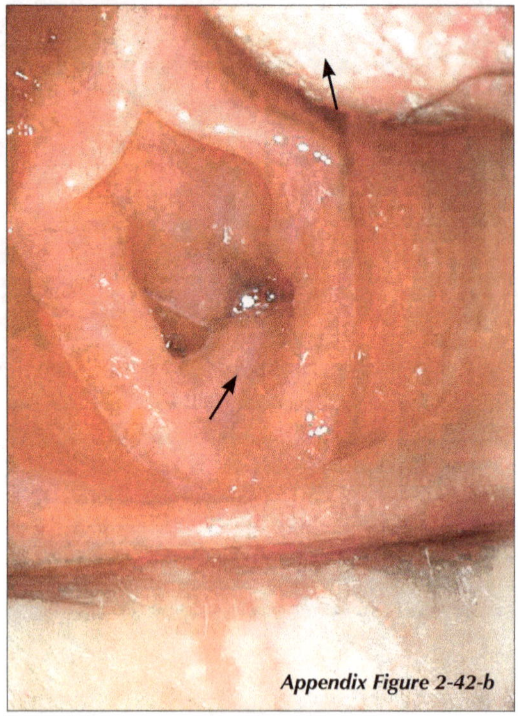

Appendix Figure 2-42-b

Appendix Figure 2-42-b. *At her follow-up examination, the child is now 11 years and 8 months old. The labium minus is thicker and darker at 3 o'clock. The intravaginal ridge is seen at the same location as in the first examination at 1 o'clock; the hymen is thicker and paler and folds outward.*

Appendix Figure 2-43-a. *An 8-year-old Mexican American girl, examined in the supine position, using labial traction. Periurethral support bands are seen bilaterally at 2 o'clock and 10 o'clock. The hymen is thick and pale at 6 o'clock, reflecting the effect of estrogen. The child has begun breast development but does not yet have pubic hair. Image reprinted with permission from eMedicine.com, 2010. Available at: https://emedicine.medscape.com/article/954024-overview.*

Appendix Figure 2-43-b. *In the prone knee-chest position, the hymen retains its thick, pale appearance.*

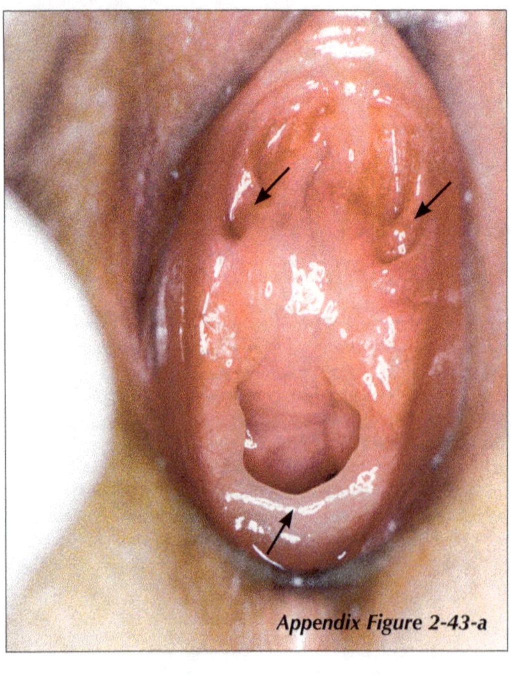

Appendix Figure 2-43-a

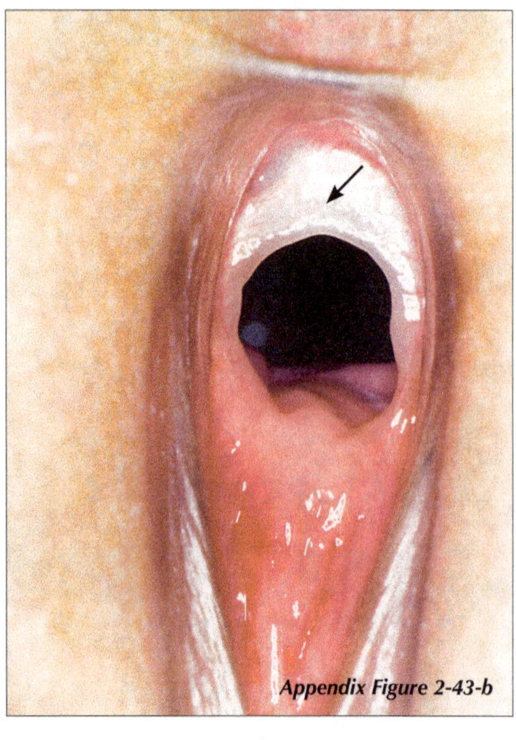

Appendix Figure 2-43-b

Appendix Figure 2-44-a. *Tulip-shaped, estrogenized hymen in a 14-year-old girl examined as part of a study of the appearance of the hymen in adolescent girls with no history of sexual activity. This girl described difficulty inserting a tampon, likely because of the shape of her hymen.*

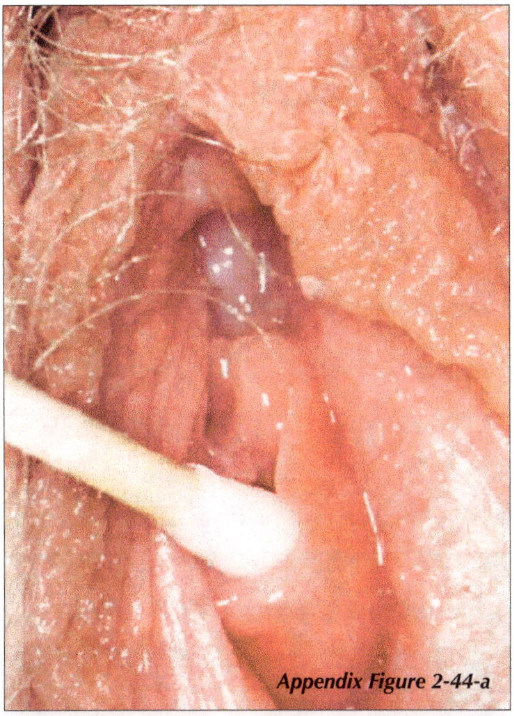

Appendix Figure 2-44-a

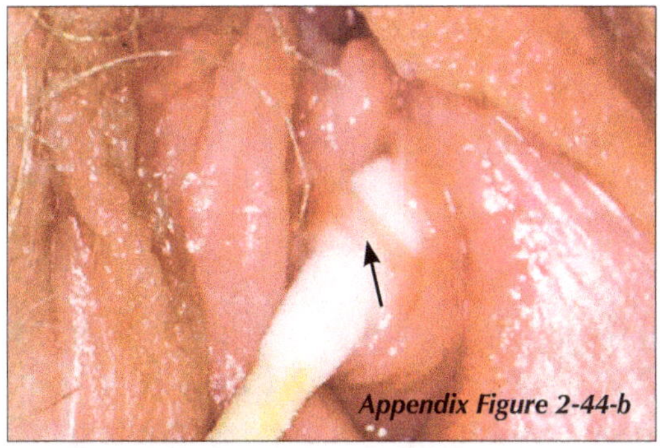

Appendix Figure 2-44-b

Appendix Figure 2-44-b. *The same 14-year-old girl with a swab showing the presence of a hymenal septum.*

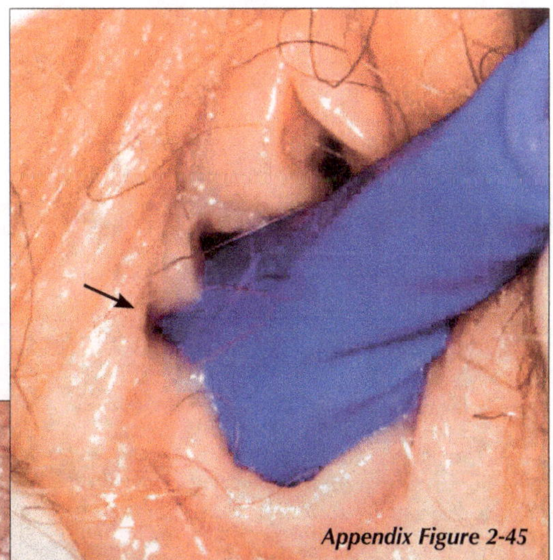

Appendix Figure 2-45

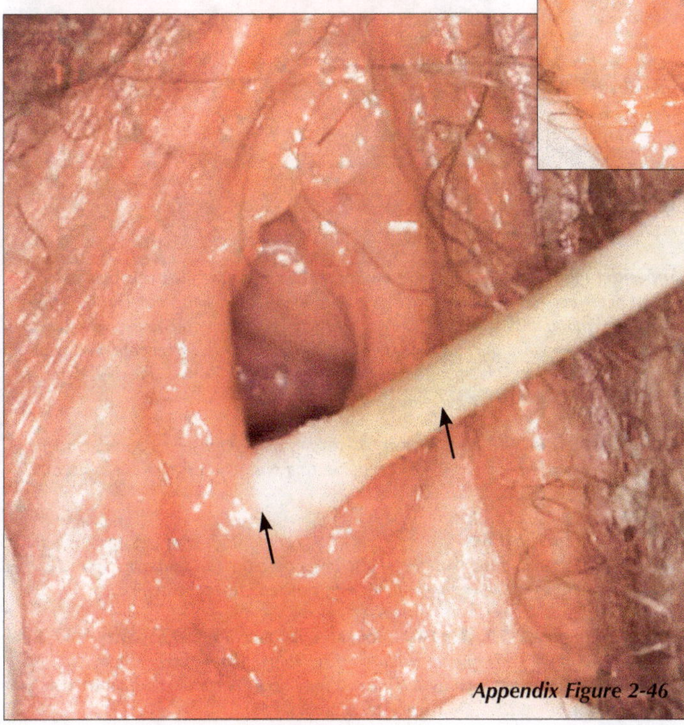

Appendix Figure 2-46

Appendix Figure 2-45. *An 18-year-old girl, consensually sexually active, with a complete cleft in the hymen at 9 o'clock. A large swab, covered by a latex balloon, provides contrast and stretches out the hymen to identify the cleft.*

Appendix Figure 2-46. *A 16-year-old girl, part of the study of the hymen in adolescents, with the hymen stretched out with a regular cotton swab. The width of the wooden handle of the swab is 2 mm, which is the same apparent width of the posterior hymen rim in this patient.*

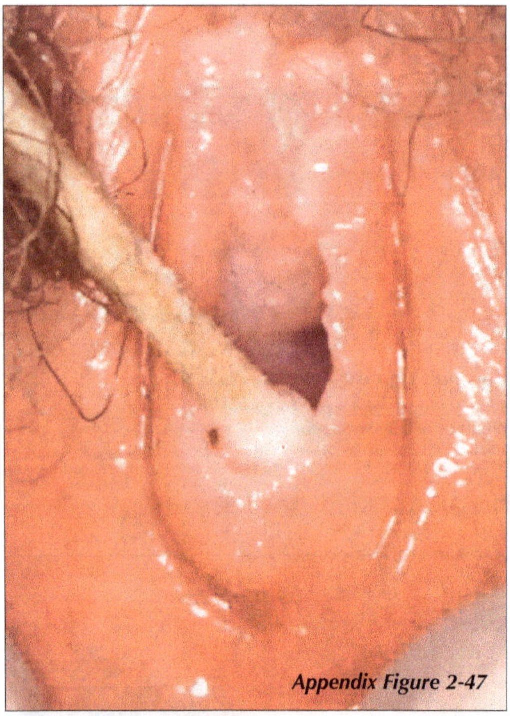
Appendix Figure 2-47

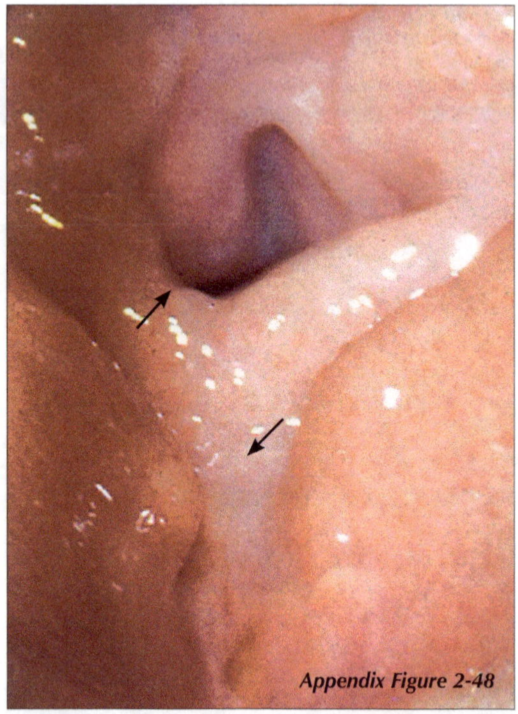
Appendix Figure 2-48

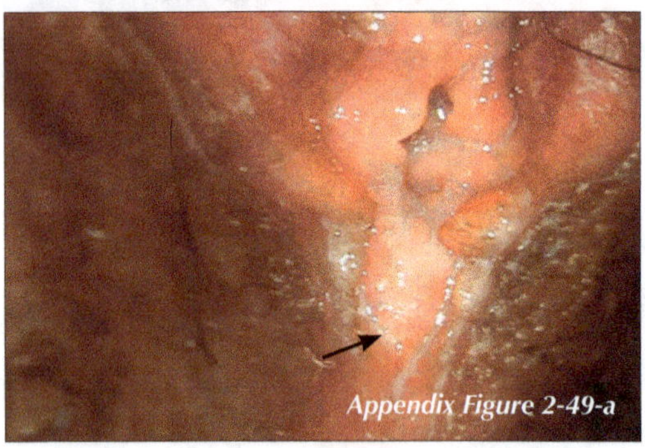
Appendix Figure 2-49-a

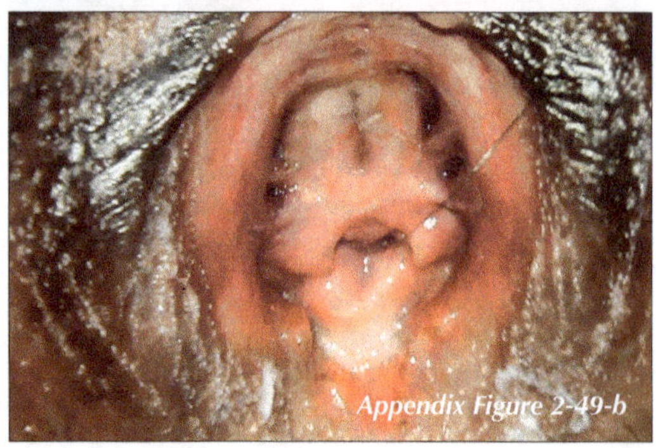
Appendix Figure 2-49-b

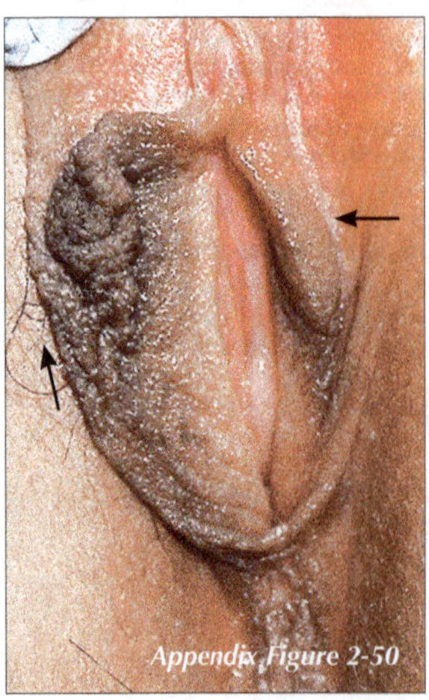
Appendix Figure 2-50

Appendix Figure 2-47. *This 14-year-old girl has a wider rim of the hymen at 6 o'clock. She denies intercourse and does not use tampons.*

Appendix Figure 2-48. *This 13-year-old girl's hymen shows the thick, pale color typical of estrogen effect at 9 o'clock. A groove in the fossa is also noted at 6 o'clock. This is a common finding in girls during the first stages of pubertal development, as the tissues of the vulva thicken in response to hormone levels. Image reprinted with permission from eMedicine.com, 2010. Available at: https://emedicine.medscape.com/article/954024-overview.*

Appendix Figure 2-49-a. *A 16 year-old-child evaluated for sexual abuse. Notice her annular estrogenized hymen. The arrow points to a posterior fossa groove, a normal finding.*

Appendix Figure 2-49-b. *The first child's 18-year-old sister who was also evaluated for suspected sexual abuse. Notice she also has a posterior fossa groove. Note also the prominent periurethral ligaments and her estrogenized crescentic hymen.*

Appendix Figure 2-50. *This 14-year-old Mexican American girl has asymmetrical development of her labia minora, with the right labium minus longer, thicker, and more pigmented than the left. Patients and parents may have concerns about their exam and need to be reassured that this asymmetry is normal.*

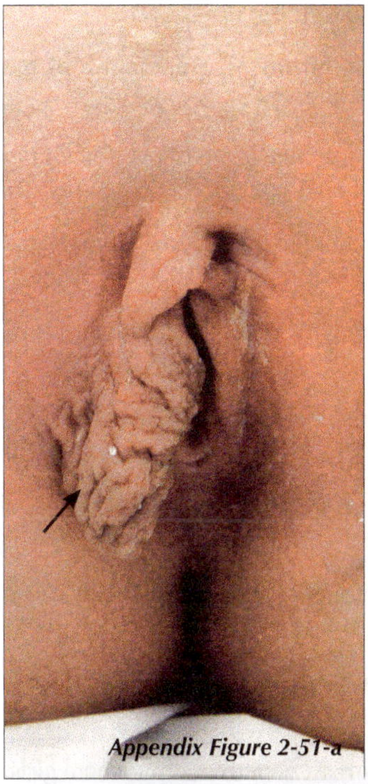
Appendix Figure 2-51-a

Appendix Figure 2-51-a. *The mother of this 11-year-old girl with Down syndrome was worried about sexual abuse because of the unusual appearance of her genital tissues. The mother had not seen the child for 2 years, and in the interval the girl had begun menstruation and needed help with hygiene. This is a dramatic example of asymmetrical development of the labia minora, with the right labium minus showing thickening, wrinkling, and hyperpigmentation caused by the androgenic hormones of puberty. On the right, the labium minus has the appearance typical of a prepubertal girl. It is not known why the tissues of the genitalia respond in this asymmetrical manner.*

Appendix Figure 2-51-b. *Using further labial traction, the estrogenized hymen is seen. Although this child had no pubic or axillary hair, she did have breast development and was having regular monthly menstrual cycles.*

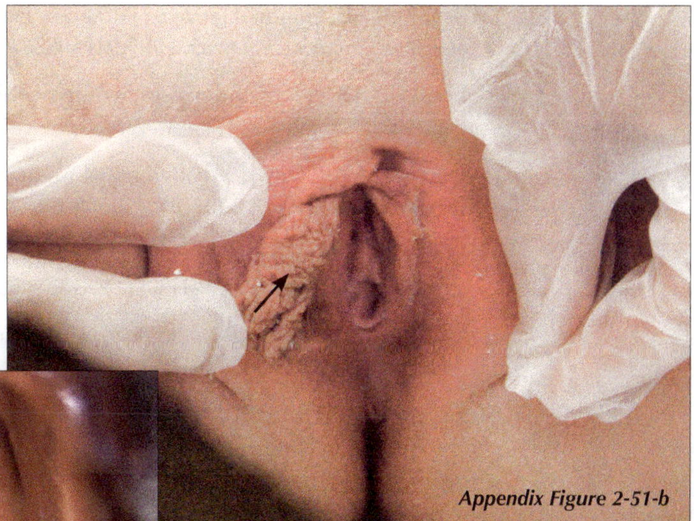
Appendix Figure 2-51-b

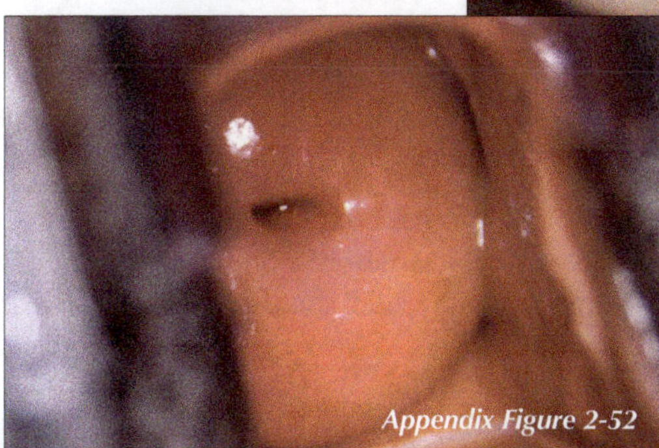
Appendix Figure 2-52

Appendix Figure 2-52. *A normal-appearing cervix with a central, round os in a 17-year-old girl.*

Appendix Figure 2-53. *A normal cervix showing cervical ectropion. This appearance is caused by the columnar epithelium of the endocervix extending outward onto the surface of the cervix in early puberty, in this case in a girl aged 14 years.*

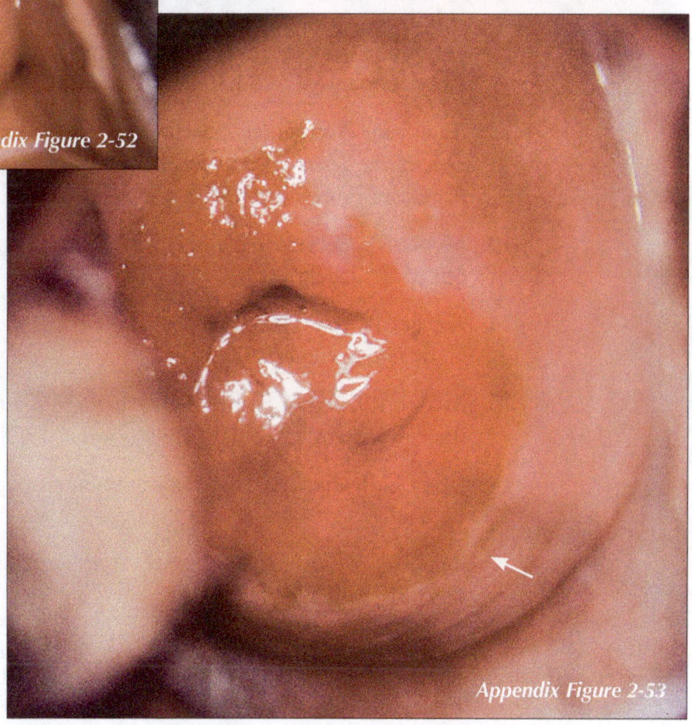
Appendix Figure 2-53

References

1. Berenson AB, Heger AH, Hayes JM, Bailey RK, Emans SJ. Appearance of the hymen in prepubertal girls. *Pediatrics*. 1992;89(3):387-394.
2. McCann J, Voris J, Simon M, Wells R. Perianal findings in prepubertal children selected for nonabuse: a descriptive study. *Child Abuse Negl.* 1989;13(2):179-193.
3. McCann J, Wells R, Simon M, Voris J. Genital findings in prepubertal girls selected for nonabuse: a descriptive study. *Pediatrics*. 1990;86(3):428-439.
4. Berenson AB. Appearance of the hymen at birth and one year of age: a longitudinal study. *Pediatrics*. 1993;91(4):820-825.
5. Berenson AB, Somma-Garcia A, Barnett S. Perianal findings in infants 18 months of age or younger. *Pediatrics*. 1993;91(4):838-840.
6. Berenson AB. A longitudinal study of hymenal morphology in the first 3 years of life. *Pediatrics*. 1995;95(4):490-496.
7. Berenson AB, Grady JJ. A longitudinal study of hymenal development from 3 to 9 years of age. *J Pediatr*. 2002;140(5):600-607.
8. Myhre AK, Bemtzen K, Bratlid D. Perianal anatomy in non-abused preschool children. *Acta Paediatr*. 2001;90(11):1321-1328.
9. Myhre AK, Berntzen K, Bratlid D. Genital anatomy in non-abused preschool girls. *Acta Paediatr*. 2003;92(12):1453-1462.
10. Starling SP, Heisler KW, Paulson JF, Youmans E. Child abuse training and knowledge: a national survey of emergency medicine, family medicine, and pediatric residents and program directors. *Pediatrics*. 2009;123(4):e595-602.
11. Makoroff KL, Brauley JL, Brandner AM, Myers PA, Shapiro RA. Genital examinations for alleged sexual abuse of prepubertal girls: findings by pediatric emergency medicine physicians compared with child abuse trained physicians. *Child Abuse Negl.* 2002;26(12):1235-1242.
12. American Professional Society on the Abuse of Children. *Practice Guidelines: Descriptive Terminology in Child Sexual Abuse Medical Evaluations*. Chicago, IL: American Professional Society on the Abuse of Children; 1995.
13. Moore KL, Persaud TVN. *The Developing Human, Clinically Oriented Embryology*. 6th ed. Philadelphia, PA: WB Saunders; 1998.
14. van der Putte SCJ. *The Development of the Perineum in the Human*. Heidelberg, Germany: Springer; 2005.
15. Merlob P, Bahari C, Liban E, Reisner SH. Cysts of the female external genitalia in the newborn infant. *Am J Obstet Gynecol.* 1978;132(6):607-610.
16. Jenny C, Kuhns ML, Arakawa F. Hymens in newborn female infants. *Pediatrics*. 1987;80(3):399-400.
17. Berenson A, Heger A, Andrews S. Appearance of the hymen in newborns. *Pediatrics*. 1991;87(4):458-465.
18. Adams JA, Kellogg ND, Farst KJ, et al. Updated guidelines for the medical assessment and care of children who may have been sexually abused. *J Pediatr Adolesc Gynecol.* 2016;29(2):81-87.

19. Adams JA, Farst KJ, Kellogg ND. Interpretation of medical findings in suspected child sexual abuse: an update for 2018. *J Pediatr Adolesc Gynecol.* 2018; 31(3):225-231.

20. Pauls RN. Anatomy of the clitoris and the female sexual response. *Clin Anat.* 2015;28(3):376-384.

21. Jarrett OO, Ayoola OO, Jonsson B, Albertsson-Wikland K, Ritzen M. Country-based reference values and international comparisons of clitoral size in healthy Nigerian newborn infants. *Acta Paediatr.* 2015;104(12):1286-1290.

22. Mondal R, Chatterjee K, Samanta M, et al. Clitoral length and anogenital ratio in Indian newborn girls. *Indian Pediatr.* 2016;53(4):299-303.

23. Brodie KE, Grantham EC, Huguelet PS, Caldwell BT, Westfall NJ, Wilcox DT. Study of clitoral hood anatomy in the pediatric population. *J Pediatr Urol.* 2016;12(3):177. e1-e5.

24. Gellis SS, Feingold M, Shaw A, Dewitt G. Picture of the month: perineal groove. *Am J Dis Child.* 1977;131(8):921-922.

25. Tanuos H, Rogers S. Index of suspicion. *Pediatr Rev.* 2001;22(11):388-393.

26. Mullassery D, Turnock R, Kokai G. Perineal groove. *J Pediatr Surg.* 2006;41(3):e41-e43.

27. Wolf RM, Long D. Pubertal development. *Pediatr Rev.* 2016;37(7):292-300.

28. Jacobs AM, Alderman EM. Gynecologic examination of the prepubertal girl. *Pediatr Rev.* 2014;35(3):97-104.

29. Adams JA, Botash AS, Kellogg N. Differences in hymenal morphology between adolescent girls with and without a history of consensual sexual intercourse. *Arch Pediatr Adolesc Med.* 2004;158(3):280-285.

Chapter 3

The Medical Evaluation of a Suspected Childhood Sexual Abuse Victim

Stephanie Anne Deutsch, MD, MS, FAAP
Martin A. Finkel, DO, FACOP, FAAP

Introduction

Sexual abuse is a common childhood experience with the potential for serious long-term physical and mental health consequences. As both awareness of sexual abuse as a pediatric problem and greater understanding of the mental health impact of sexual abuse on the child have increased, the role of the medical provider in the evaluation of sexually abused children has significantly evolved.[1] Current practice commonly employs a multidisciplinary, collaborative approach to the assessment, diagnosis, treatment, and coordination of follow-up care for children suspected of experiencing sexual abuse and may involve forensic interviewers, child protective services (CPS) and law enforcement (LE) investigators, attorneys, and medical providers working jointly to address the many legal, protective, and medical and mental health sequelae of sexual abuse victimization.[1]

Those who participate in the assessment of a child or adolescent suspected of experiencing sexual abuse must do so with knowledge, skill, and sensitivity that come from understanding the "disease of sexual victimization."[2-5] The medical evaluation in cases of suspected sexual abuse is not all that dissimilar from the evaluation of a child with an illness in that the process of coming to a diagnostic assessment incorporates all the traditional components of the evaluation of any complex medical condition. The subject matter, however, requires an understanding of the clinical expression and dynamics of sexual victimization, many features of which are unique and idiosyncratic.[6-9]

The tools to conduct a medical evaluation begin with building on this knowledge and developing the necessary skills to obtain a history from the child or adolescent victim and family in a manner that is nonjudgmental, facilitating, and empathic. The medical provider therefore assumes a unique role in the evaluation of suspected sexual abuse. Dynamics of the physician-patient relationship provide an opportunity to obtain additional historic details that may enhance understanding of the child or adolescent's experience and identify needs to be addressed from a diagnostic, treatment, and medicolegal perspective. Comprehensive medical history taking and physical examination by the medical provider afford a safe, therapeutic venue in which to address cognitive distortions that a child or adolescent might have regarding his or her experience, concerns about body intactness or appearance, and inaccurate beliefs that people can tell that inappropriate sexual contact occurred by the way he or she looks or walks. Additionally, the medical provider can encourage linkage to ongoing mental health treatment for both child victim and family, and this provision of support and reassurance is vital to initial and continued recovery from trauma related to childhood sexual abuse.

This chapter describes core elements of conducting a comprehensive evaluation, as well as the type of information to be obtained, how to obtain information, and how to document the medical history and physical examination. Intertwined throughout the chapter are several highly pertinent legal concepts that take on special significance in children suspected of having been sexually abused. Finally, the chapter provides suggestions on tying pieces together to formulate a clear and balanced diagnosis.

Presentations for Care of Suspected Child Sexual Abuse

Concern for suspected sexual abuse may arise in a variety of settings. Children and adolescents may be referred for medical evaluations from their primary care pediatrician, the emergency department (ED), CPS, children's advocacy centers (CACs), or LE investigators. Caregivers may raise concern about possible sexual abuse to the child or adolescent's pediatrician because of sexualized behaviors, concerning statements or disclosures of abuse, exposure to a known perpetrator of abuse,[1,10] behavioral changes, clinical symptoms, or nonspecific examination findings, including genital, genitourinary (GU), or gastrointestinal (GI) complaints. Caregivers and children and adolescents may present acutely to the ED after a disclosure of abuse for the treatment of injuries that may have been sustained during abuse; for evaluation of GU, GI, or acute behavioral signs and symptoms; or for forensic evidence collection, including body fluids or other evidence.

Many children and adolescents present to EDs because of concerns that something inappropriate happened and an urgent need for certainty on the part of the caregiver. Because most children who present to EDs are victims of nonacute abuse resulting from delayed disclosure, the most critical information to ascertain is the timing of the last inappropriate sexual contact. If the last inappropriate contact is beyond the window for acute injury detection, identification, and preservation of physical evidence (typically 72 hours), the medical evaluation should be deferred to the outpatient setting and performed by a medical provider with expertise in evaluation of sexual abuse. If abuse is reasonably suspected, a report should be made to CPS and/or LE to initiate investigation and ensure the child's safety.

When presenting to the primary care or ED setting, the medical provider may be the initial witness to a disclosure of abuse from the child or adolescent in the context of the therapeutic, trusted physician-patient relationship. Alternatively, when referred from a CAC, the medical provider may rely on a recorded investigative interview conducted either by CPS or LE investigators or both to obtain information regarding the suspected abusive contact. With this approach, the medical provider may enhance background information obtained from a recorded interview by asking additional, more in-depth questions of the child or adolescent to more fully understand the abusive experience, guide laboratory and diagnostic testing for sexually transmitted infections (STIs), and identify and address additional mental health and therapeutic needs.

Sources of Information in Suspected Sexual Abuse Cases

Information regarding the presenting concerns for sexual abuse will be obtained from a variety of sources, each of which must be weighed for relevance. Although information provided by CPS or LE investigators or a nonoffending caregiver regarding presenting concerns is important, it should not be relied on as the sole source of background information when formulating a diagnosis. Background information from sources other than the child or adolescent does not negate the need to speak to the child independently and can be critical to understanding the context in which a suspected event occurred.

When individuals other than the child or adolescent provide information, it will generally be considered hearsay and, therefore, should not be used in the formulation of the clinical diagnosis of child sexual abuse. The medical provider making the diagnosis preferentially relies on the interpretation and integration of the medical history, physical examination findings, and laboratory test results. When obtaining a medical history from the child and caregiver, all information is recorded verbatim. It is inadequate to simply provide a summary note because it fails to capture the nuances of the history. Documentation should reflect all introductory comments, along with the exact questions asked and the child or adolescent's verbatim responses. In part, the basis for the hearsay treatment exception is the presumption that when a patient goes to the doctor, he or she will tell the truth because it is in his or her best interest to do so. Logically, the patient will tell the truth to the doctor so the doctor can make a diagnosis and help the patient to get better more quickly. Therefore, the treatment exception allows for admissibility of the child or adolescent's description of symptoms, sensations, or pain associated with the presenting concern. The child or adolescent's description of the cause of injury or "illness" may also provide idiosyncratic details that would otherwise be difficult to explain in terms of the victim's developmentally appropriate knowledge (eg, a symptom related to a specific event without experience of the event). If the child states that the injury or contact was at the hands of a particular individual, the medical provider must explain why the identity of that individual would be important to the diagnosis at hand.[11]

Talking to Children and Adolescents About Sexual Abuse

In some communities, medical providers have been discouraged from obtaining a medical history from children and adolescents about their suspected experiences, because of a presumption that retelling will be traumatic to the child and concern for solicitation of new information that might be discrepant with the initial disclosure. In contrast, children often find it therapeutic to retell details to a medical provider who understands and can help alleviate worries or concerns. As one child stated, "I can tell you because you're a doctor."[12] The medical provider should not compromise his or her ability to conduct a complete and thorough assessment by bypassing obtaining a medical history directly from the child. If discrepancies arise, they should be addressed. Many of the questions asked by the medical provider for medical, diagnostic purposes will not have been addressed by nonmedical professionals, and the history obtained by the medical provider has the potential to enhance understanding of what a child might have experienced.

Children and adolescents respond best to, and are most likely to provide the richest contextual details when asked, questions that are developmentally appropriate and follow a nonleading, nonsuggestive style. Avoiding questions conducive to short answers and giving preference to questions that encourage a more thorough narrative response is generally recommended. As a means of simple self-test, the medical provider can review the history obtained by reading only the responses to the questions asked. If the narrative that emerges is understandable and cohesive, a limited number of leading and suggestive questions were used. There is a clear continuum regarding leading, suggestive, and coercive questioning.[11] Open-ended questions that lack suggestibility tend to provide the clearest understanding of what a child may have experienced.

The best and most valid methods to screen for a history of sexual victimization include avoidance of closed-ended questions (eg, "Have you ever been sexually abused?"), preferential use of open-ended questions, use of several screening questions to provide multiple opportunities for the respondent, use of behaviorally specific screening questions, and avoidance of vague summary terms such as *abuse* or *trauma*.[13,14] Use of a single, open-ended question (eg, "Since the last time I saw you, has anything uncomfortable, confusing, or upsetting happened to you or your family?") may provide an indication of whether or not additional screening or assessment is warranted.[13,15] More optimally, medical providers may state, "I understand that you were able to tell about something that happened to you that was confusing or upsetting, and it involved someone you knew and trusted. That happens to lots of kids. Did that happen to you?" If the child answers yes, follow up with a statement such as "You did the right thing by telling. Why did you decide to tell?" The answer to this might be followed by "What was the first thing that happened that just didn't seem okay?" Additional questions will help establish that something happened and meet the threshold to report to CPS and/or LE.

Purpose of the Medical Examination

The examination is conceptualized as serving the purposes of both diagnosing and treating abnormality (residual to sexual abuse concerns) and confirming normality (wellness). Under this rubric, all children and adolescents suspected of being abused deserve the benefit of a physical examination. For many, the issue of normality will be equal in importance to concerns about abnormality. Medical providers treat patients either through the direct provision of medicine or the time-honored benefit of reassuring patients and addressing their rational and at times idiosyncratic concerns. Reassurance by a medical provider that a child's body is okay demonstrates both to the child and caregiver that their concerns were heard and addressed and on its own can be therapeutic. When children or adolescents and caregivers can be assured that there will be no long-term adverse health consequences of the abuse, focus may be placed on addressing the mental health issues that ultimately are the key to overcoming any abuse experience.

The purpose of the examination can be explained in a variety of ways depending on the child or adolescent victim's age. The medical provider might begin with an introductory comment such as:

> You know that when you have gone to the doctor in the past and not felt well, the doctor asks you all kinds of questions, like "Does your tummy hurt? Do you have a headache or have you had a fever?" The reason the doctor asks questions is simply to understand what may have been bothering you. Then the doctor can decide what parts of your body to take a look at. The doctor can also decide whether you will need any special tests or medicines to get you better. I will be asking you some questions about what happened. The questions I am going to ask are not to embarrass you or make you uncomfortable but simply to help me understand what happened. If I understand what happened, I can do a better job of taking care of you and deciding whether you need any special tests or medicines to get you better.

Allow the child or adolescent to express any special concerns. Once it is clear that the child or adolescent understands the purpose of taking the medical history, ask the child, "Is it important to tell the doctor the truth?" The child will usually answer "yes." Follow the response by asking the child to explain why it is important to tell the truth. The child might respond by saying, "That way the doctor can help me get better." A natural transitional question will be to inquire whether the child has any worries or concerns that she or he would like to share.

Children and adolescents may appreciate the need to see a medical provider if they have been injured but may not fully understand the potential consequences of either nonconsensual or consensual sexual interactions, such as risk for STIs. Additionally, caregivers may not fully appreciate the potential consequences of the sexual interaction and should receive guidance that encourages seeking diagnostic and treatment services.

Explanation of the purpose of the examination and documentation that the child or adolescent understood that he or she is being seen for diagnosis and treatment will enhance potential admissibility of medical history under the "for purposes of medical diagnosis and treatment" exception to hearsay.[11] Admissibility of out-of-court statements is important because it allows the medical provider to fully explain the basis on which the diagnostic assessment was formulated. Many medical conditions are diagnosed without confirmatory laboratory tests or specific examination findings but rather a constellation of presenting history, symptoms, and signs.

Components of the Medical History in Cases of Suspected Sexual Abuse

Obtaining the child or adolescent's medical history is essential to comprehensive evaluation of suspected sexual abuse. The medical provider may begin with review of the child's medical history, including a detailed review of symptoms (ROS), before asking the caregiver to understand the circumstances that lead to the concern that the child may have experienced something inappropriate; discussing abuse-specific concerns is best done without the child present. Children may be spoken to independently, allowing them an opportunity to talk about their experience as well as share any worries or concerns they may have about their bodies before the physical examination. Even young children are capable of providing a narrative of an inappropriate experience if asked in a facilitating, nonjudgmental, and supportive context. Children are generally more comfortable providing details of an experience without their caregiver present because many fear that their parents may be upset about what happened and children might think they will be in trouble. When taking the history either from the child independently or the caregiver, the medical record must precisely reflect the details of the questions asked and the child's verbatim response.[11,16] The information obtained from the caregiver is important to frame the issue but generally should not be used in formulating a diagnosis because it will be considered hearsay. When hearsay is used in the formulation of a diagnosis, the use of such information should be qualified and appropriately noted. Whenever possible, information about the chief complaint or history of the possible contact should be obtained from the child alone, not from the caregiver.

The medical history should consist of the following components:

1. Birth history
2. Family history
3. Social history
4. Developmental history
5. Hospitalizations/ED visits
6. Past surgery
7. Medications/allergies
8. Review of body systems, with particular attention to GU and GI symptoms
9. Inquiry into behavioral/mental health and emotional or trauma symptoms
10. History obtained from the caregiver regarding presenting concerns
11. History obtained from the child

When a caregiver is unavailable to provide the medical history, ask the referring agency to obtain medical records for review. The history obtained from the caregiver should be structured in a way to obtain the best possible chronology of events and observations. Ask questions that encourage the caregiver to provide contextual detail regarding observations and statements. For example, if the child or adolescent made a statement to a caregiver in a manner that was spontaneous and idiosyncratic, it would be important to understand the circumstances under which the statement was made. Ask the caregiver to provide as exact a recollection of the child's disclosure or observed behavior as possible and their reaction to the disclosure. Few caregivers anticipate that their child will disclose inappropriate sexual interactions, and thus, few have developed a thoughtful response. Too often, a caregiver may respond by being upset, showing disbelief, or questioning the child in a manner that might suggest to the child that he or she was responsible for what occurred. Depending on the manner in which the caregiver responds, the child may be more or less likely to repeat the initial disclosure. The disclosure process is a process over time in which children share increasingly greater details depending on their level of comfort and perceived consequence to them and the suspected perpetrator.

Review of Systems

All body systems should be included in the medical history; however, the GU and GI review of systems will take on special importance and may provide information that has special relevance to the issue of sexual contact. The importance of the ROS stems from need to identify any current or preexisting medical conditions that should be considered when assessing GU or GI symptoms that may have an association with sexual contact; for example, when children or adolescents experience genital fondling, vulvar coitus, or coitus, they may be able to provide important historical details of postfondling dysuria, post-vulvar coital dysuria, or postcoital dysuria that can support they have experienced genital trauma.[17] Dysuria can result from rubbing, causing superficial trauma to the periurethral or vestibular structures (or both). The injuries incurred from fondling or vulvar coitus are generally superficial and heal very quickly without demonstrative residual physical examination findings.[18] When the ROS reveals a history of urinary tract infections and associated dysuria, it may be suggested that knowledge of this symptom is the result of a prior infection and not abusive contact. When considering preexisting conditions, the clinician carefully evaluates the temporal relationship between a set of symptoms and the child's symptoms referable to the contact.

Questions about the GU system should include a discussion of the following:

— History of urinary tract infections

— Vaginal discharges

— Vaginal odor

— Vaginal bleeding

— Diaper dermatitis

— Urinary incontinence

— Use of bubble baths

— Treatment for any STIs

— Menstrual history

— Use of tampons

— Abortions

— Accidental genital injuries

— Vaginal foreign bodies

— Prior examinations of the genitalia for any reason other than routine health care

— Self-exploratory activities/masturbation

The GI ROS should include the following:

— Age of toilet training

— Difficulties with toilet training

— Use of rectal suppositories, enemas, or medications for stooling

— History of constipation or painful bowel movements

— Frequency and character of stools

— History of recurrent vomiting, diarrhea, hematochezia, hemorrhoids, fecal incontinence, rectal itching, pinworms, and surgical procedures involving the GI tract

Screening for Trauma Symptoms

Sexual abuse in children and adolescents has been associated with significant mental/behavioral health and emotional comorbidities, including development of posttraumatic stress disorder (PTSD) and other anxiety disorders.[19] PTSD, an anxiety disorder following exposure to a traumatic event, involves 4 symptom clusters: intrusive thoughts, avoidance of trauma-related thoughts and feelings and/or external reminders of trauma, negative changes in mood and thoughts as a result of the trauma, and increased reactivity and physiological arousal.[19,20] PTSD diagnosis has been associated with adverse health outcomes and increased medical utilization, including reproductive health problems, pelvic pain, and dysmenorrhea.[19,21-26] PTSD after sexual abuse has been linked to a variety of somatic complaints, including dyspareunia and difficulty with orgasm,[27,28] and has also been associated with engagement in high-risk sexual behaviors.[29] Children and adolescents with PTSD may also meet criteria for other comorbid mental health disorders, including depression,[30,31] suicidality, eating disorders, anxiety, and substance abuse.[32,33] Therefore, screening for trauma and other emotional and behavioral health symptoms during the comprehensive medical evaluation after suspected sexual abuse is paramount. Although variable in their components and assessed domains, screening tools to be considered include the University of California at Los Angeles Posttraumatic Stress Disorder Reaction Index,[34] the Trauma Symptom Checklist for Children,[35] the Child PTSD Symptom Scale (CPSS),[36] the Childhood Sexual Behavior Inventory (CSBI),[37] and the Child Behavior Checklist (CBCL).[38] Children and caregivers who are identified as having trauma or emotional or other mental health and behavioral symptoms at the time of the sexual abuse evaluation should be referred for therapy by mental health clinicians who are trained in the use of evidence-based therapeutic approaches to address the unique needs of children who experience sexual abuse.

Preparing Caregiver and Child for the Physical Examination

In preparation for the examination, it is important to anticipate both fears and anxieties of the child or adolescent and the caregiver. In introductory comments to the caregiver, it is important to take time to explain what to anticipate during the evaluation. For example, the medical provider may say the following to the caregiver:

> I am a kids' doctor, and one of the things I do that is different than most kids' doctors is examine children when there has been a concern that they may have experienced something inappropriate or seen something inappropriate or both. I understand those concerns have been raised with your child. Let me tell you what we hope to accomplish today. I will review with you your child's medical history; ask you to tell me the concerns that bring you here in a chronological manner; and tell me any of your worries, concerns, or observations. I will then speak to your child alone, and when I am done speaking with your child, you will come back into the room and have your child change into a gown for a head-to-toe examination with you present throughout.

For a prepubertal female child, the medical provider should add, "I don't anticipate doing anything that is physically uncomfortable to your daughter. Because of your daughter's age, she won't experience an adult gynecologic examination as you think of it. I won't use an instrument or speculum." For male patients, the medical provider should explain that the use of an anoscope will only occur if necessary. The medical provider may sum up by saying, "If appropriate, swabbing of the vagina and/or rectum and mouth to test for STIs will be obtained. After the examination, I will meet with you again and provide my opinion, answer any questions, and discuss the next steps necessary to assess the mental health impact of what your child experienced and how to obtain appropriate mental health services."

In a developmentally appropriate way, it is equally important to anticipate and address the fears and anxieties that the child or adolescent might have before proceeding with the examination. Young children may be concerned that they are going to get a vaccination and are relieved when they find out that is not the case. Whenever possible, explain what will be happening next in the examination. If the child desires, encourage him or her to touch the instruments. This helps to demystify the examination and provides an opportunity for the child to have a sense of participation and control throughout the examination. Video colposcopy is an excellent tool that allows the child to watch the anogenital examination if he or she so desires. With young children, ask if they would like to see their belly button or finger on the television first. This serves as a means of demonstrating that there is nothing invasive about the scope. Maintain an active dialogue with the child throughout the examination, and proceed at a pace that is comfortable for the child.

The physical examination begins with a general assessment of the child's health, including vital signs and appropriate measurements. The examination will generally proceed in a head-to-toe fashion, and the record should note findings relevant to both sexual abuse concerns and general medical needs. For example, child victims of sexual abuse may also have suffered physical abuse or neglect, with demonstrative, corroborative findings on examination.

Conducting the Physical Examination

The physical examination will differ slightly depending on the time elapsed since the last episode of suspected abuse and when the child or adolescent seeks medical evaluation. In cases in which LE or another agency requests the collection of forensic evidence, a standard protocol should be followed to collect samples for analysis, sometimes called the "rape kit." For children examined outside the time frame of acute evaluation, forensic evidence collection is deferred.

The accurate interpretation of medical and laboratory findings in cases of suspected child sexual abuse requires that the medical provider be familiar with normal anatomy, congenital variations, findings caused by conditions other than abuse, and findings caused by trauma.[39] Some infections, for example, can be transmitted by sexual contact but can also be transmitted by nonsexual contact. It is essential that the medical provider have access to the latest recommendations from organizations such as the American Academy of Pediatrics (AAP) and the Centers for Disease Control and Prevention (CDC) when there is a suspicion or confirmed case of infection caused by a sexually transmissible organism.[40-45]

After the Examination: Anticipatory Guidance on Personal Space and Safety

The medical provider has an ideal opportunity to reinforce the concept of a child or adolescent's right to personal space and safety (PS&S) and provide anticipatory guidance at the conclusion of the medical evaluation for suspected sexual abuse, or sooner during routine health care visits. Because vulnerability to sexual abuse begins at an early age, it is important that caregivers and medical providers incorporate guidance about PS&S beginning when children are approximately 3 to 4 years old and continue that guidance throughout their childhood in a developmentally appropriate manner. Although it is preferential to begin this safety counseling during routine health care visits for the young child, providing anticipatory guidance to any child or adolescent regardless of age or developmental stage, and regardless of presenting medical concern, can be impactful. Although there is no guarantee that children informed about a right to PS&S will be in a position to stop their own victimization, there is the possibility that they will recognize their experience as inappropriate and tell sooner before the activities progress over time.

The medical provider can initiate anticipatory guidance around PS&S by asking caregivers if they have ever spoken to their child about "private parts" and okay and not-okay touching. If they say yes, it is appropriate to ask what they have done and provide positive reinforcement. Knowing what information the caregiver provided, and how often, is helpful. Determining what precipitated addressing PS&S with their child and what made it important for them may be critical. Some caregivers may disclose that the motivation to address the issue with their child is based on their own prior sexual abuse experiences. Depending on the caregiver response, there may be an opportunity to secure help for the caregivers themselves for their own inappropriate experience. If the caregiver has not introduced the concept of "private parts" and okay/not-okay touching to his or her child, explain that it is time to begin this discussion. Caregivers should be encouraged to teach their child that the parts of their body that are covered by their bathing suit or underwear are called private parts; that they are called that because they belong to the child; the only one who can touch their private parts is themselves, their caregivers, or a doctor; and that it is not okay for anyone to touch their private parts for any reason other than helping or to make them touch someone else's private parts. Caregivers should explain that if either of these things happens, the child needs to tell a caregiver or nonfamily caregiver, such as a teacher. The child should be told that if something happens that is not okay, it would not be his or her fault and that he or she would not be in any trouble. Caregivers should reinforce that it is never okay to have a secret and if the child is asked to keep something secret or if he or she thinks something needs to be kept secret, it is important to tell an adult.

The medical provider should encourage caregivers to teach children the appropriate names for their private parts so they have the language to communicate and be understood. Caregivers many times are uncomfortable teaching the anatomically correct terms and substitute silly words such as *peach, pocket book, diamonds,* and *kibble and bits.* If a young child tells a teacher that someone touched her "diamonds," the teacher might think the child is being silly. However, if the child said to the teacher that someone touched her vagina, there would most likely be a very different response.

The medical provider should explain that the ideal time for the continued reinforcement of the concept of PS&S is while the caregiver is supervising the child's bathing. For example, while supervising bathing the caregiver can say or ask the child the following:

— "Don't forget to wash your private parts, and when you're done, let me know and I will help you with your hair."

— "Did you wash your vagina and your butt? Let me know when you're done and I will help you with your hair."

— "Who is allowed to touch your private parts, and what do you do if someone tries to or makes you touch them?"

Over time, repetition of these queries and statements will result in the child stating, "I already know that."

Addressing the Psychological Impact of Sexual Abuse

Trauma-Focused Cognitive Behavioral Therapy

The primary impact of sexual abuse is psychological. All children and adolescents assessed for child sexual abuse should be referred to a mental health clinician skilled in using evidence-based therapies, of which the most studied is trauma-focused cognitive behavioral therapy (TF-CBT).[46-48] Originally developed to address the impact of child sexual abuse, research has now documented its effectiveness with various other types of treatment as well, including exposure to domestic violence, traumatic grief, child physical abuse, natural disasters, and war exposure. TF-CBT is the treatment for childhood trauma with the strongest research support for its effectiveness. To date, 20 randomized controlled trials—the gold standard of treatment outcome research—have been completed across the United States as well as in other countries.[46,49-53]

TF-CBT is appropriate for children aged 3 to 18 years who have experienced trauma and for their nonoffending caregivers. Caregivers learn effective parenting skills, and children and caregivers learn various other skills in parallel, including relaxation skills, affect expression and modulation skills, and cognitive coping. Additionally, there is gradual exposure to traumatic memories, including psychoeducation about the trauma and trauma reactions as well as directly discussing and processing the traumatic experiences. Children and caregivers also learn safety skills. TF-CBT has been shown to be effective with a wide range of symptoms, including symptoms of posttraumatic stress, depressive symptoms, behavioral difficulties, and sexual behavior problems.

Body Safety Education

For children in whom sexual abuse has not been substantiated but for whom concern has been raised regarding continued vulnerability, body safety education can be of value in reducing potential victimization in the future. Body safety education emphasizes a child's right to decide between comfortable and uncomfortable touching. If the child feels uncomfortable, the child reserves the right to say "no" to being touched.

Medical Record Documentation in Cases of Suspected Child Sexual Abuse

The medical record articulates the clinical encounter of medical providers, child or adolescent patient, and caregiver. The medical record of children who may have experienced abusive sexual contact shares most of the core elements of the standard medical record/consultation format found in either an office-based or a hospital-based practice. When a patient sees a medical provider, a current medical history is obtained, including a detailed ROS and appropriate developmental and social history. Verifying the medical history affords an opportunity to understand the chronology of events from the possibly abusive contact to the circumstances that resulted in disclosure.

In a review of documentation of an examination conducted on a child believed to have been sexually abused, the manner in which the record is structured and the details provided should reflect that a complete and thorough assessment was conducted. Introductory statements explain the purpose of the examination and present background information regarding how the child appeared at the time of the examination. The record should include the overall medical condition of the child, the general physical examination findings, and a detailed description of the appearance of all genital and anal structures and any relevant extragenital findings. A detailed report demonstrates that the medical provider understands the importance of being thorough and has reflected such in recording the examination findings in a precise manner.

Any physical findings interpreted to be either diagnostic or supportive of the diagnosis should have visual documentation to augment the written record. Photographic and video documentation will help eliminate the possibility that an adversary would be successful in requiring a child undergo a repeat examination if a second opinion is being sought. Any physical examination findings interpreted to support the diagnosis should be recorded either through video colposcopy or photographic documentation in anticipation of a potential defense expert challenge to an opinion. When visual evidence is available for a defense expert to review if requested, there will be no need for the child to have a reexamination. Examinations should include objective documentation of the genital and anal structures whether or not diagnostic findings are present. The justification for such is that children remain at risk for something of an inappropriate nature to occur in the future. If so, the baseline documentation of an initial examination may prove to be a useful reference should there be a concern in the future. Baseline documentation can be of particular value in those circumstances in which a child is seen in the context of a custody dispute or the allegations are unsubstantiated but are of concern. Photographic, colposcopy, and video colposcopic methods of documentation have become routine, and they are the standard of care in the evaluation of suspected sexual abuse.[54]

Because the physical examination will infrequently demonstrate physical findings that on their own are diagnostic, it is important to formulate an opinion that explains the absence of findings.[55] Although it is "normal to be normal" (as evidenced by the absence of physical findings), in most cases there are ways that this finding can be explained in a manner that informs the reader.[56,57] Rather than using truncated summary words or phrases such as "normal" examination, "no physical evidence of sexual abuse," "the examination neither confirms nor denies the history provided," or "consistent with the history of sexual abuse," the clinician should provide a clear description of the examination findings and explain the reasons for the absence of acute or chronic residual symptoms when historical details support the concern that the child experienced something of a sexually inappropriate nature. The diagnostic assessment should integrate the physical examination findings, laboratory results, and medical history in a manner that is clear and descriptive. Reliance on a diagnostic checklist that designates findings as either normal or abnormal without an opportunity to write a narrative to explain the presence or absence of findings should be avoided.

Special Medicolegal Considerations for Medical Record Documentation

In suspected sexual abuse examinations, the medical provider should presume with significant probability that CPS, LE agents, prosecutors, and defense counsel will review the medical record. In anticipation of external scrutiny, one must construct the medical record with exacting attention to detail. The medical record must be legible, well constructed, and educational, with defensible conclusions.[11] The medical record should carefully chronicle the medical history, anatomical findings (even when normal), and laboratory test results. The medical record is the instrument the clinician will use to make the diagnosis and treatment recommendations.[11] The credibility of the diagnostic assessment will be questioned if the record is incomplete or poorly formulated.[58,59]

Myers[11] has identified a number of issues that if addressed will result in a more thorough and defensible medical record. Key components of the medical record from a legal perspective are as follows:

1. Document of the child's age at the time of the statement.
2. Note the duration of elapsed time between the suspected abuse and the child's statement.
3. Specify who was present when the child made the statement, where the statement was made, and to whom it was made.
4. Document whether specific statements are made in response to questions or are spontaneous.
5. Note whether the child's responses are made to leading or nonleading questions.
6. Note whether the child's statement was made at the first opportunity that the child felt safe to talk.
7. Document the child's emotional state. Note if the child was excited or distressed at the time of the statement. If so, note what signs or symptoms of excitement or distress were observed.
8. Document whether the child was calm, placid, or sleeping before making the statement or soon thereafter.
9. Use the exact words that the child uses to describe the characteristics of the event.
10. Document the child's physical condition at the time of the statement.
11. Note any suspected incentives for the child to fabricate lies or to distort the truth.

Formulating a Diagnosis

The medical provider, when formulating a diagnosis related to suspected sexual abuse, must consider and incorporate salient aspects of each of the following:

1. Historical details and behavioral indicators reflective of the contact
2. Symptoms that can be directly associated with the contact
3. Acute and healed genital and anal injuries
4. Extragenital trauma
5. Forensic evidence
6. STIs

In formulating a diagnosis, the medical provider may need to account for (1) why there may be discrepancies between a child's perception of his or her experience and what actually happened, (2) why children who provide clear histories of pain or bleeding as a result of contact may not have diagnostic physical findings, and (3) which types of symptoms secondary to trauma might be anticipated when a child experiences genital fondling, genital-to-genital contact, or anal trauma. Throughout the diagnostic and treatment process, the medical provider must be objective, know the limitations of clinical observations, incorporate differential considerations, and formulate a diagnosis in an unbiased manner.

The following examples reflect common clinical scenarios, each of which requires the formulation of very different diagnostic assessments:

1. Inappropriate sexual contact by history and/or behaviors is described; however, there are no diagnostic physical findings on examination.
2. Diagnostic findings are present that are reflective of inappropriate contact (ie, trauma, STIs, and/or seminal products) and are supported by descriptive history or behavior.
3. Diagnostic findings are present that are reflective of inappropriate contact (ie, trauma, STIs, and/or seminal products) without descriptive history or behavior.
4. Inappropriate sexual contact can be confirmed with medical certainty without healed residual symptoms.
5. Insufficient historical or behavioral details are present to support a concern of inappropriate sexual contact, and the physical examination findings are nondiagnostic.

Although the constellation of historical, behavioral, and examination findings will vary from patient to patient, the following serve as examples of how one component of the diagnostic assessment could be formulated in each of the following common scenarios.

1. Inappropriate sexual contact by history and/or behaviors is described; however, there are no diagnostic physical findings on examination.

   Case Study 3-1

   The medical history presented by an 8-year-old girl reflects progression of a variety of inappropriate sexual activities over time that were initially represented to her in a caring and loving context. Although the initial interactions were described as playful, the activities progressed with correspondingly escalating threats to maintain secrecy. The young girl did not report experiencing any physical discomfort after the genital fondling or the stroking of her uncle's genitalia. During the medical history, she asked what that icky stuff was that came out of his "pee-pee" and explained that she had to wipe it from her "peach" by using a tissue. In addition, she said that she was worried that people could tell just by the way that they looked at her that she had to do those disgusting things. In light of the history regarding contact with genital secretions, she is at risk for contracting an STI. I have evaluated this girl for STIs. Treatment and follow-up will be initiated should any of the test results be positive. Her physical examination does not demonstrate any acute or chronic symptoms residual to the sexual contact nor would they be anticipated in light of her denial of discomfort associated with the contact. Her body image concern is common among children who experience sexual abuse. I do not believe there is any alternative explanation for this child's history of progressive engagement in sexual activities, threats to maintain secrecy, detailed description of a variety of sexually explicit interactions, and concerns about body image other than from experiencing sexual abuse. The most significant impact of her inappropriate sexual experiences is psychological. She needs to be evaluated by a clinical child psychologist to assess the impact of her inappropriate experiences, develop a therapeutic plan, and provide anticipatory guidance regarding body safety.

2. Diagnostic findings are present that are reflective of inappropriate contact (ie, trauma, STIs, and/or seminal products) and are supported by descriptive history or behavior.

Case Study 3-2

A 7-year-old girl provided a clear and detailed medical history of genital-to-genital contact with her father and being coerced into placing her mouth on her father's genitalia. She perceived the genital-to-genital contact to involve penile-vaginal penetration. She reported a history of bleeding and pain after the genital-to-genital contact. Although her disclosure occurred 1 month after the last stated contact, her physical examination demonstrated diagnostic findings that reflect sequaelae to this contact. On physical examination, a well-defined healed transection of the posterior portion of her hymen is found that extends to the base of its attachment on the posterior vaginal wall. This finding is diagnostic of blunt-force penetrating trauma and reflects the introduction of a foreign body through the structures of the vaginal vestibule, the hymenal orifice, and into the vagina. She did not report physical discomfort associated with the history of oral-genital contact, although she stated that white stuff from her father's penis got into her mouth. Her contact with ejaculate places her at risk for an STI. She has been evaluated for STIs. Should any of the tests be positive, treatment and follow-up will be initiated.

3. Diagnostic findings are present that are reflective of inappropriate contact (ie, trauma, STIs, and/or seminal products) without descriptive history or behavior.

Case Study 3-3

A 10-year-old girl was unable to provide adequate details through a history to fully understand the scope of sexually inappropriate activities for which there has been a concern. Although seminal products were found on her underwear, none were found on examination nor would be anticipated because the last suspected contact was 2 weeks earlier. This child's disclosure to her best friend regarding sexual interactions with a family "uncle" resulted in an investigation and the request for an examination to diagnose and treat any symptoms residual to the suspected sexual abuse. During attempts to obtain the medical history, this girl appeared withdrawn and would not make eye contact or engage in meaningful conversation. Throughout the examination she appeared as if she were dissociating herself from the examination process.

Her genital examination did not demonstrate any acute or chronic signs of trauma or signs of STIs. The anal-rectal examination demonstrated a well-defined linear scar at 5 o'clock in the knee-chest position. With anoscopy, the scar was observed to extend from the external anal verge tissues across the anoderm and to the pectinate line. The appearance of the scar was enhanced with the use of a red-free filter and recorded on 35-mm film and through video colposcopy.

Although this young girl appeared emotionally unavailable to provide historical details regarding inappropriate sexual activities, the recovery of seminal products in her underwear and the presence of a healed laceration of the anal tissues confirms with medical certainty that she experienced blunt-force penetrating trauma. This girl would benefit from being seen by a child psychiatrist who could assess the emotional impact of her experience, provide appropriate medication, and develop a treatment plan.

4. Inappropriate sexual contact can be confirmed with medical certainty without healed residual symptoms.

Case Study 3-4

A 9-year-old girl provided a detailed history of a variety of sexually inappropriate interactions with her stepfather spanning a 6-month time frame. The initial activities were represented to her as a special game in a loving context. The most recent event 10 days before the disclosure involved her stepfather placing his "stuff" inside her "coochie." Using an anatomically detailed model, the child clarified to me that "stuff" referred to a penis and "coochie" referred to the vagina. When asked to explain what she meant by "inside" with the use of an anatomic model of the female genitalia, she demonstrated that she thought his "stuff" was placed inside in the adult sense of penetration. On physical examination, no acute or chronic signs of trauma or STIs were found. The edge of the hymenal membrane was without interruption. The orifice diameter was 5 mm with traction and insufficient to have allowed introduction of a foreign body such as a penis into the vagina. Although this young girl perceived the genital-to-genital contact to involve penetration into the vagina, penetration was limited to the structures of the vaginal vestibule.

When asked how the genital-to-genital touching felt, she said that it hurt when he rubbed his stuff on her coochie. When asked in what way it hurt, she stated that it hurt her after her stepfather stopped touching her when she went to the bathroom afterward to "go pee." When asked to describe the discomfort she had when she went to pee, she stated that it stung. When asked if she had ever felt anything like that before, she said "no." When asked if she ever saw anything to make her know she was hurt, she responded "no." When asked how long the discomfort with peeing lasted, she said "just that day." A review of systems was negative for any alternative medical history explanation for knowledge of the symptom of dysuria. The symptom of dysuria temporally related to the genital-to-genital contact reflects trauma to the periurethral area as a result of rubbing. The only way this young girl could know about the symptom of dysuria temporally related to the genital-to-genital contact is by experiencing this condition. The trauma she incurred to the periurethral area and/or vestibular mucosa was superficial and has since healed without residual symptoms, as anticipated. The extent of genital-to-genital contact was limited to penetration within the structures of the vaginal vestibule.

5. Insufficient historical or behavioral details are present to support a concern of inappropriate sexual contact, and the physical examination findings are nondiagnostic.

   Case Study 3-5

   A 2-year-old boy was examined to address the concern that he may have been touched in a sexually inappropriate manner. This concern arose because of a diaper rash, intermittent self-stimulatory behaviors, and some resistance to having his diaper changed. His mother stated that she had been sexually abused by her father as a child and wanted to protect her son from the same. The maternal grandparents occasionally babysit her son. His physical examination is positive for diaper dermatitis caused by *Candida albicans*, and he has secondary impetiginous lesions. The historical and behavioral details that have been provided are insufficient to confirm with medical certainty that this boy has experienced anything of a sexually inappropriate nature. The constellation of behavioral changes can be attributed to his diaper dermatitis and are not the result of any sexually inappropriate contact. This child, and all children, should receive anticipatory guidance regarding body safety in a developmentally appropriate manner. I have obtained baseline documentation of the appearance of his anogenital anatomy that will serve as a reference should there be any concerns in the future. The present concerns afford an opportunity for this child's mother to address any unresolved issues concerning her own experience and exercise caution in leaving her child in the care of any individual with whom she has concern.

Less common clinical presentation scenarios may include the following:

1. A healed injury is identified on examination with no prior suspicion of abuse in the absence of historical or behavioral indicators.
2. A child is evaluated with a concern without clear historical or behavioral details to support the concern, which may be a reflection of hypervigilance as a result of a caregiver's personal experience.
3. An STI is diagnosed in a young child for whom no explanation for how the child contracted the disease is available after a complete assessment.
4. Fabricated or misinterpreted behaviors and/or history alleging sexual abuse are reported. This form of presentation may be seen in adversarial caregiver relationships, such as custody disputes.
5. An adolescent fabricates or distorts historical details.

The diagnostic assessments presented as case studies in this chapter represent a few ways in which the clinician can articulate findings and interpret them for those who will need to reference the consultative report. A clear and detailed medical record will reduce the likelihood that the clinician will need to appear in court to explain the record. The medical report should make appropriate recommendations for any follow-up medical care and mental health services.

Conclusion

When children are suspected to have experienced sexually inappropriate activities, the medical provider plays a critical role in that child's care. The medical provider's primary focus is the diagnosis and treatment of residual findings related to suspected sexual abuse. The examination is conducted both for the detection and treatment of "abnormality" with regard to injury or disease and the determination of "normality."[60] This includes anticipating and addressing anxieties and fears, providing reassurance, and treating acute injuries or STIs. Critical to the comprehensive care of the sexual abuse victim is an assessment of emotional and behavioral health needs and appropriate linkage to therapy or counseling to address trauma symptoms stemming from abuse. The unique medical provider-patient relationship can provide therapeutic value to the child and family in crisis and support the investigative process that could lead to substantiation by child protective services and the necessary steps to ensure child safety, protection, and treatment.

The evaluation of the sexually abused child dictates the need for medical providers to work in a collaborative fashion with professionals from CPS, mental health, and LE investigators. Although the examination and diagnosis may prove to have investigative value, the purpose of examining a child suspected of being abused is to diagnose and treat any medical needs that are the result of the suspected sexual contact. The medical provider's assessment should be informative for CPS and LE colleagues who must interpret the medical evaluation and consider the information within the context of a multidisciplinary perspective.

Substantiation of sexual abuse is within the purview of child protection. The medical component remains important when attempting to understand what a child might have experienced. A mental health clinician's assessment can provide additional insights into understanding a child's experience.[60-64]

The final decision regarding meeting the therapeutic and protection needs of the child and family rests on the integration of medicine, mental health, CPS, and LE collective insights. Legal outcomes whether civil or criminal are less predictable. From a medical provider's perspective, the gold standard for best outcomes focuses on meeting the medical, mental health, and protection needs of the child and family.

References

1. Newton, AW, Vandeven AM. The role of the medical provider in the evaluation of sexually abused children and adolescents. *J Child Sex Abus.* 2010;19(6):669-686.
2. Finkelhor D. Sex among siblings: a survey on prevalence, variety, and effects. *Arch Sex Behav.* 1980;9(3):171-194.
3. Finkelhor D. Boys as victims: review of the evidence. In: Finkelhor D, ed. *Child Sexual Abuse: New Theory and Research.* New York, NY: Free Press; 1984:150-170.
4. Finkelhor D, Hotaling G, Lewis IA, Smith C. Sexual abuse in a national survey of adult men and women: prevalence, characteristics, and risk factors. *Child Abuse Negl.* 1990;14(1):19-28.
5. Finkelhor D, Dziuba-Leatherman J. Children as victims of violence: a national survey. *Pediatrics.* 1994;94(4 pt 1):413-420.
6. Finkelhor D, Browne A. The traumatic impact of child sexual abuse: a conceptualization. *Am J Orthopsychiatry.* 1985;55(4):530-541.

7. Finkelhor D. The victimization of children: a developmental perspective. *Am J Orthopsychiatry*. 1995;65(2):177-193.

8. Sgroi SM. *Handbook of Clinical Intervention in Child Sexual Abuse*. Lexington, MA: DC Heath and Co; 1982.

9. Summit RC. The child sexual abuse accommodation syndrome. *Child Abuse Negl*. 1983;7(2):177-193.

10. Kellogg ND; Committee on Child Abuse and Neglect, American Academy of Pediatrics. Clinical report: the evaluation of sexual behaviors in children. *Pediatrics*. 2009;124(3):992-998.

11. Myers JEB. Investigative interviewing regarding child maltreatment. In: Myers JEB, ed. *Legal Issues in Child Abuse and Neglect Practice*. 2nd ed. Thousand Oaks, CA: Sage Publications; 1998:102-152.

12. Finkel MA. "I can tell you because you're a doctor.": commentary on girls who disclose sexual abuse: signs and symptoms following genital contact: the importance of the pediatrician's detailed medical history when evaluating suspected child sexual abuse. *Pediatrics*. 2008;122(8):422.

13. Hansen RF, Adams CS. Childhood sexual abuse: identification, screening, and treatment recommendations in primary care settings. *Prim Care*. 2016;43(2):313-326.

14. Saunders BE, Kilpatrick DG, Hanson RF, Resnick HS, Walker ME. Prevalence, case characteristics, and long-term psychological correlates of child rape among women: a national survey. *Child Maltreat*. 1999;4(3):187-200.

15. Cohen JA, Kelleher KJ, Mannarino AP. Identifying, treating, and referring traumatized children: the role of pediatric providers. *Arch Pediatr Adolesc Med*. 2008;162(5):447-452.

16. Myers JE. Role of physician in preserving verbal evidence of child abuse. *J Pediatr*. 1986;109(3):409-411.

17. DeLago C, Deblinger ED, Schroeder C, Finkel MA. Girls who disclose sexual abuse: urogenital symptoms and signs following sexual contact. *Pediatrics*. 2008;122(8):e281-e286.

18. Finkel MA. Anogenital trauma in sexually abused children. *Pediatrics*. 1989;84(2):317-322.

19. Ashby BD, Kaul P. Post-traumatic stress disorder after sexual abuse in adolescent girls. *J Pediatr Adolesc Gynecol*. 2016;29(6):531-536.

20. American Psychiatric Association. *Diagnostic and Statistical Manual of Mental Disorders*. 5th ed. Washington, DC: American Psychiatric Association; 2013.

21. Kimmerling R, Ouimette P, Wolfe J. *Gender and PTSD*. New York, NY: Guilford Publications; 2014.

22. Ouimette P, Cronkite R, Henson BR, Prins A, Gima K, Moos RH. Posttraumatic stress disorder and health status among female and male medical patients. *J Trauma Stress*. 2004;17(1):1-9.

23. Kimmerling R, Calhoun KS. Somatic symptoms, social support, and treatment seeking among sexual assault victims. *J Consult Clin Psychol*. 1994;62(2):333-340.

24. Irwin C, Falsetti SA, Lydiard RB, Ballenger JC, Brock CD, Brener W. Comorbidity of posttraumatic stress disorder and irritable bowel syndrome. *J Clin Psychiatry.* 1996;57(12):576-578.

25. Seng JS, Oakley DJ, Sampselle CM, Killion C, Graham-Bermann SA, Liberzon I. Posttraumatic stress disorder and pregnancy complications. *Obstet Gynecol.* 2001;97(1):17-22.

26. Seng JS, Graham-Bermann SA, Clark MK, McCarthy AM, Ronis DL. Posttraumatic stress disorder and physical comorbidity among female children and adolescents: results from service-use data. *Pediatrics.* 2005;116(6):e767-e776.

27. Najman JM, Dunne MP, Purdie DM, Boyle FM, Coxeter PD. Sexual abuse in childhood and sexual dysfunction in adulthood: an Australian population-based study. *Arch Sex Behav.* 2005;34(5):517-526.

28. Loeb TB, Williams JK, Carmona JV, et al. Child sexual abuse: associations with the sexual functioning of adolescents and adults. *Annu Rev Sex Res.* 2002;13:307-345.

29. Brener ND, McMahon PM, Warren CW, Douglas KA. Forced sexual intercourse and associated health-risk behaviors among female college students in the United States. *J Consult Clin Psychol.* 1999;67(2):252-259.

30. Fletcher KE. Childhood posttraumatic stress disorder. In: Mash EJ, Barkley RA, eds. *Child Psychopathology.* 2nd ed. New York, NY: Guilford Press; 2003:330-371.

31. Kilpatrick DG, Ruggiero KJ, Acierno R, Saunders BE, Resnick HS, Best CL. Violence and risk of PTSD, major depression, substance abuse/dependence, and comorbidity: results from the National Survey of Adolescents. *J Consult Clin Psychol.* 2003;71(4):692-700.

32. Reese S, Silove D, Chey T, et al. Lifetime prevalence of gender-based violence in women and the relationship with mental disorders and psychosocial function. *JAMA.* 2011;306(5):513-521.

33. Favarelli C, Giugni A, Salvatori S, Ricca V. Psychopathology after rape. *Am J Psychiatry.* 2004;161(8):1483-1485.

34. Steinberg AM, Brymer MJ, Decker KB, Pynoos RS. The University of California at Los Angeles Post-Traumatic Stress Disorder Reaction Index. *Curr Psychiatry Rep.* 2004;6(2):96-100.

35. Briere J. *Trauma Symptom Checklist for Children: Professional Manual.* Odessa, FL: Psychological Assessment Resources; 1996.

36. Foa EB, Johnson KM, Feeny MC, Treadwell KR. The child PTSD Symptom Scale: a preliminary examination of its psychometric properties. *J Clin Child Psychol.* 2001;30(3):376-384.

37. Friedrich WN. *Child Sexual Behavior Inventory.* Odessa, FL: Psychological Assessment Resources; 1997.

38. Achenbach TM, Rescorla LA. Friedrich WN. *Manual for the ASEBA Preschool Forms and Profiles.* Burlington, VT: University of Vermont, Department of Psychiatry; 2000.

39. Adams JA, Kellogg ND, Farst KJ, et al. Updated guidelines for the medical assessment and care of children who may have been sexually abused. *J Pediatr Adolesc Gynecol.* 2016;29(2):81-87.

40. Centers for Disease Control and Prevention. Sexually transmitted diseases treatment guidelines 2015. *MMWR Morbid Mortal Wkly Rep.* 2015;64(3):1-137.

41. Kellogg N; American Academy of Pediatrics Committee on Child Abuse and Neglect. The evaluation of sexual abuse in children. *Pediatrics.* 2005;116(2):506-512.

42. Siegel RM, Schubert CJ, Myers PA, Shapiro RA. The prevalence of sexually transmitted diseases in children and adolescents evaluated for sexual abuse in Cincinnati: rationale for limited STD testing in prepubertal girls. *Pediatrics.* 1995;96(6):1090-1094.

43. US Department of Justice, Office on Violence Against Women. *A National Protocol for Sexual Assault Medical Forensic Examination: Adults/Adolescents.* Washington, DC: US Department of Justice, Office on Violence Against Women; 2004.

44. Girardet RG, Lahoti S, Howard LA, et al. Epidemiology of sexually transmitted infections in suspected child victims of sexual assault. *Pediatrics.* 2009;124(1):79-86.

45. Committee on Adolescence, Society for Adolescent Health and Medicine. Screening for nonviral sexually transmitted infections in adolescents and young adults. *Pediatrics.* 2014;134(1):e302-e311.

46. Cohen JA, Deblinger E, Mannarino AP, Steer RA. A multisite, randomized controlled trial for children with sexual abuse-related PTSD symptoms. *J Am Acad Child Adolesc Psychiatry.* 2004;43(4):393-402.

47. Cohen JA, Mannarino AP, Deblinger E. *Treating Trauma and Traumatic Grief in Children and Adolescents.* 2nd ed. New York, NY: Guilford Press; 2017.

48. Deblinger E, Mannarino AP, Cohen JA, Runyon MK, Heflin AH. *Child Sexual Abuse: A Primer for Treating Children, Adolescents, and Their Nonoffending Caregivers.* 2nd ed. New York, NY: Oxford University Press; 2015.

49. Deblinger E, Lippmann J, Steer RA. Sexually abused children suffering posttraumatic stress symptoms: initial treatment outcome findings. *Child Maltreat.* 1996;1(4):310-321.

50. Deblinger E, Mannarino AP, Cohen JA, Runyon MK, Steer RA. Trauma-focused cognitive behavioral therapy for children: impact of the trauma narrative and treatment length. *Depress Anxiety.* 2011;28(1):67-75.

51. Jensen TK, Holt T, Ormhaug SM, et al. A randomized effectiveness study comparing trauma-focused cognitive behavioral therapy with therapy as usual for youth. *J Clin Child Adolesc Psychol.* 2014;43(3):359-369.

52. O'Callaghan P, McMullen J, Shannon C, Rafferty H, Black A. A randomized controlled trial of trauma-focused cognitive behavioral therapy for sexually exploited, war-affected Congolese girls. *J Am Acad Child Adolesc Psychiatry.* 2013;52(4):359-369.

53. Cohen JA, Mannarino AP, Deblinger, E. *Treating Trauma and Traumatic Grief in Children and Adolescents.* New York, NY: Guilford Press; 2006.

54. Finkel MA, Ricci LR. Documentation and preservation of visual evidence in child abuse. *Child Maltreat.* 1997;2(4):322-330.

55. Heger A, Ticson L, Velasquez O, Bernier R. Children referred for possible sexual abuse: medical findings in 2384 children. *Child Abuse Negl.* 2002;26(6-7):645-659.

56. Adams JA, Harper K, Knudson S, Revilla J. Examination findings in legally confirmed child sexual abuse: it's normal to be normal. *Pediatrics.* 1994;94(3):310-317.

57. Kellogg ND, Menard SW, Santos A. Genital anatomy in pregnant adolescents: "normal" does not mean "nothing happened." *Pediatrics.* 2004;113(1 pt 1):e67-e69.

58. Boyce MC, Melhorn KJ, Vargo G. Pediatric trauma documentation: adequacy for assessment of child abuse. *Arch Pediatr Adolesc Med.* 1996;150(7):730-732.

59. Parra JM, Huston RL, Foulds DM. Resident documentation of diagnostic impression in child sexual abuse evaluations. *Clin Pediatr (Phila).* 1997;36(12):691-694.

60. Finkel MA, Giardino AP. *Medical Evaluation of Child Sexual Abuse: A Practical Guide.* 3rd ed. Chicago, IL: American Academy of Pediatrics; 2009.

61. Friedrich WN, Beilke RL, Urquiza AJ. Behavior problems in young sexually abused boys: a comparison study. *J Interpers Violence.* 1988;3(1):21-28.

62. Friedrich WN, Grambsch P, Broughton D, Kuiper J, Beilke RL. Normative sexual behavior in children. *Pediatrics.* 1991;88(3):456-464.

63. Friedrich WN. Sexual victimization and sexual behavior in children: a review of recent literature. *Child Abuse Neglect.* 1993;17(1):59-66.

64. Friedrich WN, Jaworski TM, Huxsahl JE, Bengston BS. Dissociative and sexual behaviors in children and adolescents with sexual abuse and psychiatric histories. *J Interpers Violence.* 1997;12(2):155-171.

Chapter 4

The Medical Evaluation of Acute Sexual Abuse or Assault in Children and Adolescents

Allan De Jong, MD

Introduction

The medical evaluation of children and adolescents who are believed to have experienced acute sexual assault or abuse has 2 major components that often are concurrent: (1) providing appropriate medical care and (2) collecting and documenting evidence of a crime. The primary objective should be to provide a sensitive yet thorough evaluation of the physical and emotional needs of the victim. The examiner must be able to obtain a complete history and perform a physical examination on a child or adolescent who has recently experienced a confusing, frightening, violent, or painful event in order to decide on additional testing, treatment, and prophylaxis for injuries, infections, and pregnancy. The secondary objective of collecting forensic evidence must be accomplished parallel to the primary objective.

This chapter discusses the medical and forensic components of the evaluation process; the collection, documentation, and interpretation of historical, physical, and forensic evidence; and the medical management of children and adolescents who are victims of acute sexual assault or abuse.

Medical Evaluation Process

Medical History

The medical history of the child or adolescent who has been sexually abused or assaulted includes answers to questions of medical and forensic importance. It provides information to help direct appropriate medical care of the victim while obtaining information about the abusive events to help support forensic evidence collection, direct further criminal investigation, and aid in the interpretation of examination findings. The medical history or interview of the victim can provide a unique opportunity to get details of the abusive episode.[1-17] For children who have been victimized, the examiner must decide how much medical information should be obtained directly from the child and how much should be obtained from the child's caregivers. Before obtaining direct history from the child, information should be gathered from all other possible sources. For the adolescent who has been victimized, most of the important medical information is obtained directly from the victim, including the date and time of the assault, pertinent medical history about the anogenital area, any history of prior or subsequent sexual activity, activities since the assault, symptoms occurring at the time of the assault and since the assault, the nature of the assault itself, and information about the suspect.

How much information should be collected during the medical evaluation is debatable, and protocols that expand or restrict questioning by medical examiners vary among jurisdictions. From the medical perspective, it is always appropriate to collect enough history to allow medical personnel to provide an appropriate physical and laboratory evaluation, develop a diagnosis, and determine proper treatment of children and adolescents who have been victimized.

Pertinent medical history includes prior injuries, infections, or surgery of the anogenital area; menstrual history; and any recent or current medical treatment. The history of sexual activity before or subsequent to the sexual assault is important to the interpretation of physical findings, sexually transmitted infections (STIs), and forensic evidence. Knowledge of activities since the assault will help medical personnel determine the likelihood of finding evidence, because bathing, wiping the anogenital area, urinating, defecating, douching, removing tampons or sanitary pads, rinsing the mouth or gargling, brushing teeth, and eating or drinking can remove forensic materials. Information on whether the victim changed or did not change clothing since the assault is important because it will direct medical personnel to appropriate clothing to collect for evidence. Symptoms occurring at the time of the assault and since the assault, including anogenital pain or bleeding and nongenital pain or bleeding, are important factors that dictate medical care and evidence collection. The use of drugs or alcohol prior to the assault should prompt drug screening, and memory loss or loss of consciousness should also raise suspicion of drug use. Drug or alcohol use since the assault will alter the results and interpretation of urine or blood drug testing. The description of the nature of the assault itself is helpful for the detection, collection, and interpretation of forensic evidence, as well as for medical treatment. The history of specific types of sexual contact; types of nongenital contact (eg, kissing, licking, biting, sucking); the use of condoms, lubricants, or other contraception; ejaculation; and the location of the assault should be obtained. The history of the use of weapons, threats, and descriptions of types of force used (eg, hitting, choking, restraint) can aid in assessing nongenital injuries. Asking the victim whether the suspect may have been injured in the assault through scratching, biting, or other means may help in evidence collection. Some information about the suspect or suspects involved in the assault will help in interpretation of the forensic materials collected.[2-4,9,12,13,16]

The examiner who decides to obtain a medical history or interview about the assault directly from a young child should use appropriate interviewing techniques. There is no published data that proves that asking appropriate questions during a medical history would cause harm to the child or to the investigation.[8,12] Whenever possible, the child should be interviewed alone, because even the presence of a supportive parent may limit or otherwise influence the details disclosed by the child. Sometimes even the presence of another medical or nonmedical support person may interfere with the child's disclosure. The best interview situation is a quiet, nonthreatening environment where interviewers are able to assess the child's level of cognitive and language development and use developmentally appropriate questions. It is desirable to avoid leading and suggestive questions and to avoid showing strong emotions.[3] Nonsuggestive, open-ended questions are the best initial questions because they are designed to obtain a narrative response. Examples include (1) "Why did you come to see the doctor today?"; (2) "Why did your mother bring you to the hospital?"; (3) "Has something happened to you?"; and (4) "Has something happened to you that hurt or scared you?" Initial answers then can often be expanded by using facilitative questions, including (1) "How did that happen?"; (2) "What happened next?"; or (3) "Can you tell me more about that?" Questions that involve the use of "why" should generally be avoided as clarifying questions because the child may interpret them as suggesting blame or guilt. Multiple-choice questions may help obtain specific details; however, it is always best to include an open-ended choice as one of the answers. Such questions give the choice of 2 specific answers plus a third "or something else" option. The child is not forced to select a specific answer if the "or something else" is correct. The questions asked and the answers given should be documented in detail because information obtained through questioning by health care providers for the purpose of diagnosis and treatment may be admissible in court.[10,11]

The Physical Examination

Immediate medical evaluation for the child or adolescent victim of acute sexual assault is indicated when the victim presents with pain, bleeding, or other significant symptoms in the genital or anal area; when there is a probability of acute trauma; when there is a reasonable probability that forensic evidence may be present; and, specifically in adolescents, if the time frame for prophylactic antibiotics (up to 72 hours) or pregnancy prophylaxis (up to 120 hours) applies. The physical examination of the child or adolescent who is a victim of acute sexual assault should consist of a complete general examination and a detailed, focused anogenital examination. The examination should be performed by qualified providers with experience in child sexual abuse and assault.[1,2,5,6] Initially, the examination should be explained to the child and the general physical examination should be done first because of potential findings while allowing the child to become more comfortable with the examiner before the anogenital examination is performed. Some aspects of the general examination to record include the behavior and interaction at the time of arrival and the condition of the victim's clothing. Initial inspection should include observing and documenting foreign material including stains, secretions, grass, and soil on the clothing and body. Collection of these materials may provide useful evidence, as is further described in this chapter. The general examination also allows documentation of injuries outside the anogenital area that may be the best proof of the use of force. The location and pattern of the injuries can be used to support both their inflicted causation and the victim's description of the violence. Nongenital injuries should be preferably photographed or described in drawings and documented in the medical record.

The anogenital examination in prepubertal children is often conducted with the child in a number of examination positions including the supine frog-leg, supine knee-chest, prone knee-chest, lateral knee-chest, and modified lithotomy position (ie, positioned on the lap of a parent or other support person). There is no single examination position or combination of examination positions that provides the best visualization and the best level of comfort and cooperation for the child. The anogenital examination in adolescents is typically conducted in the lithotomy position, but visualization and documentation of genital injuries can sometimes be maximized by using additional positions as with prepubertal children. A moistened swab can be helpful to detect injuries around the hymenal rim in adolescents, and others recommend using the Foley catheter technique. The Foley catheter is inserted into the hymenal opening, the balloon is inflated inside the vaginal canal, and the balloon is positioned so that the hymen is stretched over the surface of the balloon to improve visualization. This technique is not recommended for prepubertal girls.[1,14,18] Genital injury can indicate both recent sexual contact and the use of force. Genital injury can be described in drawings and documented in the medical record, but photodocumentation has become the standard of care in many protocols.[1,5,13,14,16]

Appropriate preparation should precede the actual process of the examination. Initially, the examiner should discuss the process of the examination as well as the limits of confidentiality of the information collected because of the necessary reporting of the results to law enforcement and child protective service investigators when required by law.[2,3,14] Permission for the physical examination and the collection of forensic specimens should be obtained from the legal guardians of the children. Children and adolescents should be asked to consent or assent to the examination and be allowed to maintain control over the conduct of the examination. Children and adolescents should be allowed to choose whether or not a parent or another support person (eg, victim advocate, child life professional) is present in the examining room.

The child or adolescent should have a thorough physical examination, but the conduct of the examination should not result in additional physical and emotional trauma.[3] A slow, deliberate, nonthreatening approach maximizes cooperation and minimizes trauma. Examination of prepubertal and early pubertal females does not routinely require a speculum examination. If there is acute vaginal bleeding and the source of the bleeding is not seen on routine examination, a speculum examination may be required. In all of these cases, the examination should be done under anesthesia by using a small speculum such as the Huffman speculum. In late-pubertal adolescents, speculum examination to obtain endocervical swab specimens may be appropriate to maximize collection of spermatozoa (sperm) and seminal fluid. The examiner should take into account the adolescent's willingness and comfort with a speculum examination, and force or coercion should not be used to obtain a speculum examination.[1,6,14]

Toluidine blue dye is a vital dye used for sexual assault evaluations because it enhances injuries by staining injured skin or mucous membranes. Toluidine blue dye is not indicated in prepubertal children. There is no reason to use toluidine blue dye when a laceration is clearly visible without it. Toluidine blue can cause stinging or burning when applied, limiting the cooperation of young children.[19-20] Use of toluidine blue is controversial because it changes appearance and enhances injuries; therefore, many centers do not use it in adolescent or adult victims.[16]

Photography of both anogenital injuries and nongenital injuries can be helpful in preserving evidence that is likely to heal completely within a short time. Options involved in photographic documentation include the type of photography preferred (eg, video or still photography) and the type of equipment used to aid in the examination and photography of the anogenital area (eg, colposcopy with varying photographic formats attached or other camera systems that can provide lighting and magnification in addition to photographic documentation).[9,11,22-26]

Photographic documentation is particularly important when examination findings are being described as abnormal or indicative of injury. Not all sexual assault evaluation programs or legal jurisdictions are in agreement as to whether photographs should be used to routinely document normal anatomy, as well as all detected injuries, or whether photographic evidence should be limited to detected injuries only.[13,16] Regardless of the type of photography and the type of equipment used, certain details are important to obtain useful photographs. The photographs need to be labeled in some manner to identify the patient and the date the photographs were taken. They need to be clear and accurate, which includes proper lighting, focus, and color. A color bar standard in the photographs is helpful to ensure accurate color reproduction and a measurement standard, or ruler, is essential to determine the size of injuries. Obtaining multiple photographs of the same area of injury from varying distances may be helpful in showing the location of the injury; however, obtaining a limited number of high-quality photographs of injuries is much better than collecting numerous low-quality photographs.

Forensic Evidence Collection

Two basic types of forensic evidence are sought in sexual assault cases: transfer and identification evidence. Transfer evidence, or associative evidence, includes foreign materials found on the surface of the victim's body or clothing that are transferred to the victim from the abuser or from the crime scene itself. Identification evidence includes biological materials such as sperm, seminal fluid, or other body fluids or cellular material that contain DNA material that can be used to identify the abuser.[16]

Forensic evidence collection has traditionally been recommended when the examination occurs within 72 hours of acute sexual assault or sexual abuse.[1-4,6,13,14,16] This recommendation is based, at least in part, on research suggesting seminal fluid and other foreign substances are unlikely to be recovered in adults more than 72 hours following the last sexual contact. Clinical data from sexual assault victims is limited to support the collection of evidence beyond the 72-hour time frame, but considering that some studies conducted 4 decades ago indicate up to 50% of samples being positive for sperm 72 hours following voluntary intercourse in adults, and occasional positives up to 17 days following intercourse,[27] there is substantial historical data that supports an expanded time frame. Combined with the increasing sensitivity of DNA analysis techniques, data from samples following consensual intercourse, and the increasing importance of DNA evidence in the prosecution of acute sexual assault of adults and adolescents, the possibility of finding DNA evidence more than 72 hours following a sexual assault has prompted many centers to extend the time frame for evidence collection to 5 days or longer.[2,5,16]

Collection of forensic evidence is appropriate to consider in children presenting within 72 hours of a sexual contact that may have involved ejaculation into the vagina; when the child presents with a nonspecific history but has fluorescent material when examined using an alternative light source; if the child has been kidnapped regardless of the history; if law enforcement requests collection regardless of history; or when parents, older children, or adolescents who have been victimized request evidence collection despite absence of a clear history. The examiner should understand that the aforementioned criteria are not a mandate to collect an evidence kit. Forensic evidence is usually not found in evidence kits from young children who are victims of sexual assault.[28-36] This subject will be discussed in more detail later in the chapter. The reasons that young children do not have evidence as often as adults include differences in the dynamics of the assault and physiological differences. Child sexual abuse is more often coercive or manipulative rather than violent, and semen is less likely to be recovered from prepubertal vaginas because of the lack of estrogen, the smaller volume of the vaginal cavity itself, and the lower probability of deep penile penetration into the vaginal canal occurring during the sexual contact. For health care professionals, it is important to remember to make the medical decisions based on what is medically appropriate for the patient.

Several general guidelines about evidence collection need to be addressed before outlining a specific approach to specimen collection. First, the specific process of collection, labeling, and packaging of specimens should be consistent with the parameters established by the laboratory processing the specimens. Second, a specimen collection protocol should be used to ensure that all appropriate specimens are collected, labeled, and packaged. Third, collection kits should be standardized by providing containers, collection devices, and forms or checklists to ensure proper collection of specimens. These first 3 guidelines have prompted legal jurisdictions, ranging from individual counties to entire states, to use a common, standardized prepackaged evidence collection kit for all sexual assault cases.[4,5,13,16] Fourth, the procedures for collecting specimens should be explained in advance to the child or adolescent and their caregivers to ensure the cooperation necessary for proper specimen collection. Fifth, appropriate consent must be obtained from the parent and child before performing the examination and collecting evidence. Finally, the handling of collected specimens should be limited and clearly documented to maintain a "chain of custody (or chain of evidence)." Documentation includes limiting the number of personnel involved in handling specimens and clearly recording the specimen handlers from the time of collection through the processing of the specimens in the laboratory. Examiners of victims who have been abused should maintain control of evidence beginning with the process of collecting the samples, through the steps of appropriate drying and packaging individual samples, placing individual samples inside and sealing the container for the evidence kit, storage of the kit when necessary, and handing the sealed kit over to an appropriate law enforcement official for processing.[4,5,13,16]

General guidelines have been established, but the specific evidence collection kit and the process of collection, labeling, and packaging of specimens vary.[4,13] The specific methods used to collect and transport specimens vary, including the use of synthetic rather than cotton swabs or other minor variations in techniques. Any foreign substances introduced or used by the examiner should be documented (eg, lubricating jelly, toluidine dye, betadine) so their source can be explained if the laboratory analyzing the specimens finds these. Those collecting and handling the specimens should wear gloves to avoid exposure to potentially infectious materials and to prevent contamination of the specimens with the collector's DNA. These individuals should avoid contaminating body sites with secretions from distant sites, by collecting specimens carefully and then removing remaining secretions or stains before sampling another site. Air-drying of wet specimens and packaging them in paper envelopes or paper containers is essential to their preservation. Drying should take place at room temperature to prevent damage from high temperatures and in a clean area to prevent contamination during the drying process. Plastic bags or plastic containers retain moisture, promoting the growth of bacteria and molds that can destroy the samples. Collected "wet" evidence including urine samples, blood samples, wet clothing, tampons, sanitary napkins, diaphragms, and condoms generally should be refrigerated until released to a law enforcement representative. An outline of the basic steps in collecting and documenting forensic evidence follows.[4,13,16] Further discussion of the yield of forensic evidence in the clinical setting is included later in this chapter.

Steps in Collecting and Documenting Forensic Evidence

The collection process should follow parameters established by the forensic laboratory processing the specimens and use an established, standardized protocol and evidence collection kit. The procedure for collection should be explained to the child or adolescent and their caregivers, and appropriate consents should be obtained. The examiner should ensure a chain of custody. All steps should be documented as "performed" or "not performed," and each individual sample should be appropriately packaged, labeled, and sealed. All individual samples should be placed in a sealed container (ie, forensic evidence kit) except for toxicology and medical specimens for infections that are processed separately from the forensic evidence kit. The steps for evidence collection should consist of the following:

— Collect clothing and foreign material dislodged while the victim is undressing.

— Collect debris from the victim's body (eg, dirt, leaves, fibers, hair) on a paper collection sheet.

— Collect foreign materials from the surface of the body.

— Collect hair combings (eg, pubic, head, facial) when appropriate.

— Collect hair reference samples as needed.

— Collect oral and genital swabs and smear.

— Conduct wet mount evaluation of motile sperm if indicated.

— Collect perianal and anal/rectal samples.

— Collect known reference sources of DNA.

— Collect toxicology samples from urine and blood as indicated.

— Collect medical specimens to identify STIs.

The initial step in evidence collection is the collection of foreign material dislodged while the victim is undressing. Many protocols recommend having the victim undress over a paper collection sheet to catch any foreign material that is dislodged. This material may contain fibers or other substances that can help corroborate where the assault occurred. Routine collection of all clothing is generally not indicated; however, clothing that is stained or damaged can provide important evidence. Torn clothing can be used to support the history of a forced sexual contact. Of particular importance is underwear worn during or subsequent to the assault, because it may contain seminal fluid from the assault.[13,16] Seminal fluid or other foreign materials might persist longer on clothing than on skin or mucosal surfaces. The importance of collecting clothing in prepubertal victims has been well-documented, but the utility of routine clothing collection in adolescents is less conclusive.[28,29,34,35]

Although collected external debris is more useful in corroborating the location of the assault, collected hairs have the potential to enable identification of the assailant.[4,13,37,38] Additional materials should be collected from the body surface as indicated by a history and examination prior to collecting oral, genital, and anal samples. The collection of fingernail evidence is recommended particularly if the victim describes scratching the assailant or if material is visible under the nails. Scraping under the nails with tools included in the kit or clipping of the nails may be used to obtain samples. Fingernail clipping or scraping is not useful in most situations involving young children; however, this process can be valuable when there is evidence of physical force or violence or the child gives a history of scratching the abuser. Foreign materials from the surface of the body might include DNA-containing materials. The highest yield would be expected from any areas with suspicious stains or that fluoresce under long-wave ultraviolet light or short-wave blue light.[4,39] If visible dried secretions are present, they can be gently scraped or "flaked off" or removed with a minimally moistened swab that is air-dried before packaging. When the victim's hair is matted with foreign substances, either "flaking off" the crusted material or cutting out sections of the encrusted hair can be done to collect this material. If bite marks are present, the surface of any bite marks should be swabbed. Swabbing the areas inside and around the arches of the bite mark, rather than from the tooth marks, maximizes the yield of DNA-containing material from sites where the lips and tongue of the biter would touch during the act of biting.[40,41] Tampons or sanitary pads in menstruating females may contain seminal fluid so they should be collected and air-dried completely if possible. If they cannot be dried completely, they may need to be handled as wet evidence requiring separate packaging and alerting law enforcement to its presence and the need for special handling.[16]

Pubic hair combings are typically collected if the assault involved the patient's genital area because of a significant rate of pubic hair transfer from the assailant.[37] Head and facial hair combings should also be considered, particularly if secretions, debris, or other foreign materials are seen on the hair.[16] Experts disagree on routinely collecting any hair reference samples,[13,16] but if they are collected, cut hairs should be adequate for comparison and do not require the pain associated with plucked or pulled hairs. In reality, hair cut or pulled from the victim has become less important in identification of the suspect because of the reliance on DNA technology with much higher specificity. Hair evidence may be important in cases in which no nuclear DNA evidence is found. Although there are some data to suggest an individual's hair characteristics can change over time, there is little scientific support for collecting reference samples from the victim because hair evidence is only important in cases in which hairs are found during forensic examination but no DNA evidence is found. If reference hairs are needed, they can be collected at a later time from the victim.[16]

External genital and perianal samples should be obtained before any internal samples are collected in order to prevent contamination. The female external genitalia should be swabbed initially with at least 1 dry swab then with a slightly moistened swab. Swabbing the surface of the penis with a slightly moistened swab is reasonable, but obtaining a urethral swab for evidential purposes is not warranted.[13] If dried secretions are present in the perianal area, they can be scraped or flaked off initially, then the area can be swabbed with a slightly moistened swab.

Protocols vary as to whether collection from all 3 sites (ie, oral, genital, rectal) is done routinely or collection is done from only sites involved according to the history or from all 3 sites when the history is unclear or uncertain.[16] The number of swabs collected from each site, the type of packaging used, whether smears are made on slides in addition to the swabs, and the time frames in which samples are collected vary between protocols. Part of this variation is dependent on the laboratory processing the samples, but protocols are subject to differing interpretation of scientific data, reliance on anecdotal experience, and opinion.

The yield of oral samples is maximized when samples are obtained by swabbing between the gums and cheek and under the tongue. Oral samples only rarely yield positive results more than a few hours after the assault, but early literature suggested occasional positive results were found up to 13 hours later.[43] Internal genital samples in young girls may be limited to samples obtained from the vaginal vestibule and vaginal canal or vaginal pool samples. In older adolescents, cervical swabs should be taken in addition to the vaginal pool sample because sperm persist for a longer time in the cervix than in the vaginal canal itself.[44] Some protocols include vaginal washes to collect sperm and DNA evidence, but because of concerns about diluted evidence and the proper handling of "wet evidence," these are not commonly used.[13,16] The yield of anal and rectal samples is maximized from victims reporting anal penetration within the last 24 hours.[13,45]

Some jurisdictions recommend wet mount microscopic examination of vaginal and cervical samples to look for motile and nonmotile sperm, because detection of motile sperm is limited. Sperm can cease movement within 30 minutes and rarely past 3 hours in vaginal specimens, but they may persist for up to 7 days in cervical specimens.[43] Therefore, finding motile sperm in vaginal specimens would be a strong indicator of recent assault, but cervical specimens would be more variable. Many protocols do not rely on examiners to do wet mount evaluations despite this being the only opportunity for such an evaluation, because the experience of the individual viewing the slide is related to the ability to detect motile sperm. Putting a drop of normal saline on the slide and rolling the swab into the drop is the appropriate method to prepare wet mounts. Wet mounts should not result in any loss of evidence. If a wet mount is done, both the slide and the swab should be air-dried and placed in the evidence kit.[16]

Known reference sources of DNA include blood and buccal swabs. Buccal swabs should be taken for reference samples after rinsing the mouth. If there has been no reported oral penetration, a buccal swab should be a reasonable reference source for DNA, and blood samples from the victim as a reference are not needed. If there has been recent oral penetration, a blood sample is a more appropriate known source for DNA, and it avoids a potentially contaminated buccal swab.[4,13,16,46]

Specimens for toxicology testing and testing for STIs are typically collected during the collection of the evidence kit but are submitted for testing separate from the testing for the evidence kit itself. For suspected drug-facilitated assaults, obtain urine samples if the assault occurred within 96 hours of the examination. Some protocols also recommend obtaining a blood sample if the assault occurred within the last 24 hours, but urine samples will have positive results if the blood test has positive results and may continue to be positive for a longer period of time. The collection and handling of medical specimens used to identify STIs should follow the medical facility's policy for such specimens. A more complete discussion of testing for drugs and STIs is included later in this chapter.

Alternate Light Source Illumination

Most forensic evidence protocols recommend an alternate light source (ALS) as an aid in identifying semen stains on skin or clothing.[4,5,9,13,16,39] The fluorescing stains can be swabbed for forensic analysis. Semen may exhibit white to yellowish green fluorescence under a Wood's light; however, Wood's light examinations have limitations resulting in frequent false negative and false positive test results.

False negative tests are common because the Wood's light has low sensitivity for semen. Santucci et al[47] reported the experience of a group of physicians using a Wood's light on known semen samples and other materials. None of the semen samples fluoresced, whereas a number of ointments fluoresced. In another study, Gabby et al[48] were able to document the fluorescence of known semen samples using an ultraviolet lamp, but they noted the transience of the fluorescence. The fluorescence of semen usually faded within 28 hours, yet semen was still detectable through the use of sensitive forensic DNA tests. Standard Wood's lights produce long ultraviolet light with wavelengths within the range of 320 nm to 400 nm. Maximal semen fluorescence is produced by visible blue light at wavelengths between 450 nm and 490 nm. Ultraviolet lamps with shorter wavelengths including those with old bulbs may not produce fluorescence. Selecting alternate light sources that produce light with wavelengths of 450 nm to 490 nm will maximize sensitivity and specificity.[39,48] The visibility of fluorescence is also increased by higher concentrations of the semen on the surface inspected and by reducing the distance of the light source from the surface. Visibility is not significantly affected by the angle of the light source with respect to the surface.[49]

False positive tests are common because many substances fluoresce better than semen. Products commonly found in the perineal area in children such as A & D Ointment, Surgilube, Barrier Cream, and bacitracin will fluoresce under the Wood's light.[47] Other skin creams, lubricants, soaps, and infant formulae have also been shown to fluoresce. Urine and semen may both fluoresce with a white to yellowish green color, and urine fluorescence persists for considerably longer.[48] Recognizing these limitations, especially false negatives misdirecting evidence collection, alternate light sources may be of some help in identifying suspect areas for more definitive testing.[39,48,49]

Alternate light source illumination is typically provided by a high-intensity, tunable light source. These lighting systems typically include a number of narrow bands of light including visible blue light, and some include infrared light with wavelengths of greater than 700 nm. In addition to providing maximal fluorescence of semen, visible blue light may enhance the cutaneous and subcutaneous tissue changes associated with skin injury. Photographs of injured skin taken with narrow-band blue light may capture more clearly delineated and defined patterns of injury than those taken with broad-band white light. This process may aid in determining the specific object that produced the injury and also in recognizing subclinical injury.[50] Others have suggested the use of alternate light sources on the skin, despite its limited value, but its greatest value is in detection of foreign substances including semen on clothing.[51]

Recommended Testing for Sexually Transmitted Infections and Pregnancy

Routine STI testing of pubertal adolescents and adults who are suspected of being sexually abused should be considered.[2,3,6,7,15,52-55] Appropriate testing includes approved nucleic acid amplification tests (NAATs) or culture for *Chlamydia trachomatis* and *Neisseria gonorrhoeae* from all sites of penetration or attempted penetration, including oral and anal sites. NAATs have the benefit of having a higher sensitivity or a higher positive test rate than cultures at all sites and are the recommended test choice for adolescents including testing at extragenital sites (eg, throat and rectum).[53] Urine and vaginal NAATs can also be used in prepubertal girls. Although culture is still recommended for use in prepubertal boys and for extragenital sites in both prepubertal girls and boys, cultures are less sensitive and may no longer be available for clinical use in many hospitals.[54] NAATs or culture of vaginal specimens for *Trichomonas vaginalis* are recommended, and if vaginal discharge or odor is present, a wet mount or NAAT for bacterial vaginosis (BV) and vaginal candidiasis should be considered. A blood sample should be obtained for serologic testing for syphilis, human immunodeficiency virus (HIV), and hepatitis B and C. Routine testing for herpes virus is not recommended. Repeat testing should be considered at a 1-week to 2-week follow-up for *C. trachomatis*, *N. gonorrhoeae*, and *T. vaginalis*. Repeat serologic testing for syphilis is recommended 4 to 6 weeks, 3 months, and 6 months later.[56] Repeat testing for HIV is recommended 4 to 6 weeks and 3 months later, with repeat testing at 6 months indicated only in the event of a positive test for hepatitis C, due to delayed seroconversion.[56]

Sexually active adolescents and adults have a high baseline prevalence of STI; therefore, post-assault STI testing may enable the identification of a previously acquired STI, incubating STI infection from the assault, or pathogens (viable or nonviable) in the ejaculate itself.[2,53] Adolescents who deny prior sexual activity should be approached in the same manner as younger children in terms of routine screening for STIs, considering the significance of STI on an individual with no prior exposure to STIs, except for the sexual assault itself. The high prevalence of preexisting STIs among adults and adolescents significantly limits the forensic value of the identification of an STI in a victim. However, recent studies suggest the high prevalence of positive NAAT testing post-assault may reflect the presence of pathogens (viable or nonviable) in perpetrator secretions rather than infection in the victim.[57] Some authorities do not recommend routine testing of adolescents and adults who have been victimized who routinely receive prophylactic antibiotics because of the limited forensic value as well as concerns that information about previously acquired STIs may undermine the credibility of the victim.[2,4,13,16,57] Other authorities argue that not obtaining appropriate screening tests for STIs undermines the public health role of assessing or treating sexual contacts for infection while ignoring the fact that identification and treatment of STI among adolescent and adult assault victims is more important from a medical and psychological viewpoint rather than an evidentiary perspective.[6,7,14,52,53,57] However, prophylactic antibiotics should be offered to all adolescent victims, regardless of whether or not STI testing has been performed.

Routine STI testing of all young or prepubertal children who are suspected of being sexually abused or assaulted is not recommended. The decision to test for STIs should be made on an individual basis, weighing the risk of infection against the additional discomfort of obtaining specimens from a young child. A parent's or child's request for testing and living in a high-prevalence region for STI should be considered; otherwise, criteria for screening for STIs include a number of historical and physical parameters associated with increased risk of infection. Historical criteria include assault by multiple perpetrators, history of genital discharge, a sibling or other child in the household with a known STI, or a perpetrator with a known STI or a high risk for STIs. Testing for STIs is generally recommended if there is a reasonable disclosure by the child of genital-genital, genital-anal, or genital-oral contact. Physical criteria include the presence of genital injury, genital discharge, or genital lesions suggestive of STI[1,3,53]; it is important to remember that prepubertal children may also be asymptomatic.

The CDC recommends that selected, high-risk children who were sexually abused be tested for *C. trachomatis*, *N. gonorrhoeae*, syphilis, HIV, and hepatitis B and C. The preferred method for screening is by using the most specific tests available—either NAATs or cultures for *C. trachomatis* and *N. gonorrhoeae*. If NAATs are used, confirmatory testing should be done using either a second NAAT that targets a different genomic sequence from that used in the first NAAT or a culture before initiating treatment. In girls, vaginal secretions should be evaluated for *T. vaginalis* and BV. Children should be assessed for warts and lesions, and any ulcers or vesicles should be tested for herpes by polymerase chain reaction (PCR) or culture. Follow-up testing should be considered at a 2-week follow-up for gonococcal, chlamydial, and trichomonal infection. Repeat serologic testing for syphilis, hepatitis B and C, and HIV is recommended 4 to 6 weeks, 3 months, and 6 months later, although repeat testing for HIV at 6 months is only recommended in the event of a positive test for hepatitis C.[1,2,52,53,56] When samples for STI testing are obtained at the time of the acute evaluation in children not receiving prophylactic antibiotics, follow-up testing for STIs is recommended to maximize the identification of infected children.

Several published studies have documented the utility of NAATs at extragenital sites. A recent study by Kellogg et al[57] supports the testing using NAATs for gonorrhea and chlamydial infections at both genital and extragenital sites in children and adolescents presenting with sexual assault complaints. Only 2.4% of children younger than age 12 years had positive tests, and 16% of adolescents had positive tests. Most of the child and adolescent patients with positive tests from oral or anal sites did not provide a history of genital contact or genital penetration of that site. Of the 13 prepubertal children with positive tests, 7 (54%) were collected at sites where there was no reported sexual contact. Relying on patient symptoms, reported types of sexual contact, or selection criteria to determine need for testing may miss gonorrhea and chlamydial infections in these children. This study questions the recommended selective approach to testing for STIs in prepubertal children in particular. Although none of the commercially available NAATs are currently approved by the Food and Drug Administration (FDA) for use on extragenital sites, laboratories who establish specifications for performance characteristics in accordance with CLIA regulations can use the test results for patient management.[55,57] As a practical matter, the reader should bear in mind that many regions and, in some cases, entire states do not have access to laboratories performing cultures for STIs. Clinicians performing evaluations may have to choose the use of NAATs in non–FDA-approved roles or choose not to test for STIs at all.

Drug-Facilitated Sexual Assault

At least 20 drugs have been used to facilitate nonconsensual sexual activity and drug-facilitated sexual assault, with alcohol being the most commonly used drug. More than 40% of both adolescents who were victimized and adolescents who were assailants have reported drug or alcohol use immediately prior to sexual assault.[2] Of samples obtained from adults and adolescents who were victims of suspected drug-associated sexual assault, 46% to 67% of the samples tested positive for alcohol.[58,59] In addition to alcohol, common "recreational drugs" have been implicated in sexual assault including marijuana, benzodiazepines, cocaine, opiates, barbiturates, and amphetamines.[58,59,60,61] The typical urine toxicology screens can enable detection of recent use of most of these "recreational drugs," but confirmatory testing is recommended.[2]

Two drugs have been popularized and studied as so-called "date rape drugs," despite being documented less frequently in sexual assault than alcohol and other "recreational drugs." These 2 particular date rape drugs, flunitrazepam (Rohypnol) and gamma hydroxybutyric acid (GHB), have been used by assailants to take advantage of the amnesia and confusion they produce in victims. Alcohol potentiates their effects and often accompanies their ingestion in sexual assault cases. Rohypnol is a benzodiazepine that is colorless, odorless, and tasteless. Although it is neither manufactured nor legally sold in the United States, it is marketed by Roche Pharmaceuticals internationally, mainly in Europe and Latin America, as a hypnotic sedative for the treatment of sleep disorders, to promote musculoskeletal relaxation, and for use as a preanesthetic or agent for conscious sedation. The drug GHB is known as a behavioral depressant and hypnotic and was previously marketed in a number of health food products, with most of the currently circulating GHB being manufactured in "home-brew" laboratories with ingredients available from chemical supply houses and through recipes from the Internet.[62]

Rohypnol comes as small tablets that can be introduced into various drinks. The onset of action is within 30 minutes, with peak action at 1 hour to 2 hours after ingestion and a duration of 8 hours to 12 hours. The long half-life of 23 hours to 33 hours allows symptoms of fatigue, confusion, and inattention to persist for up to 2 days after acute ingestion. Other symptoms include drowsiness, confusion, inability to focus, memory impairment, amnesia, visual problems, urinary retention, and gastrointestinal problems. Periods of lucidity may be interspersed with confusion, and the individual may display excitability or aggressive behavior.[63] To reduce Rohypnol's use as a date rape drug, Rohypnol's manufacturer, Roche, introduced a new formulation in 1998 that dissolves very slowly in liquids and releases a blue dye. This new tablet has completely replaced the former rapidly dissolving, colorless formulation.

Usually distributed as a liquid, GHB is often mixed with strong-tasting beverages to cover up its salty taste. The onset of action is within minutes, with peak action at 20 minutes to 60 minutes. The half-life is 20 minutes to 60 minutes, and the duration of action is 4 hours to 5 hours. Most people experience nausea and vomiting, and other symptoms include visual disturbances, amnesia, and reduced inhibitions. Intense intoxication can be manifested in the victim, who appears as either a "happy drunk" or a "mean drunk."[62]

Blood test results may remain positive after Rohypnol ingestion for 5 to 7 hours and for 4 hours to 6 hours after GHB ingestion. Urine test results can remain positive for 36 hours for Rohypnol and for 12 hours for GHB. Only approximately 5% of GHB is excreted in urine. Despite low yields, urine should be collected for up to 72 hours in cases in which the ingestion of date rape drugs is suspected. Urine should be collected, refrigerated, and frozen as quickly as possible. Routine urine toxicologic tests are rarely positive for benzodiazepines with Rohypnol, and identification or confirmation can be obtained by using gas chromatography or mass spectrometry.[63]

Hindmarch et al[58] reported on the analysis of 3303 urine samples submitted from across the United States for testing because of suspicion of a drug-facilitated sexual assault. The majority of the samples were positive (61.3%) for one or more substances. More than a third of all positive samples contained multiple substances. Of the positive results, alcohol was most common (67%), marijuana was the second most prevalent drug (30.3%), and benzodiazepines were the third most common (24.8%), followed by cocaine (13.8%), amphetamines (10.8%), and opiates (4.3%). In only 4.9% of the samples was GHB present, and Rohypnol was found in only 0.5%.[58] Scott-Ham and Burton[59] studied 1014 cases of sexual assault thought to have been drug-facilitated. Alcohol was found in 46% of the cases, and 34% had taken illicit drugs, primarily marijuana or cocaine. In 2% of the cases there was clinically apparent, but hidden and deliberate, spiking of drinks with a sedative or other disinhibiting drug, and 1% reported being forced to drink liquids spiked with these drugs.[59] The data from these and other studies[60,61] lend support that there is widespread use of alcohol, marijuana, and several illicit drugs, but it does not confirm the widespread use of GHB or Rohypnol to secretly spike drinks in drug-facilitated sexual assault.

Drugs used to facilitate sexual assaults can be difficult to detect because of relatively small doses and rapid clearance from the body. Urine samples are the primary source for detecting the drugs; however, a delay in obtaining urine samples can create negative test results. A positive blood or urine test result indicates a drug's recent use, which makes it easier to associate the presence of the drug with the timing of the sexual assault.[2,58,59]

Findings and Interpretation

Physical Injury Interpretation

Nongenital injury might be the best proof of force. The location and pattern of the injuries can be used to support both the inflicted cause and the victim's description of the violence. Nongenital injuries should preferably be photographed, or described in drawings, and documented in the medical record.[13] The color of bruises should be noted, but care must be taken in interpreting the timing of injuries because injury healing and color changes in bruises take place at variable rates.[11,20] Genital injury can be used to illustrate recent sexual contact and the use of force.

Non-anogenital Trauma

Non-anogenital injury can take many forms, and the absence of non-anogenital injury does not prove consensual sexual activity. Common injuries include facial bruises, abrasions, and lacerations occasionally accompanied by tympanic membrane ruptures (**Figures 4-1** and **4-2**). Intraoral lesions resulting from penetration or attempts to prevent screaming may be seen (**Figures 4-3** and **4-4**). Neck bruising can occur with choking, biting, or sucking (**Figures 4-5** through **4-8**). Common upper extremity injuries include bruising of the lateral upper arm from grasping or punches and defensive bruises of the forearms (**Figures 4-9** through **4-11**). Punching, kicking, and grasping the lateral thighs cause common lower extremity injuries (**Figures 4-12** and **4-13**). Other common injuries include whip-like or cordlike bruises, punch bruising on the abdomen, and bruising and bite marks on the breasts (**Figures 4-14** through **4-19**).[13,65-68]

Multiple studies have revealed that the rate of non-anogenital injury in adolescents and adults who were victims of sexual assault ranges from 33% to 67%.[65-70] Rates of non-anogenital injury tended to be higher in adults who were victims (55%) than in adolescents who were victims (33%)[69]; likewise, when strangers committed the assaults, injury rates to victims were higher (61%) than when the assaults were committed by known persons (40%).[66] One explanation for these findings is that assaults involving adults who were victimized and strangers who were assailants are more violent than assaults involving ado-

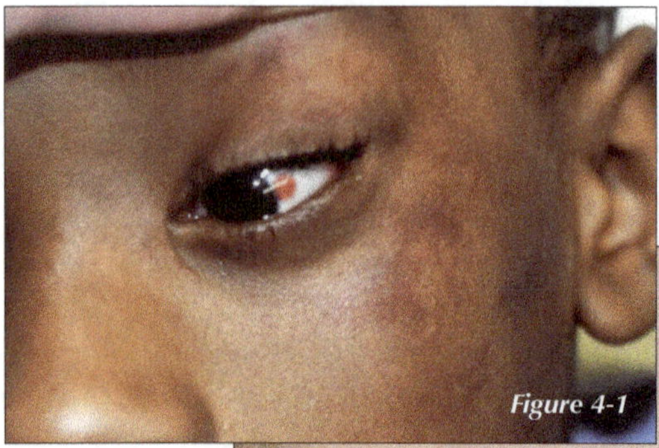

Figure 4-1. *10-year-old boy who was forced to perform oral sex on three teenagers. He was threatened, and when he refused he was slapped and punched on his face and chest. Notice the irregular bruising of his cheek and upper eyelid and a subconjunctival hemorrhage.*

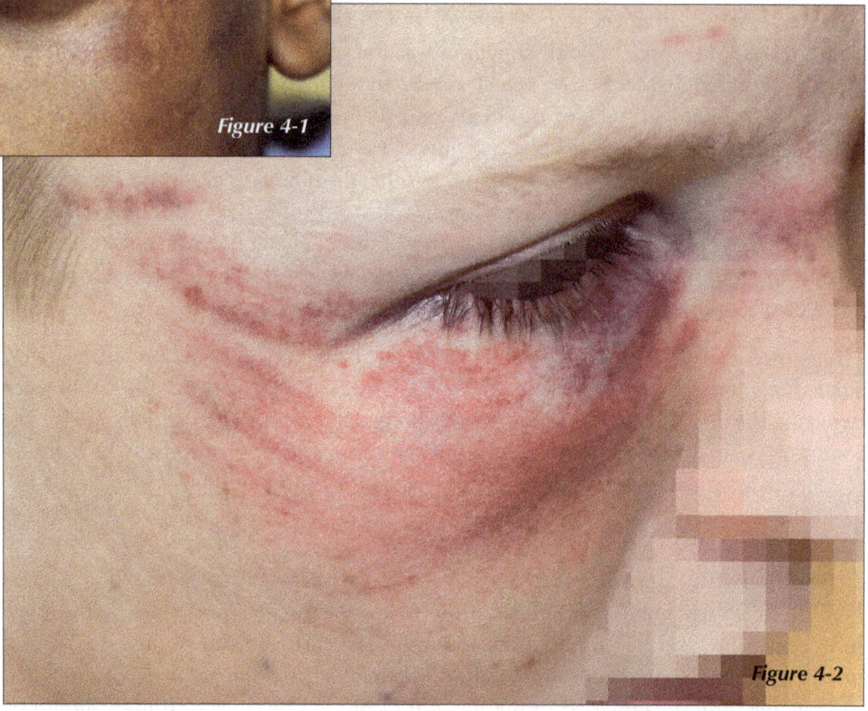

Figure 4-2. *12-year-old boy who described being struck over the side of his face with "something" by a teenager who ordered him to perform oral sex. The teenager was wearing gloves at the time. Photograph shows an abraded bruise across the boy's nasal bridge, across his lower eyelid, and extending towards the temporal area.*

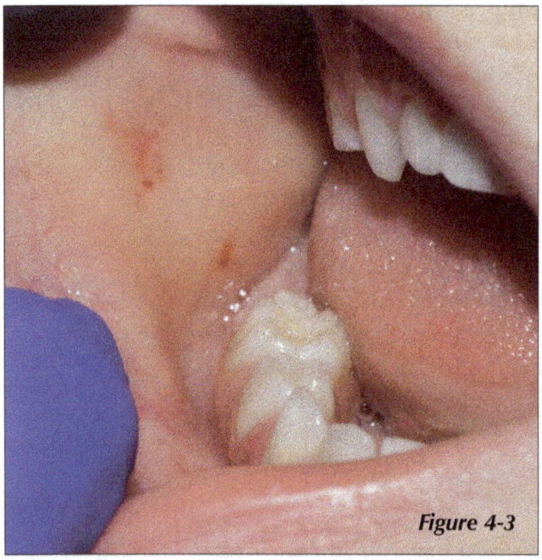

Figure 4-3. *6-year-old girl who described an older boy rubbing his hand in her genital area. She said she began to scream. Photograph shows mucosal abrasions from her teeth, caused by the boy grabbing her mouth to silence her.*

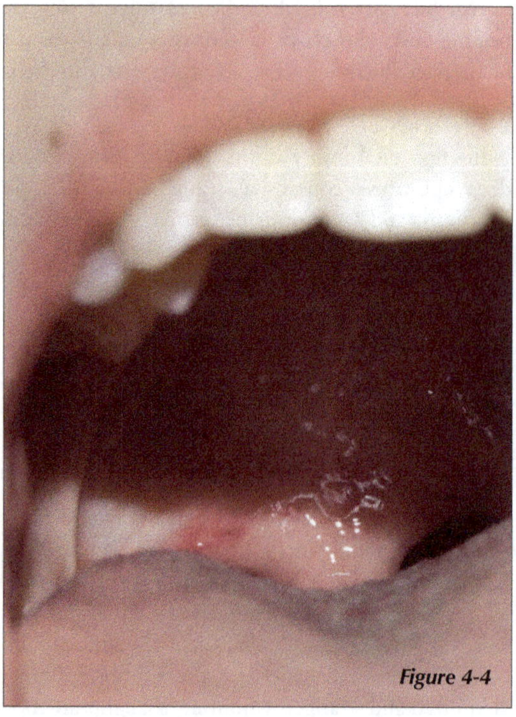

Figure 4-4. *17-year-old girl who described forced oral penetration by an unknown male. Note the bruising of her palate.*

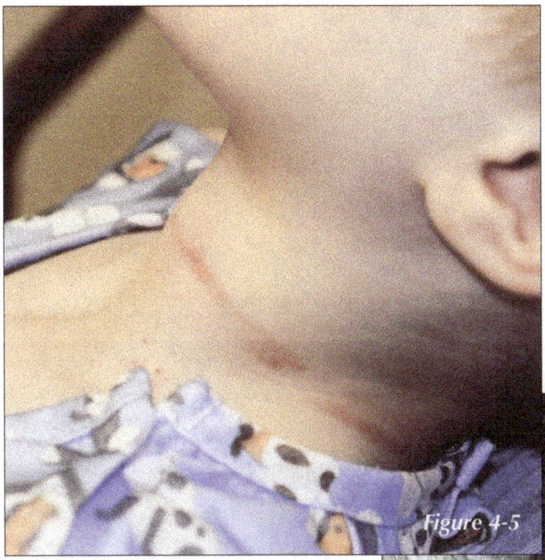
Figure 4-5

Figure 4-5. *9-year-old boy who described a teenaged boy putting a "rope" around his neck, then penetrating him anally. Photograph shows a ligature mark around his neck. An anal laceration was found as well.*

Figure 4-6. *13-year-old girl who disclosed an older teenage boy forced her to undress, then grabbed her by the neck as he penetrated her vaginally from behind. The photograph shows linear bruising over her neck that was in a similar pattern on both sides. She also had a laceration of her posterior fourchette.*

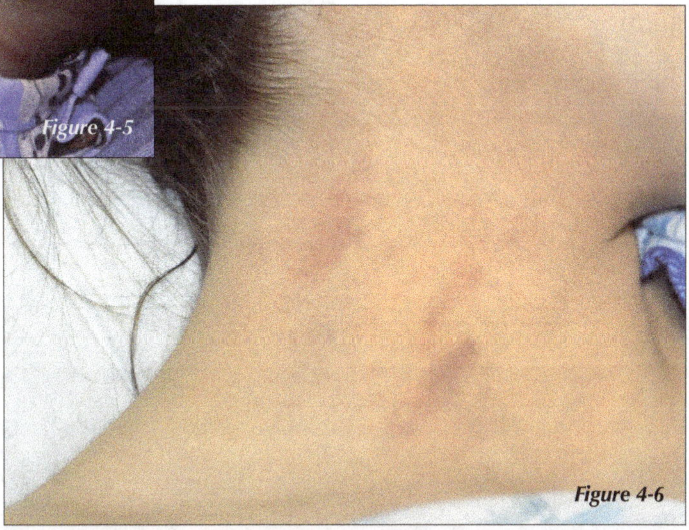
Figure 4-6

Figure 4-7. *Neck bruising present on adolescent victim of sexual assault. Photo contributed by Arne K. Myhre, MD.*

Figure 4-8. *16-year-old girl who was at a party and woke up partially clothed with genital bleeding. She had been drinking and did not know what happened. Note the suction bruise on her neck. She also had a posterior fourchette abrasion.*

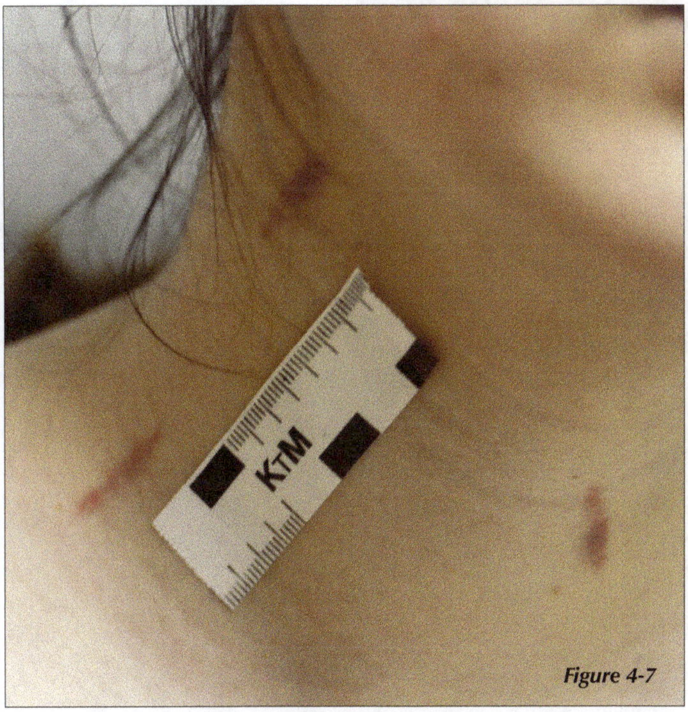

Figure 4-7

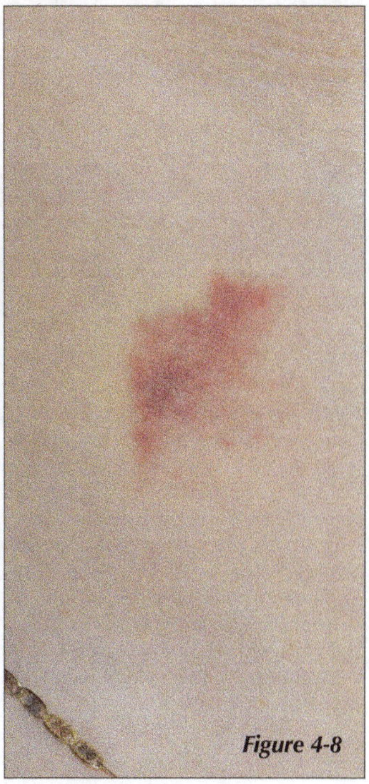
Figure 4-8

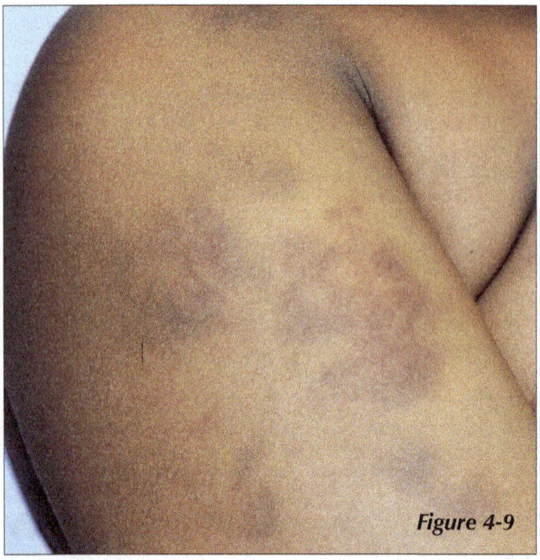

Figure 4-9. *7-year-old boy who was forced to perform oral sex on a teenage boy. The boy said he was punched multiple times until he met the teenager's demands. Photograph shows bruising of his upper arm, one of the places he was punched.*

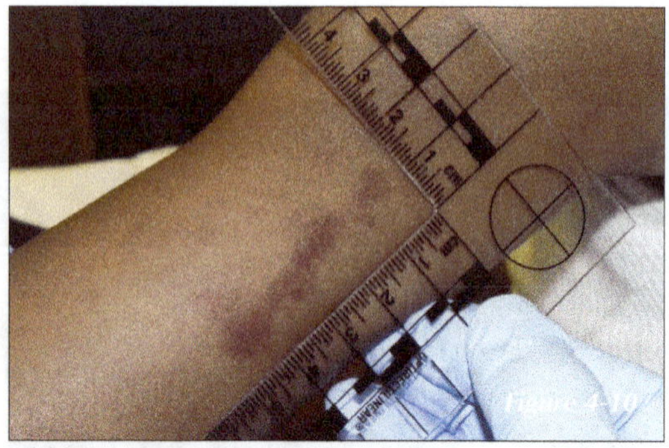

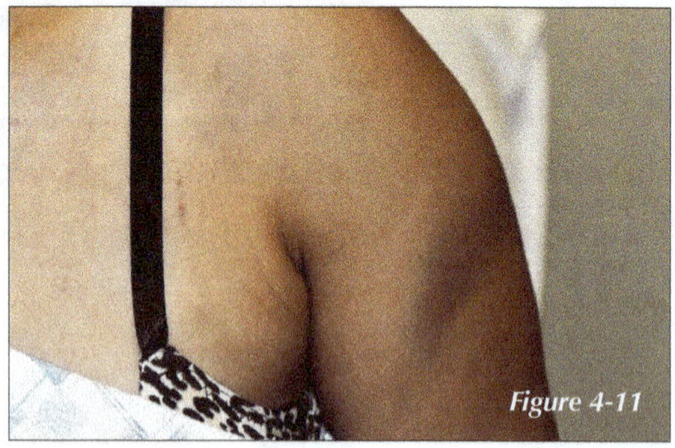

Figure 4-10. *Photograph shows a 17-year-old girl who said she was "hanging out" with an acquaintance when he grabbed her by her arms and vaginally penetrated her. Note the grasp mark bruise of her upper arm. A similar mark was seen on her other upper arm.*

Figure 4-11. *A 16-year-old girl who said an unknown male threw her to the ground, kicked her several times, then raped her. Photograph shows a bruise where he kicked her in her upper arm.*

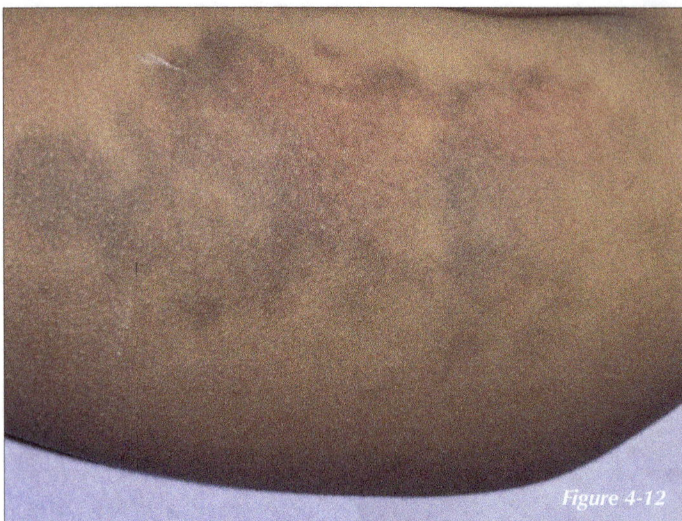

Figure 4-12. *Same girl in Figure 4-11. Photograph shows where he kicked her in her thigh.*

Figure 4-13. *9-year-old girl who disclosed her older cousin tried to put his penis in her vagina. The photograph shows a bruise on her inner thigh where she said he grabbed her to force her legs apart. She had similar bruising on her other thigh, as well as an abrasion in her fossa navicularis.*

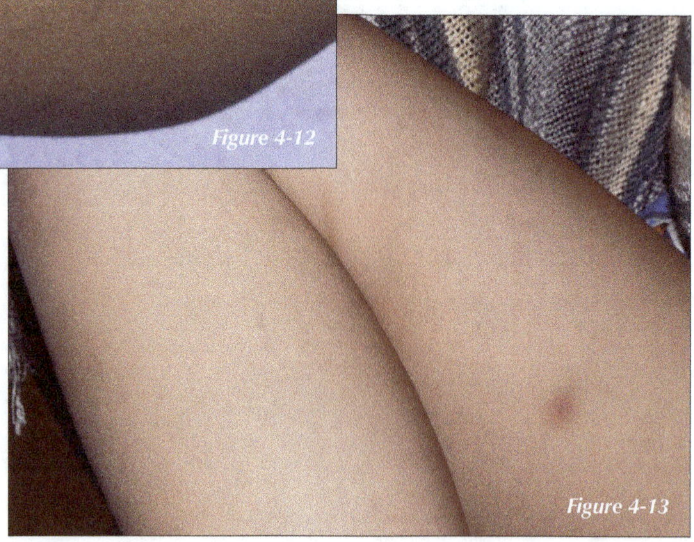

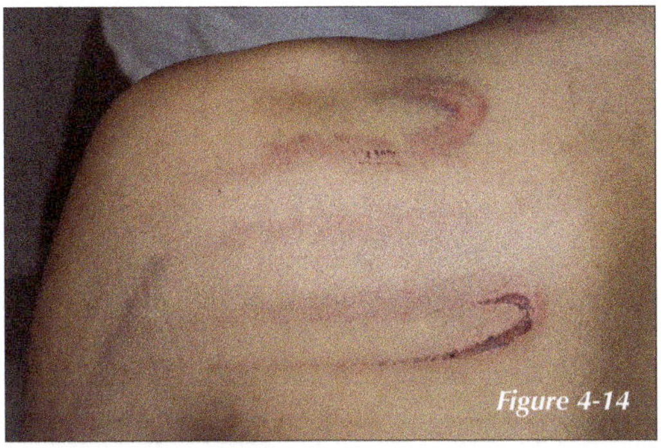

Figure 4-14

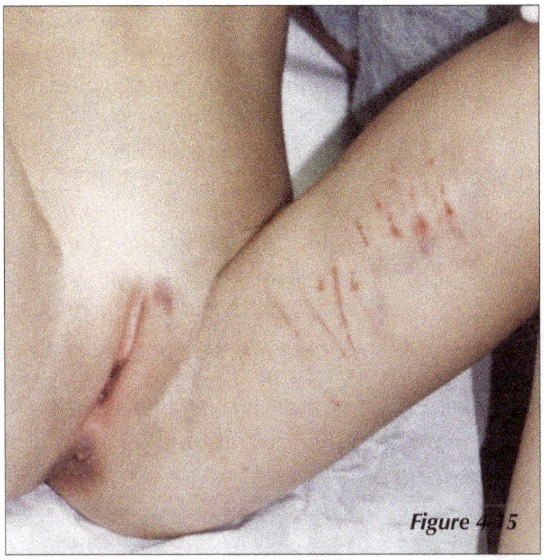

Figure 4-15

Figure 4-14. *A 15-year-old girl who described being vaginally raped by a teenage acquaintance while she was at his home. She said he asked her to have sex with him, but when she refused, he hit her multiple times with an electric cord until she acquiesced. Photograph shows several of the loop-like bruises and linear abrasions found on her back and upper arms.*

Figure 4-15. *A 6-year-old child abuse physically and sexually by her father. Child is examined the supine position. Note laceration on inner left thigh from a switch and bruise on the pelvis. There were also findings on sexual abuse, both acute and chronic, not seen in this photo. Photo contributed by Mary J. Spencer, BA, MD, FAAP.*

Figure 4-16. *An 11-year-old girl who reported being restrained by one male while another attempted to penetrate her vaginally. She said she tried to get away and one male kicked her in the abdomen. The photograph shows an abraded bruise of her lateral abdomen.*

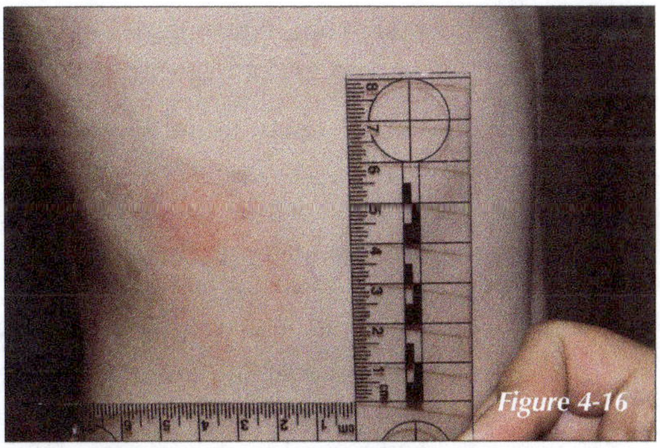

Figure 4-16

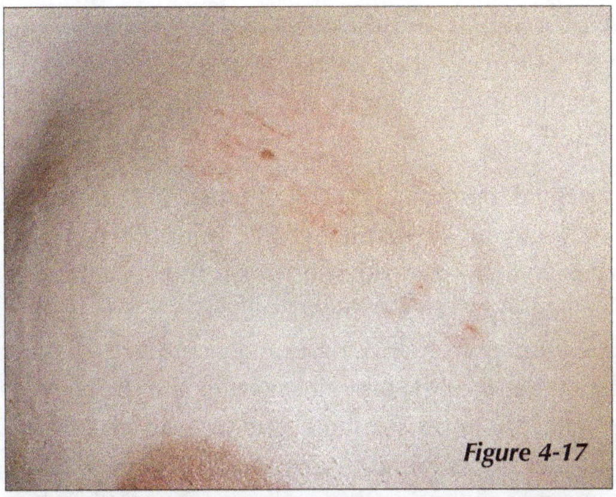

Figure 4-17

Figure 4-17. *15-year-old girl reported she had been "drinking with friends" and a teenage male she did not know forced her "to have sex." She said he bit her breast. Photograph shows faint bruising of her upper left breast with two arc shaped abrasions, consistent with superficial bite marks.*

Figure 4-18. *A 14-year-old girl who described her uncle sucking on her breast as he vaginally penetrated her. Notice the focal bruise of her right breast.*

Figure 4-19. *15-year-old girl who reported she was dragged into an alley by an unknown male and vaginally penetrated. She said he punched her several times, including in the chest. The photograph shows bruising of the lateral portion of her breast.*

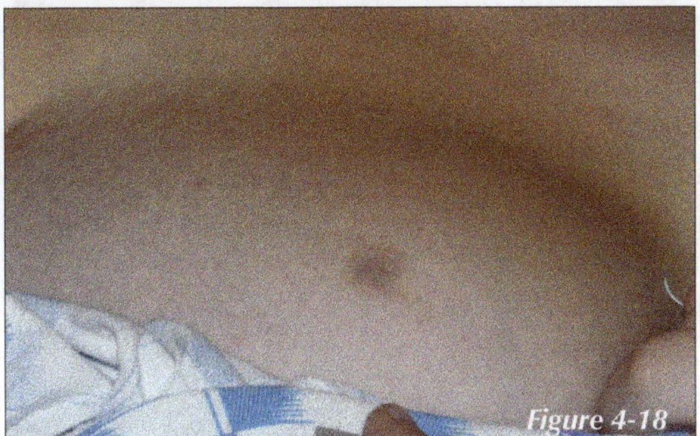

Figure 4-18

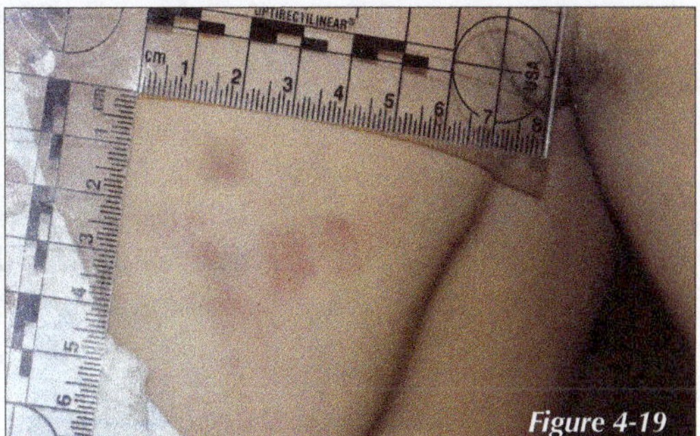

Figure 4-19

lescents who are victimized and when known persons committed the assaults. Another study found an increased rate of non-anogenital injury in assaults by strangers, when the assault did not include use of drugs or alcohol and when the victim could not remember the details of the assault.[70] The rates of anogenital injuries were higher than the rates of non-anogenital injuries in the studies reporting both types of trauma.[65-67,69,70]

Genital Trauma

Multiple studies have reported that the rate of anogenital injury in adolescent and adult sexual assault victims ranges from 12% to 83%.[22,65-81] A comparison of rates of anogenital trauma between adolescents and adults who were victims has been inconclusive. Some studies report higher rates of anogenital injury in adolescents,[69,70,71] whereas others report higher injury rates in adults.[66,72] Strickland[72] compared genital findings among adolescents and adults who were victimized. Genital trauma was found in 37% of the adults but in only 12% of the adolescents. A possible explanation was proposed: that adolescent assault may be less violent because they more frequently know their assailant (65% versus 35%). However, Jones et al[66] reported similar rates of anogenital trauma in sexual assault by strangers (77%) and by known assailants (71%). The study by Feeney et al[70] reported non–stranger-perpetrated sexual assaults were associated with more anogenital injuries in adolescents. In an earlier study, Jones et al[69] reported that adolescents had a greater frequency of anogenital injuries than adults (83% versus 64%).

Hilden et al[71] found higher rates of injury among virgins, people aged 12 years to 19 years, and those victims reporting anal penetration. Sugar et al[68] studied 819 victims of acute sexual assault who were 15 years and older and found anogenital injury was more frequent in virgins, victims younger than 20 years, victims older than 49 years, in those examined within 24 hours, and in those experiencing anal assault. Overall, 20% had anogenital injuries.[68] In support of these studies, White and McLean[73] reviewed the injury pattern found during examination of adolescent females who were virgins and nonvirgins and who had experienced acute assault. In this study, only 31% of 81 virgins had genital injury, whereas 53% of 81 nonvirgins had genital injury.[73] Zilkens et al[81] reported the genital injury rate was significantly higher in virgins when compared to nonvirgins (52.2% and 19.5% respectively).

The study by Jones et al[69] revealed anogenital injuries in 83% of 329 cases of acute sexual assault in adolescents. These researchers also noted that anogenital injuries were most frequently located at the fossa navicularis, hymen, posterior fourchette, and labia minora. Zilkens et al[81] reported that 79% of genital injury in victims were located in the same 4 sites. Adams et al[22] reviewed the medical findings from investigation of acute sexual assault of 214 adolescents and found a correlation between the time since assault and the physical findings. Only 21% had no findings, and the most common finding was tears of the posterior fourchette or fossa (40%). Erythema was found in 32%, and hymenal swelling was seen in 19%. Hymenal tears were more common in self-described virgins (19%) than in nonvirgins (3%), but other injuries were similar in type and location in both groups.[22]

Digital-vaginal penetration can also produce injury, although redness or erythema is the most common finding. Rossman et al[69] reviewed genital findings in 53 females reporting only digital-vaginal penetration. In this study, 81% had genital injuries, with 34% having only erythema; superficial tears were seen in 29% and abrasions in 21%. Lincoln et al[77] reported that a vaginal penetration scenario that included digital penetration was 4.2 times more likely to result in at least one genital injury than penetration without any finger involvement.

Consensual Sex

Several studies describe a low rate of genital injury, ranging from 9.9% to 17.8%, from consensual sexual activity; moreover, these studies describe lower injury rates with consensual sex than with sexual assault.[75,76,77] Slaughter et al[76] compared injuries in 311 rape victims with those of 75 females reporting consensual sex. Nongenital trauma was found in 57% of the rape victims. Of the rape victims, 68% had anogenital trauma, usually occurring in multiple sites, and 11% of those reporting consensual sex had genital trauma involving only a single site. The most common sites of injury in the rape victims were the posterior fourchette (70%), labia minora (53%), hymen (29%), and the fossa navicularis (25%). Lincoln et al[77] compared genital injuries in adults resulting from consensual sex and nonconsensual sex. The rate of genital injury was higher in the nonconsensual group (53.7%) than in the consensual group (9.9%). Fraser et al[75] studied 107 sexually active, otherwise healthy adult women over a 6-month period. The following changes, in order of frequency, were found in 56 of 314 (17.8%) colposcopic examinations: petechiae, erythema, abrasions, and edema. These changes were most frequently seen when examinations were done within 24 hours of intercourse or tampon use.[75] Jones et al[78] compared injuries for adolescents reporting acute sexual assault with injuries for those reporting consensual sex. The researchers in this case used toluidine blue dye to enhance the findings. Both groups had a similarly high rate of injury overall, with posterior fourchette lacerations being the most frequently seen injury in both groups. The injury rate was 85% in the group reporting nonconsensual sex and 73% in the group reporting consensual sex. Therefore, some literature suggests that the pattern of genital injury may be different in females experiencing sexual assault than in those who took part in consensual sexual activity.[75,76,78] However, Sommers et al[25] concluded in their 2005 study that "we cannot differentiate injuries that occur as the result of consent versus non-consent on the basis of visual inspection, toluidine blue dye, or colposcopy."

Anal Trauma

Anal trauma is less frequent among female sexual assault victims than are genital injuries, but this may be due to anal assault being less frequent. Slaughter et al[76] reported that 55 of 311 (17.7%) rape victims indicated anal contact and that 31 of the 55 (56.4%) examined through colposcopy had evidence of anal trauma. Zilkens et al[81] noted the 1266 women they studied reported genital assault approximately 3 times more often than anal assault. They found the genital injury rate in completed vaginal penetration was 24.5% and in attempted vaginal penetration was 15% while the anal injury rate in the completed anal penetration was 27% and in the attempted anal penetration was 9%. In their study of acute sexual assault of adolescents, Adams et al[22] found that 61% of the 214 adolescents reporting anal penetration had anal injuries. Sachs and Chu[79] reported on anal findings from a retrospective review of 548 cases. Although forced anal penetration was less frequent than vaginal rape, there was an increased severity of injury, including anal and rectal tears. Ernst et al[80] reported on anal injuries in 67 males who were sexually assaulted; on gross examination of these victims, 63% were found to have evidence of anal injury. In the study by Ernst et al,[80] the use of anoscopy and colposcopy increased the yield of cases with positive findings to 72%. There are no data comparing the prevalence of anal injury in consensual anal penetration with that in nonconsensual anal penetration.[80]

Bite Marks

Typical human bite marks are circular- or oval-patterned indentations or injuries composed of 2 opposing U-shaped arches separated by open spaces at their bases. Along the edge of the arches one frequently finds a series of small interrupted abrasions, contusions, or lacerations representing injury corresponding to individual teeth. Central bruising might be present between the arches and is caused by crush injury from jaw closure, by sucking, or by tongue-thrusting. Multiple overlapping bite marks and partial bite marks and occasional avulsive bite marks may also occur.[4,40,82]

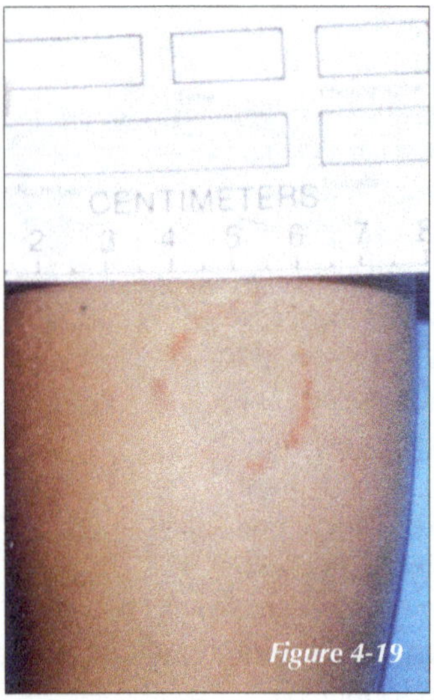

Figure 4-20.
A 5-year-old with a bite from a child on the arm. Photo contributed by Mary J. Spencer, BA, MD, FAAP.

Bite marks by adults can often be differentiated from bite marks by children based on size. The intercanine distance in adults ranges from 2.5 cm to 4.0 cm, and in children, this distance is less than 3.0 cm (**Figure 4-20**). Therefore, a bite mark with an intercanine distance of greater than 3.0 cm is strongly suggestive of an adult bite mark. Animal bite marks tend to be deeper and narrower, and the mechanism of the bite is more ripping or tearing in nature (known as ***avulsive***) than the crushing mechanism of a human bite.[40]

Bite mark identification techniques may help determine the source of bite marks on the victim's body. Bite marks are rarely present in child and adolescent sexual assault victims, and accurate sampling and analysis are difficult. High-quality photographs of bite marks can be helpful in identifying the perpetrator, and a forensic odontologist is the best resource for documenting bite mark evidence. When a forensic odontologist is not immediately available, a series of high-quality black-and-white and color photographs with assured color balance, showing overall orientation views and a series of close-ups can be interpreted at a later date. The photographs should be taken with and without a measuring scale; when a scale is used, it should be on the same plane as and adjacent to the bite mark. It should be included in the photographs, and the photographs should be taken at 90 degrees to each arch to prevent picture distortion due to the curvature of the skin.[4,40,82] However, as a result of multiple studies regarding the inconsistency of interpretation of bite marks by experts, the use of bite mark patterns for identification of specific individuals is discouraged.[41,83] Swabs from acute bite marks may contain saliva that can be analyzed for DNA, and unlike the bite mark pattern, this is very specific for identification purposes.[4,42]

Physical Injury in Prepubertal Children

There are limited data on the frequency of acute injuries in sexually abused prepubertal children. Most studies of sexually abused prepubertal girls combine data from acute and nonacute evaluations, and these studies indicate the rates of specific positive physical findings are less than 5%.[9,84] Heger et al[84] noted that many of the positive examinations were from acute assaults, but neither the percentage of acute assaults nor specific descriptions of the injuries were reported. Heppenstall-Heger et al[23] reported on the healing of acute anogenital injuries in prepubertal children. Of 6320 children evaluated, only 109 (1.7%) had acute injuries, but the percentage of the total evaluated for acute sexual assault was not reported.[23] The injuries occurred in both accidental and abusive cases, with 62 children providing a specific history of sexual abuse. Twenty-four children described penile-vaginal penetration, 19 described digital-vaginal penetration, and 19 described anal penetration. More than half of the anal injuries were anal lacerations and tears; the remainder were hematomas and abrasions. There were also 9 anal injuries found in girls who reported only penile-vaginal penetration. Of the 24 girls reporting penile-vaginal penetration, many had concurrent injuries in more than 1 site: posterior fourchette (18; 14 tears), hymen (17; 12 complete tears and 2 partial tears), perihymenal area (7), and labia minora (2). Of the 19 girls reporting digital-vaginal penetration, many had injuries in more than 1 site: posterior fourchette (6; 4 tears), hymen (7; 4 partial tears), perihymenal area (13), and labia minora (3).[23] This study describes the types of acute injuries seen in prepubertal victims of sexual abuse, but it does not allow a determination of the frequency of injuries among prepubertal victims examined acutely. Campbell et al[85] examined 209 sexual assault victims younger than age 14 years and documented that 39% had anogenital injuries. They found only redness in 13%, hymenal injury in 15%, anal injury in 3%, abrasions in 17%, and tears or lacerations in 8%. They also noted that patients examined within 24 hours of the assault were more likely to have documented injuries. Gallion et al[86] reported on findings on children younger than age 18 years and found injuries were more common in older children and in children seen acutely. Neither study differentiated between injuries seen in younger and older children.[85,86]

Two of the 5 studies evaluating forensic evidence findings in prepubertal children describe acute injuries found during medical evaluations.[29,32] Christian et al[29] reported that 62 (22.7%) of the 273 children younger than 10 years of age in their study had anogenital injuries. After the exclusion of those with erythema (redness), 13.9% were found to have injuries that were more serious. One-fourth of the injuries involved the anal tissues, and half were almost equally distributed between the posterior fourchette, labia minora, and hymen. Of those children with injuries, 88% were examined within 24 hours of their assault.[29] Palusci et al[32] reported that 25 (13.2%) of the 190 children younger than 13 years of age in their study had anogenital injuries. More than two-thirds of the injuries were hymenal lacerations, abrasions, and bruises, and one-quarter of the injuries were anal lacerations and bruises. Of those children with injuries, 56% were examined within 24 hours of their assault.[32] Two additional studies reported acute injuries in 20.8% of children and adolescents, with greater than three-quarters of the injuries found in patients examined within 24 hours[28] and in 16.6% of children and adolescents,[35] but no additional descriptions of the injuries were included in either study. Prepubertal children evaluated for acute sexual abuse within the first 72 hours have a significant rate of acute injuries, although the majority will have no injuries and the frequency of injury is much lower than reported among adult and adolescent victims of acute sexual assault. Many acute injuries heal rapidly and completely,[23,87,88] suggesting that the lower rates of injuries in nonacute evaluations is in part due to the delay of more than 72 hours in seeking medical evaluation. Immediate medical examination of prepubertal children within 72 hours of a suspected sexual abuse is appropriate for detecting injury; however, the limited data on forensic evidence in prepubertal children has supported a more selective approach for forensic evidence kit collection.[28,29,32,34,35]

Examination Findings Indicative of Abuse

Most physical findings on anogenital examination of children and adolescents evaluated for suspected sexual abuse or assault are nonspecific.[1,3,9,71,87,88] Only a limited number of findings are caused only by trauma and/or sexual contact. Evidence of acute trauma to external genital and anal tissues includes acute laceration of the posterior fourchette or vestibule, not involving the hymen, and acute lacerations or bruising of the labia, penis, scrotum, perianal tissues, or perineum (**Figures 4-21** and **4-22**). During evaluation for acute sexual assault, additional findings may be discovered that represent residual or healing injuries from prior sexual contact or other anogenital trauma. Evidence of residual healing injury to the external genital and anal areas include scars of the posterior fourchette, fossa navicularis, or perianal tissue. These injuries can be the result of physical abuse, sexual abuse, consensual sexual activity in adolescents, or accidental trauma.[1]

Other injuries are indicative of acute or healed trauma to the genital and anal tissues. These injuries include bruising, petechiae, or abrasions of the hymen (**Figures 4-23** and **4-24**); vaginal laceration or tear; acute laceration or partial or complete tear of the hymen; (**Figures 4-25** and **4-26**); perianal laceration with exposure of tissues below the dermis (**Figure 4-27**); healed hymenal transection (**Figures 4-28** and **4-29**) or a complete cleft (a defect in the hymen between 4 o'clock and 8 o'clock that extends to the base of the hymen); and/or a defect in the posterior (inferior) half of the hymen wider than a transection with the absence of hymenal tissue extending to the base of the hymen (**Figure 4-30**).[1]

When hymenal bruising or petechiae is suspected, it is important to consider possible coagulopathy or infectious process, and it is important to reexamine the child within a few days or weeks to be certain the bruise-like area has resolved, which will allow differentiation of a bruise from a hemangioma or nevus, neither of which would resolve.

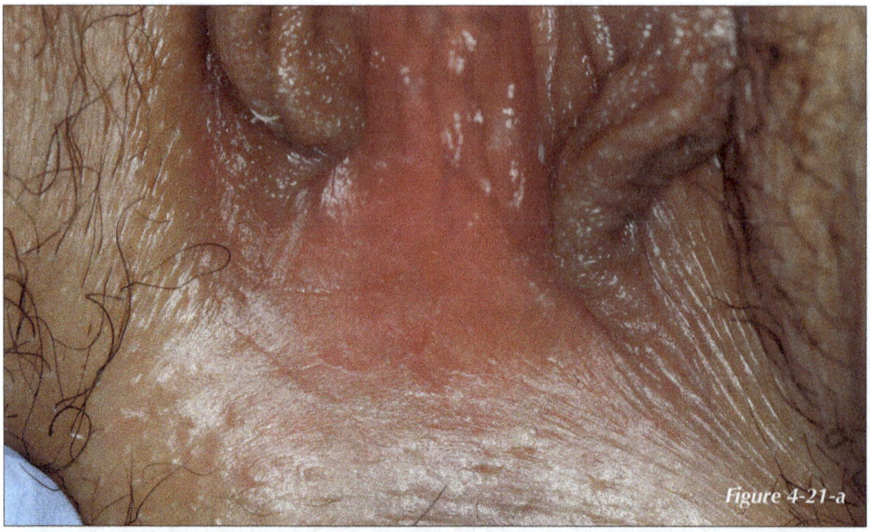

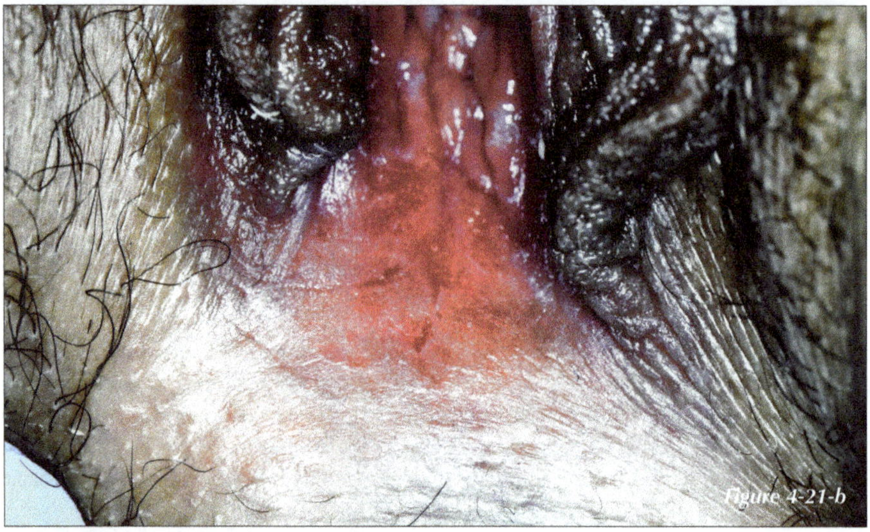

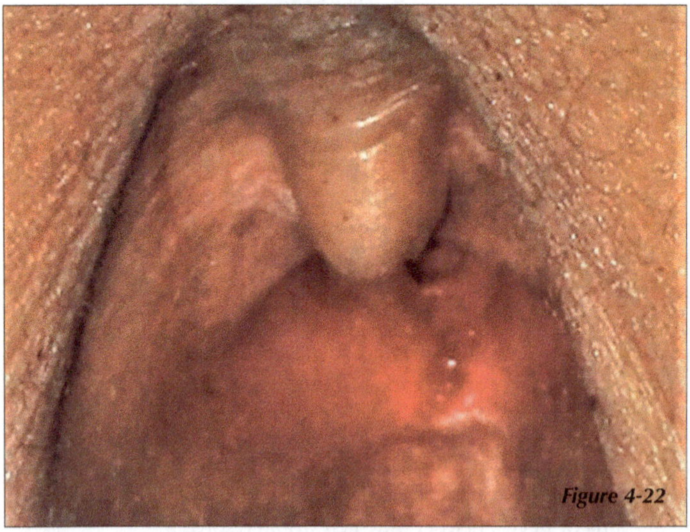

Figure 4-21-a. *A 14-year-old girl who reported being sexually assaulted by an adult male she met on the Internet. Notice the multiple lacerations to the posterior fourchette going up into the fossa navicular at 6 o'clock and 8 o'clock. Photo contributed by Diana Faugno, MSN, RN, CPN, SANE-A, SANE-P, FAAFS, DF-IAFN, DF-AFN.*

Figure 4-21-b. *Negative inverted filter of Figure 4-21-a. Injuries are easier to see. Photo contributed by Diana Faugno, MSN, RN, CPN, SANE-A, SANE-P, FAAFS, DF-IAFN, DF-AFN.*

Figure 4-22. *7-year-old girl who reported penile vaginal penetration by an 11-year-old step-brother early this morning. Photograph shows deep laceration in fossa navicularis.*

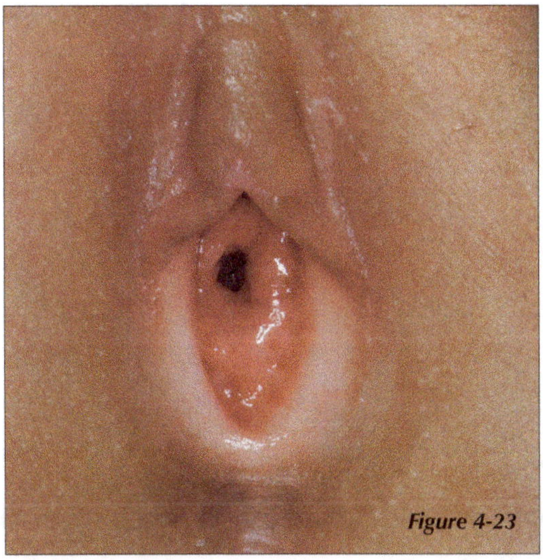
Figure 4-23

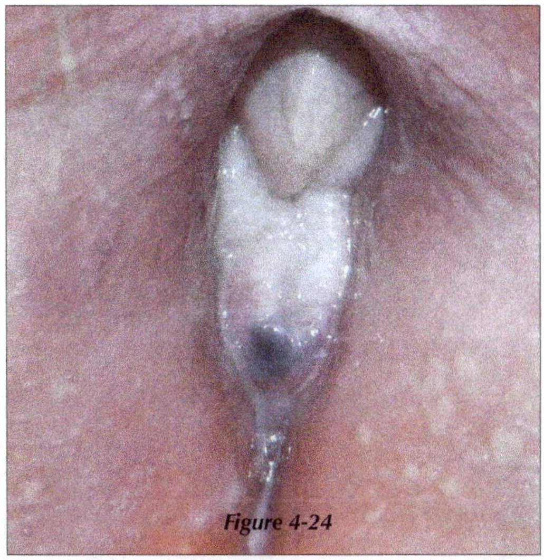
Figure 4-24

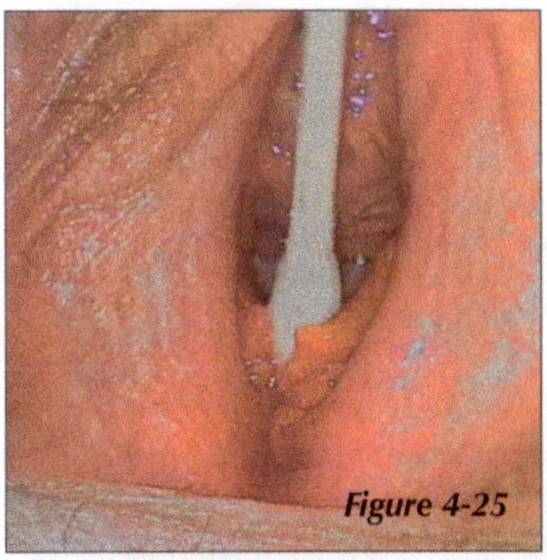
Figure 4-25

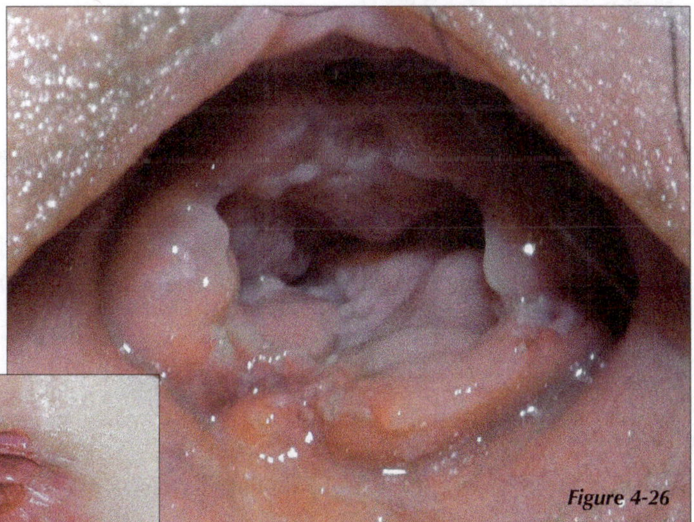
Figure 4-26

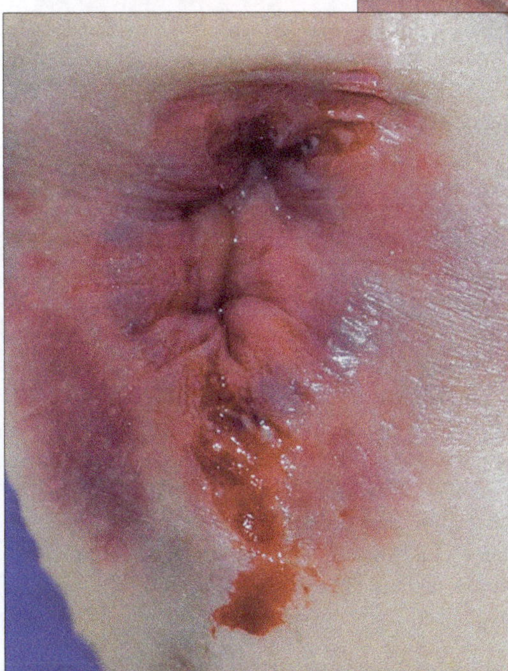
Figure 4-27

Figure 4-23. *4-year-old girl with multiple petechial bruises to the hymen. Reported acute touching 1 day before examination by an unknown family member. Photo contributed by Diana Faugno, MSN, RN, CPN, SANE-A, SANE-P, FAAFS, DF-IAFN, DF-AFN.*

Figure 4-24. *13-year-old girl who was vaginally penetrated by an adult male acquaintance. Photograph taken approximately 30 hours after the assault shows bruising of the inferior margin of the hymen. This bruise was gone 2 weeks later.*

Figure 4-25. *Photograph depicts a posterior midline acute hymenal laceration. Photo contributed by Arne K. Myhre, MD.*

Figure 4-26. *14-year-old girl disclosed being vaginally penetrated by two older adolescent males less than 24 hours ago. Photograph shows hymenal lacerations at the 3 o'clock, 6 o'clock, and 7 o'clock locations.*

Figure 4-27. *This 5-year-old boy described anal-penile penetration by an adult male occurring several hours ago. Photograph shows perianal bruising and acute anal lacerations at the 1 o'clock, 6 o'clock, 7 o'clock, and 11 o'clock locations.*

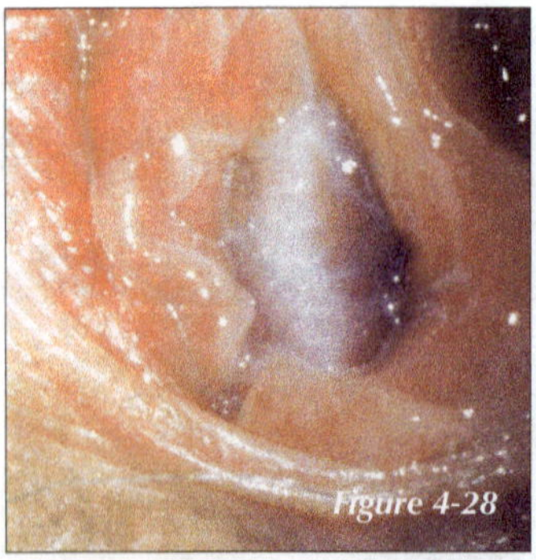

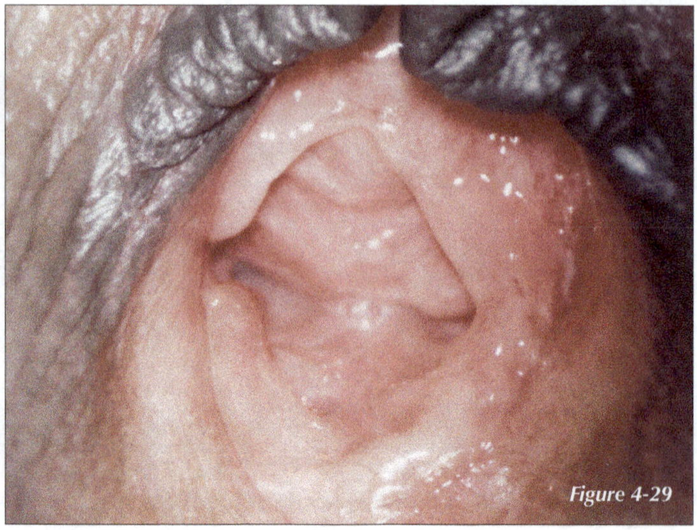

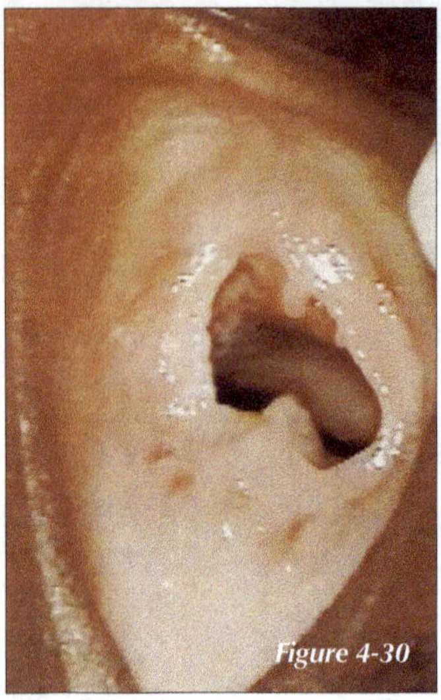

Figure 4-28. *12-year-old girl who reported forcible vaginal-penile penetration by a 17-year-old stranger. Photograph depicts a healed hymenal tear extending to the vaginal wall at 8 o'clock, 6 months after the assault. Photo contributed by Mary J. Spencer, BA, MD, FAAP.*

Figure 4-29. *12-year-old child victim of incest by her biological father. Photograph shows an old healed hymenal tear, nearly to the vaginal wall at the 9 o'clock position. There was a delay in reporting the abuse. Photo contributed by Mary J. Spencer, BA, MD, FAAP.*

Figure 4-30. *This developmentally delayed 11-year-old girl told her friend that she had "sex" with her "15-year-old boyfriend" associated with "her period" more than 2 weeks ago. Her examination showed slight irregularity in the supine position. Photograph in the prone knee chest position shows healed hymenal transection at the 12 o'clock location and a deep cleft at the 1 o'clock location.*

A detailed history is important, because these findings may be attributable to sexual abuse, consensual sexual activity, accidental injuries, or previous medical procedures. Examiners should confirm these findings by using multiple examination positions (eg, prone knee-chest) or additional techniques (eg, use of a swab or water to maximize visualization.[1]

STIs as Evidence

Sexually active adolescents and young adults have the highest rates of STIs, and STIs are more commonly identified in pubertal adolescents than in prepubertal children being evaluated for suspected sexual assault or abuse. The presence of STIs in the pubertal adolescent post-assault may represent an infection acquired through the abuse, presence of pathogens in perpetrator secretions, or infection secondary to prior sexual activity. The risk of acquiring an STI through sexual assault or abuse is directly related to the prevalence of STIs found in the adult and adolescent population from which the abuser comes.[3,9,52,53,89] One study showed that 43% of the adults and adolescents who were victims of sexual assault had at least one preexisting STI, but relatively few developed new chlamydial (2%) or gonococcal (4%) disease. However, 12% had developed trichomoniasis and 19% had developed BV as a result of their assault.[89] Several studies suggest that approximately 5% to 8% of prepubertal children evaluated for sexual abuse or assault will have an STI.[3,9,14,57,86] The incubation periods for the organisms and the timing of the examination in relation to the abuse are critically important in detecting infections.[9]

Although any sexually transmissible infection can be exchanged through sexual contact, the strength of the association between an STI and child sexual abuse is variable. Several factors must be considered when evaluating the strength of association between STI and child sexual abuse, particularly the age of the child and the specific disease identified. The physician should consider the possibility that the identified organism represents a perinatally acquired infection or an infection spread by fomites or nonsexual contact; however, the fact that an explanation of perinatal or nonsexual transmission for a specific disease is plausible does not mean that it is correct. Children with an STI may be unable or unwilling to disclose sexual abuse, and the inability to document a specific STI in a possible or suspected perpetrator does not exclude the possibility that this individual was the source of the child's infection.[3,9]

There are 5 STIs that provide strong forensic evidence in prepubertal children.[1] Infections caused by *C. trachomatis*, *N. gonorrhoeae*, *Treponema pallidum*, *T. vaginalis*, and HIV in prepubertal children are primarily sexually transmitted, and in the absence of perinatal transmission (or contaminated needles or blood transfusion for HIV), they are strong evidence of sexual abuse. Cultures have long been considered the "gold standard" for the diagnosis of *C. trachomatis* and *N. gonorrhoeae* in children; however, positive results from 2 sequential NAATs targeting different genomic sequences are considered proof of infection in genital samples.[52,53] Syphilis should be diagnosed by using standard nontreponemal serologic testing such as the Venereal Disease Research Laboratory (VDRL) test and the rapid plasma reagin (RPR) test, confirmed by specific antibody serology for *T. pallidum* such as the fluorescent treponemal antibody absorption test or the microhemagglutination–*Treponema pallidum* test.[9,53] *T. vaginalis* infections in prepubertal children beyond the first months of life are strongly suggestive of sexual contact; however, nonsexual transmission is possible theoretically.[1] *T. vaginalis* infection can be diagnosed by an experienced technician using a wet mount preparation, but specific culture media have higher sensitivity and specificity. The forensic significance of other STIs in prepubertal children is not as strong. Herpes simplex virus (HSV) infection [either type 1 HSV (HSV-1) or type 2 HSV (HSV-2) by culture] in the genital area of a child or adolescent should be considered as possible evidence of sexual abuse or sexual contact. Commercially available, type-specific serologic tests have acceptable accuracy in adults, but these tests have not been standardized in children, and even in adults, they cannot accurately distinguish HSV-1 from HSV-2. The evidence suggests that, except for transmission at birth, most HSV-2 genital infections are sexually transmitted. The source and mode of transmission in many cases of childhood human papillomavirus (HPV) infection is difficult to identify because of the lengthy and variable incubation period of HPV, the contradictory data on perinatal transmission, the possibility of nonsexual transmission, and the general prevalence of subclinical infection. The diagnosis of HPV infection is usually made clinically, but biopsy and PCR testing can be used to confirm diagnosis. When there are no data that clearly indicate perinatal transmission, every prepubertal child with genital *T. vaginalis* infection, genital HSV infection, or anogenital HPV infection should have a complete medical evaluation for sexual abuse.[3,9]

The presence of STIs has forensic significance in children, but is often not considered important forensically in older adolescents and adults.[3,13] Sexually abused children and adolescents are at risk for acquiring infections prevalent among sexually active adolescents and adults. Prepubertal children do not commonly experience STIs. Some STIs have much stronger association with sexual abuse; however, children can acquire some STIs through vertical transmission at birth and through nonsexual contact. The discovery of an STI in a child might prompt an evaluation for child sexual abuse and can be the only physical evidence of sexual abuse in some cases.[3,9,53]

Forensic Evidence Interpretation

Spermatozoa

Spermatozoa (sperm) detected in specimens taken from body orifices provide strong evidence of recent sexual contact. Live, motile sperm are detected by using a saline wet mount and are the most tangible proof of recent ejaculation into the orifice. The survival time of motile sperm is variable, depending on the body orifice in which it was deposited. Sperm motility may be present for only 30 minutes and rarely persists for more than a few hours. The mouth presents a particularly hostile environment because of the cleansing and digestive action of saliva, whereas motile sperm can persist occasionally up to 5 days in the cervix. Prepubertal girls do not produce cervical mucus, so the prepubertal female genital tract may be more destructive to semen and sperm.[9,90]

Nonmotile sperm (or "dead sperm") are detectable for a longer period than live sperm. Several studies suggest that sperm are often present for 24 hours but rarely up to 48 hours to 72 hours in the vagina after voluntary intercourse.[42] Other studies have found higher rates of positive samples, particularly in cervical samples. One study reported that sperm may be found in the endocervical canal in adults 6 days after intercourse,[91] and another study[27] involved 15 couples after voluntary intercourse and had the conclusion that sperm persists for up to 17 days. At 72 hours, sperm were still present in 50% of the vaginal specimens of the women.[27] Using vaginal and cervical scrapings for the presence of sperm, Silverman and Silverman[90] screened women who reported varying intervals between their last vaginal intercourse and their evaluation. Two-thirds of the women with a history of intercourse within that last day had sperm present, and one-third of those reporting intercourse 1 week before had sperm present.[90]

Some studies have revealed high rates of identification of sperm in samples of adolescent and adult sexual assault victims, but the researchers involved didn't specifically address the timing of samples. Riggs et al[67] described findings in 1076 victims of acute sexual assault. Sperm or seminal fluid was found in 48% of the 612 samples taken. Gray-Eurom et al[65] described findings in 801 victims examined for acute sexual assault. Sperm or seminal fluid was found in 31% of the 355 cases in which samples were processed.[65] The Tucker et al[92] study provided details on the interval between the assault and the examination in 1007 adult rape victims. A total of 919 vaginal specimens were collected and 344 (37.4%) were positive for sperm; however, 97% of the positive specimens were from women examined within 20 hours of assault. Oral and anal specimens were rarely positive. Only 1% of the oral rape cases had positive sperm results, and all positive results were examined within 3 hours of the rape. Only 2% of the anal rape cases had positive results for sperm, and all positive specimens were obtained within 4 hours of the rape. Of specimens obtained from skin surfaces, 19% yielded positive results for sperm and only 2 of 12 positive specimens were obtained more than 4 hours after the rape.[92]

Casey et al[93] evaluated forensic evidence in 1450 cases of sexual assault from a total of 3508 vaginal, 538 anal, and 849 oral swabs. The likelihood of detecting sperm from each site decreased with increasing time since intercourse. Sperm were detected in at least one-third of vaginal swabs taken within the first 18 hours, in at least one-quarter of samples taken within 18 to 48 hours, and in only 6% of samples taken after 48 hours. Of samples taken within 72 to 96 hours, 6% were positive, but there were no positive samples beyond 120 hours. Sperm were detected in approximately 20% of anal swabs taken within the first 12 hours, approximately 10% of samples taken within 12 to 48 hours, and in approximately 2% of samples taken more than 48 hours later. No samples were positive beyond 85 hours. Sperm were detected in 2.5% of oral samples taken within the first 15 hours, and only 1 of 142 samples was positive past 15 hours (detected at 27 hours).

Sperm are often found in vaginal samples during the first 48 hours, are less common in samples obtained between 72 to 96 hours, and are rarely found beyond 120 hours. Sperm are rarely present for more than 48 hours in anal specimens. Persistence of nonmotile sperm in rectal sites, however, has been documented for up to 113 hours. Sperm are rarely found in oral samples beyond 15 hours.[45,92,93] Dry specimens from any site are quite stable, and sperm can be detected in stains on clothing for 12 months or longer.[43,90,94]

Prostatic Acid Phosphatase and Other Seminal Fluid Markers

Prostatic acid phosphatase (PAP) is an enzyme secreted by the prostate gland. The concentration in semen is high, 130 IU/L to 1800 IU/L, but it is present in only very low levels (ie, less than 50 IU/L) in vaginal secretions. PAP is often considered a more sensitive indicator of recent intercourse than sperm, but it should be considered complementary to the identification of sperm.[80] In the study by Tucker et al[92] of 1007 adult rape victims, 37.4% of vaginal specimens were positive for sperm, but only 1% of the oral samples, 2% of anal samples, and 19% of skin specimens were positive for sperm. However, tests for PAP yielded positive results more frequently: that is, positive results were found in 62% of vaginal specimens, 11% of oral specimens, 12% of anal specimens, and 42% of skin specimens. Of samples positive for PAP, all were collected within 36 hours, with 88% collected within 12 hours and 68% collected within 5 hours of sexual assault. This study supports the concept of the increased sensitivity of PAP as an indicator of recent intercourse over that of sperm.[92] In individual cases PAP levels may remain elevated longer than sperm can be visualized or sperm might be detected in the absence of significant elevation of PAP levels. Two additional recent studies underline the inconsistent relationship between the presence or absence of PAP with the presence of both visible sperm and DNA.[38,93]

Enzyme levels return to normal within 72 hours, so significantly elevated PAP levels in vaginal secretions usually indicate intercourse within 24 hours to 48 hours. Half of all specimens will have negative levels within 24 hours of vaginal intercourse with ejaculation, but levels can return to normal as soon as within 3 hours of ejaculation. PAP remains elevated for an even shorter duration in the mouth (perhaps only 6 hours) and in the rectum (less than 24 hours), but limited data are available regarding these sites.[43] Anecdotal evidence supports the stability of PAP in dried seminal fluid stains on clothing for at least 3 years after the deposition of the semen, and the enzyme may persist indefinitely.[43,90,94]

Two other tests, the prostate-specific antigen (PSA, p30, semen glycoprotein of prostatic origin) and the MHS-5 antigen detection test (MHS-5 antigen, a seminal vesicle-specific protein), have been used to detect the presence of seminal fluid residues.[95,96] Any amount of PSA or p30 protein found in the vaginal fluid, urine, or saliva of females is indicative of recent sexual contact, because levels become undetectable within 48 hours of ejaculation into the vagina. The PSA test is a more sensitive test for the presence of seminal fluid than PAP in the first 48 hours, but PAP remains detectable in some vaginal specimens for longer than 48 hours. PSA can be found in other body fluids, and its presence in normal breast milk may create problems in some cases. PSA is extremely stable when dried, and therefore it may be detectable for up to 12 years in dried seminal stains on clothing.[95] The MHS-5 test uses a monoclonal antibody probe technique for the detection of a protein produced only in a male's seminal vesicles and found only in semen.[96] Although standardized laboratory kits have been developed for this test, the test has not come into general usage.[9]

Laboratory tests for the presence of seminal fluid can be interpreted properly only if certain limitations are recognized. First and most important, these tests can be negative in sample when sperm and DNA are actually present, so their use for screening samples to include or exclude samples for further forensic analysis is not appropriate.[36,93] Second, the test for sperm will yield negative results, but the PAP, PSA, and MHS-5 test may provide positive results if the alleged perpetrator has aspermia or has had a vasectomy, because seminal fluid is still produced and released. Chronic alcohol or drug abuse, chemotherapy, cancer, infection, or congenital conditions may suppress semen production.[16] Third, the tests for sperm, PAP, PSA, and MHS-5 will give negative results if ejaculation has not occurred or if a condom has prevented deposition of the ejaculate. Fourth, all tests may yield negative results, despite rapid collection of specimens, because of inadequate sampling; problems in the handling or processing of specimens; or if bathing, washing, or toileting activities have removed the ejaculate. Finally, all tests are very likely to provide negative results if they are conducted more than 48 hours to 72 hours after intercourse, because all levels fall rapidly. Clothing worn during or immediately after the abuse may test positive more than 72 hours later; however, because sperm and the seminal fluid products in dried stains can persist for a longer time.

Trace Evidence

Trace evidence pertains to the analysis of foreign materials found on the bodies of sexual assault victims, including hairs, fibers, and epithelial cells. The Locard exchange principle states that when 2 objects come into contact, material is exchanged between these objects. This principle is the scientific basis of fingerprint and trace evidence collection. Sweat and oil produced in the skin also aid in the transfer and adhesion of epithelial cells from one person's body to objects or to another person's body with physical contact.[97]

It has been estimated that the detectible primary transfer actually involves a small number of epithelial cells, approximately 20 to 1000 cells. Theoretically, a secondary transfer could take place, transferring some of those cells to a third individual or third object. A detectible secondary transfer, however, is very unlikely. Only a small amount of the primary transfer's small number of cells would be secondarily transferred, and the individual involved in the theoretical secondary transfer would be likely to leave behind a primary transfer of her own cells in a larger number than through secondary transfer. Therefore, the trace DNA identified on a surface is very likely to have come from the last individual who had contact with that surface.[97]

The average human sheds approximately 400 000 skin cells every day.[97] In addition, the secretions of the sweat glands and the oil glands carry additional cells to the surface of the body daily as they pass through the ducts and pores. Each nucleated skin cell contains approximately 5 pg (pictograms) of nuclear DNA. Multiplex PCR DNA analysis can produce full DNA profiles to identify individuals at or below 100 pg of purified DNA, so as few as 20 cells may be a sufficient source from which to produce an individual's DNA profile.[97]

The amount of DNA transferred during handling or touching is independent of the duration of contact, because the transfer would be instantaneous. However, the amount of DNA is dependent on the individual doing the transfer and the surface to which the transfer is made. Some individuals slough more epithelial cells and are better exchangers, and any exchanged cells are more likely to adhere to a porous surface than to a smooth surface.[97]

The type of DNA-containing material that is exchanged also affects the likelihood of detectible DNA transfer. Solid tissue such as skin scrapings from under victims' fingernails and seminal fluid contain the highest density of DNA. Blood is a relatively good source of DNA, but it is lower in density because only the white blood cells are nucleated. Saliva has an even lower density of DNA and the number of epithelial cells transferred by handling or touching represents the smallest reservoir of DNA-containing material.[97] Trace DNA (or "touch DNA") is associated with epithelial cell transfer by simple physical contact. Epithelial cell transfer during sexual contact has been documented between individuals. Dziegelewski et al[98] demonstrated male epithelial cells in vaginal samples up to 7 days after sexual contact by using a fluorescence in situ hybridization (FISH) Y chromosome probe.

Hair and Fiber Analysis

Body or scalp hair from the perpetrator occasionally can be found on the victim's body. Exline et al[37] studied the transfer of pubic hair during consensual sexual contact. Pubic hair combings were done immediately after intercourse, and at least one transferred hair was found in 17.3% of the 110 combings. Transfers to males (23.6%) were more common than transfers to females (10.9%).[37]

Collection of foreign hairs (human or non-human) from a victim's body might provide a link from the perpetrator to the victim. Hair analysis requires the collection of any foreign hair from the body of the victim, hairs collected from the alleged perpetrator directly, and the victim's own hair as a control. Multiple specimens from the alleged abuser and the victim must be collected from multiple sites because of the variability of hair types from different sites in one individual. Hair analysis has limited specificity, and the laboratory can conclude in the majority of cases only that the sample is consistent with, inconsistent with, or inconclusive when compared with the perpetrator's hair.[9,37] Similar microscopic comparison of foreign fibers found on the victim's body with known fibers from the perpetrator's house can help confirm the location of the abuse. Appropriate handling of fiber evidence maximizes the value of fiber analysis.[16] The forensic value of microscopic and chemical analysis of hairs and fibers has been brought under question by a lack of consistent standards and procedures and resulting lack of specificity except when combined with DNA analysis.[83]

Clothing Evidence

Clothing evidence has 3 purposes: (1) torn clothing may help provide physical proof of force, (2) stained clothing (eg, grass-stained) may suggest victim resistance or struggle, and (3) stains may provide evidence of seminal fluid or DNA of the assailant. Although some protocols suggest collection of all clothing from the victim, most recommend only selective collection of clothing with suspected stains or tears.[4,13] Protocols often recommend collection of underwear worn at the time of the assault and underwear worn since the assault.[4,5,16]

Role of Forensic Evidence in Proving the Identity of the Perpetrator

Semen, blood, saliva, body hair, bite marks, and other materials occasionally found on or in the body of the victim may help to identify the perpetrator. Proper analysis of these materials requires the expertise of a forensic pathologist or a specialized crime laboratory.

Before the development of DNA analysis, serologic genetic markers were the primary method for identifying the likely origin of body fluids in 80% of the general population who secrete these markers in all body fluids. Some subtypes of individual genetic markers are common, whereas others are rare. The frequency of particular combinations of subtypes of the genetic markers in the general population can be estimated. From this estimate, the chances of the body fluid being from a specific individual can be calculated. This calculation was perhaps more helpful for excluding suspects than identifying specific individuals.[9,38]

The typing of DNA is the most specific and important development in the identification of the perpetrator of sexual assault and has replaced conventional serologic testing.[38,46] The typing of DNA has 2 main features that make it superior to conventional serologic evaluation: better stability and higher specificity. In principle, DNA typing can enable the differentiation of one individual from all others except for an identical twin.[38]

The forensic application of DNA analysis is based on research data identifying regions of human DNA that are extremely variable among individuals. These regions, or loci, have been dubbed restriction fragment length polymorphisms (RFLPs). One particular subgroup of these RFLPs is called variable number of tandem repeats (VNTRs) loci.

A comparison of these loci in samples was the initial application of DNA typing in forensic medicine. The major advantages of VNTR loci use for DNA typing are in the large number of alleles per locus and in the fact that combining several loci provides high discrimination power among compared DNA samples. The major limitations are that a relatively large amount of high-quality (ie, not degraded) DNA is required for analysis and the process is very time-consuming.[38]

PCR amplification techniques provide the second major tool for forensic DNA typing because they allow amplification of a tiny amount of DNA into virtually any amount. Techniques of PCR amplification greatly increase the sensitivity of DNA testing because a higher number of degraded samples can be tested. This process can take advantage of considerably smaller variable areas of DNA known as short tandem repeat (STR) units, rather than the larger VNTR units. The smaller size makes them more amenable to PCR amplification, thereby increasing sensitivity, because specimens with very small amounts of DNA can be analyzed. Specificity is also increased because STR loci are more numerous than VNTR units, so comparisons can be made between larger numbers of variable DNA sequences. In addition, multiple STR loci can be analyzed simultaneously or multiplexed, which results in increased efficiency, speed, and power of analysis. The Federal Bureau of Investigation (FBI) has identified 13 specific STR loci as a core set for use in matching crime scene materials to previously typed individuals. This core set forms the basis of the Combined DNA Index System (CODIS).[38] In 2017, the core set of STR loci was expanded to 20 loci.

Autosomal STR DNA analysis is most effective for samples collected within the first 48 hours post sexual contact, and useful DNA profiles are limited beyond 72 hours. It is extremely challenging to recover a standard autosomal STR DNA profile from a sample that contains other human cellular material because the overwhelming amount of DNA from the victim obscures or masks the male perpetrator's DNA profile.[99,100]

Even smaller areas of DNA variation, or segments shorter (smaller) than STR loci, hold some potential for use in forensic DNA testing. Single nucleotide polymorphisms (SNPs) represent alterations in DNA sequence at a single nucleoside position due to changes, insertions, or deletions. These SNPs are very numerous, with millions occurring in each individual, but they typically produce only 2 alleles and, less commonly, 3 or 4 alleles. Therefore, to be of discriminating forensic value, a relatively large number of SNPs would have to be analyzed. As a result, although SNP may be more helpful in excluding suspects, ongoing research is still necessary to improve the utility of SNP testing.[38]

Mitochondrial DNA and Y chromosomal DNA also have forensic application.[38,99,100] Mitochondria contain their own small DNA genomes known as mitochondrial DNA (mtDNA). Normally, only maternal mtDNA is transmitted to children. Each cell contains only 1 nucleus, but it can contain hundreds to thousands of mitochondria. Specimens with degraded DNA or that lack nuclear DNA but contain mtDNA can be analyzed forensically. For example, a sample of hair without a root ball lacks nuclear DNA, but it still contains large amounts of mtDNA for comparison with known samples from a suspect. The limitations of mtDNA are its relatively low discriminating power and the lack of available databases compared with those available for nuclear DNA. An individual's mother, siblings, as well as all other maternally-related family members will have identical mtDNA sequences.[38]

The Y chromosome has hundreds of recognized STR loci that can be used for identification. The Y chromosome is transmitted in a single copy only from father to son, whereas mtDNA is transmitted in multiple copies from a mother to all of her children. Therefore, Y chromosomal analysis can be useful in resolving mixtures of DNA from different males, but its overall discriminating power is limited by the size of the database and the fact that all males in a paternal lineage will possess a common Y chromosomal DNA. Y chromosomal STR analysis (Y-STR) may be very useful, however, in cases in which intact sperm are no longer present but some residual DNA or seminal fluid remains. Y-STR unmasks the male perpetrator's DNA profile because it is looking specifically for DNA from males, ignoring the female victim's DNA in the process. Hanson and Ballantyne[99] demonstrated the ability to obtain full male DNA profiles from many vaginal samples within the first 5 days after voluntary intercourse in a nonclinical setting and some full and partial DNA profiles beyond the fifth day. Maiquilla et al[100] evaluated 154 children and adolescents (aged 2 to 18 years) examined within 72 hours of sexual abuse. Sperm were found in only 21% of selected samples, but full and partial Y-STR DNA profiles were identified in 42% of samples. Johnson et al[101] reported that of 45 samples that were negative for spermatozoa but positive for seminal fluid, a Y-STR profile was obtained in 86.2%. Sibille et al[102] analyzed 104 samples from 79 females testing negative for sperm. In the samples, Y-STR was present in 30% of the cases greater than 48 hours post-assault.[102] Delfin et al[103] described 112 children and adolescents (aged 2 to 17 years) testing positive for seminal fluid but negative for sperm. All were negative for autosomal DNA, but Y-STR was positive in 92.3%.

DNA is more stable than serologic testing, but degradation can occur. Factors producing degradation include exposure to sunlight and ultraviolet light, time, temperature, humidity, chemicals, and biological contamination. Mixed samples present some difficulty, but this situation is expected in sexual assault cases because both victim and assailant DNA is expected to be present. Mixed samples present greater challenges to autosomal STR analysis than Y-STR analysis. Contaminated specimens are problematic, because the addition of soaps, chemicals, bacteria, and fungi can cause degradation of the samples. Stability is improved by preventing contamination and drying, then freezing, the samples.[38,99] **Table 4-1** summarizes the types of DNA analysis and their advantages and disadvantages.

The analysis of DNA can result in 3 determinations regarding identity: exclusion, inconclusive, and match. Exclusion means that the 2 DNA samples are different, and inconclusive means that the results do not allow a determination as to whether the DNA samples are the same or different, often associated with obtaining only a partial DNA profile. A match means the DNA types are similar and there are no significant differences; therefore, the DNA samples could have the same source. The current technology for DNA typing has progressed to the point at which the reliability and validity of properly collected, properly preserved, and properly analyzed DNA data should not be in doubt.[38,99,104]

Forensic Evidence in Children

Most children evaluated for sexual abuse do not have forensic evidence. Studies focusing on highly selected groups of children and adolescents who were victims reported 14% to 30% had positive test results for sperm or PAP.[105-107] Enos et al[105] reviewed 162 cases of children who were victimized for less than 14 years, and 29 (17.9%) had positive tests for sperm or PAP. These tests were most commonly positive in the 11 to 13 year olds evaluated, but no specific age breakdown was provided.[105] Rimsza and Niggemann,[106] performed forensic tests on 50 of 311 child and adolescent victims. Sperm was found in 15 (30%), and all positives were collected within 24 hours of the sexual contact. They did not discuss whether different rates of positive tests were found among prepubertal and pubertal victims.[106] Spencer and Dunklee[107] evaluated 140 boys (aged 1 to 17 years) who were sexually abused and found that 8 of 30 boys (26.6%) examined within 72 hours had positive forensic test results; however, fluorescence with ultraviolet light alone was considered a positive test result.[107]

Table 4-1. Types of DNA Analysis for Forensic Applications

Type of DNA Analysis	Relative Loci Size	Advantages	Disadvantages
Variable Number Tandem Repeats (VNTRs) loci	Large	— Vary widely among individuals — Contains multiple alleles per unit allowing for high discrimination among individuals	— Requires relatively large amounts of high-quality, non-degraded DNA — Very time consuming analysis — Historical only (no longer used)
Autosomal nuclear short tandem repeats (STRs) DNA loci	Small	— High discriminating power when comparing 13 or more loci — Large national and international databases available — Most used DNA in forensic analysis; widely available internationally	— Requires that samples include cells that contain nuclei — Processing mixed DNA samples is more difficult — DNA degrades rapidly, limiting timeframe — Only 2 copies of DNA per nucleated cell
Mitochondrial DNA loci	Small	— Does not require nucleated cells — Thousands of copies in each cell — Exceptionally stable DNA	— Limited discriminating power because an individual's mitochondrial DNA matches all maternal relatives — Databases are currently incomplete, but are under development
Y chromosome STR loci	Small	— Mixed samples are less of a problem because male DNA (typical suspect) can be more easily separated from female DNA (typical victim)	— Limited discriminating power because an individual's Y chromosome DNA matches all paternal relatives — Databases are currently incomplete but are under development
Bi-allelic DNA loci (known as single nucleotide polymorphisms [SNP] and insertion/deletion [In-Del])	Very small	— Very numerous in all individuals — Can use degraded DNA	— Would require hundreds of loci to be compared for each analysis — No current database — Would require major shift in approach

Additional studies suggest that only 2% to 9% of all sexually abused preteen or prepubertal children evaluated have positive test results for sperm or PAP.[29-34] However, Dahlke et al[30] reported positive tests for sperm or PAP in 28% of 132 children younger than 15 years, and the percent of rape victims with positive test results increased as the age of the victims increased. Although 73% of all victims older than 14 years had positive test results, 36% of children 11 years to 14 years, only 3% of children younger than 11 years had positive tests for sperm or PAP.[30] Three additional studies focus on the results of forensic evidence collection for prepubertal children. All 3 concluded that guidelines for evidence collection in adolescents and adults who were sexual assault victims might not be appropriate for prepubertal victims.[29,32,34]

Christian et al[29] retrospectively studied 273 children younger than 10 years who selectively had evidence collection kits obtained for suspected acute sexual abuse. Some form of evidence was found in 24.9%, but only 9% had evidence found in samples from body sites. Evidence samples were most often positive for blood; moreover, only 18 (6.6%) had sperm or seminal fluid detected. All children with positive forensic evidence were seen within 44 hours, and more than 90% were examined within 24 hours of the assault. Furthermore, no swabs from any child's body were positive for blood longer than 13 hours or sperm or semen longer than 9 hours post-assault. Almost two-thirds of all evidence was found on clothing or linens, and all evidence with the exception of 1 pubic hair was found on clothing or linens when the examination was completed more than 24 hours after the sexual contact. The authors suggested that swabbing the child's body for evidence might be unnecessary after 24 hours. Because clothing and linens yielded the majority of evidence and retained the evidence for longer periods following the assault, they should be vigorously pursued for analysis.[29]

Young et al[34] retrospectively reviewed forensic evidence collected from 80 children taken to the emergency department with a history of sexual abuse or assault with genital contact occurring within the last 72 hours. The subjects were 49 children younger than 12 years and 31 children aged 12 to 16 years. Sperm or seminal fluid was found in 16 (20%) of the 80 evidence kits collected. Positive samples were correlated with the age of the victim and the length of the interval between the sexual act and evaluation in the emergency department. Only 3 of the 49 younger children (aged 11 years or younger) had positive results, and none had positive test results from samples taken from body sites. The 3 positive samples came from underwear, and one child's washcloth was also positive. In contrast, 13 of the 31 adolescents had positive results, and all 13 tested positive from samples taken from body sites. In addition, the clothing of 8 of these 13 adolescents also tested positive. Ten of these positive kits were from children who were evaluated within 6 hours, and all 16 positive kits were from children evaluated within 24 hours of the sexual contact.[34]

Palusci et al[32] retrospectively studied 122 children younger than 13 years who had evidence collection kits done within 72 hours of suspected acute sexual abuse. Specimens were initially evaluated for acid phosphatase, and positive results were further assessed with microscopic examination for sperm and immunoassay for p30 antigen (PSA). Of the children, 69% were evaluated within 24 hours of sexual contact. Only 9% of the children had positive forensic evidence from body sites or from clothing. Pubertal children, or those having physical injury at the time of evaluation, were more likely to have positive forensic results. Children who bathed, changed clothing, or who were examined later within the 3-day period were less likely to have positive test results. Nearly twice as many positive results were obtained from clothing as from samples from body sites. Semen or sperm was identified from body swabs only from unbathed, female children older than 10 years of age or on clothing and other objects.[32]

All 3 studies[29,32,34] emphasize the importance of the collection of clothing, and all underscore the limited yield from specimens collected from the bodies of prepubertal victims. All 3 studies also have a similar limitation in that they all used microscopic examination for the detection of sperm and assays for either PAP or PSA, rather than DNA analysis, to identify seminal fluid.

Published data assessing the usefulness of assays for DNA in prepubertal or young pubertal children are limited. Two studies reported forensic evidence in children younger than 10 years of age presenting within 72 hours of an acute sexual assault.[28,35] They found 8.9%[28] and 9.3%.[35] of these children had positive DNA testing evidence. Thackeray et al[28] examined 124 children and reported 18 positive kits (20 positive samples). Positive results were from samples from the victim's body (9), from clothing (4), and from both (7). Of the 20 positive samples, 17 were collected within 24 hours of the incident. Of 11 children with positive DNA evidence, 9 were examined within 24 hours, 1 between 24 and 48 hours, and 1 at 54 hours after the incident. Girardet et al[35] examined 151 children, and DNA was obtained in 14 cases: from the body in 3, clothing in 9, and both body and clothing in 2. Of the 5 positive DNA samples from the body, 1 was collected within 7 hours, 1 at 35 hours, 1 at 66 hours, 1 at 96 hours, and 1 at an unknown time interval from the acute assault. Two additional studies sought DNA evidence in acute sexual assault in children using Y-STR DNA analysis. Delfin et al[103] reported that 4 of 4 victims younger than 11 years of age were positive for Y-STR DNA but noted the samples were all collected within 24 hours of the assault. Maiquilla et al[100] reported that 4 of 29 children younger than 10 years of age evaluated for acute sexual assault were positive for Y-STR DNA. All samples were collected within 24 hours of the assault.

Sperm and PAP are usually not detected in young children who were acute sexual abuse victims, and positive DNA results are relatively uncommon. Much of the evidence collected is not found on body sites, and certainly, the collection of clothing and linens should be performed.

Some studies report occasional positive tests for DNA from samples obtained from the victim's body beyond the first 24 hours post-assault, but there are no clear predictors for this infrequent DNA detection. The questions remain, however, whether forensic specimens should be collected from the body cavities of all prepubertal children, unless one is absolutely certain the tests will be negative, or whether one should consider the absence of data in support of this approach while remembering that the primary goal is to provide sensitive, supportive clinical care to these children. Ultimately, the appropriate timing for forensic evidence collection may be more a philosophical decision than a scientific one.

Relationship of Physical and Forensic Evidence to Successful Prosecution

Tintinalli and Hoelzer[108] reviewed the legal outcomes of 67 prosecuted cases involving adult and adolescent victims and found no correlation between physical and forensic evidence and legal outcome. In contrast, Rambow et al[109] reviewed cases of 182 victims who had forensic examinations performed and concluded that forensic findings were significantly associated with successful prosecution. Three more recent studies of adult and adolescent victims sought association between physical evidence of sexual contact and the filing of charges and successful prosecution.[61,110,111] Gray-Eurom et al[61] reviewed 801 forensic evaluations. In 355 cases a suspect was identified. Evidence of trauma was found in 202 (57%), and sperm was found in 110 (31%) cases in which a suspect was identified. When the authors looked for correlation between evidence and successful prosecution, the presence of trauma was correlated but the presence of sperm was not. Victims younger than 18 years of age and the use of a weapon were also associated with successful prosecution. Successful prosecution was related to evidence of force or lack of consent (ie, trauma), rather than the evidence of a sexual act itself (eg, sperm).[61] In the second study,[110] the extent of injury was associated with the filing of charges and rates of conviction. McGregor et al[110] also reported greater than a threefold increase in filing charges in the presence of forensic specimens being collected, irrespective of the test results. This suggests that the victim's willingness to submit to forensic evaluation appears to provide some validation of the victim's reported sexual assault.[110] The third study[111] reported that only 15% of the 888 girls and women older than 15 years evaluated for sexual assault had charges filed. Characteristics positively associated with prosecution were examination within 24 hours of the assault, assault by a partner or spouse, oral assault, and anogenital trauma.[111] Cross et al[112] note that biological evidence may help lead to an arrest in some sexual assault cases involving adults; however, the impact of biological evidence on arrest and prosecution is likely to be limited by the fact that the most common defense to charges of sexual assault is consent rather than denial of sexual contact.

Studies of features related to prosecutorial outcomes in child sexual abuse cases generally include more nonacute cases than cases of acute sexual assault. The likelihood of cases being accepted for prosecution has been associated with perpetrator confessions and physical injury. Cross et al[113] reviewed 431 cases referred for prosecution and found that confessions and medical evidence were the strongest predictors of prosecution. Stroud et al[114] reported that slightly more than half the cases involving 1043 children completing a forensic interview were accepted for prosecution. Cases with children who had mild to no injury were more likely to result in acceptance, but for some unknown reason, cases with children who had the most severe injuries were less likely to be prosecuted.[114] Brewer et al[115] reviewed 200 cases and found prosecution was more likely when (1) the perpetrator abused multiple victims, (2) the perpetrator was not a nuclear family member, (3) when the abuse involved older children, or (4) when the abuse involved acts that were more serious (with the presence of physical evidence). Most cases involved nonacute sexual abuse, and prosecutorial outcomes were not discussed in these studies.

Kerns and Ritter[116] compared the frequency of abnormal genital findings in 83 girls examined following perpetrator confessions and 583 girls who reported abuse but whose cases did not have perpetrator confessions. There was no significant difference in the likelihood of abnormal genital findings between the 2 groups. Neither the number of girls evaluated for acute assault nor the prosecutorial outcomes were reported.[116] Muram[91] reviewed 31 cases with perpetrator confessions of sexual abuse. Significant examination findings were observed in 11 of 18 (61%) girls with admitted vaginal penetration but were also found in 3 of 13 (23%) girls when penetration was denied. Hymenal or vaginal tears were reported in 9 of 17 girls evaluated within 72 hours of sexual abuse. The prosecutorial outcomes were not reported.[91]

De Jong and Rose[31] reviewed 115 cases of child sexual abuse prosecuted for felony charges. Medical evidence of injury or seminal fluid was present in only 23% of cases that resulted in felony convictions, but the overall conviction rate was 76%. Convictions occurred in 67 of 85 cases (79%) without medical evidence, whereas only 20 of 30 cases (67%) with medical evidence resulted in convictions. The felony conviction rate was significantly lower among 23 children who were younger than 7 years of age (52%), despite a higher rate of physical evidence (56%). This study suggests that the verbal evidence may have been more critical than physical evidence in many cases.[31] Adams et al[117] analyzed 236 cases in children younger than 18 years of age with perpetrator conviction for sexual abuse. Most of the legal cases were decided by guilty pleas, and only 14% were decided by trials. Abnormal genital findings were present in 14%, and abnormal anal findings were present in 1%. Only 10% of the children were examined acutely within 72 hours of sexual contact, and they had a significantly higher rate of abnormal examinations.[117] Palusci et al[118] studied the relationship of physical findings and prosecution outcome in 497 children having nonacute examinations for sexual abuse. Overall, 17% of the children had significant physical findings. Those cases involving positive findings were 2.5 times more likely to result in successful prosecution; however, 67% of children with positive physical findings had either no prosecution or unsuccessful prosecutorial outcomes. Positive physical findings were better than disclosure of abuse to predict acceptance for prosecution and successful prosecution, but a lack of disclosure was the best predictor of not seeking prosecution and unsuccessful prosecution.[118] Therefore, most of the data on prosecuted cases involving children of sexual abuse focus on nonacute sexual abuse rather than acute sexual assault. These authors[31,117,118] emphasize the importance of verbal evidence, history, or disclosure in studies primarily reporting nonacute sexual abuse. DNA evidence was not available in almost all of these children, which may have affected their cases. Verbal evidence is expected to be important in acute cases, based on the relatively low rates of documentation of specific injuries, STIs, and forensic evidence in acute child sexual assault cases.

Medical Management Considerations

The major medical interventions required for children and adolescents who are sexual assault victims involve therapy for STIs, emergency contraception, treatment of injuries, certification of physical health, and recommendations for counseling. These interventions are often initiated at the first medical evaluation, but medical follow-up is recommended to maximize the effect of the interventions.[2,4-7,14-16,53]

Prophylactic antibiotic therapy for children who were sexually abused is a controversial subject, but routine prophylaxis is not generally recommended for prepubertal children.[3,5,6,9,14,52,53] Routine prophylaxis for *C. trachomatis*, *N. gonorrhoeae*, and *T. vaginalis* is commonly offered to adolescents and adults as follows: ceftriaxone 250 mg intramuscularly in a single dose, plus azithromycin 1 g orally in a single dose, plus metronidazole or tinidazole 2 g orally in a single dose.[6,14,52,53] Oral cephalosporins can be substituted for ceftriaxone and doxycycline 100 mg orally twice a day for 7 days may be substituted for azithromycin, but due to antibiotic resistance, the substitutions may not have equal efficacy.[52] If the individual is not previously immunized for hepatitis B, a first dose of vaccine is recommended, with follow-up doses to be given 1 to 2 months and 4 to 6 months after the initial dose. Routine prophylactic use of hepatitis B immune globulin (HBIG) is not recommended, but HBIG is recommended as an adjunct to initiating hepatitis B immunization when the perpetrator of the sexual assault is known to be positive for hepatitis B surface antigen.[6,14,52,53] Given the high prevalence of HPV, initiating HPV immunization should be considered at the time of the acute evaluation in previously unimmunized female victims aged 9 to 26 years and male victims aged 9 to 21 years.[2,5,14,52] Selective testing should be done for STIs in younger children as previously outlined. An individually tailored therapy should be initiated if this testing reveals specific infections.

Initiating HIV postexposure prophylaxis (PEP) for acute sexual assault victims is not universally recommended but encouraged for selected individuals despite unknown efficacy. The CDC states that there is a lack of data on the risk of HIV transmission from a single sexual assault and the efficacy of antiretroviral agents to reduce HIV transmission after a possible nonoccupational exposure. The CDC recommends considering the use of PEP for HIV in sexual abuse or assault cases when the perpetrator is known to be HIV-infected, the exposure event presents a substantial risk of transmission, and treatment can be initiated within 72 hours. If the perpetrator's HIV status is unknown, PEP should be considered on a case-by-case basis. Exposure risk factors include local

HIV prevalence; involvement of multiple perpetrators; likelihood of ejaculation occurring on mucous membrane; mucosal lesion on mucous membranes; and oral, vaginal, and/or anal trauma or penetration. HIV PEP is not recommended if there is "negligible exposure risk."[2,6,14,52,53] Examiners should discuss the risk of acquiring HIV, the potential benefits of PEP and its unknown efficacy in this setting, and in the case of children, discuss known toxicity of PEP with the victim and parents. A highly active antiretroviral therapy (HAART) 3-drug combination is recommended, including 2 nucleotide analog reverse transcriptase inhibitors (NRTIs) plus one protease inhibitor. The current preferred regimen is tenofovir, emtricitabine, and raltegravir initiated within 72 hours of exposure and continued daily for 28 days.[6,52,56] Clinicians involved in acute sexual abuse evaluations of children and adolescents should establish a protocol that includes the approach to discussing PEP for HIV, the immediate availability of a 3-day to 7-day starter kit of the PEP drugs, and follow-up in consultation with a pediatric infectious disease specialist.[6,52,56]

Pregnancy risk and pregnancy prevention should be considered in all pubertal girls and young adults. The chance of pregnancy after a single instance of unprotected intercourse is estimated to be 2% to 5%, 20% to 30% during the midcycle, and 2% to 4% anywhere else in the cycle. The actual risk for many adolescents is difficult to determine because many have irregular cycles and few can pinpoint their ovulation days. Therefore, all pubertal girls should have a pregnancy test and be offered pregnancy prophylaxis.[2,6,7,14,119] Emergency contraception should be discussed with the adolescent if she is not pregnant and if less than 120 hours have elapsed since the assault. Emergency contraception (EC) will prevent approximately 80% to 90% of expected pregnancies if taken appropriately. Emergency contraception using combination estrogen and progestin "birth control pills" (ie, the Yuzpe method) combines relatively low efficacy with high risk of side effects and is no longer recommended. There are 3 recommended regimens for emergency contraception. The first regimen uses a progestin, levonorgestril (Plan B) with a total dose of 1.5 mg of levonorgestril in 2 pills. The total dose can be given at one time; alternatively, one pill is given, and 12 hours later, the second pill is given. The second regimen is an antiprogestin—ulipristal acetate (UPA)—taken as a single 30 mg dose. The third regimen is insertion of a copper intrauterine device (IUD), the most effective of all EC options. Levonorgestril is the most widely available option and is effective up to 120 hours after intercourse, but its efficacy declines over time. UPA is somewhat less available, but its efficacy does not decline over the 120-hour window for EC. The efficacy of any oral EC medication is reduced in obese women. Levonrogestril becomes less effective for women with a body mass index (BMI) of > 25 and ineffective at BMI > 30. UPA becomes less effective at BMI > 30 and ineffective at BMI > 35. The efficacy of copper IUDs is not effected by BMI; however, availability or victim acceptability in the setting of acute sexual assault may be an issue. If a copper IUD is not available or acceptable to the victim, UPA is the best option in women with a BMI of > 25.[119] Nausea and vomiting are common side effects of oral emergency contraception. Oral antiemetics, including meclizine and metoclopramide, can be helpful when given 1 hour before the initial dose. Menstruation occurs within 21 days in more than 95% of patients receiving emergency contraception. If menstruation does not occur, both physiologic and psychological factors should be assessed.[9,16]

Most acute genital and perianal injuries do not require surgical intervention. The primary therapy for acute injuries is maintaining proper hygiene in the anogenital area. Sitz baths can be initiated, after specimens for evidence and culture are collected, to promote healing and to prevent secondary infections. Prophylactic broad-spectrum antibiotics are not generally indicated in wound care. Topical or oral antibiotics may be recommended for extensive injuries, but few data support their efficacy. Lubricating ointments or diaper creams may be helpful to reduce irritation. Nonstick dressings or absorbent pads may help, but frequently changed cotton underwear may be sufficient. Small vulvar or perianal hematomas may be treated with pressure and ice packs. Large hematomas or lacerations may require a surgical or gynecologic consultation, with surgical repair done (when necessary) with the patient under general anesthesia.[9]

A mental health professional should evaluate all children and adolescents for posttraumatic disorders subsequent to their evaluation for acute sexual abuse or assault.[2,3,9,14] This assessment is both to determine the need for counseling for the child who has been victimized and the child's parents and to evaluate the level of family support for the child. Sexual assault can trigger significant acute and chronic emotional trauma. One must remember that the role of the medical provider is primarily promoting the child's physical and emotional well-being; with that said, the management of both the physical and emotional trauma begins at the time of the acute medical evaluation of the abused or assaulted child or adolescent. The parents and child need reassurance regarding physical and emotional concerns. When the child's examination reveals no physical trauma, both need reassurance that the child is physically normal and can grow and develop into a physically normal adult despite this experience. If the child has injuries, reassurance can be given that most injuries heal rapidly and completely and, once healed, should have no physical effects on the functioning of the genital and anal areas. Acknowledge that the child and the parents may experience a number of emotional reactions, including anger, humiliation, guilt, blame, and sadness. Counseling should help manage these symptoms. Reassure the child and parents that, regardless of events leading to the abuse or assault itself, the child is not responsible for being sexually assaulted; the assailant is responsible for abusing the child.[3,9]

Most victims will not return for follow-up care, with many factors affecting the likelihood that they will.[120] In a study of 727 child and adolescent victims returning for follow-up care, Gavril et al[121] reported that the interpretation of trauma likelihood changed in 17.7% of returning patients, and additional STIs were identified in 6.5%, altering both interpretation of initial examination findings and identification of patients requiring additional medical treatment. The physical and emotional needs of the child should be addressed, whenever possible, in coordination with the child's primary medical care provider.[3] Girardet et al[122] found that 8% of children who had been victimized had significant unmet health care needs identified during their medical evaluation that needed intervention which could result in patient morbidity unrelated to sexual abuse. All children should have a follow-up appointment whether or not an acute injury or infection is present. In children without initial injury or infection or with minor acute injury, this examination allows time to reassure the child and the parents that no permanent physical damage has occurred. This "certification of physical wellness" may help some of the children avoid the "damaged goods" feelings commonly experienced by abused children. Posttraumatic emotional symptoms can also be assessed during the follow-up appointment. The unmet health care needs can also be addressed at this time. Children with more severe injury should be carefully followed up until healing is complete. They need assurance that any residual scarring should not affect their health and functioning as adults.

Conclusion

All children and adolescents being evaluated for suspected acute sexual assault or abuse should have a medical evaluation that incorporates the major objectives of providing appropriate medical care while collecting and documenting evidence of sexual contact. The medical history or interview can help direct the medical care of the child and provide a unique opportunity to obtain important evidence in the form of the history of the sexual assault. The majority of acute examinations in prepubertal children will not disclose physical trauma, STIs, or positive forensic medical evidence that sexual contact has occurred. Many physical examinations in adolescents will yield some physical injury evidence or positive forensic evidence, with higher rates reported when evaluations occurred within the first 24 hours to 48 hours after the assault. Identification of certain STIs in prepubertal children is forensically important, but the forensic value of these infections is more limited in adolescents. The quality of forensic evidence is maximized by following an appropriate protocol for evidence collection and the documentation of proper handling of all evidence. Analysis of DNA provides a more sensitive and more specific approach to the identity of the offender than conventional serologic testing, but there are few published data about the performance of DNA analysis in child and adolescent sexual assault cases. The history of the abuse or assault is the most important evidence in victims of prepubertal sexual assault. Physical evidence of force, injury, or sexual contact is helpful, but it is neither necessary nor sufficient for conviction of the perpetrator of acute sexual assault. The major medical interventions required involve prophylactic and therapeutic antibiotics for STIs, emergency contraception, treatment of injuries, certification or reassurance of physical health, and recommendations for counseling.

References

1. Adams JA, Kellogg ND, Farst KJ, et al. Updated guidelines for the medical assessment and care of children who may have been sexually abused. *J Pediatr Adolesc Gynecol.* 2016;29(2):81-87.

2. Jenny C, Crawford-Jakubiak JE; Committee on Child Abuse and Neglect; American Academy of Pediatrics. The evaluation of children in the primary care setting when sexual abuse is suspected. *Pediatrics.* 2013;132(2):e558-e567.

3. Kellogg N; American Academy of Pediatrics Committee on Child Abuse and Neglect. Clinical report: the evaluation of sexual abuse in children. *Pediatrics.* 2005;116(2):506-512.

4. American College of Emergency Physicians. *Evaluation and Management of the Sexually Assaulted or Sexually Abused Patient.* 2nd ed. Dallas, TX: American College of Emergency Physicians; 2013.

5. US Department of Justice, Office on Violence Against Women. *A National Protocol for Sexual Abuse Medical Forensic Examinations: Pediatric.* Washington, DC: US Department of Justice, Office on Violence Against Women; 2016.

6. Mollen CJ, Goyal MK, Frioux SM. Acute sexual assault: a review. *Pediatr Emerg Care.* 2012;28(6):584-590.

7. Schilling S, Samuels-Kalow M, Gerber JS, Scribano PV, French B, Wood JN. Testing and treatment after adolescent sexual assault in pediatric emergency departments. *Pediatrics.* 2015;136(6):e1495-e1503.

8. Finkel MA, Alexander RA. Conducting the medical history. *J Child Sex Abus.* 2011;20(5):486-504.

9. Finkel MA, De Jong AR. Medical findings in child sexual abuse. In: Reece R, Ludwig S, eds. *Child Abuse: Medical Diagnosis and Management.* 2nd ed. Philadelphia, PA: Lippincott Williams & Wilkins; 2001:207-286.

10. Frasier LD. The pediatrician's role in child abuse interviewing. *Pediatr Ann.* 1997;26(5):306-311.

11. Giardino AP, Finkel MA. Evaluating child sexual abuse. *Pediatr Ann.* 2005;34(5): 382-394.

12. Schaeffer P, Leventhal JM, Asnes AG. Children's disclosures of sexual abuse: learning from direct inquiry. *Child Abuse Negl.* 2011;35(5):343-352.

13. Ledray LE. *Sexual Assault Nurse Examiner Development and Operation Guide.* Washington, DC: Office for Victims of Crime, US Department of Justice; 1998.

14. Trotman GE, Young-Anderson C, Deye KP. Acute sexual assault in the pediatric and adolescent population. *J Pediatr Adolesc Gynecol.* 2016;29(6):518-526.

15. Goyal MK, Mollen CJ, Haynes KL, et al. Enhancing the emergency department approach to pediatric sexual assault care: implementation of a pediatric sexual assault response team program. *Pediatr Emerg Care.* 2013;29(9):969-973.

16. US Department of Justice, Office on Violence Against Women. *A National Protocol for Sexual Assault Medical Forensic Examinations: Adults/Adolescents.* 2nd ed. Washington, DC: US Department of Justice, Office on Violence Against Women; 2013.

17. Greenbaum J, Crawford-Jakubiak JE; Committee on Child Abuse and Neglect. Child sex trafficking and commercial sexual exploitation: health care needs of victims. *Pediatrics.* 2015;135(3):566-574.

18. Starling SP, Jenny C. Forensic examination of adolescent female genitalia: the Foley catheter technique. *Arch Pediatr Adolesc Med.* 1997;151(1):102-103.

19. Jones JS, Dunnuck C, Rossman L, Wynn BN, Nelson-Horan C. Significance of toluidine blue positive findings after speculum examination for sexual assault. *Am J Emerg Med.* 2004;22(3):201-203.

20. McCauley J, Gorman RL, Guzinski G. Toluidine blue in the detection of perineal lacerations in pediatric and adolescent sexual abuse victims. *Pediatrics.* 1986;78(6):1039-1043.

21. Mears CJ, Heflin AH, Finkel MA, Deblinger E, Steer RA. Adolescents' responses to sexual abuse evaluation including the use of video colposcopy. *J Adolesc Health.* 2003;33(1):18-24.

22. Adams JA, Girardin B, Faugno D. Adolescent sexual assault: documentation of acute injuries using photo-colposcopy. *J Pediatr Adolesc Gynecol.* 2001;14(4):175-180.

23. Heppenstall-Heger A, McConnell G, Ticson L, Guerra L, Lister J, Zaragoza T. Healing patterns in anogenital injuries: a longitudinal study of injuries associated with sexual abuse, accidental injuries, or genital surgery in the preadolescent child. *Pediatrics.* 2003;112(4):829-837.

24. Ricci L. Photodocumentation in child abuse cases. In: Jenny C, ed. *Child Abuse and Neglect Diagnosis, Treatment and Evidence.* Saint Louis, MO: Elsevier Saunders; 2011:215-221.

25. Sommers MS, Fisher BS, Karjane HM. Using colposcopy in the rape exam: health care, forensic, and criminal justice issues. *J Forensic Nurs.* 2005;1(1):19, 28-34.

26. Woodling BA, Heger A. The use of the colposcope in the diagnosis of sexual abuse in the pediatric age group. *Child Abuse Negl.* 1986;10(1):111-114.

27. Soules MR, Pollard AA, Brown KM, Verma M. The forensic laboratory evaluation of evidence in alleged rape. *Am J Obstet Gynecol.* 1978;130(2):142-147.
28. Thackeray JD, Hornor G, Benzinger EA, Scribano PV. Forensic evidence collection and DNA identification in acute child sexual assault. *Pediatrics.* 2011;128(2):227-232.
29. Christian CW, Lavelle JM, De Jong AR, Loiselle J, Brenner L, Joffe M. Forensic evidence findings in prepubertal victims of sexual assault. *Pediatrics.* 2000;106(1 pt 1):100-104.
30. Dahlke MB, Cooke C, Cunnane M, Chawla J, Lau P. Identification of semen in 500 patients seen because of rape. *Am J Clin Pathol.* 1977;68(6):740-746.
31. De Jong AR, Rose M. Legal proof of child sexual abuse in the absence of physical evidence. *Pediatrics.* 1991;88(3):506-511.
32. Palusci VJ, Cox EO, Shatz EM, Schultze JM. Urgent medical assessment after child sexual abuse. *Child Abuse Negl.* 2006;30(4):367-380.
33. Tilelli JA, Turek D, Jaffe AC. Sexual abuse of children: clinical findings and implications for management. *N Engl J Med.* 1980;302(6):319-323.
34. Young KL, Jones JG, Worthington T, Simpson P, Casey PH. Forensic laboratory evidence in sexually abused children and adolescents. *Arch Pediatr Adolesc Med.* 2006;160(6):585-588.
35. Girardet R, Bolton K, Lahoti S, et al. Collection of forensic evidence from pediatric victims of sexual assault. *Pediatrics.* 2011;128(2):233-238.
36. Gringas F, Paquet C, Bazinet M, et al. Biological and DNA evidence in 1000 sexual assault cases. *Forensic Sci Int Genet.* 2009;2(1):138-140.
37. Exline DL, Smith FP, Drexler SG. Frequency of pubic hair transfer during sexual intercourse. *J Forensic Sci.* 1998;43(3):505-508.
38. National Commission on the Future of DNA Evidence. *The Future of Forensic DNA Testing: Predictions of the Research and Development Working Group.* Washington, DC: US Department of Justice, National Institute of Justice; 2000.
39. Nelson DG, Santucci KA. An alternate light source to detect semen. *Acad Emerg Med.* 2002;9(10):1045-1048.
40. Sweet DJ. Bitemark evidence: human bitemarks: examination, recovery, and analysis. In: Bowers CM, Bell GL, eds. *Manual of Forensic Odontology.* Colorado Springs, CO: American Society of Forensic Odontology; 1995:151-188.
41. Reesu GV, Brown NL. Inconsistency in opinions of forensic odontologists when considering bite mark evidence. *Forensic Sci Int.* 2016;266:263-270.
42. Sweet D, Lorente JA, Valenzuela A, Lorente M, Villanueva E. PCR-based DNA typing of saliva stains recovered from human skin. *J Forensic Sci.* 1997;42(3):447-451.
43. Allard JE. The collection of data from findings in cases of sexual assault and the significance of spermatozoa on vaginal, anal and oral swabs. *Sci Justice.* 1997;37(2):99-108.
44. Sharpe N. The significance of spermatozoa in victims of sexual offences. *Can Med Assoc J.* 1963;89(10):513-514.
45. Enos WF, Beyer JC. Spermatozoa in the anal canal and rectum and in the oral cavity of female rape victims. *J Forensic Sci.* 1978;23(1):231-233.

46. Annas GJ. Setting standards for the use of DNA-typing results in the courtroom--the state of the art. *N Engl J Med.* 1992;326(24):1641-1644.

47. Santucci KA, Nelson DG, McQuillen KK, Duffy SJ, Linakis JG. Wood's lamp utility in the identification of semen. *Pediatrics.* 1999;104(6):1342-1344.

48. Gabby T, Winkleby MA, Boyce WT, Fisher DL, Lancaster A, Sensabaugh GF. Sexual abuse of children: the detection of semen on skin. *Am J Dis Child.* 1992;146(6):700-703.

49. Mackenzie B, Jenny C. The use of alternate light sources in the clinical evaluation of child abuse and sexual assault. *Pediatr Emerg Care.* 2014;30(3):207-210.

50. West MH, Barsley RE, Hall JE, Hayne S, Cimrmancic M. The detection and documentation of trace wound patterns by the use of an alternative light source. *J Forensic Sci.* 1992;37(6):1480-1488.

51. Wawryk J, Odell M. Fluorescent identification of biological and other stains on skin by the use of alternative light sources. *J Clin Forensic Med.* 2005;12(6):296-301.

52. Seña AC, Hsu KK, Kellogg N, et al. Sexual assault and sexually transmitted infections in adults, adolescents, and children. *Clin Infect Dis.* 2015;61(suppl 8):S856-S864.

53. Centers for Disease Control and Prevention. 2015 sexually transmitted diseases treatment guidelines. *MMWR Recomm Rep.* 2015;64(RR-3):1-140.

54. Black CM, Driebe EM, Howard LA, et al. Multicenter study of nucleic acid amplification tests for detection of *Chlamydia trachomatis* and *Neisseria gonorrhoeae* in children being evaluated for sexual abuse. *Pediatr Infect Dis J.* 2009;28(7):608-613.

55. Centers for Disease Control and Prevention. Recommendations for the laboratory-based detection of *Chlamydia trachomatis* and *Neisseria gonorrhoeae*—2014. *MMWR Recomm Rep.* 2014;63(RR-2):1-19.

56. Centers for Disease Control and Prevention, US Department of Health and Human Services. *Updated Guidelines for Antiretroviral Postexposure Prophylaxis After Sexual, Injection Drug Use, or Other Nonoccupational Exposure to HIV—United States, 2016.* Atlanta, GA: Centers for Disease Control and Prevention; 2016.

57. Kellogg ND, Melville JD, Lukefahr JL, Nienow SM, Russell EL. Genital and extragenital gonorrhea and *Chlamydia* in children and adolescents evaluated for sexual abuse. *Pediatr Emerg Care.* 2018;34(11):761-766.

58. Hindmarch I, ElSohly M, Gambles J, Salamone S. Forensic urinalysis of drug use in cases of alleged sexual assault. *J Clin Forensic Med.* 2001;8(4):197-205.

59. Scott-Ham M, Burton FC. Toxicological findings in cases of alleged drug-facilitated sexual assault in the United Kingdom over a 3-year period. *J Clin Forensic Med.* 2005;12(4):175-186.

60. Juhascik MP, Negrusz A, Faugno D, et al. An estimate of the proportion of drug-facilitation of sexual assault in four U.S. localities. *J Forensic Sci.* 2007;52(6):1396-1400.

61. Beynon CM, McVeigh C, McVeigh J, Leavey C, Bellis MA. The involvement of drugs and alcohol in drug-facilitated sexual assault: a systematic review of the evidence. *Trauma Violence Abuse.* 2008;9(3):178-188.

62. Snead OC III, Gibson KM. Gamma-hydroxybutyric acid. *N Engl J Med.* 2005;352(26):2721-2732.

63. Anglin D, Spears KL, Hutson HR. Flunitrazepam and its involvement in date or acquaintance rape. *Acad Emerg Med.* 1997;4(4):323-326.

64. Schwartz AJ, Ricci LR. How accurately can bruises be aged in abused children? Literature review and synthesis. *Pediatrics.* 1996;97(2):254-257.

65. Gray-Eurom K, Seaberg DC, Wears RL. The prosecution of sexual assault cases: correlation with forensic evidence. *Ann Emerg Med.* 2002;39(1):39-46.

66. Jones JS, Wynn BN, Kroeze B, Dunnuck C, Rossman L. Comparison of sexual assaults by strangers versus known assailants in a community-based population. *Am J Emerg Med.* 2004;22(6):454-459.

67. Riggs N, Houry D, Long G, Markovchick V, Feldhaus KM. Analysis of 1,076 cases of sexual assault. *Ann Emerg Med.* 2000;35(4):358-362.

68. Sugar NF, Fine DN, Eckert LO. Physical injury after sexual assault: findings of a large case series. *Am J Obstet Gynecol.* 2004;190(1):71-76.

69. Jones JS, Rossman L, Wynn BN, Dunnuck C, Schwartz N. Comparative analysis of adult versus adolescent sexual assault: epidemiology and patterns of anogenital injury. *Acad Emerg Med.* 2003;10(8):872-877.

70. Feeney H, Chiaramonte D, Campbell R, Greeson MR, Fehler-Cabral G. Anogenital and physical injuries in adolescent sexual assault patients: the role of the victim-offender relationship, alcohol use, and memory impairment. *J Forensic Nurs.* 2017;13(2):52-61.

71. Hilden M, Schei B, Sidenius K. Genitoanal injury in adult female victims of sexual assault. *Forensic Sci Int.* 2005;154(2-3):200-205.

72. Strickland JL. Adolescent acute sexual assault: contrasting with adult experiences. *Obstet Gynecol.* 2001;97(4 suppl 1):S6.

73. White C, McLean I. Adolescent complainants of sexual assault; injury patterns in virgin and non-virgin groups. *J Clin Forensic Med.* 2006;13(4):172-180.

74. Rossman L, Jones JS, Dunnuck C, Wynn BN, Bermingham M. Genital trauma associated with forced digital penetration. *Am J Emerg Med.* 2004;22(2):101-104.

75. Fraser IS, Lähteenmäki P, Elomaa K, et al. Variations in vaginal epithelial surface appearance determined by colposcopic inspection in healthy, sexually active women. *Hum Reprod.* 1999;14(8):1974-1978.

76. Slaughter L, Brown CR, Crowley S, Peck R. Patterns of genital injury in female sexual assault victims. *Am J Obstet Gynecol.* 1997;176(3):609-616.

77. Lincoln C, Perera R, Jacobs I, Ward A. Macroscopically detected female genital injury after consensual and non-consensual vaginal penetration: a prospective comparison study. *J Forensic Leg Med.* 2013;20(7):884-901.

78. Jones JS, Rossman L, Hartman M, Alexander CC. Anogenital injuries in adolescents after consensual sexual intercourse. *Acad Emerg Med.* 2003;10(12):1378-1383.

79. Sachs CJ, Chu LD. Predictors of genitorectal injury in female victims of suspected sexual assault. *Acad Emerg Med.* 2002;9(2):146-151.

80. Ernst AA, Green E, Ferguson MT, Weiss SJ, Green WM. The utility of anoscopy and colposcopy in the evaluation of male sexual assault victims. *Ann Emerg Med.* 2000;36(5):432-437.

81. Zilkens RR, Smith DA, Phillips MA, Mukhtar SA, Semmens JB, Kelly MC. Genital and anal injuries: a cross-sectional Australian study of 1266 women alleging recent sexual assault. *Forensic Sci Int.* 2017;275:195-202.

82. American Board of Forensic Odontology. ABFO reference manual. American Board of Forensic Odontology Web site. https://abfo.org/resources/abfo-manual/. Accessed April 30, 2018.

83. Committee on Identifying the Needs of the Forensic Sciences Community, National Research Council. *Strengthening Forensic Science in the United States: A Path Forward.* National Academies Press, Washington, DC; 2009.

84. Heger A, Ticson L, Velasquez O, Bernier R. Children referred for possible sexual abuse: medical findings in 2384 children. *Child Abuse Negl.* 2002;26(6-7):645-659.

85. Campbell R, Patterson D, Dworkin E, Diegel R. Anogenital injuries in childhood sexual abuse victims treated in a pediatric Forensic Nurse Program (FNE) program. *J Forensic Nurs.* 2010;6(4):188-195.

86. Gallion HR, Milam LJ, Littrell LL. Genital findings in cases of child sexual abuse: genital vs vaginal penetration. *J Pediatr Adolesc Gynecol.* 2016;29(6):604-611.

87. McCann J. The appearance of acute, healing, and healed anogenital trauma. *Child Abuse Negl.* 1998;22(6):605-615.

88. McCann J, Miyamoto S, Boyle C, Rogers K. Healing of hymenal injuries in prepubertal and adolescent girls: a descriptive study. *Pediatrics.* 2007;119(5):e1094-e1106.

89. Jenny C, Hooton TM, Bowers A, et al. Sexually transmitted diseases in victims of rape. *N Engl J Med.* 1990;322(11):713-716.

90. Silverman EM, Silverman AG. Persistence of spermatozoa in the lower genital tracts of women. *JAMA.* 1978;240(17):1875-1877.

91. Muram D. Child sexual abuse: relationship between sexual acts and genital findings. *Child Abuse Negl.* 1989;13(2):211-216.

92. Tucker S, Claire E, Ledray LE, Werner JS, Claire E. Sexual assault evidence collection. *Wis Med J.* 1990;89(7):407-411.

93. Casey DG, Domijan K, MacNeill S, Rizet D, O'Connell D, Ryan J. The persistence of sperm and the development of time since intercourse (TSI) guidelines in sexual assault cases at Forensic Science Ireland, Dublin, Ireland. *J Forensic Sci.* 2017;62(3):585-592.

94. Ricci LR, Hoffman SA. Prostatic acid phosphatase and sperm in the post-coital vagina. *Ann Emerg Med.* 1982;11(10):530-534.

95. Graves HC, Sensabaugh GF, Blake ET. Postcoital detection of a male-specific semen protein: application to the investigation of rape. *N Engl J Med.* 1985;312(6):338-343.

96. Keil W, Bachus J, Tröger HD. Evaluation of MHS-5 in detecting seminal fluid in vaginal swabs. *Int J Legal Med.* 1996;108(4):186-190.

97. Wickenheiser RA. Trace DNA: a review, discussion of theory, and application of the transfer of trace quantities of DNA through skin contact. *J Forensic Sci.* 2002;47(3):442-450.

98. Dziegelewski M, Simich JP, Rittenhouse-Olson K. Use of a Y chromosome probe as an aid in the forensic proof of sexual assault. *J Forensic Sci.* 2002;47(3):601-604.

99. Hanson EK, Ballantyne J. A Y-short tandem repeat specific DNA enhancement strategy to aid the analysis of late reported (≥ 6 days) sexual assault cases. *Med Sci Law.* 2014;54(4):209-218.

100. Maiquilla SM, Salvador JM, Calacal GC, et al. Y-STR DNA analysis of 154 female child sexual assault cases in the Philippines. *Int J Legal Med.* 2011;125(6):817-824.

101. Johnson CL, Giles RC, Warren JH, Floyd JI, Staub RW. Analysis of non-suspect samples lacking visually identifiable sperm using a Y-STR 10-plex. *J Forensic Sci.* 2005;50(5):1116-1118.

102. Sibille I, Duverneuil C, Lorin de la Grandmaison G, et al. Y-STR DNA amplification as biological evidence in sexually assaulted female victims with no cytological detection of spermatozoa. *Forensic Sci Int.* 2002;125(2-3):212-216.

103. Delfin FC, Madrid BJ, Tan MP, De Ungria MC. Y-STR analysis for detection and objective confirmation of child sexual abuse. *Int J Legal Med.* 2005;119(3):158-163.

104. National Academy of Science. The evaluation of forensic DNA evidence: excerpt from the Executive Summary of the National Research Council Report. *Proc Natl Acad Sci U S A.* 1997;94(11):5498-5500.

105. Enos WF, Conrath TB, Byer JC. Forensic evaluation of the sexually abused child. *Pediatrics.* 1986;78(3):385-398.

106. Rimsza ME, Niggemann EH. Medical evaluation of sexually abused children: a review of 311 cases. *Pediatrics.* 1982;69(1):8-14.

107. Spencer MJ, Dunklee P. Sexual abuse of boys. *Pediatrics.* 1986;78(1):133-138.

108. Tintinalli JE, Hoelzer M. Clinical findings and legal resolution in sexual assault. *Ann Emerg Med.* 1985;14(5):447-453.

109. Rambow B, Adkinson C, Frost TH, Peterson GF. Female sexual assault: medical and legal implications. *Ann Emerg Med.* 1992;21(6):727-731.

110. McGregor MJ, Du Mont J, Myhr TL. Sexual assault forensic medical examination: is evidence related to successful prosecution? *Ann Emerg Med.* 2002;39(6):639-647.

111. Wiley J, Sugar N, Fine D, Eckert LO. Legal outcomes of sexual assault. *Am J Obstet Gynecol.* 2003;188(6):1638-1641.

112. Cross TP, Alderden M, Wagner A, Sampson L, Peters B, Lounsbury K. Biological evidence in adult and adolescent sexual assault cases: timing and relationship to arrest [published online ahead of print April 20, 2017]. *J Interpers Violence.* doi:10.1177/0886260517704229.

113. Cross TP, De Vos E, Whitcomb D. Prosecution of child sexual abuse: which cases are accepted? *Child Abuse Negl.* 1994;18(8):663-677.

114. Stroud DD, Martens SL, Barker J. Criminal investigation of child sexual abuse: a comparison of cases referred to the prosecutor to those not referred. *Child Abuse Negl.* 2000;24(5):689-700.

115. Brewer KD, Rowe DM, Brewer DD. Factors related to prosecution of child sexual abuse cases. *J Child Sex Abus.* 1997;6(1):91-111.

116. Kerns DL, Ritter ML. Medical findings in child sexual abuse cases with perpetrator confessions. *Am J Dis Child.* 1992;146:494.

117. Adams JA, Harper K, Knudson S, Revilla J. Examination findings in legally confirmed child sexual abuse: it's normal to be normal. *Pediatrics.* 1994;94(3):310-317.

118. Palusci VJ, Cox EO, Cyrus TA, Heartwell SW, Vandervort FE, Pott ES. Medical assessment and legal outcome in child sexual abuse. *Arch Pediatr Adolesc Med.* 1999;153(4):388-392.

119. Society for Adolescent Health and Medicine. Emergency contraception for adolescents and young adults: guidance for health care professionals. *J Adolesc Health.* 2016;58(2):245-248.

120. Ackerman DR, Sugar NF, Fine DN, Eckert LO. Sexual assault victims: factors associated with follow-up care. *Am J Obstet Gynecol.* 2006;194(6):1653-1659.

121. Girardet R, Giacobbe L, Bolton K, Lahoti S, McNeese M. Unmet health care needs among children evaluated for sexual assault. *Arch Pediatr Adolesc Med.* 2006;160(1):70-73.

122. Gavril AR, Kellogg ND, Nair P. Value of follow-up examinations of children and adolescents evaluated for sexual abuse and assault. *Pediatrics.* 2012;129(2):282-289.

Chapter 5

THE SEXUAL ABUSE POSTEXAMINATION CONFERENCE WITH FAMILIES

Karen J. Farst, MD MPH
Jerry G. Jones, MD

CHARACTERISTICS AND GOALS OF THE POSTEXAMINATION CONFERENCE

The characteristics of a postexamination conference, which takes place after the medical evaluation for suspected sexual abuse, vary and are driven by the age of the child, the perpetrator's relationships and means of engagement with the child, and the duration of contact. Throughout this chapter, ***parent(s)*** refers to the nonoffending custodial conference participants. The conference procedures are not different for other guardians as long as they have a legal right to the information.

The goals of the medical evaluation of child sexual abuse go far beyond an evidentiary examination.[1] The goals include: obtaining relevant medical history, documenting injuries or infections related to abuse, identifying medical conditions unrelated to the abuse event that may need treatment, assessing the safety of the child, screening for emotional and behavioral issues in the child that may require referral for further evaluation and treatment, and reassuring the child and family about the child's health when appropriate. Because most examination findings are normal, parents usually can be reassured their children have no residual injuries or infections related to the abuse event, allowing them to focus on safety and psychological needs.[2,3] Parents should also understand the importance of meeting their own emotional needs, because each person in the family is a victim. They should understand the community system for investigation and management, how to access it, and what to expect from it. If possible, they should be empowered to become informed and involved case managers for their children.

CONFERENCE PARTICIPANTS

The child sexual abuse examiner should participate in these conferences. Beyond the explanation of the medical findings, the examiner should be prepared to address some of the surrounding psychosocial issues of the child and parents. Differing levels of support personnel may be available to participate with the medical provider, depending on the resources of the medical facility and whether the examination is occurring within an entity such as a children's advocacy center (CAC), which has a formalized role for an advocate for the patient and family. Social workers, nurses, family advocates, child protective services workers, law enforcement investigators, and mental health and other professionals may contribute in their areas of expertise. The examiner may not need to be present during the entire postexamination conference if other participants are available. If others are not available, however, the examiner should be prepared to lead the conference, still functioning within a team structure that includes other professionals readily available for assistance when needed.[4]

Ideally both parents are present, although fathers are commonly absent despite staff encouragement to attend. Child victims old enough to receive information may also participate. Younger children may be involved only for reassurance of overall good health, because the sexual abuse examination is conducted in the context of a general examination. Parents should have time without their children present so they can discuss adult concerns or issues that may cause distress to the child if present. Older children deserve a conference without their parents to allow for a more open exchange of information.

Conference Procedures

The postexamination conference should be held in a comfortable room large enough to accommodate the participants without being intimidating in size. It should not be held in an examination or waiting room. Appropriate informational booklets for child and adult victims, printed material regarding referral resources, and paper for providing written instructions should be available. All participants should be present and introduced at the beginning of the conference. The examiner and other staff should be seated in a manner to allow eye contact among the participants to facilitate a conversation style encounter as opposed to the examiner or staff standing in the room with family and patient seated.

The components of the postexamination conference are summarized in **Table 5-1**. The conference can be divided into 2 fields of health care: medical and psychosocial. The order of their discussion is dictated by the parents' perceived reason for presentation and the professional with whom they have had the most contact. If the parents brought their child for a medical evaluation, the examiner should generally proceed first to meet their medical expectations. The transition from one component of the conference to the next should be stated clearly. The parents should be told the reasons for discussion of concerns that the parents did not vocalize, such as a wish to be certain a child will grow up to be emotionally healthy.

Medical Aspects

The examiner should explain the physical findings and their significance in lay terms. It is generally appropriate to assume the parents have little knowledge of genital anatomy. Parental understanding of the medical information is essential, whether or not findings of sexual abuse are present. Many patients and parents enter the medical evaluation with the belief that the examiner will be able to determine the presence, type, and severity of abuse that has (or has not) occurred. The examiner must be able to clearly communicate to lay people the results and limitations of the examination findings with rationale.

The reasons and research supporting an absence of physical findings indicative of abuse are covered in other chapters of this text. Some parents may use a lack of physical findings to decide the validity of their child's allegation of abuse. A parent's negative reaction to a child's disclosure may be heightened with the information that physical proof of the abuse is absent. The child who has made a credible disclosure that is not believed by the parent is at risk for re-exposure to the abuser, lack of support in working through the victimization, and endorsing self-blame.[5] Emotional support from a significant figure in a child's life is an important factor in development of resilience in the aftermath of sexual abuse.[6,7] A careful explanation of the implications of normal examination findings may prevent some of these safety and psychological risks.

The significance of abnormal findings should be explained. Parents need to understand that examinations are performed for both health and forensic purposes. Healed genital and anal injuries with forensic significance seldom have health significance. An explanation of the genital anatomy may help parents understand the location of an injury and

Table 5-1. Outline of the Sexual Abuse Postexamination Conference

STEP	DESCRIPTION
Introduction	— Provide an appropriate room. — Have all participants present and introduced at onset. — Provide seating for all participants.
Medical Component	— Describe and explain all findings. — Explain tests that were obtained, timeline for results to return, and how family will be notified of results. — Provide the forensic and/or health significance of the absence or presence of findings of sexual abuse. — Validate the child's feelings regarding the examination. — Provide information that will alleviate medical fears and address poor body image. — Make follow-up recommendations.
Psychosocial Assessment and Referrals	— Identify and alleviate sources of confusion, stress, fear, guilt, and shame. — Identify children who need referral for counseling, possibly using a child symptom report tool. — Identify parents' needs for counseling for stress, unresolved personal abuse issues, intimate partner violence, and substance abuse, possibly using a parent symptom report tool. — Make reassessment and referral recommendations.
Closure	— Summarize findings and reinforce recommendations. — Provide written recommendations and resource material.

the reasons for normal findings on examination of a young child said to have been penetrated genitally. The analogy of a teacup can be useful in distinguishing penetration of the labia from penetration of the hymen. The rim and bowl of the cup are analogous to the separated labia and vestibule, and the hymen is at the bottom of the vestibule/cup. Just as penetration of the bowl may not reach the bottom of the cup, penetration of the vestibule may not include penetration of the hymen. However, penetration of the labia majora meets the legal definition of "rape" in most jurisdictions. Penetration of the labia to the level of the hymen without vaginal penetration can cause the child to report an event as something going "in" and causing discomfort or pain.[8] This is especially true in prepubertal girls with unestrogenized hymens. It is important for caregivers to understand that the mucosal skin of the anal and genital areas can distend or stretch without necessarily tearing and that injuries to mucosal skin typically heal quickly and without visible findings of residual injury.[9,10]

Parents should be encouraged to ask questions about the medical evaluation. Verification of the history of sexual abuse may occur at this time or before the examination, depending on the clarity and accuracy of the information initially available to the examiner. The child should not be reinterviewed for forensic details of the event if a coordinated, detailed forensic interview has already been performed.[11] Information from the forensic interview should be shared with the examiner as part of a coordinated community response. Because the examiner is providing a medical evaluation rather than a focused forensic examination, a complete medical history, including family history, and system review should be performed to gather information that would not be collected in the forensic interview.[1] The examiner may uncover unmet health needs and other forms of abuse or neglect. The examiner is also in a unique position to relate symptoms of trauma (physical or emotional) to the abuse event. This could be pertinent to how the child has disclosed the abuse event (such as painful contact against an unestrogenized hymen with residual dysuria)[12] and can also serve as an opportunity to impress upon the family the importance of having the child assessed for the most appropriate form of trauma-focused therapy.[13,14]

Children's roles in accomplishment of their examinations should be praised and perhaps reinforced by asking them to provide a rating of the experience. Several standard measures have been suggested.[15] This expression of a child's feelings about the examination validates the child and gives some sense of control. Children's responses to appropriately performed examinations are usually positive, providing relief to parents.[16,17] Children should be firmly reassured that their examination findings are normal when that is true. Shame and poor body self-esteem can be harmful sequelae in the child who has been sexually abused.[18,19] For many children reassurance by a doctor or nurse that their body is normal and not damaged is the first step toward healing from the emotional trauma of the abuse.

When developmentally appropriate, postexamination explanations to children alone regarding the health of their bodies may answer questions that are too difficult for them to ask the examiner in the presence of their parents.[3] Many children have fears about their bodies that may or may not be rational, such as irreparable damage, pregnancy, future inability to have children, and sexually transmitted infections. These fears may be elicited during the conference alone with the child and should be addressed. Information provided to children should be provided to the parents as well, so they can reinforce the information in the recovery process. If the parent or caregiver was not with the child during or after the examination when these subjects were discussed, the provider should clarify with the child if this information can be shared with the parent or caregiver as part of their ongoing care, or if that would raise concern to the patient. If the child is struggling with sharing information related to sexuality or sexual health with their parent, the provider could offer to meet with the child and parent to facilitate the conversation and advocate for the child's concerns.

Psychosocial Aspects and Crisis Intervention

The children and family victims of sexual abuse are almost always in crisis. The onset of the crisis for the child may be when the sexual event occurred or began, and it may be intensified or diminished after disclosure. For the family, the crisis begins when the sexual abuse is disclosed. Although the crisis event and disclosure are commonly of a circumscribed duration, the responses of the child, family members, and community agencies are not.

Child sexual abuse examiners must have knowledge of common psychosocial factors and be prepared to offer guidance and referral; however, the psychosocial component does not involve psychotherapy. Crisis intervention in a single visit cannot substitute for the multiple visits commonly required for such treatment. Although medical professionals may perceive this aspect of the conference to be the responsibility of mental health or social work professionals, families in crisis look to medical providers for leadership. Sometimes the examiner may be the only child abuse professional available for the conference.

Crisis intervention historically has been designed to accomplish a single goal: the facilitation of recovery of relatively normal people after a single traumatic event. Similarly, a one-time postsexual abuse examination conference must have focused psychosocial goals to be effective. The family in crisis should not be overwhelmed with information. Generally, 2 goals are sufficient. A goal for the parents and older children is to *identify and alleviate sources of confusion, concerns, and stress*. A goal for all is to identify those children and parents who require referral to mental health services.

Some family concerns are commonly expressed and the examiner must be prepared to address them. Usual questions and potential responses, to be adapted to the context and psychological status of the parents, include the following.

Disclosure and Its Reliability

These frequently asked questions relate to the disclosure and its reliability:

1. Why did I not realize the sexual abuse was occurring?
2. Why did it take so long for my child to tell anyone?
3. Why did my child tell someone else and not me?
4. My daughter loves and misses her [father] and he loves her. Doesn't that indicate that he could not have sexually abused her?

The answers to these questions are based on the dynamics of child sexual abuse. Parents may not realize that sexual abuse is occurring because it is secretly performed by people the parents and children trust. Children may fail to recognize that an abusive relationship is wrong.[20] Delay in disclosure is also common if a child fears their disclosure could result in retribution or anger directed at them or harm to someone else.[20-22] Although the parent may be angry with the alleged offender, children who provide a reliable disclosure of sexual abuse may still love and miss the perpetrator. They simply want the sexual abuse to stop.

The answers to these questions may provide clues that a parent does not believe a child's credible disclosure, and they warrant exploration with the parent. A parent's denial of the validity of a credible disclosure may be based on general distrust of the child's truthfulness, allegiance to the alleged perpetrator, or fear of consequences. The provider should attempt to ascertain whether the caregiver will protect the child from the alleged perpetrator during the investigation. If it appears likely the child will not be protected, the appropriate child protection agency should be contacted for a safety disposition. Beyond the immediate safety of the child, parental denial of the sexual abuse and anger at the child for having disclosed the abuse can have significant negative effects on the child's well-being, including accepting self-blame for the event[5] and increasing risk of suicide.[23,24] Mothers who are unsupportive of a child's disclosure of abuse have been found to have more problems with substance abuse, criminal behaviors, and problematic relationships with their male partners compared with supportive parents.[25]

Conflict With Relatives

Questions regarding conflict with relatives are common:

1. My parents say I should not have reported the sexual abuse by my [brother], and they are attempting to get my daughter to change her disclosure. What should I do?
2. Does this mean my child cannot visit her [grandparents]?

Parents should be praised for supporting their child in the face of pressure from family members. Children should never be subjected to adults who try to change their disclosure, and any exposure to them should be with strict supervision. Parents often become estranged from relatives who choose to believe the denial of an offender over the disclosure of a child, resulting in loss of family support for one of the parents. The parent who loses family support often requires counseling to deal with this loss as well as the sexual abuse of the child.

Safety of the Child

The following 3 questions relate to the safety of the child or family:

1. What can I do about court-ordered visitation with the alleged perpetrator this weekend?
2. He has a history of violence. How can I protect myself and my child?
3. The offender is my teenaged son. He has nowhere to live but in our home. How can I protect my daughter?

Protection of the child and family must be a priority. Visitation with an alleged perpetrator should cease until an investigation has been completed. However, the parent could become in violation of a court order if a visitation is denied. In many states, an order of protection is easily obtained and will prevent a parent from being held in contempt. A parent should also consult the child protective services investigator, who may be able to obtain the alleged perpetrator's agreement to forgo court-ordered visitation until an investigation is completed. An attorney should also be consulted. The parent who fears violence from an alleged perpetrator should receive recommendations similar to those for battered spouses. If possible, the parent should seek a place of shelter. If that is not a realistic option, the parent's locks should be changed and the concern reported to law enforcement for additional advice. When the perpetrator is a sibling of the child, the children must be separated. The offender should be taken into state custody, admitted for a psychiatric evaluation, or live with a family member who has no children and can provide appropriate supervision. When a sibling who has perpetrated abuse remains in the home, concerns should be expressed to child protective services and another arrangement should be encouraged.

The Child's Behavior

Parents commonly ask at least 2 questions regarding their child's behavior:

1. Should I let my child talk about the sexual abuse?
2. Why did my child touch another child's genital area at childcare?

Some parents hope their child will forget the abuse. Other parents have personal fears about confronting the abuse. However, parents should listen to the child who wishes to talk and acknowledge that their child's ability to speak about the abuse is brave. The child who asks questions deserves age-appropriate answers. Parents should be encouraged to avoid asking the child in-depth questions while an investigation is in progress, and allow the investigators time to gather needed information. Repeated questioning of a child with pressure to provide details of the event could be perceived as coaching the child to provide information. The child's spontaneously expressed feelings should be validated. Sexually abused children often feel guilt, and they should be reassured that the abuse is not their fault. Most importantly, parents should reassure their children that they believe the disclosure and will work to keep them safe.[5] Some children find the sexual abuse to be a secret too emotion-laden to articulate to a parent, perhaps because of feelings of guilt, fear of punishment, or a wish to protect the offender or parent. A parent's anger toward the alleged offender can cause increased stress in the child.

A more appropriate response to questions about whether the alleged offender will be punished might be to explain that the alleged offender needs time or assistance to get help for his or her problem. A parent's persistent silence may reinforce the child's perception that the subject is off-limits or that the parent holds the child partially responsible for causing the family stress. The appropriate management, based on child and parental factors, can be recommended by the child's therapist.

Parents need to know that young sexually abused children may reenact the sexual act with toys, other children and adults, and themselves. Even highly focused behavior may resolve relatively soon after the sexual abuse ceases. If not, parents will need counseling in its management, and the child will need treatment if age appropriate. A common concern of parents is that their children may begin acting out sexually although they did not display such behavior at the time of the medical evaluation. The parents may become confused in attempting to differentiate between healthy and problematic sexual behaviors. Parents in general have been found to be in need of education on the range of age-appropriate sexual behaviors,[26] and they have voiced a desire to discuss the subject with their child's pediatrician.[27] The examiner should be prepared to describe the normal range of child sexual behaviors in relation to the developmental level of the child at the time of the examination.[28] Although no scale clearly defines normal and abnormal behavior, tools such as the Child Sexual Behavior Inventory have been normalized between sexually abused and nonabused groups to provide reference ranges for clinicians and parents.[29]

The Investigation

Parents commonly ask the following questions about the investigation:

1. How can I learn the status of the investigation?
2. My child would not talk to the investigator. Will that result in unsubstantiation of the abuse?

The multijurisdictional nature of a child abuse investigation can be confusing and stressful to a family that is already in crisis. A brief account of the local child protection and law enforcement and judicial structure can be helpful to the caregivers as they attempt to navigate an unfamiliar process. Studies of investigations performed with a coordinated, multidisciplinary approach versus segregated agencies show that both patient satisfaction[30] and legal outcomes are better with a coordinated response.[31,32] This may be partially attributable to the level of support the family unit receives in the coordinated process. Providing a summary of the investigation process and status, as well as resources such as investigator or victim advocate contact telephone numbers, may help bridge gaps between the family in crisis and the system.

If a child does not disclose abuse to an investigator, the likelihood that sexual abuse will be substantiated may be diminished unless other evidence exists. If a child has disclosed abuse to a parent but not to an investigator trained to interview children, an age-appropriate counseling referral may be helpful. The child may disclose more in the course of therapy.

Examination Findings

Parents may ask questions pertaining to the examination:

1. Will normal examination findings prevent prosecution?
2. Is my daughter still a virgin?

Normal medical evaluation findings alone should never prohibit prosecution.[33,34] However, it is likely that supporting evidence, such as a child who is able to provide credible testimony in court, another eyewitness, or a perpetrator's confession, will be needed. Most prosecutors are aware that child victims of sexual abuse commonly have normal examination findings, which the medical report should also state. The medical provider will be able to provide this information in court if needed. Emphasize that the priority at the time of the conference is protection of the child and emotional healing of the child and family.

The question regarding virginity is more difficult to answer. It is open to interpretation, depending on the beliefs and culture of parents and other participants in the postexamination conference. If the hymen is normal, the examiner can reassure the parents that physical evidence of sexual intercourse is absent (although a normal hymen does not rule out the occurrence of hymenal penetration). An explanation of the anatomy may help parents understand the difference between labial and hymenal penetration. Reinforcing to the parent that the child did not "give his or her virginity away" in an abuse or assault situation may provide some distinction to the issue as well.

In addition to identifying and alleviating sources of confusion, concerns, and stress, another psychosocial goal of the postexamination conference is to *identify those children and parents who need referral for mental health services.* This goal requires the assessment of the intensity of the effects of the sexual abuse and related events on the child as well as an assessment for co-occurring stress in the parent and potential dysfunction in the family unit.

The multifaceted psychological needs of the child must be identified and managed, because sexual abuse is associated with negative outcomes in childhood and adulthood. These negative outcomes include the following:

— High-risk sexual behaviors[35,36]

— Suicidality[37,38]

— Depression[39]

— Occurrence of other adverse childhood experiences[40]

— Teen pregnancy[41]

— Sexually transmitted diseases later in life[42]

— Early initiation of illicit drug use and later addiction[43]

— Eating disorders[44]

— Regular smoking and drinking in adolescence[45]

— Poor adult physical and mental health outcomes[46-48]

Evaluation of the Child's Psychological Distress

Although sexually abused children commonly experience fears, behavior problems, sexualized behaviors, poor self-esteem, depression, and posttraumatic stress disorder (PTSD), parents sometimes underestimate mental health issues in their children until asked about specific symptoms. Many tools are available to assess the presence of stress-related behaviors in children, including the Children's Depression Inventory,[49] Mood and Feelings Questionnaire,[50] Pediatric Symptom Checklist,[51] Trauma Symptom Checklist for Children,[52] University of California at Los Angeles (UCLA) Posttraumatic Stress Disorder Reaction Index,[53] and others (**Table 5-2**). Most of these validated screening instruments are time consuming to administer and require training or licensing in administration and scoring.

Table 5-2. Screening Tools for Behaviors in Children

CHECKLIST	LOCATION
— Child Sexual Behavior Inventory — Trauma Symptom Checklist for Children — Trauma Symptom Checklist for Young Children	— Available for purchase from Psychological Assessment Resources, Inc. (copyrighted materials) — 1-800-331-8378 — https://www.parinc.com/
— Children's Depression Inventory-2 (CDI2)	— Available for purchase from Pearson Education (copyrighted material) — https://www.pearsonclinical.com/
— Mood and Feelings Questionnaire	— Available for download with registration at http://devepi.duhs.duke.edu/mfq.html
— Pediatric Symptom Checklist	— Available for download from https://www.brightfutures.org/mentalhealth/pdf/tools.html
— UCLA PTSD Reaction Index	— Available for download with licensing agreement at https://www.reactionindex.com/index.php

A formal psychological screening evaluation is usually unnecessary at the level of the postexamination conference. Parents should be encouraged to accept referral to an appropriate mental health professional for assessment regardless of the presence or absence of reported symptoms. A brief, self-report questionnaire that includes somatic and emotional symptoms of distress (including suicidal ideations) may assist in separating those requiring emergent referral versus a scheduled appointment. These questions may include the following:

—Does your child have frequent headaches or stomachaches?

—Does your child have nightmares or difficulty going to sleep?

—Does your child have fear of a specific person or place?

—Has your child had a change in appetite or weight (loss or gain)?

—Has your child become aggressive or withdrawn (change from baseline)?

—Have you (has your child) talked about or caused harm to self?

—Have you (has your child) talked about or attempted suicide?

Family Support Structure

Although addressing the child's mental health issues in a postexamination conference is important, an assessment of the stability of the family support structure is equally necessary. Negative reactions to a child's disclosure of abuse can have harmful effects on the adult's well-being.[23] Parents may not volunteer information regarding their own disturbing mental health symptoms, but they usually provide compelling information when asked how they are handling their stress. They commonly report symptoms of PTSD, especially when told that parents who had bad experiences growing up often have difficulty with problems such as a recurrence of flashbacks when they learn their children have been sexually abused. Mothers who are still experiencing symptoms of trauma from their own past abuse are much more likely to have children with behavioral issues than mothers without a history of abuse.[54] A parent's unresolved mental health problems, including depression, may be exacerbated by a child's disclosure. Answering *yes* to the following 2 questions on a self-report questionnaire has been found to detect more than 70% of women with depressive symptoms[55]:

— Lately, do you feel down, depressed, or hopeless?

— During the past month, have you felt very little interest or pleasure in the things you used to enjoy?

Adverse Childhood Experiences

Child sexual abuse has been defined as an ***adverse childhood experience (ACE).*** Other ACEs, including physical abuse and neglect, are also commonly found in the homes of sexually abused children.[40] ACEs involving the family support structure include intimate partner violence (IPV) and substance abuse.[22] The examiner should ask about these issues during the postexamination conference and make appropriate referrals, if needed, because these issues can affect family functioning beyond parental health issues. All conference professionals should have information about and be prepared to identify and manage IPV and substance abuse.

Intimate Partner Violence

IPV is commonly found in families where children are reported as victims of abuse or neglect.[56] Also, children have been found to be at higher risk for an ACE such as abuse or neglect if IPV is present in the home.[57,58] Children of mothers who have been victims of IPV are more likely to have behavioral problems than children of nonabused mothers.[59-61] The American Academy of Pediatrics (AAP) has provided guidance for the clinician with suggestions for introducing the topic of IPV with parents[62]:

— We all have disagreements at home. What happens when you and your partner disagree?

— Is there shouting, pushing, or shoving? Does anyone get hurt?

— Has your partner ever threatened to hurt you or your children?

— Do you ever feel afraid of your partner?

Care must be taken when exploring the possibility of IPV. The parent's safety may be jeopardized if the offender finds shelter or hotline information in support material or in the patient's medical record.[62]

Parental Substance Abuse

Parental substance abuse is often associated with poor parenting, physical abuse, psychological abuse, and neglect, and often results in ACEs.[63,64] Substance abuse and IPV are often intertwined.[65] Parents may be asked if there is a personal or family history of illegal drug use. Screening questions such as the CAGE questionnaire and CAGE Adapted to Include Drugs[66] may be useful for inclusion on a self-report questionnaire.[67] A positive response to 1 or more of the following questions can be used as a positive screen.

— Have you ever felt you should cut down on your drinking or drug use?

— Have people annoyed you by criticizing your drinking or drug use?

— Have you ever felt bad or guilty about your drinking or drug use?

— Have you ever had a drink or used drugs first thing in the morning (eye-opener) to steady your nerves or to get rid of a hangover?

Ending the Conference

The stress of a child's disclosure and ensuing investigation may impede the family's ability to recall information from the conference. Written information should be available for the family to take home. The information should address follow-up, such as repeat blood tests, prescriptions, order of protection, examinations of siblings, or counseling. Other support information that may be provided, depending on issues identified during the conference, includes brochures; Internet sites; and telephone numbers for legal services, victim advocates, domestic violence shelters, and support groups such as Alcoholics Anonymous (AA), Narcotics Anonymous (NA), and parent and child sexual abuse support groups. The sexual abuse examiner should be prepared to provide resources and referral numbers to caregivers and iterate the importance of following through with the referrals.

The conference should be concluded with a verbal summary of information and recommendations. Parents should be commended for any actions warranting praise, and the examiner should offer to be available for questions that may arise later.

Prevention of Conference Problems

Postexamination conferences are often more difficult than expected. Although the psychosocial aspects of sexual abuse have been more researched than the physical aspects, gaps in information remain. A family's dysfunction can create a sense of chaos or futility, which is compounded by the flagging efforts of overburdened agencies. It is not surprising that new challenges regularly arise in these conferences. Perhaps the most troubling to professional participants is their vulnerability to questions and family issues for which they are not prepared. The most emergent may be the child who is at risk for suicide. Conference participants should establish a relationship with an appropriate mental health provider to deal with such cases promptly. Other issues such as the child's safety may require consultation with investigators, prosecutors, child protective services, or attorneys ad litem. Such resources should be established before problems arise.

Follow-up

A telephone call to the family within a few days after the conference can be beneficial. Parents often do not understand or recall information provided at medical visits, and this is likely a greater problem for emotionally charged families dealing with sexual abuse. Many parents are in denial or have difficulty focusing on meeting their needs and those of their children. Almost all families need additional encouragement or the opportunity to reaffirm the information and recommendations given in the postexamination conference.

Depending on the issues that need to be addressed, a social worker, family advocate, or other professional who was present at the initial conference can make this follow-up call instead of the medical provider. The caller should ask how the parents and children are handling stressors identified in the conference and ask about symptoms of anxiety, stress, and depression. The caller should also ask the parents if there are new concerns regarding themselves, their children, and the agency investigation. Prior recommendations should be reinforced. Parents should be given the results of tests that were performed at the initial visit. If the family members appear to be doing well, they should be encouraged to call if future concerns develop. Generally, no additional follow-up should be initiated unless requested, since it may appear intrusive.

Research Needs

Published studies regarding crisis intervention have primarily involved psychiatric and critical incident situations. Rigorous evaluations of postsexual abuse examination conferences appear to be absent in the published literature, and little has been written on the subject. Areas in need of research include the usefulness of screening measures for child and family stressors, the effectiveness of crisis intervention, parental understanding of information provided, and compliance with recommendations and referrals. Use of control groups is confounded by possible ethical issues, difficulty in matching subjects, and the potential availability of other sources of information and intervention.

Conclusion

The medical evaluation of a child victim of sexual abuse should encompass more than a forensic examination and provision of results to a family and agencies. Medical needs should be identified. A parent-completed report that includes the child's behavior symptoms and the parent's stress, depression, past physical and sexual abuse, neglect, IPV, and substance abuse can be a helpful adjunct to the postexamination conference. The examiner should determine that the child likely will be safe, supported, and provided needed medical and mental health treatment. Family members should receive support, intervention, and referrals for their stress, as well as enhancement of their ability to help their child. They should leave the medical evaluation process functioning more confidently and effectively than when they entered.

References

1. Adams JA, Kellogg ND, Farst KJ, et al. Updated guidelines for the medical assessment and care of children who may have been sexually abused. *J Pediatr Adolesc Gynecol.* 2016;29(2):81-87.

2. Jenny C, Crawford-Jakubiak JE; American Academy of Pediatrics. Committee on Child Abuse and Neglect. The evaluation of children in the primary care setting when sexual abuse is suspected. *Pediatrics.* 2013;132(2):e558-e567.

3. Leventhal JM, Murphy JL, Asnes AG. Evaluations of child sexual abuse: recognition of overt and latent family concerns. *Child Abuse Negl.* 2010;34(5):289-295.

4. Mitchell JT. Characteristics of successful early intervention programs. *Int J Emerg Ment Health.* 2004;6(4):175-184.

5. Melville JD, Kellogg ND, Perez N, Lukefahr JL. Assessment for self-blame and trauma symptoms during the medical evaluation of suspected sexual abuse. *Child Abuse Negl.* 2014;38(5):851-857.

6. Rosenthal S, Feiring C, Taska L. Emotional support and adjustment over a year's time following sexual abuse discover. *Child Abuse Negl.* 2003;27(6):641-661.

7. National Council on the Developing Child. Young children develop in an environment of relationships. Harvard University Center on the Developing Child Web site. https://developingchild.harvard.edu/resources/wp1/. Accessed August 10, 2017.

8. Anderst J, Kellogg N, Jung I. Reports of repetitive penile-genital penetration often have no definitive evidence of penetration. *Pediatrics.* 2009;124(3):e403-e409.

9. Heppenstall-Heger A, McConnell G, Ticson L, Guerra L, Lister J, Zaragoza T. Healing patterns in anogenital injuries: a longitudinal study of injuries associated with sexual abuse, accidental injuries, or genital surgery in the preadolescent child. *Pediatrics*. 2003;112(4):829-837.

10. Berkowitz CD. Healing of genital injuries. *J Child Sex Abuse*. 2011;20(5):537-547.

11. National Children's Alliance. Standards for accredited members. National Children's Alliance Web site. http://www.nationalchildrensalliance.org/ncas-standards-for-accredited-members/. Accessed August 10, 2017.

12. DeLago C, Finkle MA, Clarke C, Deblinger E. Urogenital symptoms after sexual abuse vs irritant contact in premenarchal girls. *J Pediatr Adolesc Gynecol.* 2012;25(5):334-339.

13. The National Child Traumatic Stress Network. Trauma types. National Child Traumatic Stress Network Web site. https://www.nctsn.org/what-is-child-trauma/trauma-types. Accessed August 10, 2017.

14. Cohen JA, Deblinger E, Mannarino AP. Trauma-focused cognitive behavioral therapy for children and families. *Psychother Res*. 2018;28(1):47-57.

15. Dubowitz H. Children's responses to the medical evaluation for child sexual abuse. *Child Abuse Negl.* 1998;22(6):581-584.

16. Marks S, Lamb R, Tzioumi D. Do no more harm: the psychological stress of the medical examination for alleged child sexual abuse. *J Paediatr Child Health.* 2009;45(3):125-132.

17. Palusci VJ, Cyrus TA. Reaction to videocolposcopy in the assessment of child sexual abuse. *Child Abuse Negl.* 2001;25(11):1535-1546.

18. Negrao C 2nd, Bonanno GA, Noll JG, Putnam FW, Trickett PK. Shame, humiliation, and childhood sexual abuse: distinct contributions and emotional coherence. *Child Maltreat.* 2005;10(4):350-363.

19. Eubanks JR, Kenkel MY, Gardner RM. Body-size perception, body-esteem, and parenting history in college women reporting a history of child abuse. *Percept Mot Skills*. 2006;102(2):485-497.

20. Schaeffer P, Leventhal JM, Asnes AG. Children's disclosures of sexual abuse: learning from direct inquiry. *Child Abuse Negl.* 2011;35(5):343-352.

21. Goodman-Brown TB, Edelstein RS, Goodman GS, Jones DP, Gordon DS. Why children tell: a model of children's disclosure of sexual abuse. *Child Abuse Negl.* 2003;27(5):525-540.

22. Kellogg ND, Menard SW. Violence among family members of children and adolescents evaluated for sexual abuse. *Child Abuse Negl.* 2003;27(12):1367-1376.

23. Ullman SE. Social reactions to child sexual abuse disclosures: a critical review. *J Child Sex Abus*. 2003;12(1):89-121.

24. Plunkett A, O'Toole B, Swanston H, Oates RK, Shrimpton S, Parkinson P. Suicide risk following child sexual abuse. *Ambul Pediatr*. 2001;1(5):262-266.

25. Leifer M, Kilbane T, Grossman G. A three-generational study comparing the families of supportive and unsupportive mothers of sexually abused children. *Child Maltreat.* 2001;6(4):353-364.

26. Pullins LG, Jones JD. Parental knowledge of child sexual abuse symptoms. *J Child Sex Abus.* 2006;15(4):1-18.

27. Thomas D, Flaherty E, Binns H. Parent expectations and comfort with discussion of normal childhood sexuality and sexual abuse prevention during office visits. *Ambul Pediatr.* 2004;4(3):232-236.

28. National Child Traumatic Stress Network. Sexual abuse: understanding and coping with sexual behavior problems in children. National Child Traumatic Stress Network Web site. https://www.nctsn.org/sites/default/files/resources//understanding_coping_with_sexual_behavior_problems.pdf. Accessed August 10, 2017.

29. Friedrich WN, Fisher JL, Dittner CA, et al. Child Sexual Behavior Inventory: normative, psychiatric, and sexual abuse comparisons. *Child Maltreat.* 2001;6(1):37-49.

30. Jones LM, Cross TP, Walsh WA, Simone M. Do children's advocacy centers improve families' experiences of child sexual abuse investigations? *Child Abuse Negl.* 2007;31(10):1069-1085.

31. Joa D, Edelson MG. Legal outcomes for children who have been sexually abused: the impact of child abuse assessment center evaluations. *Child Maltreat.* 2004;9(3):263-276.

32. Smith DW, Witte TH, Fricker-Elhai AE. Service outcomes in physical and sexual abuse cases: a comparison of child advocacy center-based and standard services. *Child Maltreat.* 2006;11(4):354-360.

33. Frasier LD, Makoroff KL. Medical evidence and expert testimony in child sexual abuse. *Juv Fam Court J.* 2006;57(1):41-50.

34. Finkel MA. Putting it all together. *J Child Sex Abus.* 2011;20(6):643-656.

35. Hillis SD, Anda RF, Felitti VJ, Marchbanks PA. Adverse childhood experiences and sexual risk behaviors in women: a retrospective cohort study. *Fam Plann Perspect.* 2001;33(5):206-211.

36. Bensley LS, Van Eenwyk J, Simmons KW. Self-reported childhood sexual and physical abuse and adult HIV-risk behaviors and heavy drinking. *Am J Prev Med.* 2000;18(2):151-158.

37. Bergen HA, Martin G, Richardson AS, Allison S, Roeger L. Sexual abuse and suicidal behavior: a model constructed from a large community sample of adolescents. *J Am Acad Child Adolesc Psychiatry.* 2003;42(11):1301-1309.

38. Dube SR, Anda RF, Felitti VJ, Chapman DP, Williamson DF, Giles WH. Childhood abuse, household dysfunction, and the risk of attempted suicide throughout the life span: findings from the Adverse Childhood Experiences Study. *JAMA.* 2001;286(24):3089-3096.

39. Chapman DP, Whitfield CL, Felitti VJ, Dube SR, Edwards VJ, Anda RF. Adverse childhood experiences and the risk of depressive disorders in adulthood. *J Affect Disord.* 2004;82(2):217-225.

40. Dong M, Anda RF, Dube SR, Giles WH, Felitti VJ. The relationship of exposure to childhood sexual abuse to other forms of abuse, neglect, and household dysfunction during childhood. *Child Abuse Negl.* 2003;27(6):625-639.

41. Hillis SD, Anda RF, Dube SR, Felitti VJ, Marchbanks PA, Marks JS. The association between adverse childhood experiences and adolescent pregnancy, long-term psychosocial consequences, and fetal death. *Pediatrics.* 2004;113(2):320-327.

42. Hillis SD, Anda RF, Felitti VJ, Nordenberg D, Marchbanks PA. Adverse childhood experiences and sexually transmitted diseases in men and women: a retrospective study. *Pediatrics.* 2000;106(1):e11.

43. Dube SR, Felitti VJ, Dong M, Giles WH, Anda RF. The impact of adverse childhood experiences on health problems: evidence from four birth cohorts dating back to 1900. *Prev Med.* 2003;37(3):268-277.

44. Ackard DM, Neumark-Sztainer D, Hannan PJ, French S, Story M. Binge and purge behavior among adolescents: associations with sexual and physical abuse in a nationally representative sample: the Commonwealth Fund survey. *Child Abuse Negl.* 2001;25(6):771-785.

45. Simantov E, Schoen C, Klein JD. Health-compromising behaviors: why do adolescents smoke or drink? identifying underlying risk and protective factors. *Arch Pediatr Adolesc Med.* 2000;154(10):1025-1033.

46. Dong M, Giles WH, Felitti VJ, et al. Insights into causal pathways for ischemic heart disease: adverse childhood experiences study. *Circulation.* 2004;110(13):1761-1766.

47. Felitti VJ, Anda RF, Nordenberg D, et al. Relationship of childhood abuse and household dysfunction to many of the lauding causes of death in adults: the Adverse Childhood Experiences (ACE) Study. *Am J Prev Med.* 1998;14(4):245-258.

48. Dube SR, Felitti VJ, Dong M, Chapman DP, Giles WH, Anda RF. Childhood abuse, neglect, and household dysfunction and the risk of illicit drug use: the adverse childhood experiences study. *Pediatrics.* 2003;111(3):564-572.

49. Timbermont B, Braet C, Dreessen L. Assessing depression in youth: relation between the Children's Depression Inventory and a structured interview. *J Clin Child Adolesc Psychol.* 2004;33(1):149-157.

50. Daviss WB, Birmaher B, Melhem NA, Axelson DA, Michaels SM, Brent DA. Criterion validity of the Mood and Feelings Questionnaire for depressive episodes in clinic and non-clinic subjects. *J Child Psychol Psychiatry.* 2006;47(9):927-934.

51. Reijneveld SA, Vogels AG, Hoekstra F, Crone MR. Use of the Pediatric Symptom Checklist for the detection of psychosocial problems in preventive child healthcare. *BMC Public Health.* 2006;6:197.

52. Briere J, Johnson K, Bissada A, et al. The Trauma Symptom Checklist for Young Children (TSCYC): reliability and association with abuse exposure in a multi-site study. *Child Abuse Negl.* 2001;25(8):1001-1014.

53. Steinberg AM, Brymer MJ, Decker KB, Pynoos RS. The University of California at Los Angeles Post-Traumatic Stress Disorder Reaction Index. *Curr Psychiatry Rep.* 2004;6(2):96-100.

54. Paredes M, Leifer M, Kilbane T. Maternal variables related to sexually abused children's functioning. *Child Abuse Negl.* 2001;25(9):1159-1176.

55. Dubowitz H, Feigelman S, Lane W, et al. Screening for depression in an urban pediatric primary care clinic. *Pediatrics.* 2007;119(3):435-443.

56. Hazen AL, Connelly CD, Kelleher K, Landsverk J, Barth R. Intimate partner violence among female caregivers of children reported for child maltreatment. *Child Abuse Negl.* 2004;28(3):301-319.

57. Dube SR, Anda RF, Felitti VJ, Edwards VJ, Williamson DF. Exposure to abuse, neglect, and household dysfunction among adults who witnessed intimate partner violence as children: implications for health and social services. *Violence Vict.* 2002;17(1):3-17.

58. Ernst AA, Weiss SJ, Enright-Smith S. Child witnesses and victims in homes with adult intimate partner violence. *Acad Emerg Med.* 2006;13(6):696-699.

59. McFarlane JM, Groff JY, O'Brien JA, Watson K. Behaviors of children who are exposed and not exposed to intimate partner violence: an analysis of 330 black, white, and Hispanic children. *Pediatrics.* 2003;112(3 pt 1):e202-e207.

60. Kernic MA, Wolf ME, Holt VL, McKnight B, Huebner CE, Rivara FP. Behavioral problems among children whose mothers are abused by an intimate partner. *Child Abuse Negl.* 2003;27(11):1231-1246.

61. Hazen AL, Connelly CD, Kelleher KJ, Barth RP, Landsverk JA. Female caregivers' experiences with intimate partner violence and behavior problems in children investigated as victims of maltreatment. *Pediatrics.* 2006;117(1):99-109.

62. Thackeray JD, Hibbard R, Dowd MD; American Academy of Pediatrics. Clinical report—intimate partner violence: the role of the pediatrician. *Pediatrics.* 2010;125(5):1094-1100.

63. Barnard M, McKeganey N. The impact of parental problem drug use on children: what is the problem and what can be done to help? *Addiction.* 2004;99(5):552-559.

64. Walsh C, MacMillan HL, Jamieson E. The relationship between parental substance abuse and child maltreatment: findings from the Ontario Health Supplement. *Child Abuse Negl.* 2003;27(12):1409-1425.

65. Cohen JB, Dickow A, Horner K, et al; Methamphetamine Treatment Project. Abuse and violence history of men and women in treatment in treatment for methamphetamine dependence. *Am J Addict.* 2003;12(5):377-385.

66. Brown RL, Rounds LA. Conjoint screening questionnaires for alcohol and other drug abuse: criterion validity in a primary care practice. *Wis Med J.* 1995;94(3):135-140.

67. Mdege ND, Lang J. Screening instruments for detecting illicit drug use/abuse that could be useful in general hospital wards: a systematic review. *Addic Behav.* 2011;36(12):1111-1119.

Chapter 6

Non-Emergent Medical Examination Procedures and Techniques

Nancy D. Kellogg, MD
Natalie N. Kissoon, MD, FAAP

Introduction

When sexual abuse is first reported, medical staff should determine when and where the medical evaluation should be conducted. Some communities have a single program or facility that provides evaluations for all victims regardless of when the abuse occurred, whereas other communities have one program for victims with recent or acute injuries and another for victims who were abused several days or more prior to clinical presentation. Victims of recent abuse are likely to require forensic evidence collection, photodocumentation, or treatment for injuries. Victims of chronic or remote abuse usually do not have emergent medical or forensic needs and their medical evaluations can occur in an outpatient setting. Child advocacy centers and outpatient facilities often provide a child-friendly, calm, safe, and supportive setting for non-emergent medical evaluations, victim assistance, counseling, and other services.

Indications for a Medical Assessment

Because the majority of examinations for sexual abuse do not show signs of trauma, some experts question the need for medical examinations, especially when the last incident of abuse occurred some time prior to examination. There are several reasons why the medical assessment is recommended:

— The child may not provide a full disclosure of the abusive act(s) and the examination may reveal evidence of penetrative trauma.

— The child and family are often concerned about whether the child's body is normal and, more specifically, whether the hymen is undamaged.

— Reassuring the child and family that the examination findings are normal may reduce anxiety and make the child feel less stigmatized by the abuse. Some cultures place value on the virginity of young females and may even deny certain celebrations (eg, a quinceañera) if a girl's virginity is in question.

— In court proceedings, jurors and judges may perceive the lack of a medical assessment as an incomplete investigation, negating the importance of the victim's statement.

— Some children are victims of repeated sexual abuse. Examinations with photodocumentation allow for detection and comparison of changes that can occur over time.

— The presence of a previously undiagnosed sexually transmitted infection (STI) such as *Chlamydia* or gonorrhea may be detected.

The need for an emergent examination is not solely dependent on the time frame of the last sexual abuse. Situations that may require an emergent examination more than 72 hours after the last abusive incident include:

— Anal or genital pain or bleeding

— Emergency contraception or postexposure prophylaxis for STIs[1]

— Penetrative trauma occurring within the last 7 days: Although forensic evidence is generally not collected more than 72 hours after the last abusive incident, acute injuries are sometimes visible for several days following abuse. Because injuries are likely to resolve completely within days, it is important to photodocument them for legal purposes.

— Submission of items, such as clothing and linens, for forensic analysis: These items can be collected and packaged in accordance with chain of custody procedures by either hospital personnel equipped for and trained in forensic evidence collection or by law enforcement.

— Psychological emergencies such as suicidal ideation[1]

— Safety concerns such as suspected human trafficking[1]

— Family or child request: Parents will have concerns when they learn their child has been sexually abused, even in cases in which the last episode of abuse occurred months earlier. A medical assessment conducted in the hospital can provide answers to common questions (eg, "Is my child OK?"; "Was my child penetrated?") and alleviate parents' fears expeditiously.

The Medical Examination: Setting the Scene

The medical examination of a suspected victim of sexual abuse should not cause the victim additional psychological or physical trauma. The keys to a successful genital examination of a child or teenager are:

— Adequate preparation of the child (and often the parent) for the examination

— Familiarity with and facility for various examination techniques and positions

— A confident yet sensitive approach

Overall, the clinician should prioritize the patient's need for respect, privacy, and control, especially if the patient is an adolescent. The goal of preparation is to reduce anxiety and to promote the child's sense of control. Ideally, patient preparation will be performed by a nurse or another qualified support practitioner. Preparation can be performed in the presence of parents to reduce their anxiety, as well. The child or adolescent should be shown the examination room and equipment prior to the medical evaluation. It may be helpful to show the patient a cotton-tipped applicator used for sample collection and let the patient touch the cotton tip to appreciate how soft it feels. With adequate preparation, most examinations can be completed without sedation.

If an examiner appears nervous or anxious, his or her patient is more likely to feel nervous and anxious. The child's privacy and need for control should be respected. The examiner should explain everything that is about to occur. Raising the head of the examination table allows the child to see the examiner and allows the examiner to gauge the child's reactions and anxiety during the examination. Children should be allowed to change into the examining gown in private and keep all other areas of their bodies that are not being examined draped. Children and adolescents should be allowed to choose whether they want a support person to be with them during the examination, although many adolescents prefer not to exercise this option. The examiner should avoid "shop talk" and move quickly and gently through the examination. When using any examination techniques, constant, even, gentle pressure should be applied, and groping and sudden movements should be avoided. Encouraging the child to talk during the examination may serve as an effective distraction. Some photocolposcopes use a digital system that captures and displays images on a computer. Children and their families may or may not wish to view such images; therefore, they should be informed ahead of time in the event that such images will appear on-screen during the examination.

A knowledgeable medical assistant or nurse can greatly enhance the examination. An assistant can show the child the examination room and orient the child to the various positions and equipment used during the examination. The assistant can also help position the child and provide distractions that may assist in relaxing younger children during the examination. By handing the examiner specula or swabs for specimen collection, ensuring that the child is adequately draped at all times, and capturing images as needed, the assistant can ensure that the examination is more efficient and more comfortable for the child.

If an adolescent or an older child adamantly refuses an examination, the examination can be delayed, barring immediate medical or forensic needs. In this situation, the clinician should clarify examination procedures and clearly explain what information the examination might provide. Doing so allows the adolescent to make a more informed decision about whether or not to undergo the examination. The following are common reasons that adolescents refuse examinations, followed by appropriate clinician responses:

1. ***Concern that a speculum will be used*:** In most instances, a speculum examination is not required. Vaginal swabs may provide adequate samples when the patient is reluctant to undergo a speculum examination. The physician should strive to minimize the trauma of the sexual abuse examination by utilizing less traumatic sampling techniques, such as using smaller swabs and using urine samples to test for STIs, in lieu of vaginal samples for adolescents who cannot tolerate vaginal sampling.
2. ***"I don't feel comfortable with anyone looking down there."***: The physician should clearly describe the examination techniques and explain the use of draping to reassure the adolescent that only one area of the body will be uncovered at a time. Additionally, the physician should emphasize the benefits of ensuring the patient's health.
3. ***"I know I am okay."***: The physician should explain that the only way to make sure someone is okay is through examination. Many, if not most, individuals with STIs have no noticeable symptoms.

Speculum examinations should not be conducted on the prepubertal child unless there is a need to establish and/or treat a source of bleeding or to identify a vaginal foreign body and should only be done with sedation. Digital examinations of the rectum are not informative and, therefore, not necessary.

Because children and adolescents are often victims of more than one type of abuse, suspected victims of sexual abuse should be examined carefully for any signs of physical abuse and neglect. A head-to-toe examination with careful and thorough inspection of all body surfaces may reveal inflicted injuries incurred either during the sexual abuse or as a result of the sexual abuse. For example, some adolescents who are sexually abused by strangers or peers are blamed for their assault and beaten by their parents. Additionally, signs of self-injurious behaviors (eg, cutting) may be found on the arms, legs, or abdomen. A treatment plan should ensure that these patients receive appropriate mental health services and that caregivers are aware and vigilant of these behaviors.

Victims of sex trafficking sometimes present in outpatient settings for evaluation and treatment. In such cases, it is important to document any tattoos, brands, or other body markings observed on examination. (Refer to Chapter 14, "Child Sexual Abuse: An International Perspective," for more information on the trafficking of children and adolescents.)

Examination Positions and Techniques

Practitioners who examine sexually abused children must be familiar with various examination positions (ie, patient placement) to ensure complete visualization of anogenital anatomy and the techniques (ie, examiner manipulation) required to perform a comfortable and thorough examination. These skills can be improved through numerous examinations of nonvictimized children and adolescents.

Examination Positions

There are 5 positions that may be helpful during the medical examination. Most examinations require only 2 of these positions: (1) either the supine frog-leg position or the supine lithotomy position, depending on the child's age and size, and (2) the prone or supine knee-chest position. For males, the genitalia may be examined with the patient lying supine on the examination table. Although the legs need to be parted during the testicular examination, a frog-leg position is not necessary. If testicles are difficult to palpate, the testicular examination should be conducted with the patient sitting up in a tailor position. The prone or supine knee-chest position is still recommended for males as this position provides the best visualization of the perianal structures.

Supine Frog-Leg Position

This position is used for smaller, prepubertal female children. The child places the soles of the feet together, with knees flexed laterally (**Figure 6-1-a**). Placing the feet on a pull-out shelf at the base of the examination table may allow for better manipulation and visualization of the genitals, especially if the shelf is slightly below the level of the table. Some clinicians allow the child to adopt a modified version of this position, with the child sitting in the mother's lap (**Figure 6-1-b**). This position usually provides an adequate view of the vulva, hymen, and vestibule. If abnormalities of the hymen are observed, examination in the prone knee-chest position is essential to confirm these findings (**Figure 6-2**). In the supine position, the normal hymen sometimes folds on itself, creating an artificial abnormality (ie, thickening, irregularity) that unfolds or normalizes in the prone knee-chest position. Additionally, hymenal hemorrhages may intensify and become more apparent in the prone knee-chest position.

Supine Lithotomy Position

This position is used for larger, prepubertal female children and all female adolescents. The feet are first placed in the examination table stirrups. The child then moves or slides the hips and buttocks to the end of the table and flexes the knees outward. This position provides an adequate view of the vulva, hymen, and vestibule.

Prone Knee-Chest Position

This position provides the best view of the perianal area. The child's shoulders, elbows, and forearms are placed on the table in order to make the lower back lordotic and to extend the hips upward. The knees are placed about 18 inches apart. The knees should be set at an approximate 90-degree angle. This position can be used to confirm irregularities of the hymen observed in the supine position. In the prone knee-chest position, it is possible to visualize the vaginal walls and cervix without inserting a speculum.

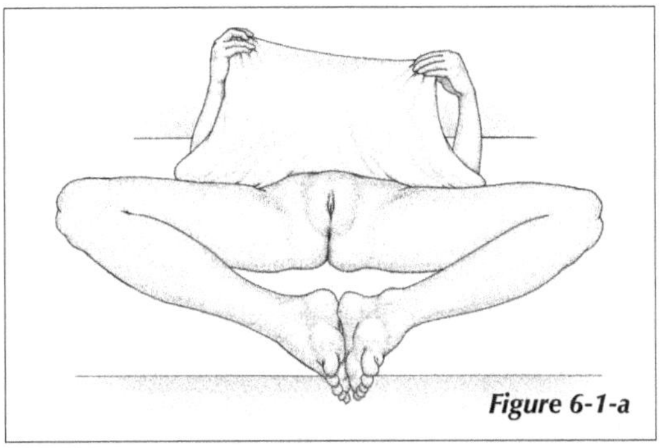

Figure 6-1-a

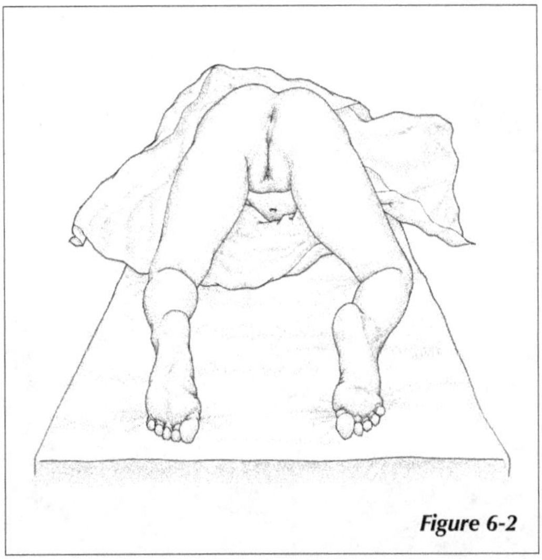

Figure 6-2

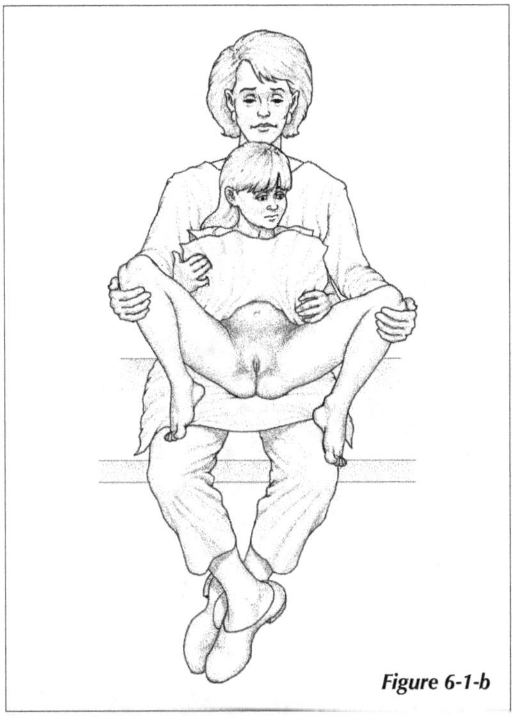

Figure 6-1-b

Figure 6-1-a. *A child in the supine frog-leg position.*

Figure 6-1-b. *A child in the supine knee-chest position while sitting on a caregiver's lap.*

Figure 6-2. *A child in the prone knee-chest position.*

Supine Knee-Chest Position

This position is generally used for anal examinations in infants and small, prepubertal children. The knees are drawn up to the chest in order to visualize perianal structures. This position is sometimes considered a less compromising position than prone knee-chest, and it allows the examination to be completed more quickly. The lateral decubitus position may be used instead of the supine knee-chest position, particularly when trauma to the anus is of low concern based on patient history.

Lateral Decubitus Position

This position can be used to examine the anus in all age groups. The knees should be placed together and drawn up to the chest, such that the anus can be visualized with minimal gluteal separation or distortion of the tissue. This position does not provide the optimal visualization accomplished with the prone knee-chest position; however, it is a good transition position between the supine and prone knee-chest placements, and it is preferable to the knee-chest position for gathering samples for evidence or STI testing.

Examination Techniques

For female patients, the examiner should begin with labial separation. With the patient in the supine position, the examiner moves the labia majora laterally and inferiorly, using the ventral/distal aspects of 2 to 3 fingers placed just below the inferior margins of each labium minus (**Figure 6-3**). Proceeding to labial traction, the examiner grasps the labia majora just above the posterior commissure, with the ventral aspects of the thumb placed medially and the lateral aspect of the first digit flexed at both joints. The examiner gently pulls the

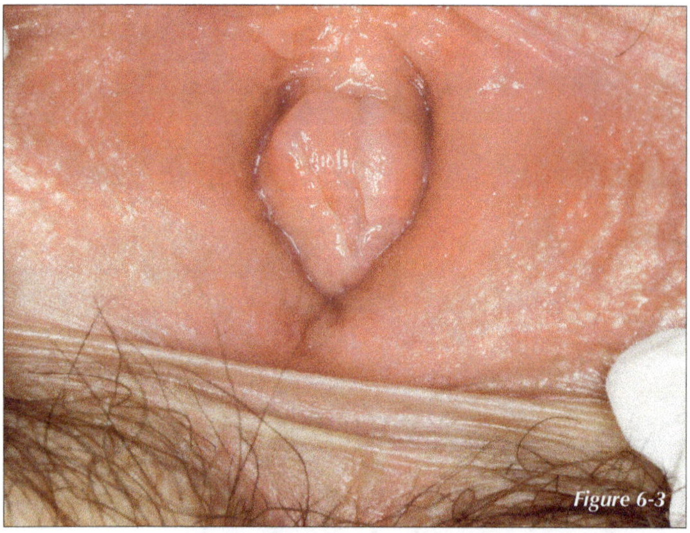

labia in the anteriorly (ie, toward the examiner). This technique often causes the folds of the hymen to separate and the opening of the hymen to become apparent (**Figures 6-4-a** and **b**). Moving the fingers superiorly and posteriorly affords the examiner several views of the vestibule and hymen.

The lateral decubitus position should follow the supine position. The examiner gently separates the buttocks, allowing some visualization of the anal folds. The examiner should be aware that applying excessive or uneven pressure

Figure 6-3. *Appearance of the hymen and vestibule, utilizing labial separation in the supine lithotomy position.*

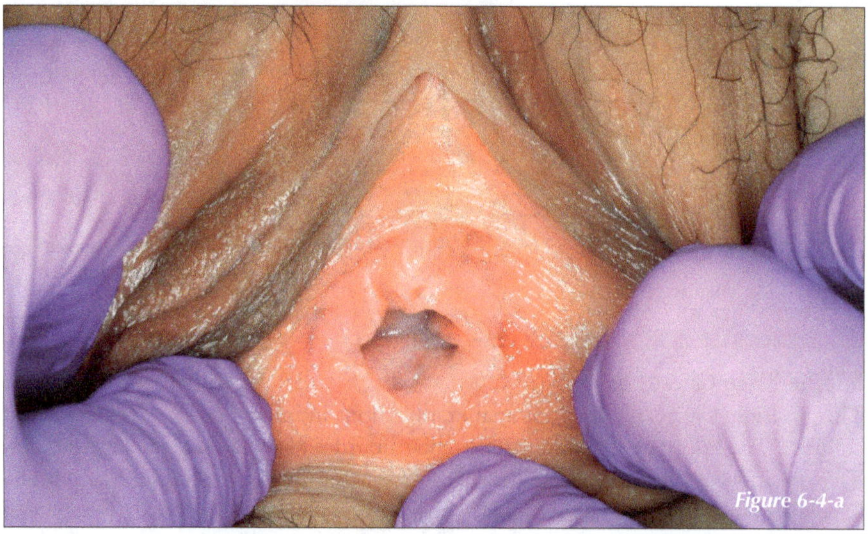

Figure 6-4-a. *Labial separation in an adolescent who is in the supine lithotomy position.*

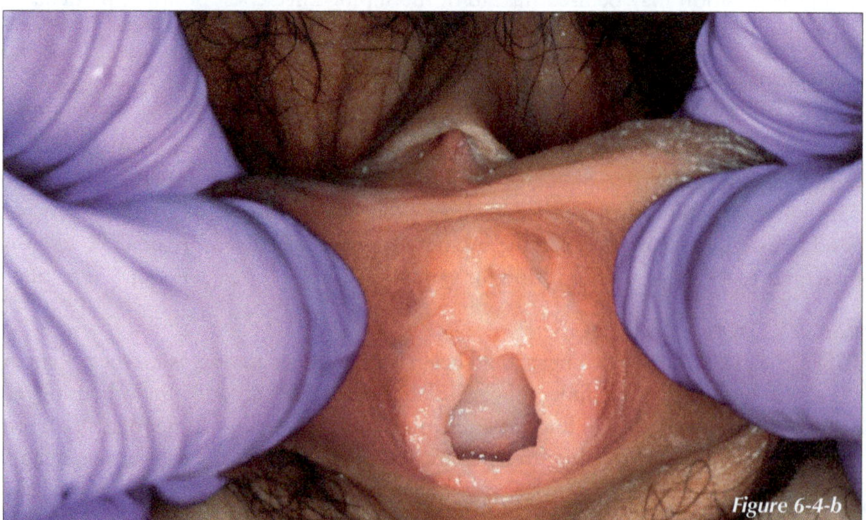

Figure 6-4-b. *The same adolescent, with the examiner using the labial traction technique in the supine lithotomy position.*

can potentially distort the anatomy. This position is primarily used prior to examination in the prone knee-chest position when there is little or no concern for sexual contact involving the anus or for collecting samples for forensic and infectious disease testing.

The final position is the prone knee-chest position. This position can be particularly embarrassing for the child, so the examiner should work quickly, keeping the child draped appropriately throughout this portion of the examination. The examination sheet should be draped over the child's hips and waist, and the edges brought down and together to form a small circular drape that uncovers first the anus and then the genitalia. An assistant or support person should hold the drape so it does not fall and cause undue embarrassment to the child. After the child is properly positioned, the examiner should visualize the anus and perianal tissues without tissue traction, then gently apply traction to the anal folds to reveal any excoriations, fissures, or scars. Significant anal findings are usually, but not always, visible without traction. After moving the drape downward to expose the genitalia, the examiner places the dorsal aspects of each thumb at the 2 o'clock and 10 o'clock positions of the posterior labial commissure (**Figure 6-5**). The examiner lifts the gluteus muscles upward while keeping fingers firmly placed on the buttocks superior to the thumbs, exposing the rim of the hymen. Complete visualization of the posterior rim of the hymen may require viewing each posterior third in sequence by lifting first with the left thumb, then straight up with both thumbs, and finally, lifting with the right thumb only. Apparent hymenal notches and clefts seen and/or demonstrated with cotton-tipped applicators should be confirmed in the prone knee-chest position (**Figures 6-6** through **6-9**).

Common examination position and technique errors include:

— Applying labial traction insufficient to adequately visualize the hymenal margins and vestibule

— Inadequate lower back lordosis while in the prone knee-chest position

— Inadequate lifting of the gluteus muscles with the examiner's thumbs during examination in the prone knee-chest position

Figure 6-5. *A child in the prone knee-chest position.*

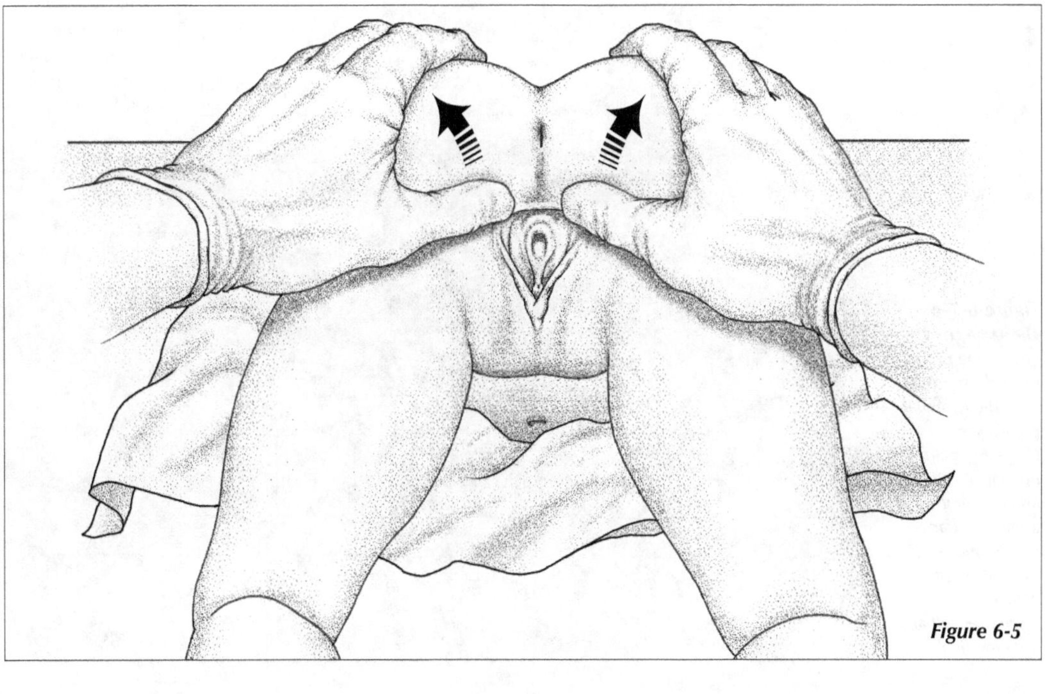

Figure 6-5

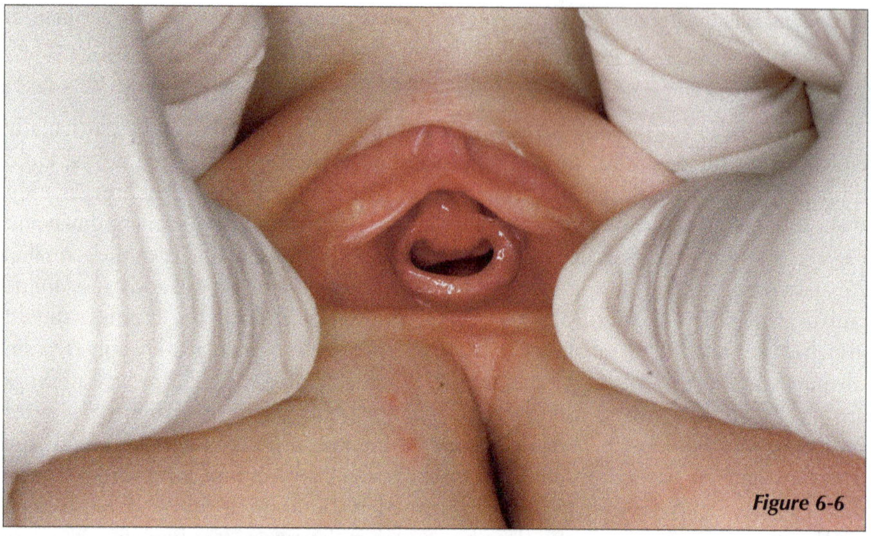
Figure 6-6

Figure 6-6. *Appearance of the hymen and vestibule, with the child in the supine lithotomy position and the examiner using the labial traction technique. The margins of the hymen are easily visualized from 1 o'clock to 11 o'clock.*

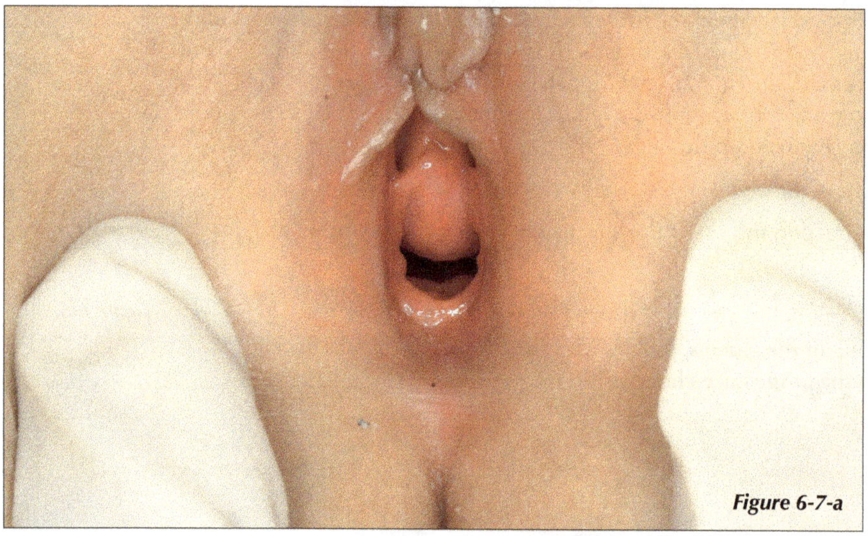
Figure 6-7-a

Figure 6-7-a. *Labial separation, with the child in the supine position. Note the bumps at 3 o'clock and 9 o'clock.*

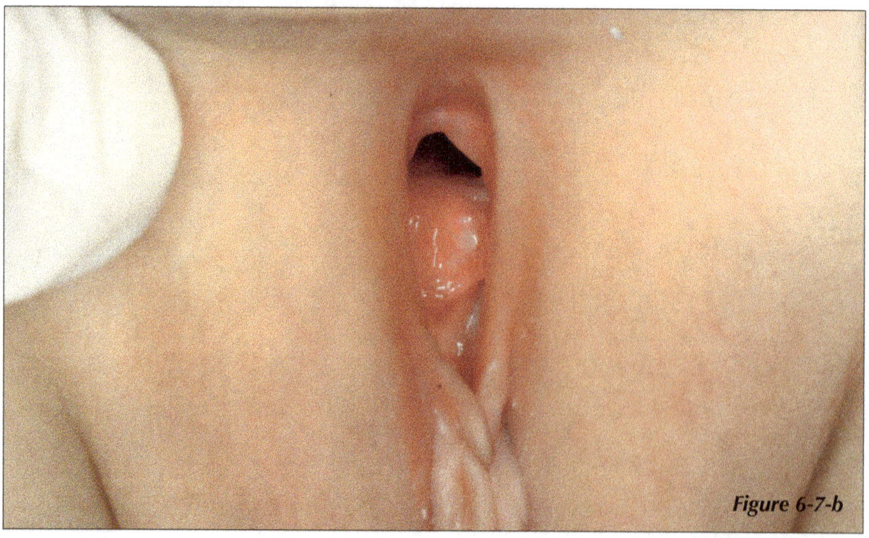
Figure 6-7-b

Figure 6-7-b. *The same child, now in the prone knee-chest position. The hymenal bumps seen in Figure 6-7-a are no longer visible, and due to the additional traction to one side, the child's left hymenal area is more exposed and asymmetrical.*

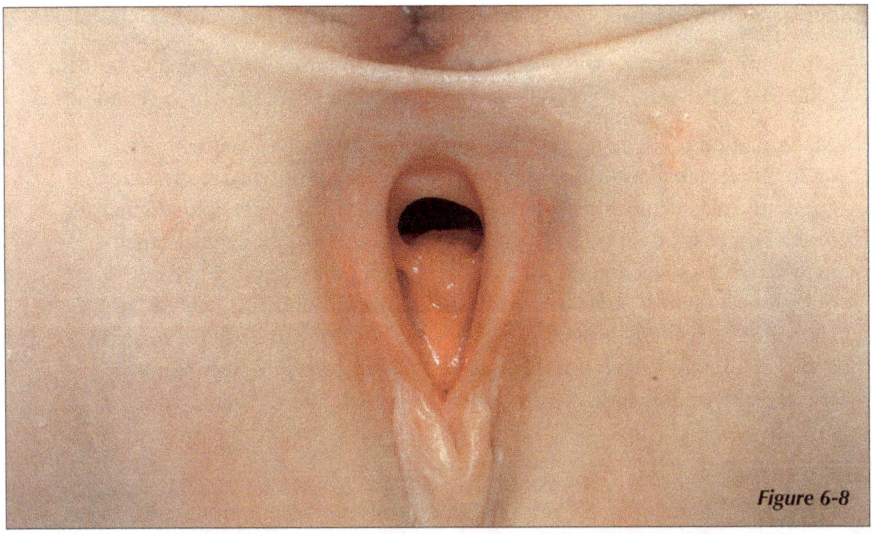

Figure 6-8.
Appearance of the hymen and vestibule, using knee-chest position. They hymen is crescentic and thin. The anus is also visible.

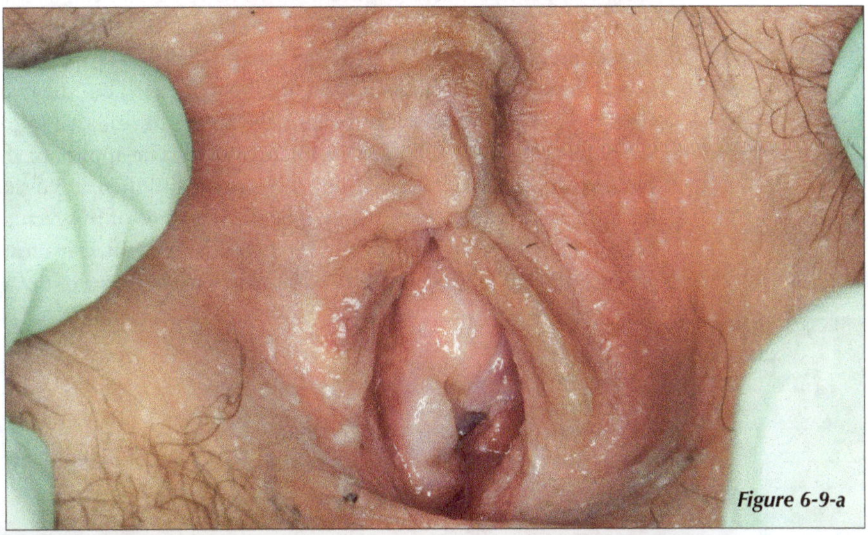

Figure 6-9-a.
A demonstration of labial separation showing hymenal injury, with the child in the supine lithotomy position.

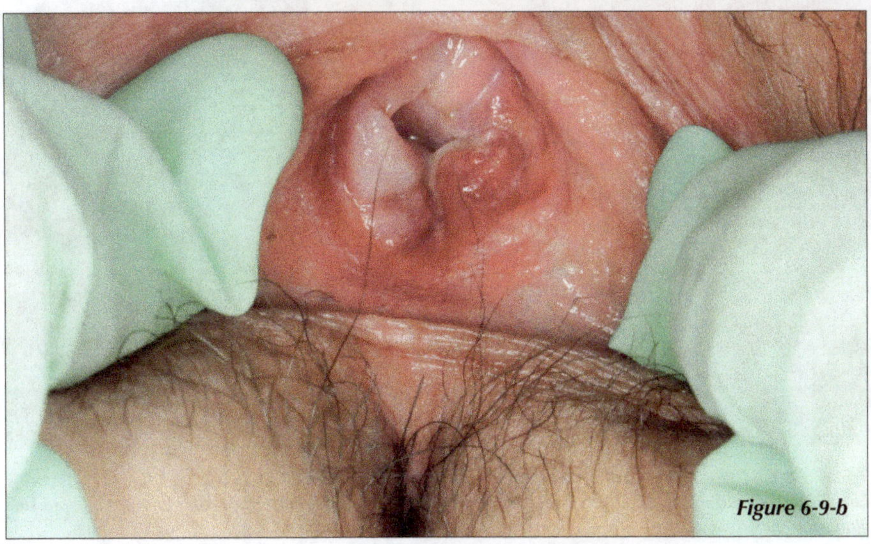

Figure 6-9-b.
A demonstration of labial traction showing hymenal injury, with the child in the supine lithotomy position.

Additional techniques that enhance visualization of genital structures include the following:

— Moistening the hymen with water or nonbacteriostatic saline so that redundant folds that adhere to the vestibule or vaginal structures are straightened and freed.

— Manipulation of the hymenal edges with a Foley catheter filled with water[2] or air[3]; a large, balloon-covered cervical swab[4]; or a moistened, cotton-tipped applicator may demonstrate clefts that are obscured by overlapping hymenal folds (**Figure 6-10**). The Foley catheter is inserted into the vaginal canal, inflated with a small amount of water, and then pulled gently in an external direction so that the edges of the hymen are splayed over the inflated catheter balloon. The balloon-covered swab is placed just inside the vaginal opening and then used to stretch out the hymen. Problems with this technique are considerable and include discomfort to the patient and the potential to misinterpret the hymen as missing or the hymenal rim as too narrow when the Foley catheter balloon flattens the hymen during extraction.

— Demonstration of hymenal rim integrity can also be accomplished utilizing a cotton-tipped applicator (**Figure 6-11**). The applicator can be used to reflect the folds of the hymen both externally and internally to allow for complete inspection of all surfaces. This is particularly useful to reveal occult hymenal hemorrhages. The examiner should attempt to stretch out the hymenal rim from 6 o'clock to 9 o'clock by placing the applicator internal to the hymen at 9 o'clock and gently pulling the hymen upward. The applicator should then be placed just inside the hymenal rim at 6 o'clock and then at 3 o'clock, stretching outward then upward respectively. The disadvantage of this technique is occasional patient discomfort and the potential to artificially create a defect or obscure a defect in the hymen due to incorrect placement of the applicator.

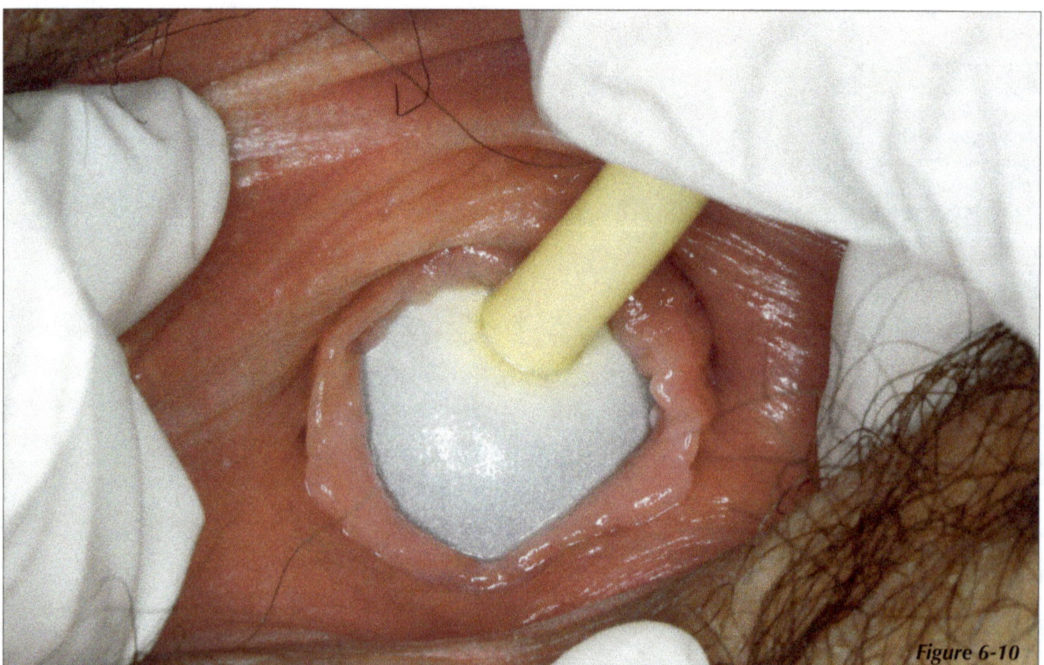

Figure 6-10. *This picture shows the Foley catheter balloon technique (using air) in an adolescent in the supine lithotomy position. The examiner placed the catheter into the vaginal vault and inflated the balloon with air. The examiner placed firm but gentle pressure close to the inflated balloon and pulled the catheter upward to allow for the display of the hymen's edges around the balloon.*

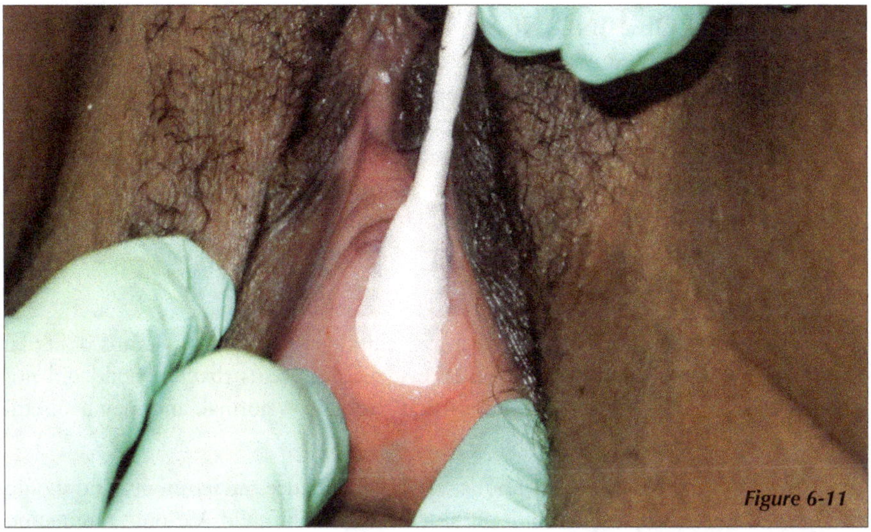

Figure 6-11. *Demonstration of the hymenal rim from 3 o'clock to 10 o'clock in an adolescent, using a large cotton-tipped applicator. There are no defects or transections present in the hymen.*

Photodocumentation

Photodocumentation of anal and genital examination findings, regardless of whether such findings are interpreted as normal or abnormal, is an accepted standard of care in the medical assessment of suspected sexual abuse. Additionally, equipment that magnifies and illuminates the genitalia and perianal tissues should be used during the examination.[5,6] Photodocumentation has become integral to peer review and quality assurance as the range of knowledge and expertise has broadened,[7] and it has provided a valuable adjunct for many studies of abnormal and normal anogenital findings. There are several additional advantages to photodocumentation.

— Photographs, video clips, and slides are valuable teaching aids.

— Changes in the examination findings over time may be accurately documented in some cases of repeat victimization.

— Images of trauma may be effectively presented in legal proceedings.

— Images of examination findings may obviate the need for repeated examinations when there is clinician difference in opinion.

— Photodocumentation allows for peer review and, when needed, mentoring.

Methods of Photodocumentation

There are a variety of methods for photodocumentation. Examination findings can be documented using a 35 mm camera with a ring flash, a digital camera, or a photocolposcope with a video or still camera attachment. Photocolposcope systems provide additional features that facilitate examinations, (eg, foot pedal shutter release and hands-free visualization, systems that incorporate patient record information with image captures, encryption features), but they are considerably more expensive than a camera-only system. During the examination, the photocolposcope or camera should be placed between the examiner and the patient, at a right angle to the plane of the anatomy being examined. In a 2003 study of 122 experienced clinicians (averaging 1700 examinations apiece), 85% used photocolposcopes.[4] In this study, photocolposcope use was significantly associated with a greater number of correct interpretations of anal and genital findings.

Images taken during a sexual abuse evaluation can be scanned into the computer or captured directly during the examination. Software programs are available to archive such data and create patient files. Images can then be encrypted and sent (or received) via electronic mail.

Discussion of Findings With Children and Parents

After completing the examination, the child should sit up and be adequately draped or changed into clothing before discussing the results of the examination. In a brief, age-appropriate way, the child should be addressed first about the examination findings. Children should be reassured that they are normal and healthy, and that even if minor injuries are found, they will heal quickly and completely. After discussing the examination with the child, a separate and more comprehensive discussion can be held with the caretaker(s).

Conclusion

A medical assessment is recommended for all children who may be victims of sexual abuse. The medical evaluation may reveal evidence of events that the child did not disclose, can reassure the child and family that the child is normal, and may be useful in court proceedings.

The medical evaluation should be conducted with confidence and sensitivity, and should not cause additional psychological or physical trauma to the child. Various examination positions and techniques are used, and photodocumentation should be used whenever possible. The results should be discussed with children and caretakers, and children should be reassured that they are normal and healthy.

References

1. Adams JA, Kellogg ND, Farst KJ, et al. Updated guidelines for the medical assessment and care of children who may have been sexually abused. *J Pediatr Adolesc Gynecol.* 2016;29(2):81-87.
2. Persaud DI, Squires JL, Rubin-Remer D. Use of Foley catheter to examine estrogenized hymens for evidence of sexual abuse. *J Pediatr Adolesc Gynecol.* 1997;10(2):83-85.
3. Jones JS, Dunnuck C, Rossman L, Wynn BN, Genco M. Adolescent Foley catheter technique for visualizing hymenal injuries in adolescent sexual assault. *Acad Emerg Med.* 2003;10(9):1001-1004.
4. Kellogg ND, Adams, J. The role of clinician expertise and training in the interpretation of examination findings in suspected victims of child sexual abuse. *SCAN.* 2003;15(4):1-2.
5. Jones JG, Lawson LL, Rickert CP. Use of optical glass binocular magnifiers in the examination of sexually abused children. *Adolesc Pediatr Gynecol.* 1990;3(3):146-148.
6. Bays J, Chadwick D. Medical diagnosis of the sexually abused child. *Child Abuse Negl.* 1993;17(1):91-110.
7. Adams JA. The role of photo documentation of genital findings in medical evaluations of suspected child sexual abuse. *Child Maltreat.* 1997;2(4):341-347.

Chapter 7

Evidence-based Approach to Child Sexual Abuse Examination Findings

Kelly Liker, MD, FAAP
Jonathan Thackeray, MD
Robert A. Shapiro, MD
Anthony C. Leonard, PhD
Kathi L. Makoroff, MD

Introduction

Competent clinical decision-making and treatment require knowledge of the published literature specific to the field in which one practices and the skills to critically assess the methodology behind these studies. Original studies must be carefully reviewed so that limitations, methodological errors, and unrecognized biases are identified before determining whether the stated conclusions are justified and whether the studies provide strong evidence that can be incorporated into patient diagnoses and care. Evidence-based medicine (EBM) stresses the examination of evidence from clinical research and from other sources by giving the practitioner a set of guidelines for use in interpreting available medical literature. Patient values, benefits, and risks must also be factored into the clinical decision-making process. There are many good resources available on the use of EBM and critical assessment of the literature.[1,2] This chapter provides a background on and examples of EBM relating to the diagnosis of children who have been sexually abused.

EBM uses the best combination of research evidence and clinical experience to optimize clinical diagnoses. In full, EBM consists of 5 steps: (1) formulating an answerable question, (2) finding the best evidence to answer the question, (3) critically appraising the evidence for validity, (4) integrating the critical appraisal with clinical experience and other patient circumstances, and (5) evaluating steps 1 through 4 to continually improve the process.[3] In part, the remainder of this chapter will address step 3, critically appraising the evidence for validity, by presenting the classic properties of diagnostic tests, which can also be applied to issues that are not generally thought of as diagnostic tests but that involve the prevalence of some trait across a group with or without a diagnosis. When assessing original research that pertains to interpreting diagnostic test results, it is useful to consider these 3 questions: (1) "Is the methodology sound and are the results valid?"; (2) "Does this test enable differentiation between patients with and without the condition?"; and (3) "How can the study results be applied to patient care?"

Methodology Soundness and Result Validity

The diagnostic validity of examination findings and laboratory test results must be determined through the study of subjects whose test results (ie, examination findings) and true disease statuses (ie, conditions) are known. The most appropriate study designs used to assess the diagnostic validity of examination and test findings are case-control studies and cross-sectional studies. Case reports or case series can be informative or suggestive, but the information derived from them cannot be used to rigorously establish the rates and proportions associated with a test. Although the double-blind, randomized, controlled study is often thought to produce the "strongest" evidence, it is not typically used to answer questions concerning the accuracy and usefulness of examination findings or tests, because neither the test results nor the conditions for which they test are under experimenter control. Well-designed and well-executed case-control and cross-sectional studies can provide valid and useful information by preventing or minimizing methodological errors that can cause bias and unjustified conclusions. Understanding the strengths and limitations of different study designs is necessary to critically assess methodology and results.

Case-Control Studies

The case-control study typically compares 2 groups to each other: cases and controls. The groups compared in many child abuse studies are children who have been abused (ie, cases) and children who have not been abused (ie, controls or "control subjects"). Cause and effect cannot be determined from the case-control study, and caution is always in order when conclusions are extrapolated beyond the population and conditions for observation from which the data were sampled. A limitation of case-control studies is that they cannot establish population rates for a condition, because the researcher sets the rate of sampled cases. A related strength of these studies is that they often require far fewer subjects than do cross-sectional studies, especially when the conditions or diseases studied are rare.

A common cause of bias in case-control studies is the failure to accurately select which patients should be considered cases and which controls. This type of bias is particularly prevalent in child abuse literature, because there is no gold standard available to accurately differentiate controls from cases. Without a gold standard, study designers must use a methodology that will minimize this type of error. If serious methodological limitations or errors exist, the resulting bias may lead to unjustified or incorrect study conclusions. Poor study design may also fail to remove the examination findings, test findings, or other study variables from case or control determination. For example, a study that is designed to identify examination findings in children who were abused but that also uses specific examination findings in selecting cases versus controls introduces this type of error. A less obvious design flaw that introduces the same error results when outcome data, such as court proceedings, are used to determine which patients are cases (ie, in the abuse group). The study variable, such as an examination or test finding, would likely have influenced the court's decision, thus causing this circular type of error. These methodological errors can invalidate the study's results.

Bias can also be introduced into a case-control study if the researchers who are measuring or assessing the study findings are not blinded to which patients are cases and which are controls. This type of bias, although unintentional, is not uncommon. Blinding will strengthen the conclusions of a case-control study.

Cross-Sectional Studies

A cross-sectional study examines a specific group of patients at a single point in time. This study design is applicable when asking questions such as "What is the normal configuration of the newborn hymen?" or "What is the appearance of the pregnant adolescent hymen?" The prevalence of disease or examination findings can be determined through the cross-sectional study. As in case-control studies, effective patient selection is critical to the study methodology and must be clearly understood before applying study conclusions to clinical scenarios. Cause and effect cannot be determined from the cross-sectional study, but this kind of study can provide information regarding findings in a specific population (eg, abused or not). For example, a cross-sectional study that examines the hymenal findings of pregnant adolescents may demonstrate that a certain percentage of adolescent girls have no hymen transections. It would, in that case, be reasonable to conclude that transections are not always found in the hymenal examination following vaginal penetration. The same study may find that a certain percentage of teens have transections of the hymen. However, a cause-and-effect relationship should not be assumed based on this study, and it would not be reasonable to conclude that transections are caused by vaginal penetration.

Case Reports and Case Series

A case report is a descriptive study of a single patient's clinical course, history, and findings. A case series is a descriptive study of more than 1 patient. Case series are useful when reporting rare events or events that have clear causation. A case report is typically published when it will provide new information or supportive evidence that will help professionals in the field. Examples of case reports include children who have sustained known genital trauma and how their injuries heal or reports of unusual events that result in mimics of abuse.

Review Articles and Summary Reports

Review articles summarize the available original research for the reader. The authors take responsibility for finding and critically assessing the research relevant to the topic. Although some summary reports provide more supportive documentation regarding research methodologies than others, reading and critiquing the original research will often provide the reader with a better understanding of the literature.

A meta-analysis is a specific type of summary report analyzing the mathematical data from numerous original studies. The meta-analysis combines studies that use quantitative methods to summarize results and, by combining data, the meta-analysis may be able to demonstrate a level of certainty increased beyond that of any of the individual studies. Meta-analyses are limited by the quality of the original research as well as issues that arise when combining studies that may use different patient populations.

Assessing Study Validity

Regardless of the type of study design, an assessment of the study population and the research methods is required to determine the validity of the study results. Research findings may be invalid because of bias in the study design, which can be introduced by poor patient selection (ie, selection bias) or lack of researcher blinding to patient characteristics (ie, measurement bias), as discussed in the previous sections. The following questions should be considered when assessing the validity of original research:

Regarding Study Population

— Who comprised the study population?

— How were they recruited?

— Was the selection of control subjects and cases appropriate?

— What bias may have been introduced by this selection and exclusion?

— Were patients who may have similar findings included in the study?

— Was an appropriate standard used to identify cases?

— Does this study population represent a general group of patients or only a small subset?

— Was the study population large enough to allow for the discovery of meaningful differences?

Regarding Study Methodology

— Were the study methods appropriate for addressing the stated hypothesis?

— Was circular reasoning excluded (ie, was the outcome made independent of any study variables)?

— Were measurement error and differences between examiners prevented? If not, were these factors assessed and accounted for in the statistical analyses?

— Was examiner bias reduced by including blinding in the methodology?

— Are examination findings well-defined and reproducible by other examiners in different settings?

— Have the study results been independently confirmed by another study?

Useful Patient Differentiation

A thorough understanding of research findings often requires knowledge of the statistical processes through which those findings are expressed. One particular set of statistical processes, those used to generate the properties of a diagnostic test, are sometimes especially relevant to studies of sexual abuse. The diagnostic test situation, in which a test with a dichotomous (ie, yes-or-no) outcome is used to predict a likewise dichotomous disease state, parallels the situation in which a dichotomous clinical finding is used to ascertain whether sexual abuse has occurred. The clinical finding acting as a diagnostic test for the condition of having been sexually abused is shown in the study by Berenson et al,[4] which is further discussed later in this chapter. A number of important numerical qualities of such a test can be calculated by using **Table 7-1** and the following formulae. The value of *a* is the number of patients who have the disease and test positive (ie, the number of children who have been abused and who have a specific examination or test finding). The value of *b* is the number of patients who do not have the disease and test positive. The value of *c* is the number of patients who do have the disease and test negative. The value of *d* is the number of patients who do not have the disease and test negative.

Table 7-1. Possible Relationships Between a Diagnostic Test Result and the Condition for Which It Tests

Status of Test	Positive for Disease/Condition	Negative for Disease/Condition
Positive Test Result/Finding	*a* (true-positive)	*b* (false-positive)
Negative Test Result/Finding	*c* (false-negative)	*d* (true-negative)

— ***Disease prevalence (ie, pretest probability)*** = $(a + c)/(a + b + c + d)$: Defined as the proportion of people who have the disease or condition and is sometimes simply referred to as prevalence. The posttest probability will be affected by the disease prevalence in the tested population. The posttest probability of a test is discussed later in this chapter.

— ***Odds ratio*** = $(ad)/(bc)$: Defined as the measure of the overall strength of the relationship between the test and the condition for which it tests. An odds ratio of 1 indicates that the test and the condition are unrelated (ie, the probability of having the condition is the same for those whose test results are positive as for those whose test results are negative). The odds ratio increases as the test and condition become more strongly linked, whereas an odds ratio between 0 and 1 would indicate that a negative test result was more predictive of the condition than was a positive test result. A useful property of the odds ratio is that it remains constant if the prevalence is artificially changed or specified, as occurs in a case-control study. In such a study, the research design dictates the prevalence of the disease, often requiring 1 case (ie, a patient with the disease condition) for every 1 control (ie, a control subject without the disease being studied). The odds ratio from the resulting table will match the odds ratio from the population as a whole, in whom the disease is far less prevalent than in the research sample. Note that when rows or columns of the table are reversed, the odds ratio becomes its own multiplicative inverse (*bc/ad*), indicating the odds in favor of negative test results. For this reason, a clear statement about the odds ratio takes the following form: "the odds ratio in favor of positive test results and existence of the disease condition is *X*, where an *X* greater than 1 indicates an association of positive test results and the condition or disease, and an *X* less than 1 indicates that a negative test result is associated with the condition or disease."

A shortcoming of the odds ratio as a summary statistic is that it does not enable differentiation between the 2 types of errors from the diagnostic test (ie, a positive test result in a study subject without the condition or a negative test result in a patient in whom the condition is actually present). These 2 errors may have very different consequences, so it is important to consider statistics that focus on one or the other.

— ***Sensitivity*** = *a/(a + c):* Defined as the proportion of patients with the target disorder or condition who have a positive test result or examination finding. A test with a high sensitivity will have few false-negative results (ie, negative test results for patients who actually have the condition), so that a negative test result should indicate with high probability that the condition is absent.

— ***Specificity*** = *d/(b + d):* Defined as the proportion of patients without the target disorder or condition who have a negative test result or examination finding. A test with a high specificity has few false-positive results (ie, positive test results for study subjects who do not actually have the condition), so that a positive test result should indicate with high probability that the condition is present.

It is assumed for the remainder of this discussion that sensitivity and specificity are fixed qualities of a test, invariant to changes in prevalence or to use of the test in different populations. In the real-life use of diagnostic tests, this is generally a reasonable assumption.

— ***Positive predictive value (ie, PPV, or posttest probability)*** = *a/(a + b):* Defined as the proportion of patients with a positive test result or examination finding who have the target disorder or condition. The complementary value is b/(a + b), the proportion of patients with positive test results who do not actually have the condition. The sum of these 2 values is 1. Given a particular sensitivity and specificity of a test, PPV is dependent on the prevalence of the condition. It is very important to keep in mind that, for rare conditions, a test with excellent (ie, very high) sensitivity and specificity can still have a high number of false positives, even to the point that most of the patients with positive test results do not actually have the condition. The dependence of PPV and NPV on prevalence means that unless a test enables flawless prediction, its usefulness is always dependent dependent on properties of the population in which it will be used.

— ***Negative predictive value (NPV)*** = *d/(c + d):* Defined as the proportion of patients with a negative test result or examination finding who do not have the target disorder or condition. The complementary value is c/(c + d), the proportion of patients with negative test results who actually have the condition. The sum of these 2 values is 1. As with PPV, given a particular sensitivity and specificity of a test, NPV is dependent on the prevalence of the condition.

The PPV and NPV are both dependent on prevalence, also referred to as pretest probability. If the prevalence of a condition is low, PPV becomes lower and, therefore, less useful, whereas the NPV becomes higher. This becomes an important factor when critiquing the literature and applying it to clinical child abuse decision-making. For example, when reviewing an article regarding the use of a new laboratory test designed to diagnose a sexually transmitted infection (STI), if the values given for PPV and NPV pertain to a population with a high incidence of disease (eg, an adolescent population), the PPV and NPV must be recalculated to take into account the low prevalence of STIs in the child abuse population. In a description of the qualities of a test, independent of any population to which it might be applied, it is informative to cite the likelihood ratios (LRs) of the test.

— ***Positive likelihood ratio (LR+)*** = sensitivity/(1 – specificity) = *[a/(a + c)] / [b/(b + d)]:* The positive likelihood ratio (LR+) represents the probability that someone with the condition will have a positive test result, divided by the probability that someone without the condition will have a positive test result. The LR+ is sometimes simply referred to as the ***likelihood ratio*** of the test, and it is desirable that a test have a high positive likelihood ratio. Because LR+ is dependent solely upon a test's sensitivity and specificity, the LR+ does not change when the population or prevalence changes; that is, LR+ is a property of the test alone.

— ***Negative likelihood ratio (LR–)*** = (1 – sensitivity)/specificity = *[c/(a + c)] / [d/(b + d)]:* The negative likelihood ratio (LR–) represents the probability that someone with the condition will have a negative test result, divided by the probability that someone without the condition will have a negative test result. It is desirable that this be a small number, much less than 1. Like LR+, it is a property of the test, independent of prevalence or population.

The LR of a test can be used to determine the relationship between the pretest probability (ie, prevalence) and the posttest probability (ie, PPV, or the proportion of patients testing positive who actually have the condition). The relationship makes use of the concept of ***odds***, where the odds of something happening is equal to its probability divided by 1 minus that probability. For example, something that happens 4 times out of 5 has a probability of 0.8 and odds of 4 divided by 1, or 4. The pretest odds of having a condition (ie, prevalence divided by 1 minus the prevalence) multiplied by LR is equal to the posttest odds, or the odds that someone has the condition, given that they tested positive. Those odds can be reverse-transformed into the posttest probability by the following transformation: probability = odds / (odds + 1). A likelihood ratio of 1.0 means that the posttest and pretest probabilities are exactly the same and that the positive test result is uninformative. In other words, having a positive test result does not make one any likelier to have the condition than that person was before taking the test (ie, the population prevalence). Two aids to making this transformation from pretest to posttest probabilities using odds and LR are the nomogram [ie, a slide rule-like chart that has the intervening calculations built in (see **Figure 7-1**)] and a table linking possible pretest and posttest probabilities (**Table 7-2**).

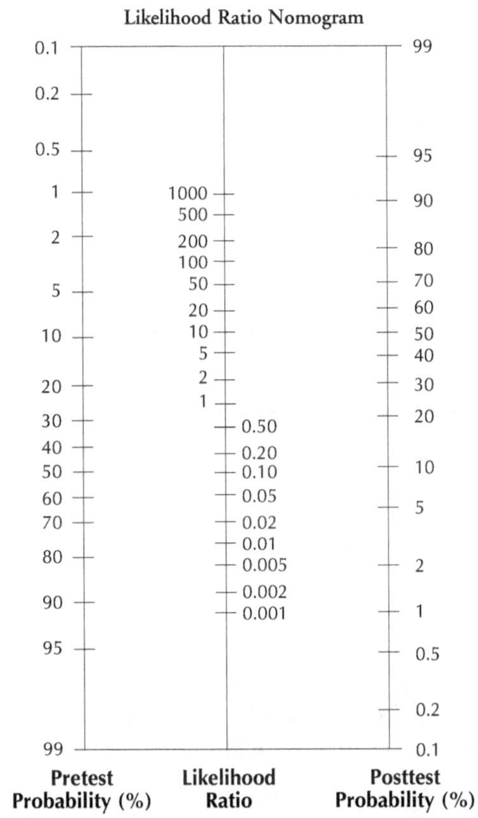

Figure 7-1

Table 7-2. Posttest Probabilities for Pairs of Likelihood Ratios and Pretest Probabilities

Likelihood Ratio	Pretest Probability					
	1%	**2%**	**10%**	**25%**	**50%**	**70%**
50	34%	51%	85%	94%	98%	99%
10	9%	17%	53%	77%	91%	96%
5	5%	9%	36%	63%	83%	92%
1	1%	2%	10%	25%	50%	70%
0.5	1%	1%	5%	14%	33%	54%
0.1	0%	0%	1%	3%	9%	19%
0.05	0%	0%	1%	2%	5%	10%

Figure 7-1. *Likelihood ratio nomogram. Adapted with permission from Centre for Evidence-Based Medicine.*[5]

— ***P values, hypothesis testing, and confidence intervals:*** The reporting of many statistics includes reporting of their associated *P* values, but evaluations of diagnostic tests are sometimes reported without *P* values. This is because *P* values usually address a null hypothesis of "no difference" or "no relationship." In the diagnostic test situation, this is a hypothesis that the test is worthless, or stated another way, patients with positive test results will have the same probability of having the condition as those with negative test results. Rejecting that null hypothesis and establishing that the test is probably not worthless meets a very low standard. The evaluators of the test are usually interested in establishing how good the test is, not whether it is any good at all. A different null hypothesis could be tested (eg, that the odds ratio is 3), but the selection of which odds ratio or other measure of the strength of the test/condition relationship to test tends to be arbitrary. For these reasons, statistics associated with test properties are often reported with confidence intervals (CIs) rather than with *P* values. The ***confidence interval*** quantifies the precision or uncertainty of a study result. A 95% CI is the range of values within which we can be 95% certain that the true value for the whole population lies. Another way of thinking about a CI is that 95% of such intervals will contain the true population value. As with *P* values, a larger sample size allows for more precision in estimates, shrinking the size of the CI.

The computation and use of many of the statistics just discussed can be illuminated through examination of a particular example. Data provided by the study performed by Berenson et al[4] shows the association between female children who have been abused sexually and the putative indicators of sexual abuse. In this study, a sample of 192 children who had been abused was compared to a similar sample of 200 children believed not to have been abused. Vaginal discharge was evaluated as an indicator of previous sexual abuse. The raw numbers from the study are presented in **Table 7-3**.

In the sample populations represented in **Table 7-3**, the prevalence of the condition of having been sexually abused is 192/392 = 0.49, or 49%. This prevalence is, of course, set by the researchers and is not informative concerning the prevalence of sexual abuse in the population at large. Most of the statistics derived from the table, however, are invariant across changes in population prevalence.

Table 7-3. Vaginal Discharge As an Indicator of Previous Sexual Abuse

Presence/Absence of Discharge	Abused Patient Population	Nonabused Patient Population	Abused plus Nonabused
Discharge Present (+)	21	8	29
No Discharge Present (-)	171	192	363
Total	192	200	392

The table has an odds ratio of (21·192)/(8·171) = 2.95 and an associated *P* value of 0.01, the derivation of the *P* value not being shown. The odds ratio indicates that the odds of experiencing discharge is almost 3 times as high in children who were abused as in children who were not abused.

The sensitivity of the test is 21/192 = 0.109, or 10.9%, meaning that only 10.9% of children who were abused were found to have vaginal discharge. The specificity is 192/200 = 0.96, or 96%, meaning that for children who were not abused, only 4% had vaginal discharge.

The PPV is 21/29 = 0.724, or 72.4%, meaning that a positive test result (ie, the presence of vaginal discharge) indicates, for this sample, a 72.4% probability of having been abused. The complement of this is 1 – 0.724 = 0.276, or 27.6%, meaning that if one assumes that a positive test result (ie, discharge) indicates previous abuse, one would be wrong 27.6% of the time. These numbers are dependent on the overall prevalence of child abuse in the sample (eg, the population at large). For example, in a population where abuse is much less frequent, most cases of vaginal discharge would occur in girls who had not been previously abused.

The NPV is 192/363 = 0.529, or 52.9%, meaning that among girls with no vaginal discharge, 52.9% had not been abused. The complementary rate of 47.1% indicates that if one assumes the lack of discharge indicates that no abuse has occurred, one would be wrong 47.1% of the time. Again, these numbers are dependent on the prevalence of abuse in the sample under consideration, which is a sample intentionally rich in abuse cases. These numbers would be far better (ie, with a higher NPV) if figured from the prevalence of abuse in the population at large and not only from the sample of sexually abused girls.

The positive likelihood ratio, or LR+, is 0.109/(1 – 0.96) = 2.7, meaning that abused girls had almost 2.75 times the probability of discharge as did the girls believed not to have been abused.

The negative likelihood ratio, or LR–, is (1 – 0.109)/0.96 = 0.93, meaning that the abused girls had a probability of not showing discharge that was just 7% lower (1 – 0.93) than that of girls believed not to have been abused.

Applying Study Results to Patient Care

The numbers reported above tell us many things about the use of vaginal discharge as a sign that sexual abuse has occurred. The odds ratio of 2.95 and its associated *P* value of 0.01 indicate that vaginal discharge is almost certainly associated with earlier abuse, but that the association is far from perfect. Only 10.9% of abused girls have discharge, meaning that we would not want to interpret a lack of discharge as indicating the nonexistence of abuse. The specificity of 96% means that among girls believed not to have been abused, only 4% will have discharge, indicating that perhaps discharge is a strong indicator of earlier abuse, because so few girls who have not been abused have it. It is also true, however, that because only 10.9% of the abused girls have discharge, a fair portion of girls with discharge have not been abused. That portion goes up as the prevalence of abuse goes down, to the point that if only 5% of a population of girls had been abused, 7 out of 8 girls with positive tests results actually would not have been abused. Thus, vaginal discharge should never be used as forensic evidence of abuse, and even in a clinical setting, one should (1) view discharge as a very weak indicator of possible abuse and (2) view a lack of discharge as a weak indicator of the absence of abuse.

Reviewing the Literature Regarding Child Sexual Abuse Examination Findings

The following sections contain a review of 3 original research articles to assess the research methodology and validity (ie, methods), to discern the usefulness of a diagnosis of child sexual abuse (ie, results), and to analyze the application of the research results to patient care.

Review of Cross-Sectional Study

Methods

In this cross-sectional study, Smith et al[6] describe the anogenital examination findings in nearly 3600 pediatric patients who were evaluated for suspected sexual abuse or assault. Examiners retrospectively reviewed examination photographs and patient files to determine examination findings. Examination findings were classified as normal, indeterminate, or diagnostic for trauma and/or sexual abuse/assault. The classifications were further defined in the article. For cases in which medical records were ambiguous or unclear, and in all cases in which findings were determined to be diagnostic, 2 research team clinicians independently reviewed the written documentation and photodocumentation for accuracy. The sample population included all children and adolescents younger than the age of 18 who underwent evaluation for suspected sexual abuse/assault and for whom an anogenital examination was performed and documented.

Methods Discussion

The authors designed this study to address a specific question encountered by many child abuse physicians: In what proportion of pediatric patients who undergo anogenital examination for suspected sexual abuse/assault are findings determined to be diagnostic? The additional goals of the study were to characterize these diagnostic findings and to analyze whether the identification of diagnostic findings is affected by variables of age, gender, or timing of examination. This population is suitable to answer the primary study question because it represents a large sample size of children and adolescents who receive anogenital examinations for suspected sexual abuse/assault. Bias caused by population selection is not an issue, and because this is a cross-sectional study, there are no control subjects. The selection of study population is appropriate to test the study hypothesis.

A significant limitation to this study, as stated by the authors, is that the Adams et al[7] approach to the interpretation of findings has been revised and updated since data analysis was completed. Specifically, 1 parameter pertaining to the interpretation of a healed hymenal transection was changed, which could have affected the classification of findings in this study. There were 22 patients for whom this finding was identified, and there was insufficient detail to distinguish which classification they might have received under the updated interpretation criteria. Additionally, photodocumentation was only reviewed for findings determined to be diagnostic; therefore, it is possible that patients determined not to have diagnostic findings were misclassified. Finally, it is not stated whether reviewers were blinded to the determinations made by the treating provider at the time the photodocumentation was reviewed by the research team clinicians.

Results

Examination documentation from 3569 pediatric patients was reviewed. Of the anogenital examinations, 87.3% were classified as normal, 6.9% were classified as indeterminate, and 4.8% were classified as diagnostic for trauma and/or sexual abuse/assault (excluding accidental trauma). Additionally, 0.9% of examinations were determined to be diagnostic of trauma from accidental causes. Factors that increased the likelihood of diagnostic findings included adolescence (ie, being aged 12 to 18 years), female gender, and examinations performed within 72 hours of sexual contact. The authors conclude that the prevalence of diagnostic findings in children and adolescents evaluated for sexual abuse/assault is low, especially for younger children and male children, and that timely examination from reported sexual contact is important. They also state that the study results support that medical findings should not be relied on to confirm or refute an allegation of sexual abuse/assault.

In regard to using this data in clinical practice, this study provides evidence that a majority of children and adolescents evaluated for sexual abuse/assault will not have diagnostic physical findings upon anogenital examination. To improve validity, future studies could use the updated criteria for interpreting findings, require photodocumentation review for *all* examinations, and could blind reviewers to the original determinations made by the treating physicians. The authors used a classification scale to define the examination finding categories of normal, indeterminate, and diagnostic. Readers should be familiar with this classification system and might need to consider how this study's findings would change should another classification system be used.

Review of Case-Control Study

Methods

Adams et al[8] designed this study to determine the frequency of hymenal notches and clefts and mean width of the hymen at the midline, comparing adolescent subjects who reported and those who denied having experienced penile-vaginal intercourse. Both case and control subjects (females aged 13 to 19 years) were recruited from a university adolescent medicine practice. Inclusion criteria for both groups included gender, age, established history of menstruation, and having a parent present to consent if the patient was younger than 18 years. Exclusion criteria for both groups included a history of past pregnancy or abortion, past episodes of forced sexual intercourse, and diagnoses of anorexia nervosa or anxiety disorder. Case subjects were those patients who reported a history of penile-vaginal intercourse and control subjects were those patients who denied a history of penile-vaginal intercourse. A history of penile-vaginal intercourse was determined via patient completion of a survey which included questions concerning home, education, history of abuse, drug use, behavioral health concerns, and sexual activity.

A complete physical examination by a child abuse pediatrician was completed in the office setting. Using a cotton-tipped swab moistened with water, the edge of the hymen was gently stretched to clearly define the amount of tissue present at the 6 o'clock position of the posterior rim of the hymen. Any areas that appeared to be notches or clefts were examined further. Photographs were taken using a 35 mm camera attached to a colposcope at 6x or 10x magnification and converted to slides. All slides were reviewed by one of the authors. Measurements of the width of the hymenal rim at the 6 o'clock position were taken using a calibrated measuring device. Slides from all subjects whose photographs clearly showed the entire hymenal rim were sent to 2 additional experts in adolescent gynecology. The reviewers were blinded to the patients' sexual histories and were asked to describe the location of any deep notches or complete clefts in the hymen, using a standardized definition. The student's t-test was used to compare continuous variables between subjects who said they had engaged in intercourse involving penile-vaginal penetration and those who said they had never experienced such contact.

Methods Discussion

The methods for this case-control study certainly allow for discussion of validity and application of the findings to larger populations. As the authors identify, the primary limitation of this study is a reliance on the subjects to accurately report a history of (or absence of) penile-vaginal intercourse. However, in the absence of a gold standard to diagnose previous sexual activity, studies such as these must rely on self-report. As such, the authors attempted to incorporate sexual history questioning into a larger survey to validate the results. A significant number of subjects approached refused to participate. Furthermore, more than 20% of images were lost to technical issues. How these limitations affect the study findings is unclear. Additionally, the original examiner was not blinded to the subject's sexual history, but the high inter-rater agreement on findings suggests that this did not affect the results. Their methods for the collection of study material (ie, diagnostic-quality photographic documentation, review of examination findings) seem sufficient; therefore, this study seems well designed and should provide valid results.

Results

Because of space limitations, only a few results will be discussed. It is estimated that only 1 patient in 10 approached agreed to participate in the study. A total of 85 subjects were recruited, with a mean age of 16.5 years. Twenty-seven subjects (cases) reported a history of consensual penile-vaginal intercourse, and 58 subjects (controls) denied such history. Due to poor-quality photographs, 18 subjects were excluded, resulting in 22 cases and 45 controls for further analysis. Using the Cohen's kappa statistic, a measure of inter-rater agreement, agreement between the examiner and each reviewer for findings ranged from 0.71 (substantial) to 0.85 (almost perfect).

The authors demonstrated significant differences in the examination findings between the case and control groups. Although the mean width of the hymenal rim between cases (2.5mm) and controls (3.0mm) lacked statistical significance, there were significantly more cases [6 out of 27 (22%)] than controls [3 out of 58 (3%)] with a posterior hymenal rim measurement of less than or equal to 1 mm wide. Additionally, when examining the 18-year-old to 19-year-old subjects, the authors found that lateral deep notches or complete clefts were significantly more common in cases [7 out of 11 (63%)] than controls [1 out of 10 (10%)]. Likewise, posterior deep notches were significantly more common in cases [7 out of 11 (63%)] than controls [2 out of 10 (20%)]. Perhaps most importantly, the authors found that upon examination, 14 out of 27 cases (52%) had normal hymens.

As with many case-control studies, there were no findings in this study exclusive to the case group (ie, posterior deep notch) that were not also seen in at least 1 subject of the control group. Even when a study reports a finding of interest seen only in cases and not controls, the reader is urged to resist the temptation to claim "certainty" about the finding. One must always consider the possibility that chance may account for the lack of findings in one group. For example, if one were to sample a random population of 200 in which a dichotomous (ie, yes or no) trait has a rate of 2 out of 200 (1%), the chance that one would find no cases in this sample is 13.4%. If the rate of occurrence is only 1 in 200, as seen in the some of the results of this study, the chance of finding no cases in this random population is 36.7%.

Nevertheless, this study contributes significantly to the literature, providing evidence that certain hymenal findings, such as lateral deep notches, complete clefts, and posterior deep notches may be more commonly seen in adolescents with a self-reported history of penile-vaginal intercourse. This study also reminds us that penile-vaginal intercourse often may not result in any abnormal physical examination findings.

Although the study incorporated strong methodology to minimize patient bias and interpretation bias, there are inherent limitations in the case-control design that cannot be avoided. Further research with a larger sample of subjects may support these findings.

Review of Case Series

Methods

Abraham et al[9] present a case series of well-documented vaginal rupture injuries following sexual assault. The case histories of 3 children and 1 adolescent who presented to the emergency department with these injuries are described. The authors provide detailed descriptions of presenting complaints, examination findings, surgical interventions, and investigative outcomes. High-resolution photographs of external genital and vaginal injuries are reproduced in the article.

Methods Discussion

There is no apparent bias in this study, and the investigators present data about each of the 4 cases sufficient to allow the reader to determine whether the case reports are valid. Although this case series involves only 4 patients, the data is useful for clinical practice because the study provides clinicians with a report of an unusual, but important, traumatic finding that may be seen in children and adolescents following sexual assault.

Conclusion

Understanding medical literature requires study using informed methodologies. Medical professionals involved in the medicolegal outcomes that often follow reports of child sexual abuse should be familiar with the original research that supports or refutes accusations of abuse. Detailed analysis of the original research is needed before making conclusions about a study's utility and applicability for a specific clinical question.

References

1. The Centre for Evidence-Based Medicine. Home Page. Centre for Evidence-Based Medicine Wed site. https://www.cebm.net/?o=1014. Accessed February 19, 2019.

2. Cochrane AL. *Effectiveness and Efficiency: Random Reflections on Health Services.* London, England: Nuffield Provincial Hospitals Trust; 1972.

3. Sackett DL, Straus SE, Richardson WS, Rosenberg W, Haynes RB. *Evidence-Based Medicine: How to Practice and Teach EBM.* 2nd ed. Edinburgh, Scotland: Churchill Livingstone; 2000.

4. Berenson AB, Chacko MR, Wiemann CM, Mishaw CO, Friedrich WN, Grady JJ. A case-control study of anatomic changes resulting from sexual abuse. *Am J Obstet Gynecol.* 2000;182(4):820-834.

5. Centre for Evidence-Based Medicine. Likelihood ratios. Centre for Evidence-Based Medicine Web site. https://www.cebm.net/2014/02/likelihood-ratios/. Accessed February 19, 2019.

6. Smith TD, Raman SR, Madigan S, Waldman J, Shouldice M. Anogenital findings in 3569 pediatric examinations for sexual abuse/assault. *J Pediatr Adolesc Gynecol.* 2018;31(2):79-83.

7. Adams JA, Farst KJ, Kellogg ND. Interpretation of medical findings in suspected child sexual abuse: an update for 2018. *J Pediatr Adolesc Gynecol.* 2018;31(3):225-231.

8. Adams JA, Botash AS, Kellogg N. Differences in hymenal morphology between adolescent girls with and without a history of consensual sexual intercourse. *Arch Pediatr Adolesc Med.* 2004;158(3):280-285.

9. Abraham M, Kondis, J, Merritt DF. Case series: vaginal rupture injuries after sexual assault in children and adolescents. *J Pediatr Adolesc Gynecol.* 2016;29(3):e49-e52.

Chapter 8

Interpretation of Genital and Anal Findings in Children and Adolescents With Suspected Sexual Abuse: State of the Science

Joyce A. Adams, MD

Introduction

The identification and interpretation of medical and laboratory findings in children with possible sexual abuse requires an evaluation by a health care provider who has a high level of knowledge, clinical expertise, and familiarity with the research studies describing findings in nonabused and abused children.

This chapter will review the changes in interpretation of medical and laboratory findings with respect to sexual abuse that have resulted from the publication, between 1989 and 2016, of cross-sectional, case control, and longitudinal studies of abused and nonabused children. An updated approach to the interpretation of findings in children with suspected abuse will be presented. This approach was developed as a collaborative project by a group of physician specialists who met to update and revise a classification system first proposed by Adams and colleagues in 1992.[1]

History

In the early 1980s, as the magnitude of the problem of child sexual abuse was becoming apparent, child protection and law enforcement agencies began to refer more children for medical examinations as part of the investigation of abuse allegations. The physicians who performed these examinations were handicapped, however, by a lack of data concerning normal anatomical variations in the appearance of the genital and anal tissues in children of different ages. As most children were not examined within hours or days of an episode of violent sexual assault, but weeks or months after the most recent molestation, signs of acute injury, such as bleeding or bruising, were often absent. Because most of the physicians who examined these children had not previously used magnification and specialized techniques to study the detailed appearance of children's genitalia, findings such as a hymenal opening appearing "too big" or dilation of the child's anus during the examination, among many others, were taken to be signs of abuse.

Studies in Genital and Anal Findings in Children and Adolescents With Suspected Sexual Abuse

Between 1989 and 1991, 3 studies that describe genital or anal findings in nonabused children were published. McCann et al[2] described anal findings in 267 prepubertal children who were carefully screened and found to have no suspicion of abuse. Of these 267 children, they obtained photographs of genital findings in 93 girls between 10 months and 10 years of age examined using a camera attached to a colposcope.[3] Another study, which describes the appearance of the hymen in newborn infants, provided additional normative data.[4] Data from these studies, along with recommendations from the American Academy of Pediatrics,[5] were used to develop the first version of a table describing an approach to classifying anogenital and laboratory findings in children with suspected sexual abuse.[1] This approach was not presented as a consensus document, but as a tool that might be helpful in descriptive studies concerning frequency of genital findings in studies of abused children. Many findings that had previously been interpreted as resulting from abuse, but were commonly documented in the studies of newborn infants and nonabused children, were listed as "normal" or "nonspecific." In the "suspicious" and "suggestive" categories, findings were listed that had been described in a small percentage of nonabused children but were also described in children giving a history of abuse. Findings in the "clear evidence of penetrating injury" category were all characteristic of trauma or the residua of trauma.

Between 1991 and 2003, additional studies were published, describing the appearance of genital findings in nonabused girls. Berenson et al[6] described the appearance of the hymen in 211 girls between the ages of 1 month and 7 years. Many of the features noted by McCann et al[3] were also seen in this study. Berenson's group later reported on a longitudinal study of hymenal development, following girls aged newborn to 9 years.[7-9] Several important changes were noted in the appearance of the hymen in girls over time: The horizontal width of the hymen opening increased with age, and the amount of tissue measured (from magnified photographs) at the 6 o'clock location decreased.

The table listing the different categories of physical findings has been revised several times since 1992. As additional cross-sectional studies reporting genital findings in nonabused prepubertal girls and healing of injuries have been published, findings have been added or reclassified.[10-13] Until 2005, versions of the table included 2 separate sections: "classification of findings" and "overall assessment of the likelihood of abuse." After consultation with colleagues, the table was condensed to focus on physical and laboratory findings only. The revised table was first published in the *APSAC Advisor* in the summer of 2005.[14]

Table 8-1 was collaboratively developed by a group of expert physicians, with support from the Midwest Regional Children's Advocacy Center. Between 2004 and 2006, this group developed guidelines for the medical care of children who may have been sexually abused. The guidelines were first published in 2007 and included an updated table listing suggested interpretation of medical and laboratory findings.[15] The members of this group updated the guidelines and table again between 2011 and 2018.[16,17] The updated table (Table 8-1) has been modified based on feedback from colleagues.

In 2016, a survey was sent to members of the Ray Helfer Society, an honorary society of specialist physicians in the field of child abuse evaluation. Participants were asked to list their level of agreement on how the medical findings listed in the table published in 2016 should be interpreted. The level of agreement with the listing of findings was between 89% and 100%, but several suggestions were made about the format of the interpretation of findings table. Some of the suggested changes are incorporated into the table below.

Research

The "gold standard" for research design in a study that tries to determine cause and effect is a randomized, double-blind control study, in which subjects are randomly selected to receive or not receive treatment or intervention and neither the subjects nor the researchers know who is receiving the treatment or intervention. This is obviously

Table 8-1. 2018 Updated Approach to Interpretation of Medical Findings in Suspected Child Sexual Abuse*

Section I: Physical Findings

A. Findings documented in newborns or commonly seen in nonabused children: These findings are normal and are unrelated to a child's disclosure of sexual abuse.

Normal variants

1. Normal variations in appearance of the hymen
   a. Annular: Hymenal tissue present all around the vaginal opening, including at the 12 o'clock location
   b. Crescentic hymen: Hymenal tissue is absent at some point above the 3 o'clock to 9 o'clock locations
   c. Imperforate hymen: Hymen with no opening
   d. Microperforate hymen: Hymen with 1 or more small openings
   e. Septate hymen: Hymen with 1 or more septae across the opening
   f. Redundant hymen: Hymen with multiple flaps folding over each other
   g. Hymen with tag of tissue on the rim
   h. Hymen with mounds or bumps on the rim at any location
   i. Any notch or cleft of the hymen (regardless of depth) above the 3 o'clock and 9 o'clock locations
   j. A notch or cleft in the hymen, at or below the 3 o'clock location or 9 o'clock location, that does not extend nearly to the base of the hymen
   k. Smooth posterior rim of hymen that appears to be relatively narrow along the entire rim (may give the appearance of an "enlarged" opening)
2. Periurethral or vestibular band(s)
3. Intravaginal ridge(s) or column(s)
4. External ridge on the hymen
5. Diastasis ani (smooth area)
6. Perianal skin tag(s)
7. Hyperpigmentation of the skin of the labia minora or perianal tissues in children of color
8. Dilation of the urethral opening
9. Normal midline anatomic features
   a. Groove in the fossa, seen in early adolescence
   b. Failure of midline fusion (also called perineal groove)
   c. Median raphe (has been mistaken for a scar)
   d. Linea vestibularis (midline avascular area)

(continued)

Table 8-1. 2018 Updated Approach to Interpretation of Medical Findings in Suspected Child Sexual Abuse* *(continued)*

10. Visualization of the pectinate/dentate line at the juncture of the anoderm and rectal mucosa (seen when the anus is fully dilated)
11. Partial dilatation of the external anal sphincter, with the internal sphincter closed, causing visualization of some of the anal mucosa beyond the pectinate line, which may be mistaken for anal laceration

B. Findings commonly caused by medical conditions other than trauma or sexual contact: These findings require that a differential diagnosis be considered, as each may have several different causes.

12. Erythema of the anal or genital tissues
13. Increased vascularity of vestibule and hymen
14. Labial adhesion
15. Friability of the posterior fourchette
16. Vaginal discharge that is not associated with a sexually transmitted infection
17. Anal fissures
18. Venous congestion or venous pooling in the perianal area
19. Anal dilatation in children with predisposing conditions, such as current symptoms or history of constipation and/or encopresis, or children who are sedated, under anesthesia, or with impaired neuromuscular tone for other reasons, such as post-mortem

C. Findings due to other conditions, which can be mistaken for abuse

20. Urethral prolapse
21. Lichen sclerosus et atrophicus
22. Vulvar ulcer(s), such as aphthous ulcers or those seen in Behçet's disease
23. Erythema, inflammation, and fissuring of the perianal or vulvar tissues due to infection with bacteria, fungus, viruses, parasites, or other infections that are not sexually transmitted
24. Rectal prolapse
25. Red/purple discoloration of the genital structures (including the hymen) from lividity postmortem, if confirmed by histological analysis

D. No expert consensus regarding degree of significance: These physical findings have been associated with a history of sexual abuse in some studies, but at present, there is no expert consensus as to how much weight they should be given, with respect to abuse. Findings 27 and 28 should be confirmed using additional examination positions and/or techniques, to ensure they are not normal variants (findings 1.i, 1.j) or a finding of residual traumatic injury (finding 37).

(continued)

Table 8-1. 2018 Updated Approach to Interpretation of Medical Findings in Suspected Child Sexual Abuse* *(continued)*

26. Complete anal dilatation with relaxation of the internal and external anal sphincters, in the absence of other predisposing factors such as constipation, encopresis, sedation, anesthesia, and neuromuscular conditions

27. Notch or cleft in the hymen rim, at or below the 3 o'clock or 9 o'clock location, which extends nearly to the base of the hymen but is not a complete transection. This is a very rare finding that should be interpreted with caution unless an acute injury was documented at the same location.

28. Complete cleft/suspected transection to the base of the hymen at the 3 o'clock or 9 o'clock location

E. Findings caused by trauma: These findings are highly suggestive of abuse, even in the absence of a disclosure from the child, unless the child and/or caretaker provides a timely and plausible description of accidental anogenital straddle, crush or impalement injury, or past surgical interventions that are confirmed from review of medical records. Findings that may represent residual/healing injuries should be confirmed using additional examination positions and/or techniques.

Acute trauma to genital/anal tissues

29. Acute laceration(s) or bruising of labia, penis, scrotum, or perineum

30. Acute laceration of the posterior fourchette or vestibule, not involving the hymen

31. Bruising, petechiae, or abrasions on the hymen

32. Acute laceration of the hymen, of any depth (partial or complete)

33. Vaginal laceration

34. Perianal bruising or perianal laceration with exposure of tissues below the dermis

Residual (healing) injuries to genital/anal tissues

35. Perianal scar (a very rare finding that is difficult to diagnose unless an acute injury was previously documented at the same location)

36. Scar of posterior fourchette or fossa (a very rare finding that is difficult to diagnose unless an acute injury was previously documented at the same location)

37. Healed hymenal transection/complete hymen cleft—a defect in the hymen below the 3 o'clock to 9 o'clock location that extends to or through the base of the hymen, with no hymenal tissue discernible at that location

38. Signs of female genital mutilation (FGM) or cutting, such as loss of part or all of the prepuce (clitoral hood), clitoris, labia minora or labia majora, or vertical linear scar adjacent to the clitoris (Type 4 FGM)

(continued)

Table 8-1. 2018 Updated Approach to Interpretation of Medical Findings in Suspected Child Sexual Abuse* *(continued)*

Section II: Infections

A. Infections not related to sexual contact

39. Vaginitis caused by fungal infections such as *Candida albicans*, or bacterial infections transmitted by nonsexual means, such as streptococcus type A or type B, *Staphylococcus sp.*, *Escherichia coli*, *Shigella*, or other gram-negative organisms

40. Genital ulcers caused by viral infections such as Epstein-Barr virus

B. Infections that can be spread by nonsexual as well as sexual transmission: Interpretation of these infections may require additional information, such as mother's gynecologic history [human papillomavirus (HPV)] or child's history of oral lesions [herpes simplex virus (HSV)], or presence of lesions elsewhere on the body (molluscum contagiosum) which might clarify likelihood of sexual transmission. After complete assessment, a report to child protective services may be indicated in some cases. Photographs or video recordings of these findings should be taken then evaluated and confirmed by an expert in sexual abuse evaluation to ensure accurate diagnosis.

41. Molluscum contagiosum in the genital or anal area. In young children, transmission is most likely nonsexual. Transmission from intimate skin-to-skin contact in the adolescent population has been described.

42. Condyloma acuminatum (HPV) in the genital or anal area. Warts appearing for the first time after age 5 years may be more likely to have been transmitted by sexual contact

43. Herpes simplex type 1 or 2 infections in the oral, genital, or anal area

C. Infections caused by sexual contact, if confirmed by appropriate testing, and perinatal transmission has been ruled out

44. Genital, rectal, or pharyngeal *Neisseria gonorrhoeae* infection

45. Syphilis

46. Genital or rectal *Chlamydia trachomatis* infection

47. *Trichomonas vaginalis* infection

48. HIV, if transmission by blood or contaminated needles has been ruled out

Section III: Findings diagnostic of sexual contact

49. Pregnancy

50. Semen identified in forensic specimens taken directly from a child's body

**This table lists medical and laboratory findings; however, most children who are evaluated for suspected sexual abuse will not have physical signs of injury or infection. The child's description of what happened and report of specific symptoms in relationship to the events described are both essential parts of a full medical evaluation.*

not an option when trying to study the changes in genital and anal anatomy caused by sexual abuse. The next best method is the case-control study. In 2000, Berenson et al[18] published the first case-control study of genital findings in nonabused girls between 3 and 8 years of age compared to girls who described digital or penile-vaginal penetration. The subjects in the nonabused group had the most complete screening available to ensure their nonabused status, including interviews of the child and parents, record review, and completion of behavioral surveys by the parents. The selection of subjects was not random; for each child evaluated for suspected sexual abuse at one center who agreed to participate in the research study, a child of the same age and ethnicity was recruited from a population of children receiving well-child examinations at another site. The researchers were blinded as much as possible by using the same examination methods, photographic equipment, and number and type of photographs taken, such that when blindly reviewing the photographs, the site where the child had been examined could not be determined. Details in the appearance of the genital tissues were carefully recorded and compared between 2 groups: (1) those who described having experienced vaginal penetration and (2) those who were determined to be nonabused after careful screening. There were very few significant differences between the 2 groups. Vaginal discharge was more common in the abused group, although no cultures were taken to determine the cause of the discharge. As compared to their nonabused controls, labial adhesions were more common in Caucasian girls who had been abused, but that was not the case for Mexican American or African American girls.

Hymenal Data

Berenson et al[18] found that superficial notches in the hymen (arbitrarily defined as extending through up to 50% of the width of the hymen) located below the 3 o'clock to 9 o'clock line were equally common in abused and nonabused girls, which threw doubt on the connection between this finding and trauma to the hymen. It is important to note that when a mound or bump was noted on the edge of the hymen, the area next to the bump, even if it gave the impression of being an indentation, was not counted as a notch. The authors only identified notches through more than 50% of the width of the posterior hymen (deep notches) in girls who described digital- or penile-vaginal penetration (only 2 out of 192 girls between the ages of 3 and 8 years alleging penetration). Distinguishing between superficial notches (through 50% or less of the width of the hymen) and deep notches (through more than 50% of the width of the hymen) can be extremely difficult, and is not possible in clinical practice.

Myhre and associates[10] found that only 1 of 175 nonabused girls aged 5 to 7 years in their study had a superficial notch in the hymen, and none were found to have a deep notch, using the same definitions as Berenson et al.[18] However, they described bumps (mounds) on the hymen in 21% to 23% of subjects, depending on examination position. The researchers in the Myhre study followed the same convention as described in the Berenson case-control study and did not identify a narrowing in the hymen next to a bump as a notch.

In a study of the appearance of the hymen in adolescent girls admitting consensual intercourse compared to girls who denied such contact, there was no statistically significant difference in the frequency of deep notches in the posterior rim of the hymen below 3 o'clock to 9 o'clock.[19] However, deep notches and complete clefts in the hymen in a lateral location (ie, 3 o'clock and 9 o'clock) were both significantly more common in girls admitting vaginal intercourse than in girls who denied intercourse (26% vs 5%, $p < .01$ for each). The fact that these features were identified in 5 out of 58 adolescent girls denying intercourse suggests that notches or clefts at the 3 o'clock or 9 o'clock position might represent normal variants, but they could also be the result of previous penetration.

A posterior rim of hymen that measures less than 1 millimeter in width was not reported in prepubertal girls selected for nonabuse in 5 separate studies in which measurements were taken from magnified photographs using a calibration method.[3,6,7,10,18] In another study, a posterior hymenal rim estimated to be less than 1 to 2 millimeters wide was found in 22% of girls referred for gynecologic examination for other reasons and had no history or suspicion of abuse.[20] Most experts acknowledge that it is very difficult to measure the width of the posterior rim of hymen in many cases, and that estimates of rim width are often inaccurate. Any attempts at measurement, in clinical practice, are discouraged.

If magnified photographs are taken using a camera with a macro lens or a camera attached to a colposcope and a photograph is taken of a millimeter ruler at the same magnification and same focal length, the printed photograph of the ruler can be held next to the printed photograph of the hymen in order to take measurements. This was the method used in the research studies mentioned above. The problem arises in determining exactly how to measure the width of the posterior hymenal rim. One can start to measure, from a photograph, at the inner edge of the hymen if it is fully visualized, but it is difficult to determine from a 2-dimensional image where the lower edge of the hymen attaches to the muscular portion of the introitus, adjacent to the fossa navicularis.

The hymen may appear very narrow in the posterior/inferior rim in children when it has folded out or folded inward. This phenomenon was documented in Myhre's study of nonabused girls in Norway,[10] in which the use of water instilled during the examination of the child in the supine position caused the rim to "float" up and be seen more clearly. In the longitudinal follow-up study by Berenson et al, girls examined at age 3 years were re-examined at 5, 7, and 9 years of age.[9] Measurements of the width of the hymen at the 6 o'clock position, with the patient supine, showed a significant decrease in hymenal width as the child aged and a significant increase in the width of the hymenal opening.

Sexually Transmitted Infections

Warts, vesicles, and ulcers in the genital or anal area may cause concern for the possible sexual transmission of infections such as condyloma accuminata, herpes simplex, or syphilis. Wart-like lesions in the genital or anal area may be skin tags or warts not of the genital type, or they may be condyloma acuminata acquired from perinatal transmission or other nonsexual transmission. Although genital warts can also be transmitted by sexual contact, it is difficult to determine whether or not sexual abuse should be suspected in a child who is too young to give a history or who has denied that he or she has experienced any type of sexual contact or sexual abuse.

A recent study from Greece examined prevalence of HPV infection in prepubertal girls, sexually active adolescents, and non-sexually active adolescent girls, as determined by the detection of HPV by DNA testing.[21] The rates of detecting HPV from vaginal swabs were 47% of sexually active adolescent girls, 28% of non-sexually active girls, and 34% of prepubertal girls. These results support the conclusion that HPV in children and adolescents is likely transmitted by means other than sexual contact.

Vesicular lesions or ulcers in the genital or anal area can have infectious and noninfectious causes.[22] These include herpes, syphilis, varicella, or other viruses; Behçet's disease[23]; Crohn's disease; and idiopathic causes such as aphthous ulcers.[24,25] Viral cultures or polymerase chain reaction (PCR) analysis are needed to diagnose herpes infection. Serologic tests must be done to diagnose syphilis. It is recommended that these tests be performed and the results received before reporting possible sexual abuse unless a child has given a disclosure of abuse.

Mimics

The most common medical findings that are mistaken for signs of sexual abuse include the following:

- Redness of the genital or anal tissues
- The appearance of a "dilated" hymen, urethra, or anal opening felt by caretakers to be "too big"
- A concern for an "absent" hymen because of a relatively narrow posterior hymenal rim when labial traction is applied in a relaxed child
- Mistaking the presence of labial adhesions as "scars" in the genital area
- Mistaking the iatrogenic breakdown of a labial adhesion as a tear of the posterior fourchette caused by abuse, mistaking the irregular appearance of the pectinate line as scars or tears of the anus
- Mistaking the blue coloration around the anus caused by venous congestion for anal bruising

Other rarer conditions, such as the congenital failure of midline fusion (or perineal groove), hemangiomas of the hymen or labia, urethral prolapse, and lichen sclerosus, can also be confused with signs of sexual abuse trauma. Examples of normal variations in the appearance of the hymen and anus and other conditions that may be mistaken for abuse are shown in **Appendix Figures 8-1-a** through **8-43-b**.

Anal Dilation

Total anal dilation, with relaxation of both internal and external anal sphincters, is a finding that has been documented in both abused and nonabused children. In Myhre's study of nonabused children in Norway,[26] 4.7% of the children had dilation when the child was examined in the prone knee chest position, but less than 1% had this finding when examined in the left lateral position. In McCann and associates study of nonabused children,[2] 14.7% of the children had this finding within 30 seconds of being examined in the prone knee-chest position.

In a retrospective study of 1115 children evaluated for suspected sexual abuse in one center,[27] total anal dilation was found significantly more often among children with probable anal penetration (primarily determined by child's disclosure) than in those without probable anal penetration (12% vs 3.7%, $p = .000$). However, anal dilation was also more common in girls than boys, in children examined in the prone knee-chest position, and in children with anal symptoms of constipation, encopresis, or diarrhea. After controlling for those variables, anal dilation was still significantly associated with anal penetration. This association was seen in both pubertal and prepubertal children and in children seen acutely and nonacutely.

Anal dilation can be caused by chronic constipation, sedation, anesthesia, neuromuscular conditions, and can be seen during the autopsy.[28] No consensus currently exists among experts as to how this finding should be interpreted in the absence of a history of anal penetration given by the child. If a child has anal symptoms, anal dilation can be considered a finding commonly caused by other conditions (as indicated in Table 8-1). However, in a child without any anal symptoms, anal dilation can be considered supportive of abuse if the child makes a clear disclosure of anal penetration.

Anal dilation in children with suspected sexual abuse is viewed differently in the United Kingdom, where anal examinations are performed with the child lying in the left-lateral position (ie, on his or her side, with knees to chest) rather than the supine or the prone knee-chest position, as is common in the United States. This examination technique may contribute to the United Kingdom's higher reported rate of anal dilation in children who describe anal penetration. In a study published in 2014, Hobbs and Wright[29] reported that "reflex anal dilatation" was observed in 41 of 184 (22%) of children reporting anal penetration, as compared to 0 of 179 children without suspicion of sexual abuse examined in the same manner. However, it should be noted that constipation was not addressed as a possible contributing factor. This rate (22%) is much higher than the rate found by Myhre et al[27] in 2013 (12%). In the Hobbs study, in which examinations were performed with the child lying in the left-lateral position, the buttocks were separated for 30 seconds in order to see if dilation would occur. In the Myhre study, the medical records and photodocumentation of the examinations do not clearly indicate how long the examiner waited before photographing anal dilation, as it was not standardized in that center for examiners to wait a full 30 seconds to look for anal dilation.

Injuries

As mentioned earlier, signs of acute trauma, such as bruising, abrasions, and lacerations are rare in children who are examined for possible sexual abuse. In a review of findings in more than 2000 children presenting for examinations for suspected abuse to one large urban center, 96% of the children had normal or nonspecific findings upon examination.[30] As several case reports have demonstrated, lacerations of the posterior fourchette, fossa, hymen, and anus can also be caused by accidental injuries.[31-33] The history from the child, as well as a thorough investigation of the setting in which the accident is alleged to have occurred, are essential to determine whether or not the injuries could have been caused by the described accident.

A recent study by Gallion et al[34] documenting injuries in girls evaluated for possible sexual abuse was designed to determine whether injuries were more common when the child described vaginal penetration, as opposed to genital contact. The authors also compared the rate of "diagnostic findings" of genital trauma (eg, bruises, abrasions, lacerations) in girls who were examined acutely (within 72 hours of the abuse) and nonacutely (after more than 72 hours post abuse). They found that only 2.2% of girls examined nonacutely had diagnostic genital findings, as opposed to 21.4 % of those examined acutely. They also found that injuries were more common in adolescents than in prepubertal girls. When controlling for age and time post-assault, the most significant factor associated with injuries was whether the girl said that she felt something went "inside" or "both inside and outside" her genitals during the abuse. Diagnostic findings were 12 times more likely to be found in girls who said something went "inside" or "both inside and outside" during the abuse. Before their examinations, the examiners asked every girl the following question: "When you wipe after you go pee, do you feel like you are wiping inside, outside, or both?" This is clearly an imperfect tool for determining what a young girl means by "inside," and young girls certainly don't wipe inside their vagina, past the hymenal opening, after urinating. Adolescent girls were found to be more likely to answer "inside" than prepubertal girls.

A multicenter study by McCann and associates[35-37] of the healing of genital injuries in prepubertal and adolescent girls provided new information on the rates of healing of different types of injury. In this study, colleagues were invited to submit cases, with photodocumentation, of children with acute genital injuries who had at least 1 follow-up visit to show healing of the injuries. Team members reviewed the photodocumentation and analyzed findings from the photographs. Among prepubertal girls, a total of 40 lacerations were identified (35 in the posterior location), and among pubertal girls, 80 hymenal lacerations were identified (50 in the posterior location, 18 lateral, and 12 anterior). The difference in location was statistically significant, with adolescents showing a higher proportion of lacerations at 3 o'clock or 9 o'clock than prepubertal girls. As the timing of follow-up examinations was not standardized, it was not possible to say how long, on average, it took for the lacerations to heal. However, it was noted that lacerations that did not extend through more than 50% of the width of the hymen generally healed to less than a deep notch, some healing to such a degree that they became undetectable. Of the lacerations extending to or through the base of the hymen, most healed as transections. This was true in cases of prepubertal and adolescent girls.

Although data indicate that complete lacerations of the hymen in prepubertal girls will, if not repaired, usually heal to a deep notch or transection, the absence of a transection in an adolescent patient does not rule out the possibility that vaginal penetration occurred. In a study by Adams et al,[19] fewer than half of adolescent girls who described consensual penile-vaginal intercourse had complete clefts in the hymen. In another study reviewing the appearance of the hymen in pregnant adolescent girls, only 2 of 36 girls had genital findings indicative of previous vaginal penetration.[38] These results are explained by the fact that the hymen in adolescent girls is fully estrogenized and can stretch to accommodate penile-vaginal penetration without tearing.

In 2003, Jones et al[39] reported that posterior fourchette lacerations highlighted by toluidine blue dye in adolescents brought for sexual abuse examinations, were not significantly more common in girls who said the intercourse was consensual than in girls who described forced intercourse. Because the dye is taken up by nucleated cells and only the very top layer of the epidermis is made up of cells without nuclei, anything that disrupts the superficial epidermis will allow dye uptake by the cell layer just below. There have been no studies of prepubertal or adolescent girls with genital irritation or discharge and without a history of recent sexual abuse or intercourse. Therefore, it is difficult to say with certainty that superficial abrasions or fissures in the skin of the vulva or anus are associated with sexual contact or may have other possible explanations.

Conclusion

The overall rate of diagnostic findings in children evaluated for suspected sexual abuse is between 3% and 5%, but it is important to recognize the impact of other factors. Research shows that the rate of abnormal findings is much higher in acute examinations.[34] With regard to interview techniques, examining professionals need to develop a method to more accurately interpret children's descriptions of abusive events (eg, what a child might mean by a statement such as "It went inside my front private."). Going forward, examiners will also require a means of determining degree of penetration when penile-anal contact is described by both boys and girls. Perhaps a variation of the "When you wipe…" question employed by Gallion et al[34] could be applied to anal contact as well. If children were asked the "When you wipe…" question during medical history taking, it might also be helpful to ask the following question after the examination: "When [the abusive event] happened, did it feel like it does when you wipe after you go pee?" Readers should bear in mind that in many jurisdictions, penetration is not legally defined as "penetration beyond the hymen" or "beyond the external anal sphincter." It is usually defined in terms similar to "penetration of the female genitalia or the anus, however slight." Therefore, penetration beyond the labia majora is sufficient to make a legal determination of rape or sexual assault.

It should be noted that few children evaluated for suspected sexual abuse will have an STI. The child or adolescent who is confirmed to have an infection caused by a sexually transmitted organism has most likely acquired that infection through sexual contact if perinatal transmission and autoinoculation have been ruled out. Recommendations regarding testing for STIs, interpretation of the significance of positive tests, and treatment are discussed in detail in Chapter 10.

Appendix 8-1: Normal Variations and Forensic Photography

The following photographs are examples of some of the findings listed in Table 8-1. For examples of normal anatomic variants, see Chapter 2.

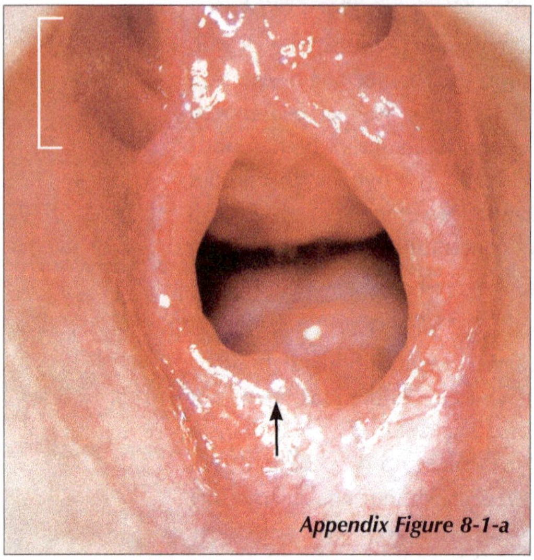

Appendix Figure 8-1-a

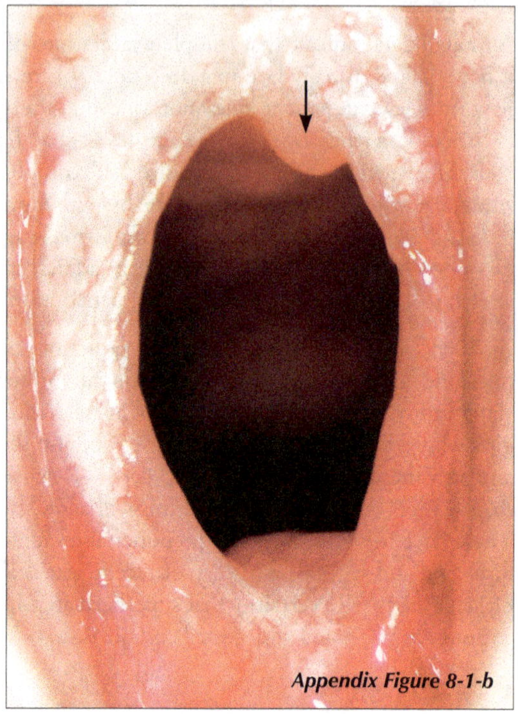

Appendix Figure 8-1-b

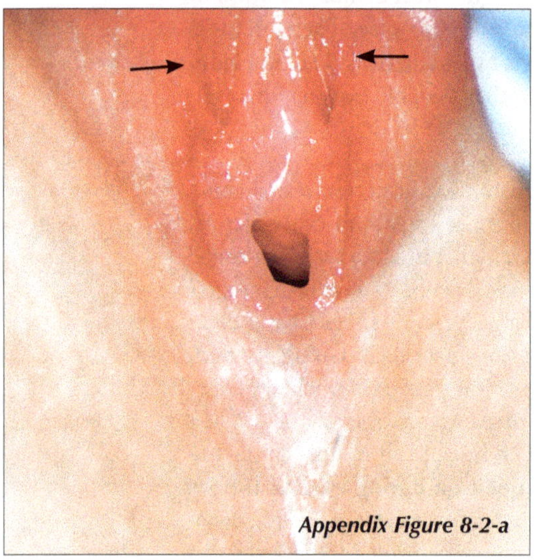

Appendix Figure 8-2-a

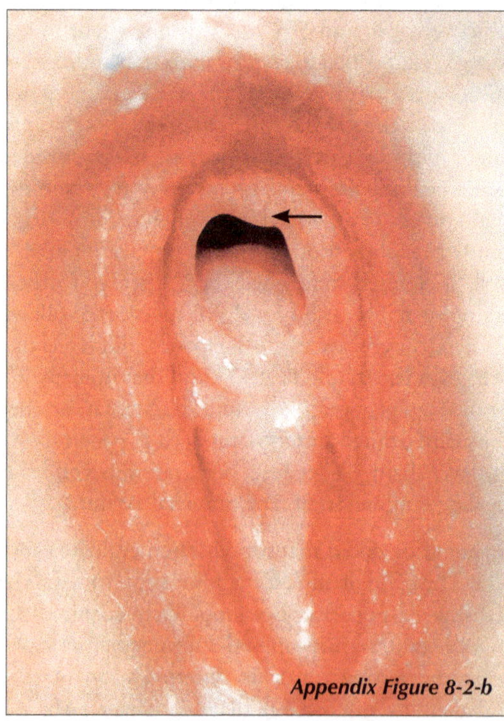

Appendix Figure 8-2-b

Appendix Figure 8-1-a. *This 8-year-old girl described an attempted fondling. Hymen is normal, showing periurethral bands and a mound on the hymen at 7 o'clock.*

Appendix Figure 8-1-b. *The same child, examined in the prone knee-chest position. A mound on the hymen is still present at 12 o'clock, likely attached to an intravaginal ridge behind the mound.*

Appendix Figure 8-2-a. *This 6-year-old female described fondling 1 week prior to examination. This is a normal hymen, showing periurethral bands at 1 o'clock and 11 o'clock.*

Appendix Figure 8-2-b. *In the prone knee-chest position, the hymen is smooth, with a mound noted in the midline at 1 o'clock.*

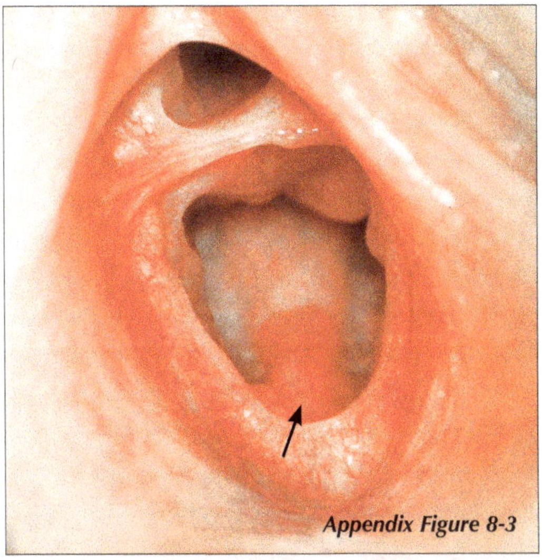

Appendix Figure 8-3

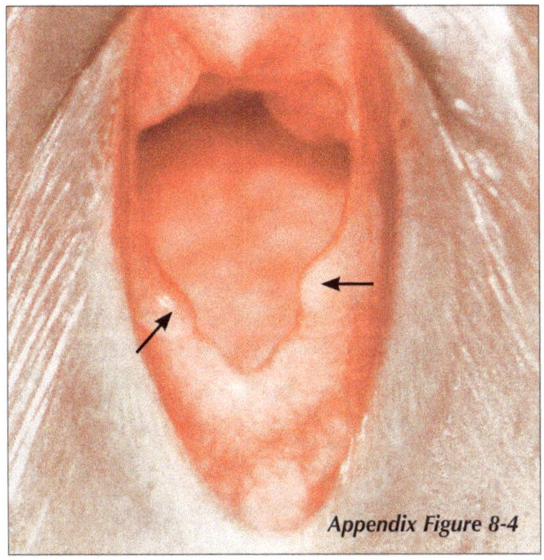

Appendix Figure 8-4

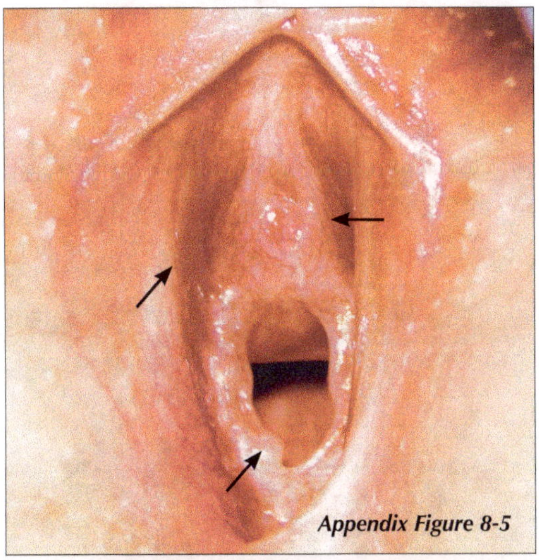

Appendix Figure 8-5

Appendix Figure 8-3. *A 6-year-old girl, examined using labial traction. The urethral opening is dilated, and there is an intravaginal column on the posterior vaginal wall in the midline at 7 o'clock. Both of these findings are normal.*

Appendix Figure 8-4. *This is a 7-year-old African-American girl, examined using separation. There are 2 mounds at 4 o'clock and 7 o'clock on the crescentic hymen. Mounds are commonly seen in girls of this age and are not indicative of trauma.*

Appendix Figure 8-5. *A 6-year-old girl with a normal hymen. There is a mound at 7 o'clock and a normal, hypervascular appearance of the vestibular tissues in the sulci between the hymen and the inner labia minora bilaterally at 2 o'clock and 9 o'clock. The hymen on either side of a mound can appear relatively narrow but should not be mistaken for a notch or cleft.*

Appendix Figure 8-6-a. *This 5-year-old girl presents with vaginal discharge and increased vascularity of the vestibule and hymen. She has what appears in this photograph to be a notch at 6 o'clock and a mound between 3 o'clock and 5 o'clock.*

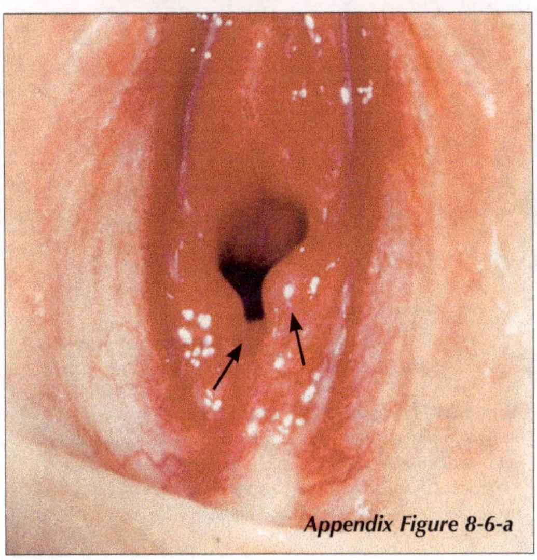

Appendix Figure 8-6-a

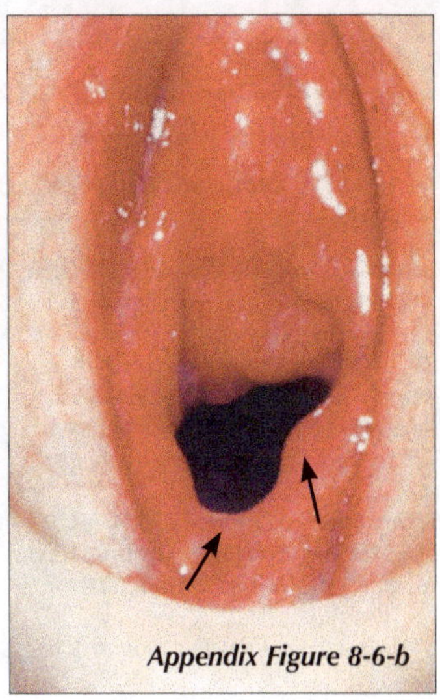

Appendix Figure 8-6-b

Appendix Figure 8-6-b. *With additional labial traction, the posterior hymen smoothes out at 7 o'clock, and the mound is visible again at 3 o'clock to 5 o'clock. The "pseudo-notch" has disappeared. All cultures were negative. Even though this girl eventually gave a history of molestation, there is no sign of trauma to her hymen. Multiple examination techniques are needed if there appears to be an abnormality in 1 view.*

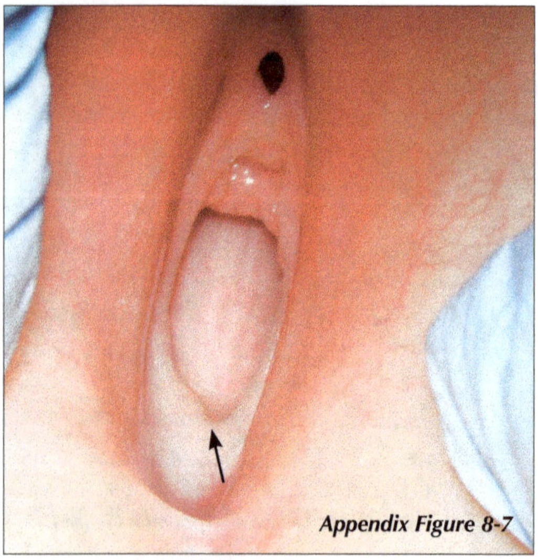

Appendix Figure 8-7

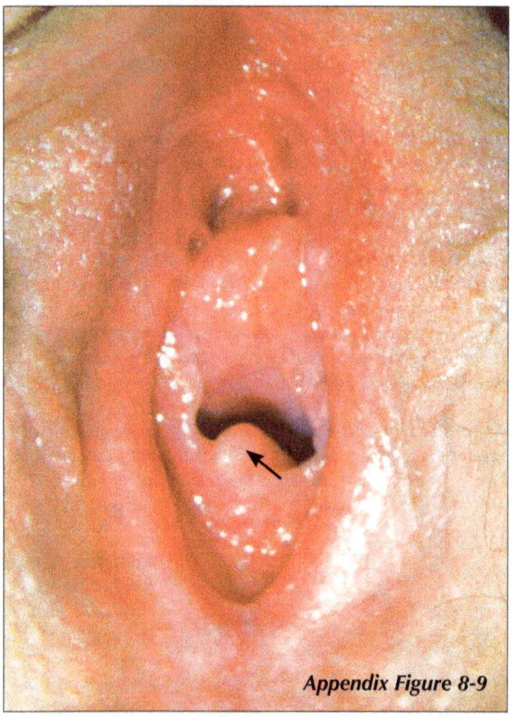

Appendix Figure 8-9

Appendix Figure 8-7. *An 8-year-old, developmentally delayed, and obese female with an elongated hymenal opening and a very shallow indentation in the hymen at 5 o'clock. Another interpretation of this finding is that there is a mound on the hymen at 6 o'clock, and the area at 5 o'clock is only a "pseudo-notch." However, because both shallow notches and mounds are seen in nonabused children, neither finding is concerning for trauma.*

Appendix Figure 8-8. *This 7-year-old girl described a history of fondling over her clothes. The hymen is normal, with a mound at 9 o'clock and an intravaginal ridge behind the mound.*

Appendix Figure 8-9. *A 12-year-old girl with a mound and ridge at 6 o'clock.*

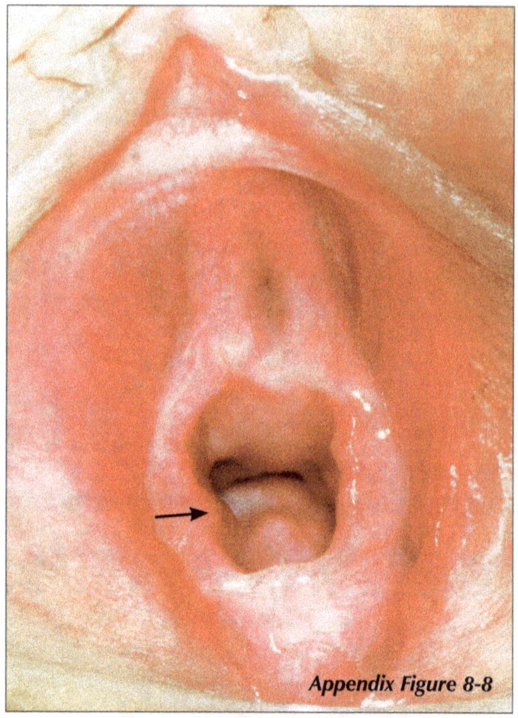

Appendix Figure 8-8

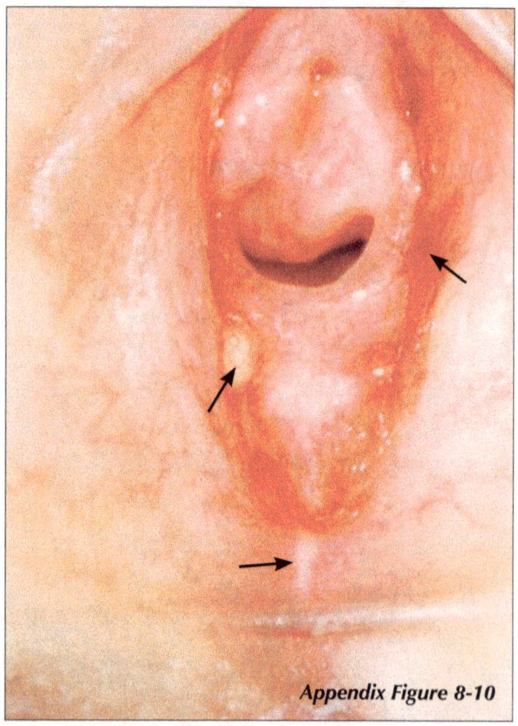

Appendix Figure 8-10

Appendix Figure 8-10. *A 6-year-old girl with increased redness in the vestibule at 3 o'clock to 5 o'clock, a small follicle in the vestibule at 8 o'clock, and a midline avascular area at 6 o'clock. Follicles are probably mucosal inclusion cysts and are seen in both prepubertal and adolescent girls.*

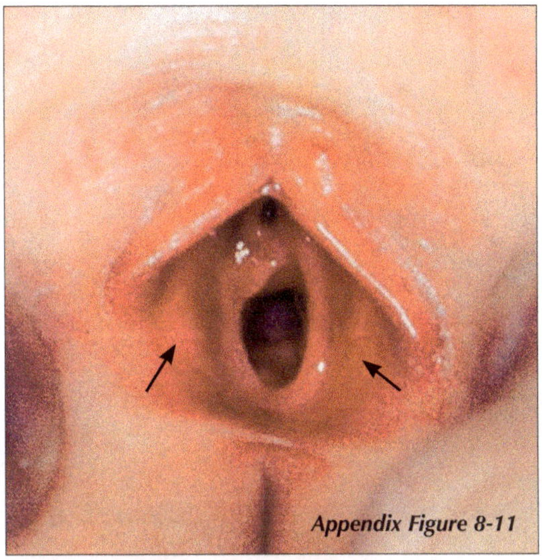

Appendix Figure 8-11

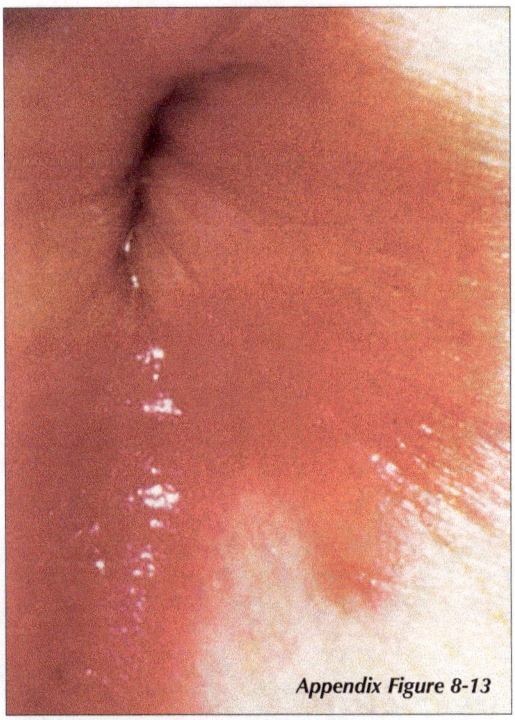

Appendix Figure 8-13

Appendix Figure 8-11. *This 3-year-old girl has confluent, marked erythema in the vestibule and inner labia minora at 4 o'clock and 9 o'clock. Her cultures were positive for Group A beta hemolytic streptococci, a non-sexually transmitted infection.*

Appendix Figure 8-12. *A prepubertal girl with redness around the anus due to venous congestion. This is a common finding unrelated to trauma.*

Appendix Figure 8-13. *This 4-year-old boy has marked erythema around the anus and complains of pain. The cultures were positive for Group A beta hemolytic streptococci, and he responded well to oral antibiotics.*

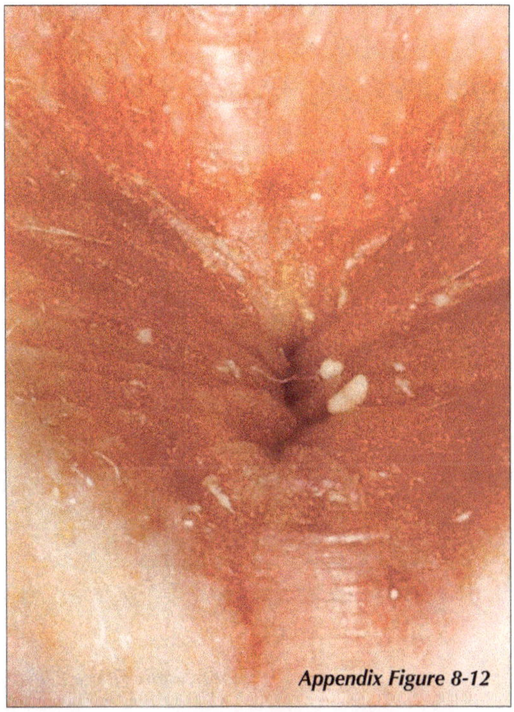

Appendix Figure 8-12

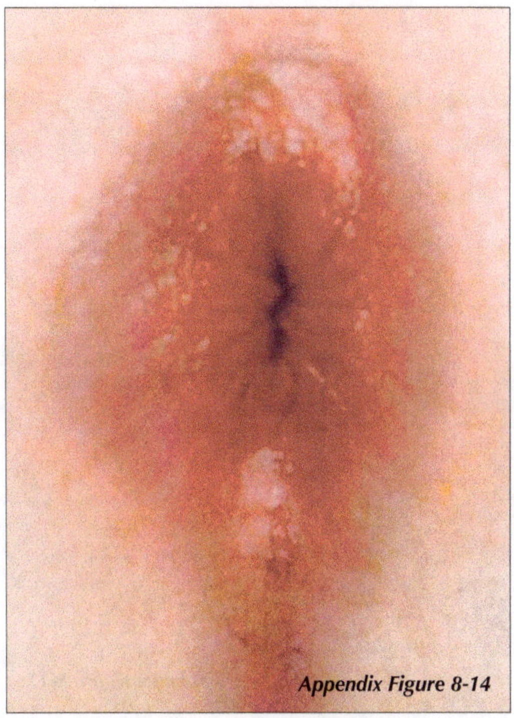

Appendix Figure 8-14

Appendix Figure 8-14. *This 3-year-old boy complained of pain due to inflammation of the perianal skin. There is also streptococcal cellulitis. Children may complain of pain and even say that someone (often a caretaker) hurt their bottom, since wiping or cleaning such irritated tissue can be painful.*

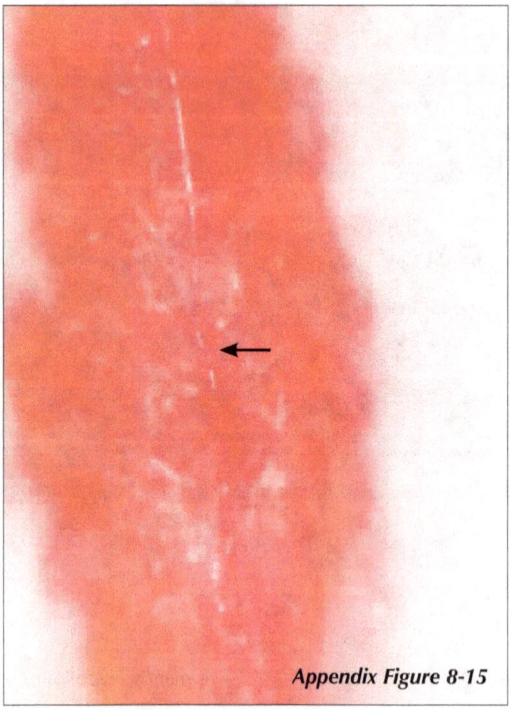
Appendix Figure 8-15

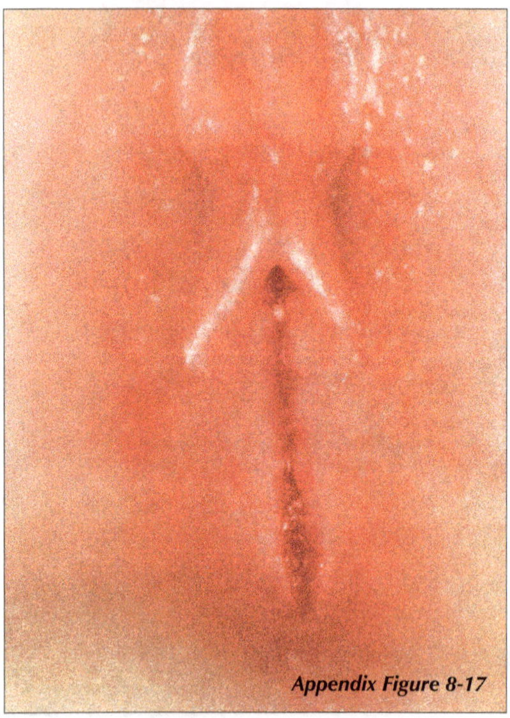
Appendix Figure 8-17

Appendix Figure 8-15. *This 3-year-old boy said "Big Momma hurt my cookie." His babysitter had wiped his bottom after having diarrhea, and he complained of pain. Cultures were positive for* Streptococcus *in this case.*

Appendix Figure 8-16. *A 4-year-old girl with posterior labial adhesion at 6 o'clock and no history of sexual abuse.*

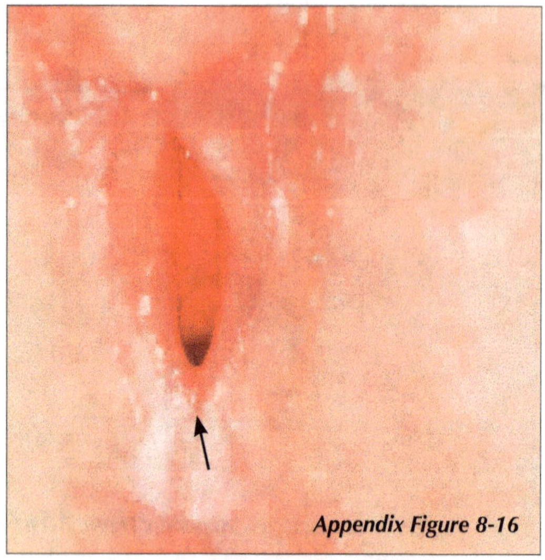
Appendix Figure 8-16

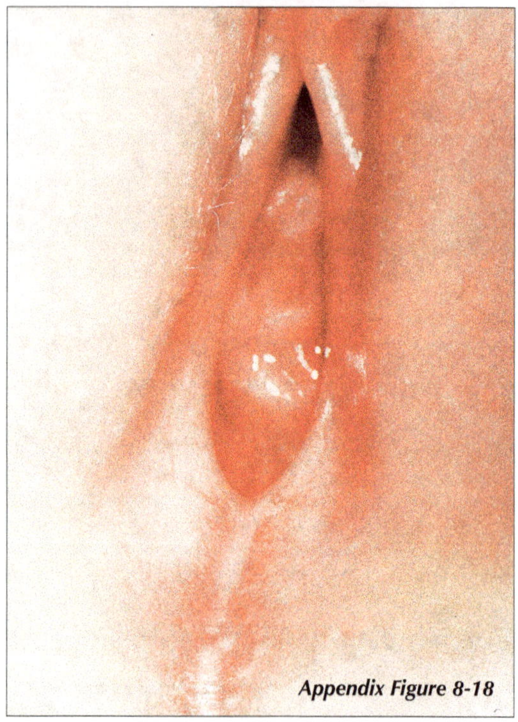
Appendix Figure 8-18

Appendix Figure 8-17. *A 2-year-old in diapers had spots of blood on diaper causing concern. She has an almost total adhesion of her labia minora. The anterior opening is not visible on this photograph, but she has been having normal passage of urine with no obvious discomfort.*

Appendix Figure 8-18. *A 30-month-old girl examined in the supine position. Posterior fusion of the labia is seen clearly in this photograph as a pale, midline avascular area. This can break down with labial separation, causing slight bleeding.*

Appendix Figure 8-19-a. *This 6-year-old girl gave a history of 1 episode of genital fondling. There is a large labial adhesion, with a small opening just under the clitoral hood and another opening inferiorly. She was treated with estrogen cream.*

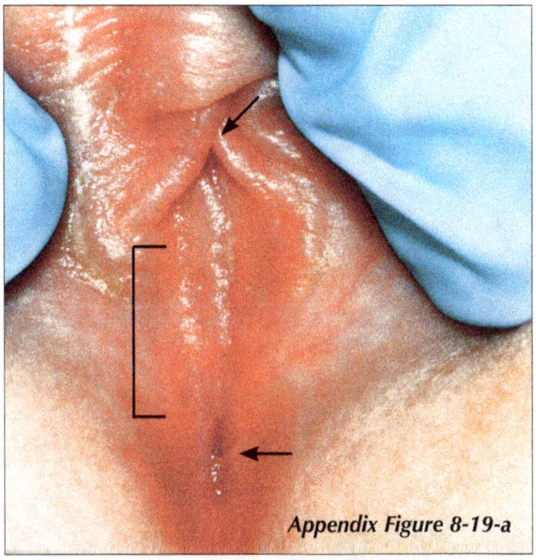

Appendix Figure 8-19-a

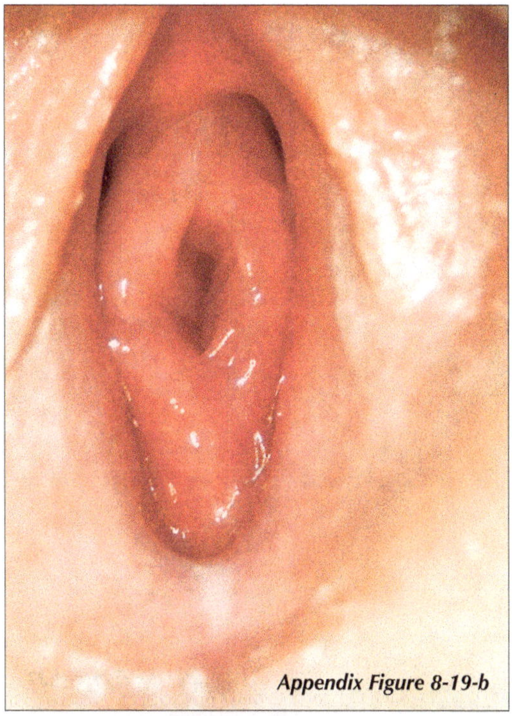

Appendix Figure 8-19-b

Appendix Figure 8-19-b. *One month later, after treatment with topical estrogen cream, the adhesion is almost completely resolved. The hymenal tissue is thickened and pale as a result of the effects of the estrogen cream.*

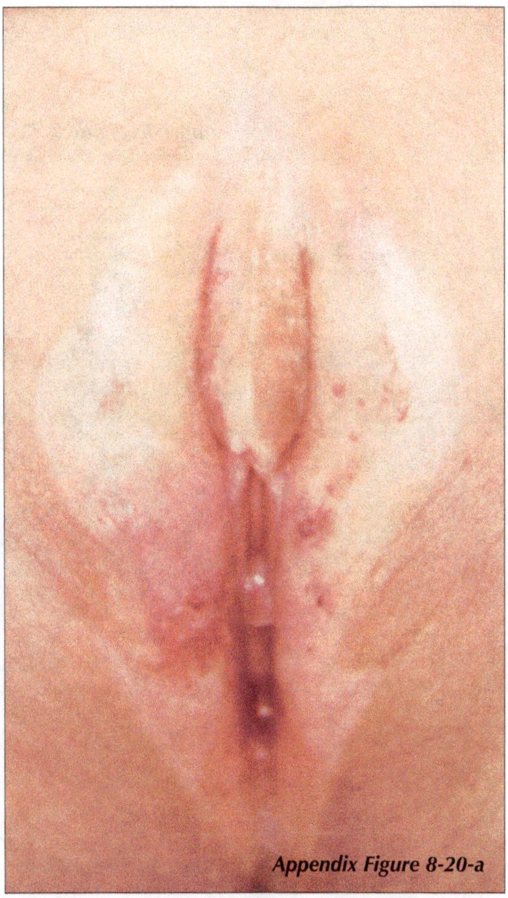

Appendix Figure 8-20-a

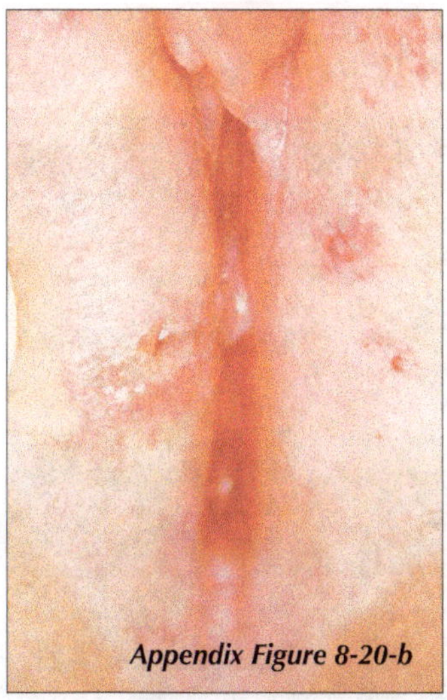

Appendix Figure 8-20-b

Appendix Figure 8-20-a. *7-year-old Mexican-American girl presented with genital itching and spots of blood on her underwear. There is hypopigmentation and thinning of the skin of the vulva, with small areas of excoriation. This is lichen sclerosus, a condition of unknown etiology that causes signs and symptoms that may be mistaken for trauma. Image reprinted with permission from eMedicine.com, 2010. Available at: https://emedicine.medscape.com/article/954024-overview.*

Appendix Figure 8-20-b. *A close-up view of the atrophic, hypopigmented skin. Note the very clear line of demarcation between the normal and affected skin.*

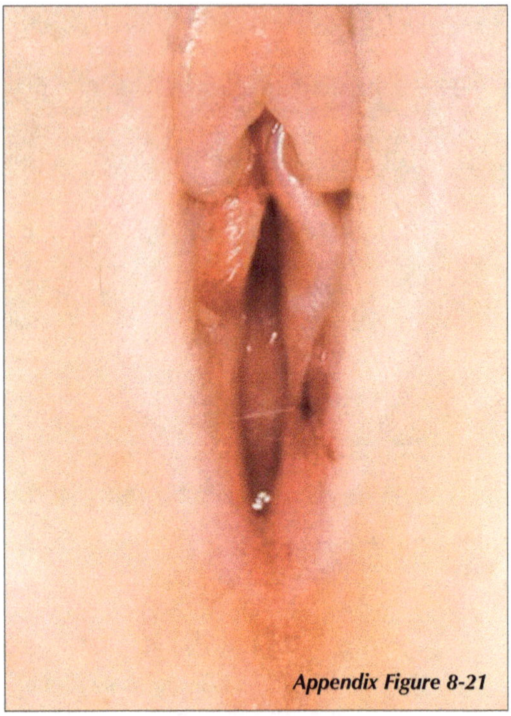

Appendix Figure 8-21

Appendix Figure 8-21. *This 7-year-old Caucasian girl also has lichen sclerosus. The hypopigmentation is a little harder to see, but the atrophic skin demonstrates the bleeding caused by minor rubbing or wiping. Using a red-free (green) filter on the colposcope can sometimes accentuate hypopigmentation.*

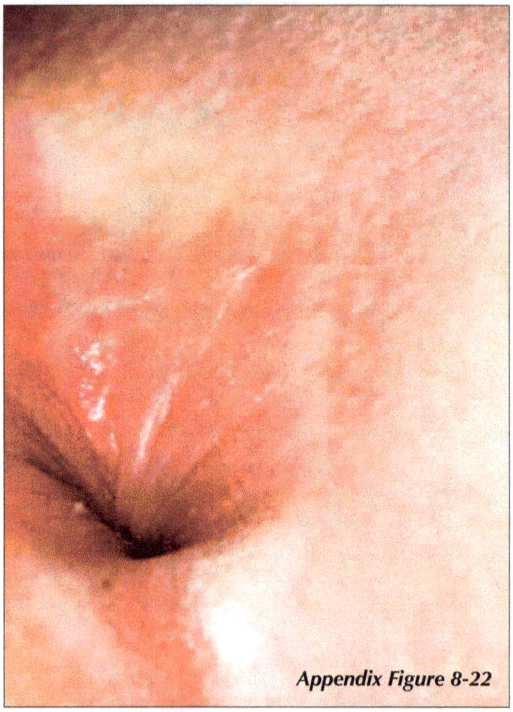

Appendix Figure 8-22

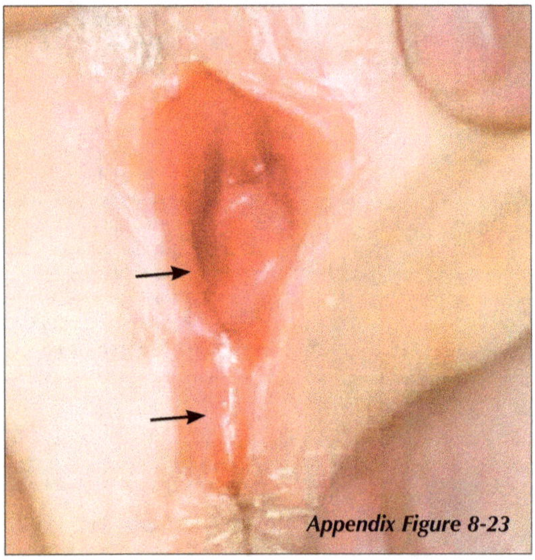

Appendix Figure 8-23

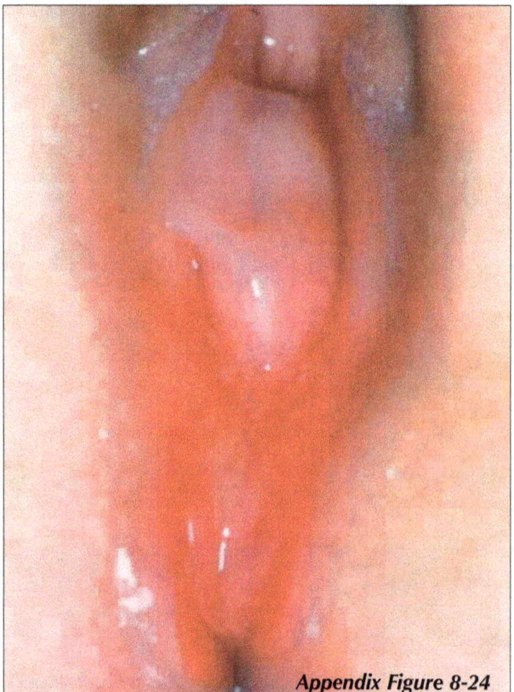

Appendix Figure 8-24

Appendix Figure 8-22. *Lichen sclerosus affecting the perianal skin. The same pattern of hypopigmented, atrophic, easily abraded skin is evident in this photograph.*

Appendix Figure 8-23. *A 16-month-old girl referred for unusual appearance of the genital tissues. There was no history suggestive of injury or abuse. There is a mucosal defect extending from the fossa to the anus in the midline. This is failure of midline fusion, also called perineal groove. It did not change in appearance over a period of 6 months, ruling out trauma.*

Appendix Figure 8-24. *This is a 4-month-old infant with the same condition. At the time she was evaluated, the condition of failure of fusion had not been recognized, and there was a concern for possible abuse. The child's family did not bring her back for a follow-up visit.*

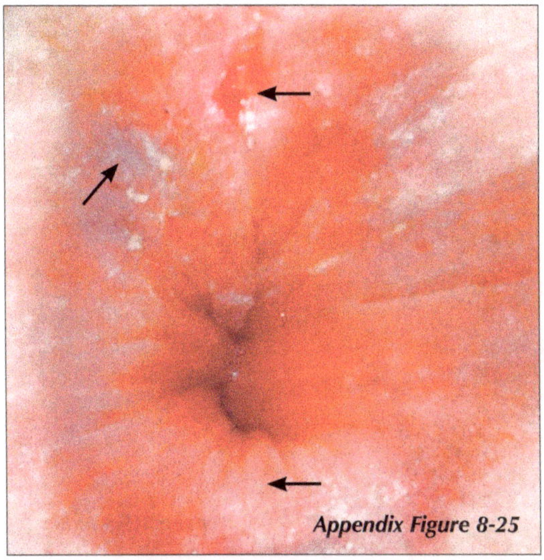

Appendix Figure 8-25

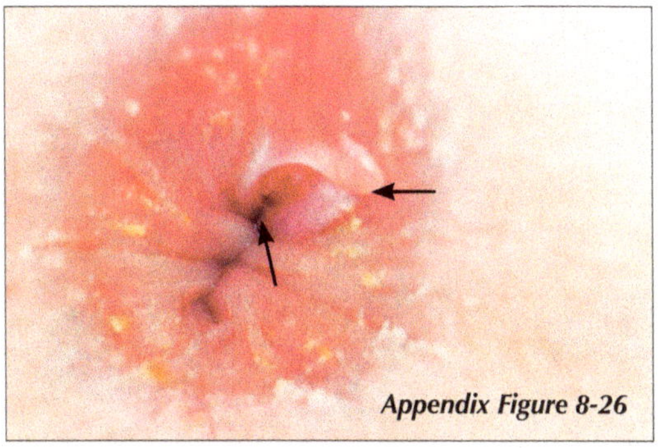

Appendix Figure 8-26

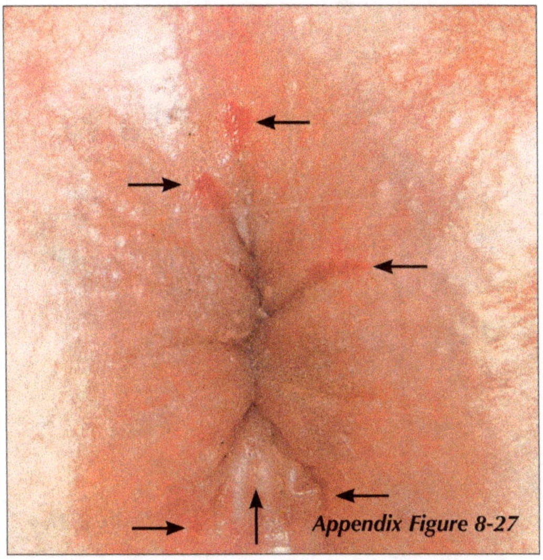

Appendix Figure 8-27

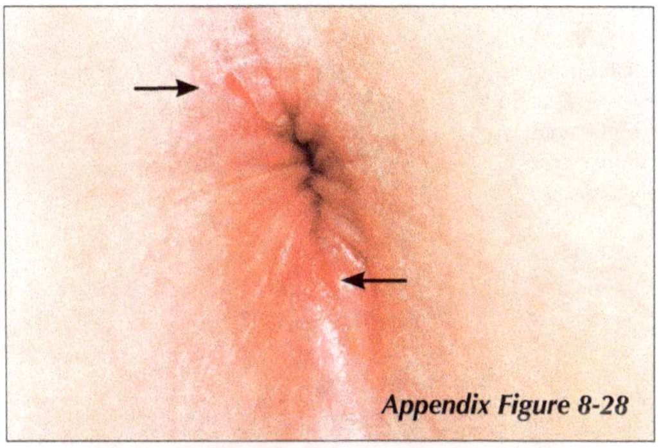

Appendix Figure 8-28

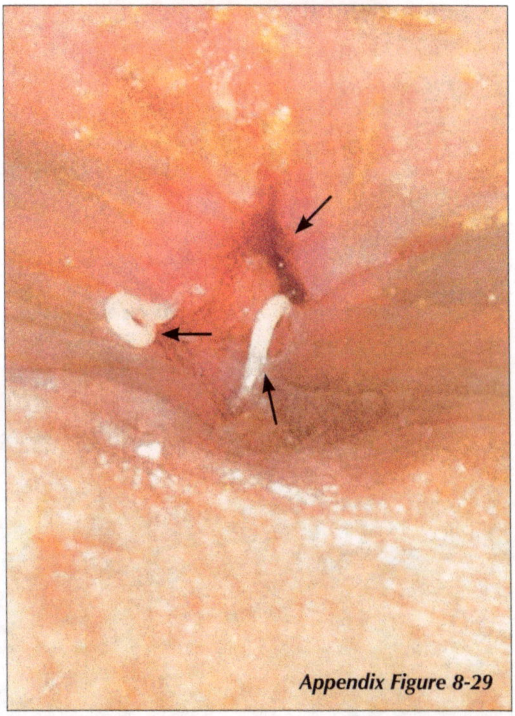

Appendix Figure 8-29

Appendix Figure 8-25. *A 6-year-old boy with a history of constipation who denied any anal trauma. There is an anal fissure at 12 o'clock and venous pooling at 1 o'clock. The area at 7 o'clock is called the anal verge.*

Appendix Figure 8-26. *An 8-month-old infant with an anal fissure at 12 o'clock and an anal tag at about 1 o'clock. The most common cause of anal fissures is constipation, and tags may form at the site of the fissure.*

Appendix Figure 8-27. *This 9-month-old male was being cared for by an uncle while the child's mother was away from home. When the mother came back, she found blood in the baby's diaper and became alarmed. The uncle explained that the baby had been screaming in pain while passing a stool earlier that day. The mother recovered a used diaper with a large (4 cm diameter), rock-hard bowel movement in it, which she brought along to the doctor. The baby has venous congestion and multiple small anal fissures caused by the passage of the large, hard stool.*

Appendix Figure 8-28. *This 6-year-old girl has a history of hard stools and no history of molestation. There are fissures at 6 o'clock and 11 o'clock.*

Appendix Figure 8-29. *This child complained of anal itching. On examination, the anus is partially dilated at 1 o'clock, and there are 2 pinworms coming out of the opening at 6 o'clock and 9 o'clock.*

Appendix Figure 8-30. *Anal polyp in an infant. These are large anal tags that sometimes also contain veins. They require no treatment.*

Appendix Figure 8-31-a. *A 2-year-old female with a red bottom after coming back from a visit with her father. The child's parents are divorced, and her mother worries about the possibility of abuse.*

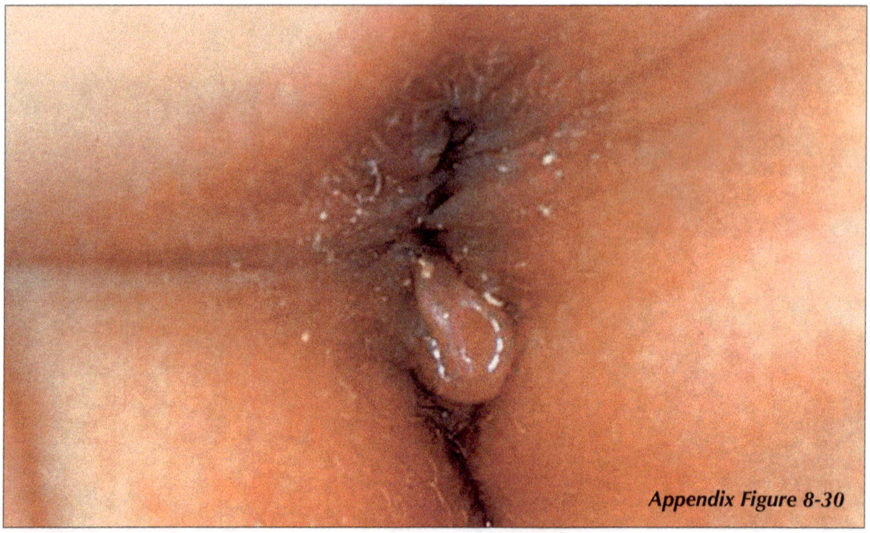

Appendix Figure 8-30

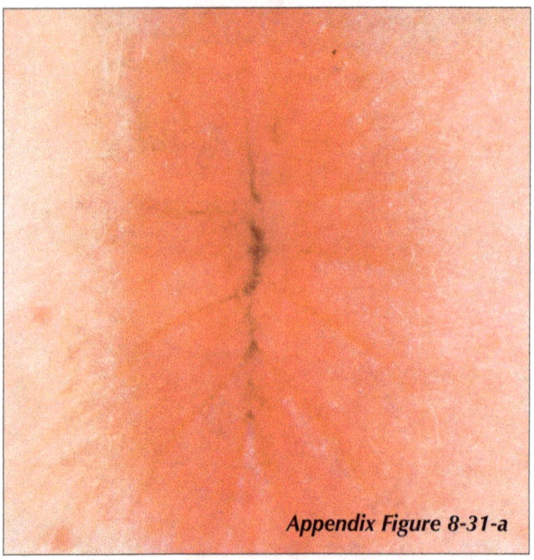

Appendix Figure 8-31-a

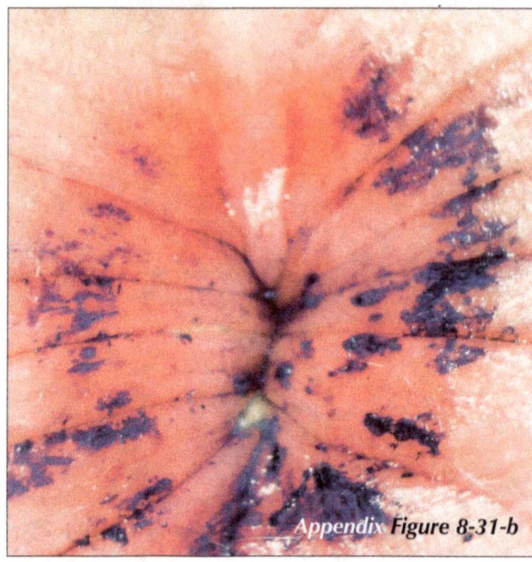

Appendix Figure 8-31-b

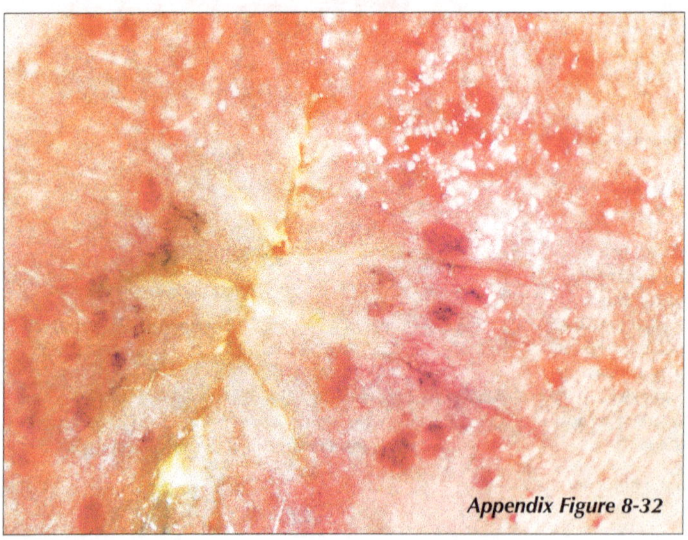

Appendix Figure 8-32

Appendix Figure 8-31-b. *An application of toluidine blue dye highlights superficial abrasions around the anus caused by diaper dermatitis. Positive dye uptake is only indicative of disruption of the superficial layer of the epidermis, which can be caused by minor rubbing, scratching, or dermatitis.*

Appendix Figure 8-32. *A 4 month old with diaper dermatitis. The uptake pattern, highlighted by toluidine blue dye, is not typical of lacerations.*

Appendix Figure 8-33. *Normal anal folds in an 11-year-old girl examined in the prone knee-chest position.*

Appendix Figure 8-34. *This 8-year-old girl, examined in the prone knee-chest position, has a partially relaxed anal sphincter, with a deep fold at 6 o'clock that should not be mistaken for a laceration. By allowing the child to further relax, the sphincter will usually dilate fully, and the folds, including deep folds, will smooth out.*

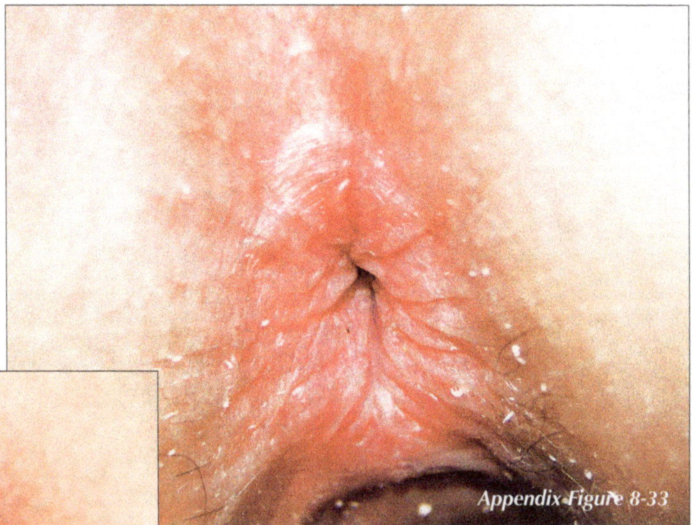

Appendix Figure 8-33

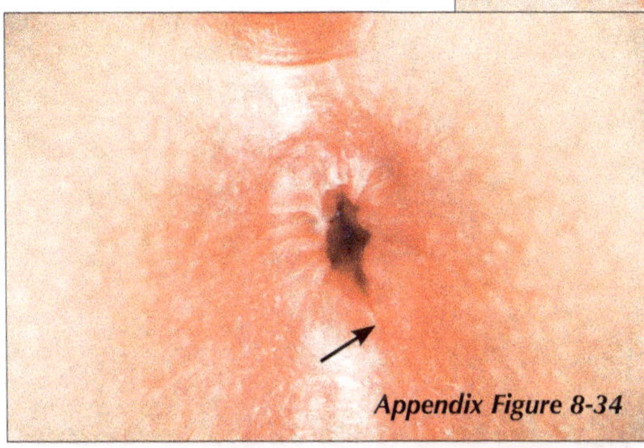

Appendix Figure 8-34

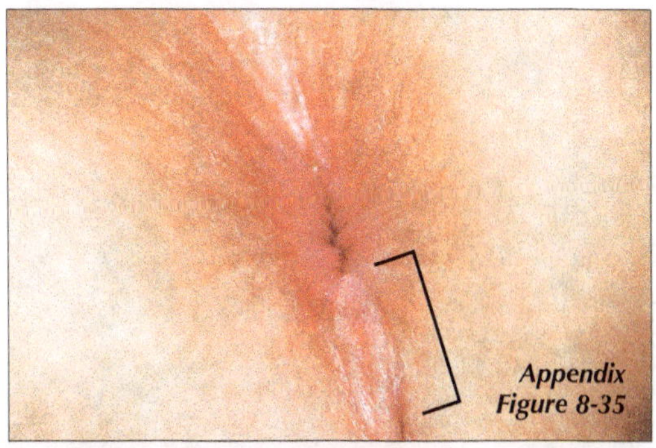

Appendix Figure 8-35

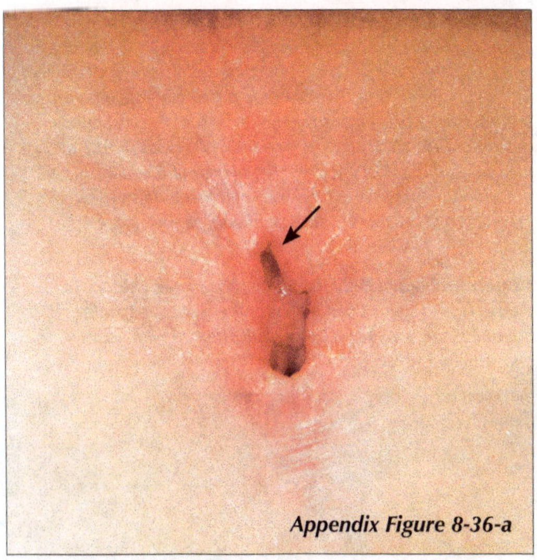

Appendix Figure 8-36-a

Appendix Figure 8-35. *This boy has a thick fold of skin in the median raphe, which is a normal finding.*

Appendix Figure 8-36-a. *Partial dilation of the external anal sphincter with a deep groove seen at the 12-o'clock position.*

Appendix Figure 8-36-b. *With more complete relaxation of the external and internal anal sphincters, stool is visible in the rectal vault at 2 o'clock, and the deep fold has disappeared.*

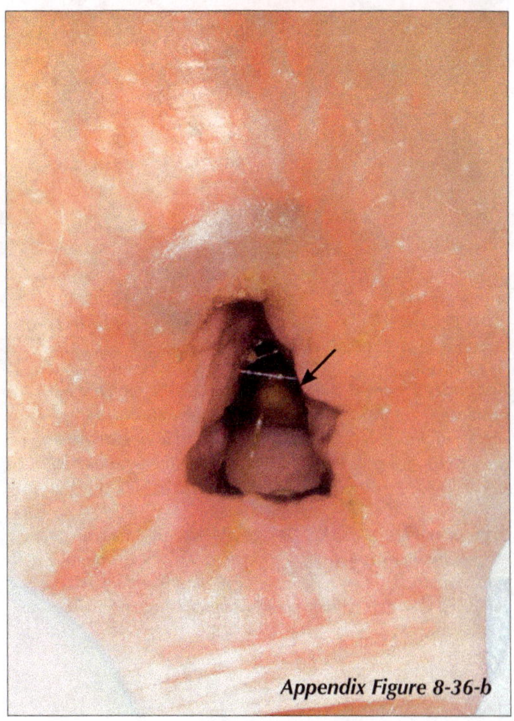

Appendix Figure 8-36-b

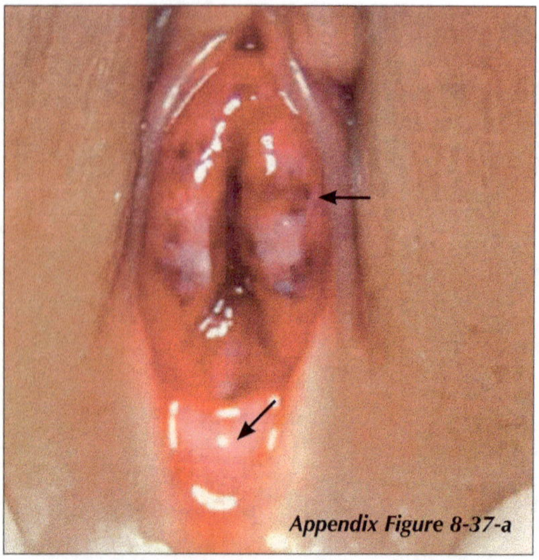
Appendix Figure 8-37-a

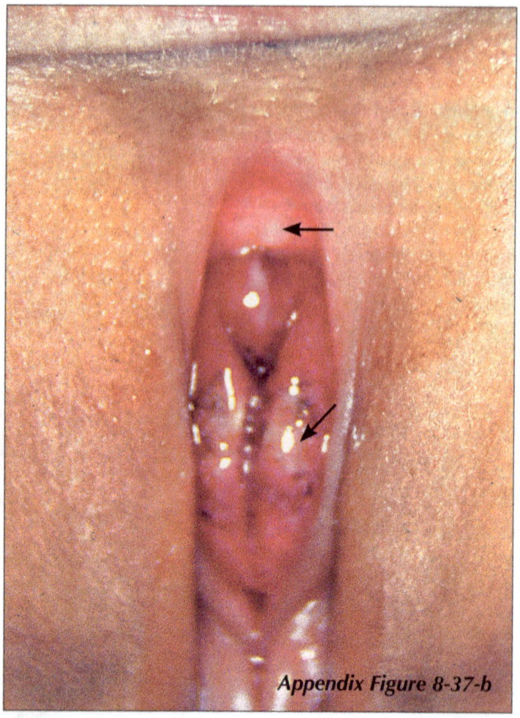
Appendix Figure 8-37-b

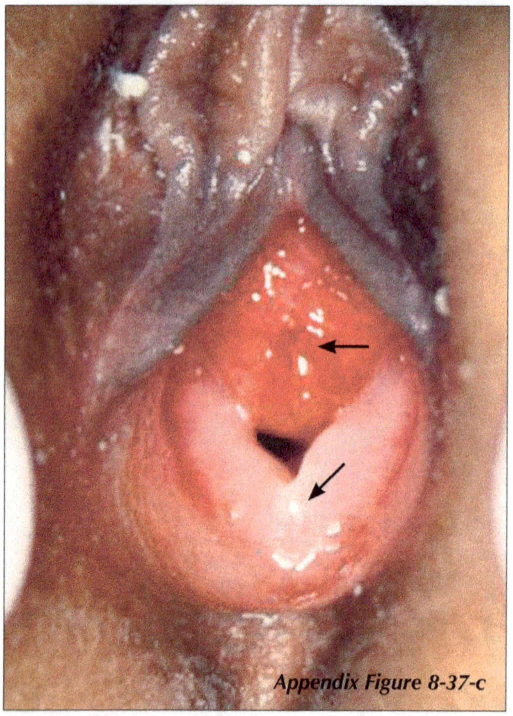
Appendix Figure 8-37-c

Appendix Figure 8-37-a. *This 3-year-old girl presented with blood in her underwear and a history of having pulled out a Foley catheter during a recent hospitalization. She is examined in the supine position. The bleeding is coming from a prolapsed urethra, the swollen tissue taking up most of the vestibule in this photo. The dark areas at 3 o'clock, 5 o'clock, and 7 o'clock may be early signs of necrosis. The hymen at 6 o'clock is pale and smooth. Image reprinted with permission from eMedicine.com, 2010. Available at: https://emedicine.medscape.com/article/954024-overview.*

Appendix Figure 8-37-b. *In the prone knee-chest position, the prolapsed urethra still occludes the hymenal opening. This condition can usually be successfully treated with warm soaks and watchful waiting.*

Appendix Figure 8-37-c. *After 2 weeks, the prolapse has significantly resolved. The hymen at 6 o'clock is now better visualized. Image reprinted with permission from eMedicine.com, 2010. Available at: https://emedicine.medscape.com/article/954024-overview.*

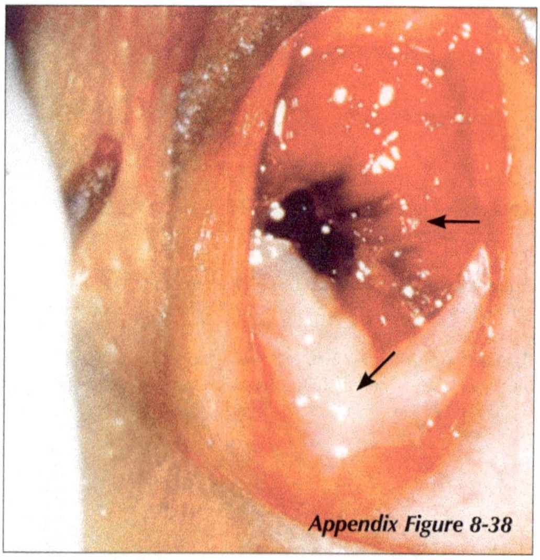
Appendix Figure 8-38

Appendix Figure 8-38. *A 4-year-old African-American girl with urethral prolapse from 3 o'clock to 9 o'clock superiorly and a normal, thick hymen below 3 o'clock and 9 o'clock inferiorly. The black area at 9 o'clock could represent early necrosis.*

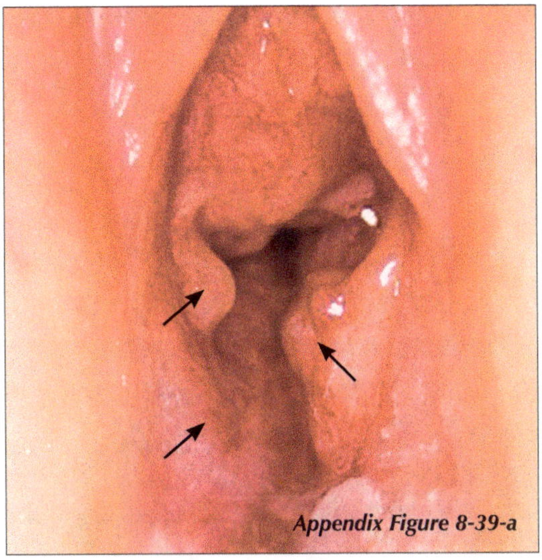

Appendix Figure 8-39-a

Appendix Figures 8-39-a *through* **8-39-g.** *This 9-year-old girl was sexually assaulted by her stepfather 6 days prior to evaluation. She disclosed the abuse to a school nurse after the nurse noted that the girl was bleeding.*

Appendix Figure 8-39-a. *With minimal labial separation, a laceration of the posterior fourchette is seen at 6 o'clock, and a loss of hymenal tissue is seen between 4 o'clock and 9 o'clock.*

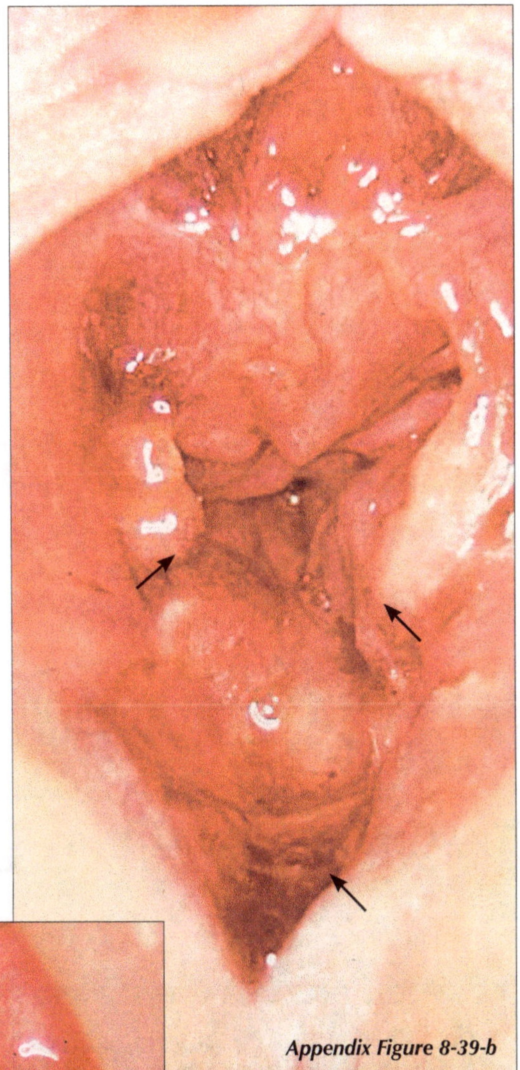

Appendix Figure 8-39-b

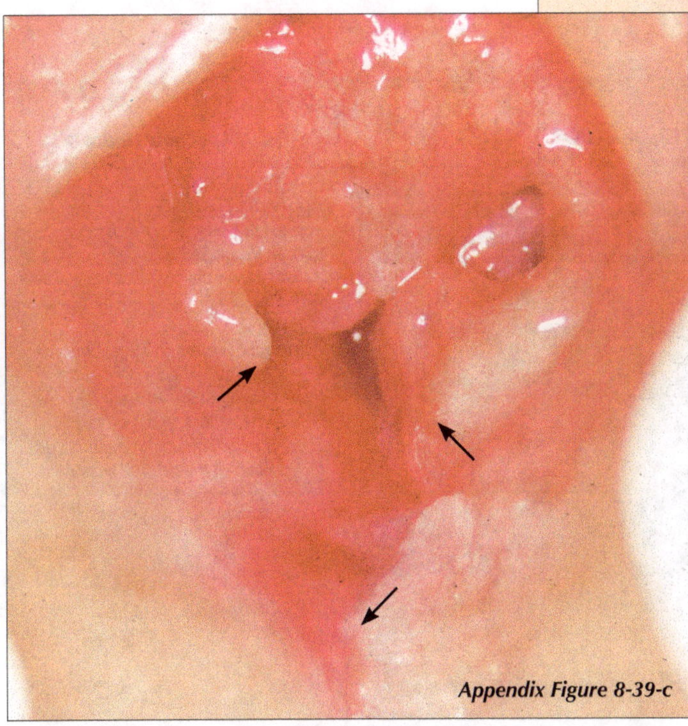

Appendix Figure 8-39-c

Appendix Figure 8-39-b. *With additional labial separation, the hymen is completely transected, with the torn edges indicated at 5 o'clock and 9 o'clock. The deep laceration of the fossa and posterior fourchette at 6 o'clock began to ooze blood when the labia were separated by the examiner. Image reprinted with permission from eMedicine.com, 2010. Available at: https://emedicine.medscape.com/article/954024-overview.*

Appendix Figure 8-39-c. *At 13 days after the assault, the posterior fourchette tear is beginning to heal. There is a loss of hymen tissue between 5 o'clock and 8 o'clock. Some healing of the posterior fourchette laceration can be seen at 6 o'clock.*

Appendix Figure 8-39-d. *At 13 days post assault, the loss of hymen in the midline between 2 o'clock and 11 o'clock is clearly evident, with the child in the knee-chest position.*

Appendix Figure 8-39-e. *One month post assault, the posterior fourchette tear has healed, leaving a midline scar at 6 o'clock. The 2 sections of the hymen are seen again, with a loss of hymenal tissue between 5 o'clock and 8 o'clock. An adhesion has developed anteriorly between the labia minora at 12 o'clock.*

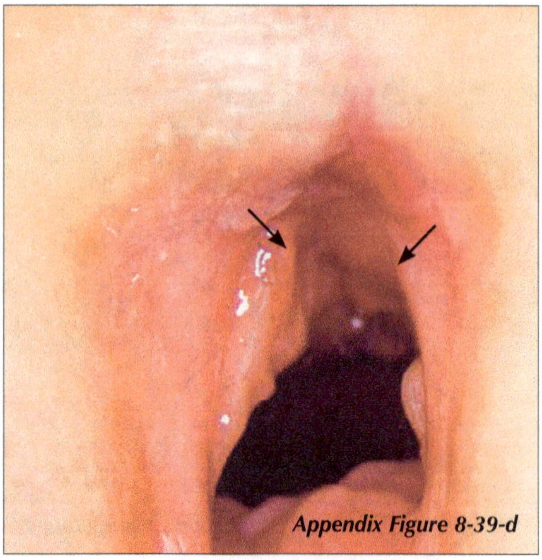

Appendix Figure 8-39-d

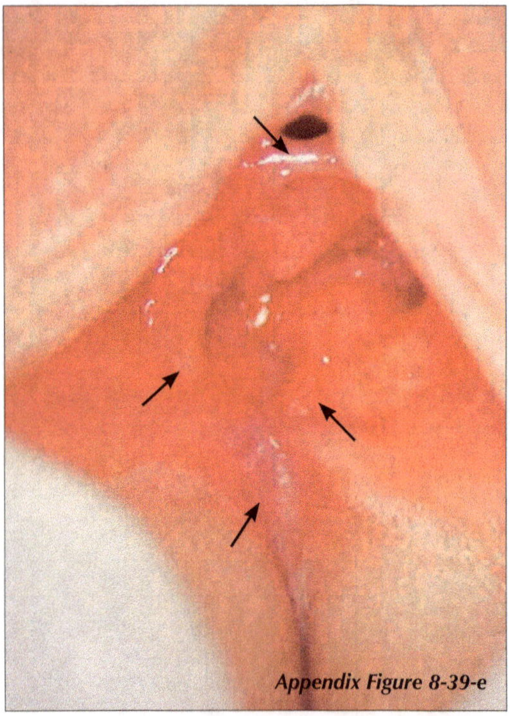

Appendix Figure 8-39-e

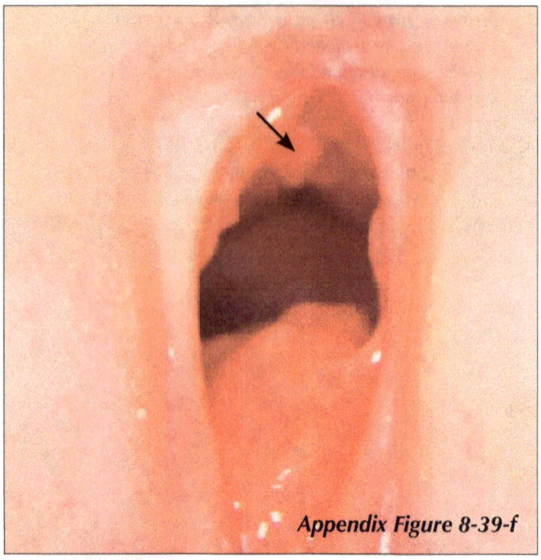

Appendix Figure 8-39-f

Appendix Figure 8-39-f. *One month post-assault, reactive scar tissue appears to have developed within the vagina at 12 o'clock on the posterior vaginal wall, with the child in the knee-chest position.*

Appendix Figure 8-39-g. *One year after the assault, the 2 edges of the hymen have not grown back together between 5 o'clock and 7 o'clock. There is a midline scar of the fossa at the location of the original laceration (shown at 6 o'clock).*

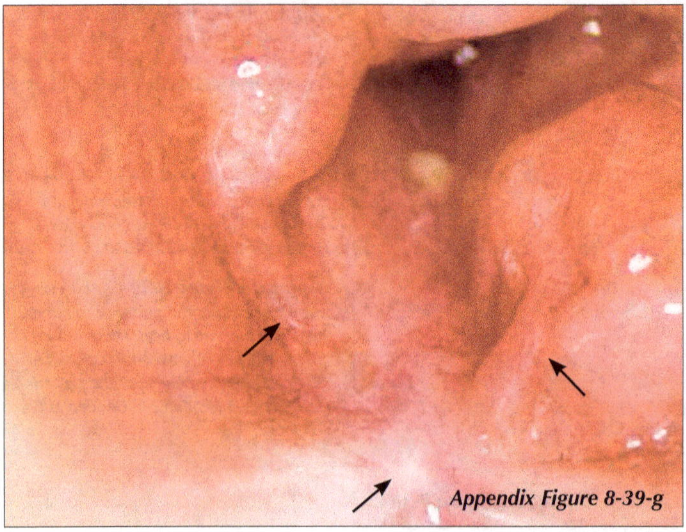

Appendix Figure 8-39-g

Appendix Figures 8-40-a *through* **8-40-h.** *This 9-year-old girl was abducted and raped by a stranger. She was found walking along the highway and given a ride to the hospital. After the girl identified the assailant's truck, he was arrested, charged, and convicted.*

Appendix Figure 8-40-a. *This photo was taken 3 days after surgical repair of a deep laceration of the posterior fourchette that extended across the perineum, almost to the anal verge. The 2 parts of the transected hymen were overlapped (upper arrow), when the posterior fourchette tear was sutured (shown at 6 o'clock).*

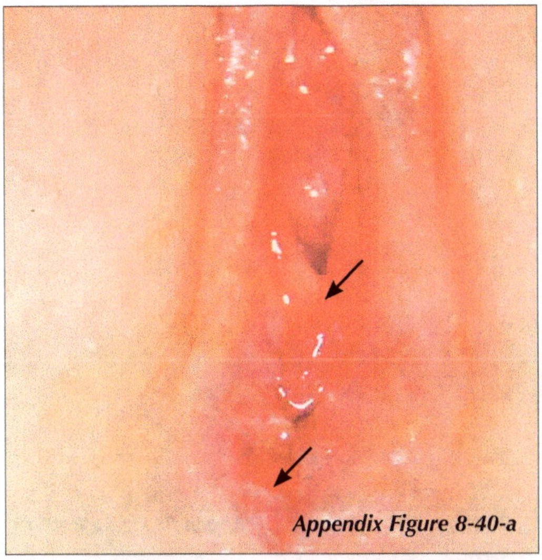

Appendix Figure 8-40-a

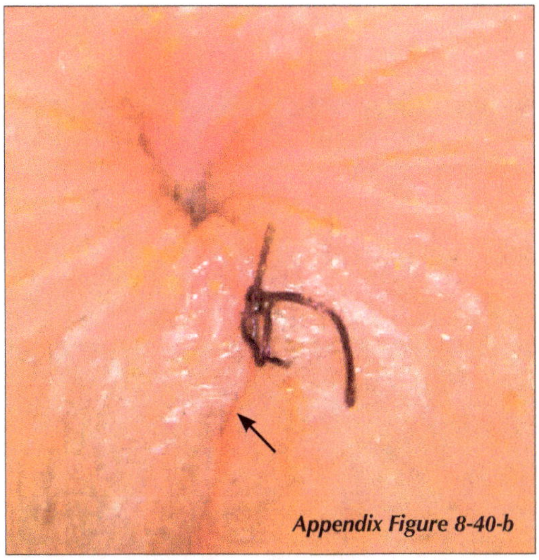

Appendix Figure 8-40-b

Appendix Figure 8-40-b. *This photograph shows the extent of the laceration and the suture repair at 6 o'clock, extending almost to the anal verge.*

Appendix Figure 8-40-c. *16 days after the assault, the repaired posterior fourchette laceration is healing well. The 2 halves of the hymen, shown at 7 o'clock and 5 o'clock, are joined by a small band of scar tissue at 6 o'clock.*

Appendix Figure 8-40-d. *At 16 days post-assault, the left half of the torn hymen is bound down to the fossa with scar tissue (top arrow). The thin line across the perineum is the scar from the repaired laceration at 6 o'clock.*

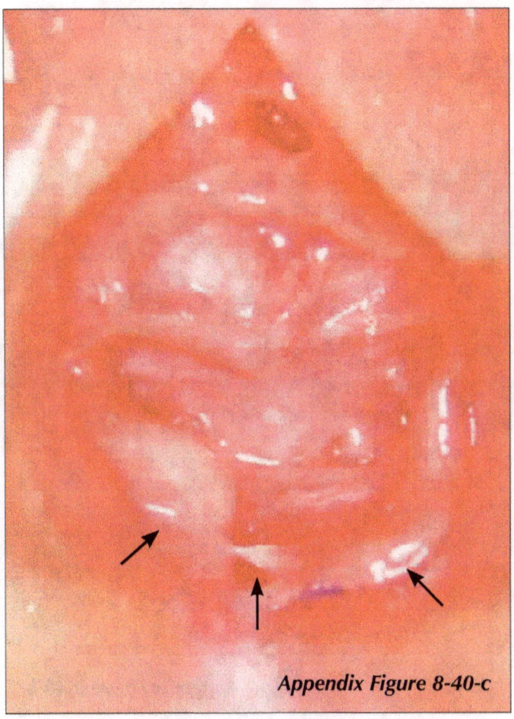

Appendix Figure 8-40-c

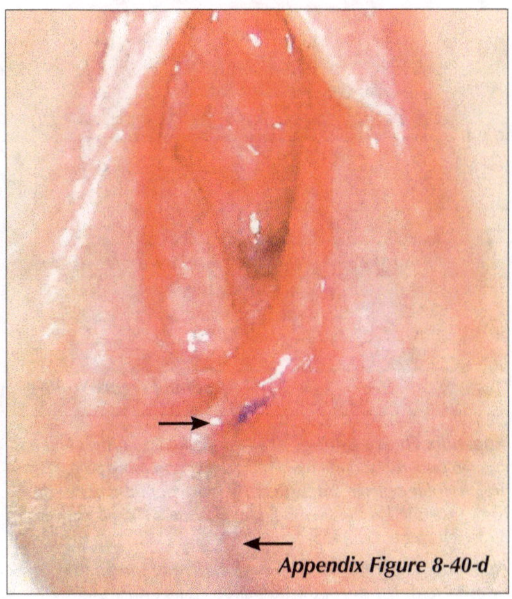

Appendix Figure 8-40-d

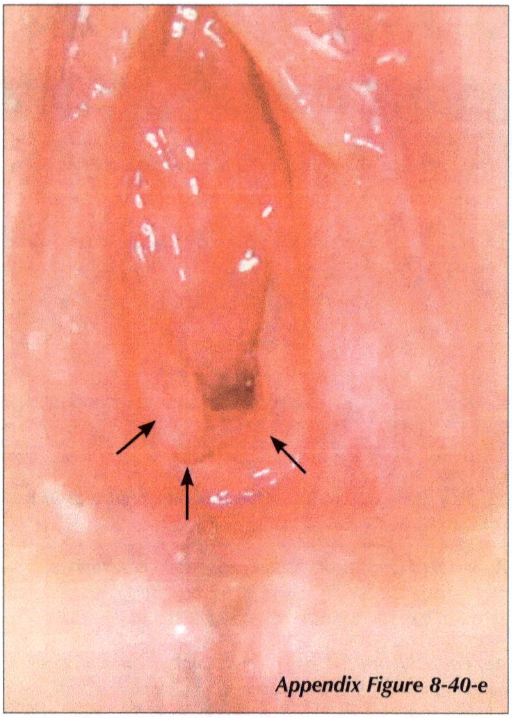

Appendix Figure 8-40-e

Appendix Figure 8-40-e. *One month post-assault, there is still a small band of scar tissue connecting the 2 halves of the hymen (shown at 6 o'clock).*

Appendix Figure 8-40-f. *Six months post-assault, the white, flat scar tissue has developed in the fossa at 5 o'clock to 6 o'clock, adjacent to the site of the hymenal laceration.*

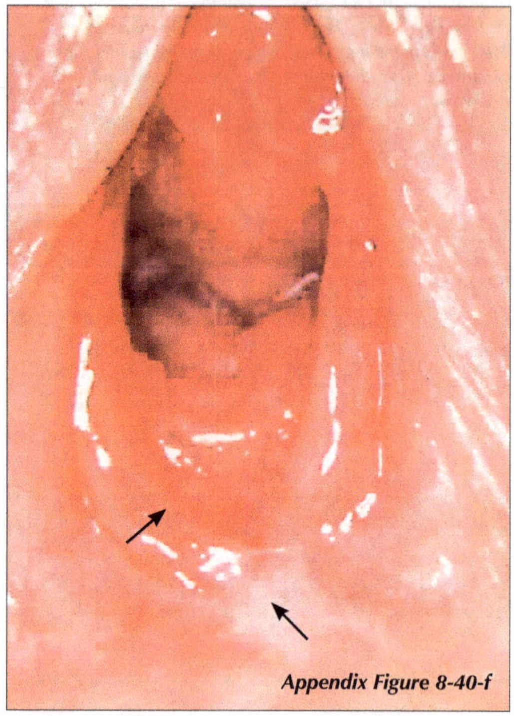

Appendix Figure 8-40-f

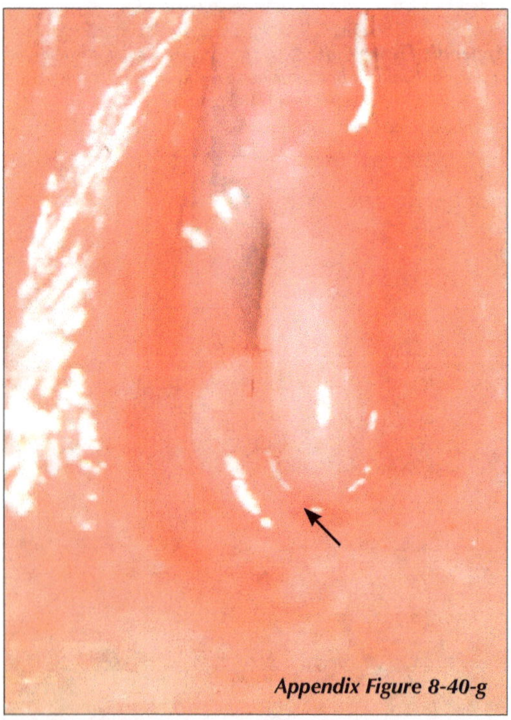

Appendix Figure 8-40-g

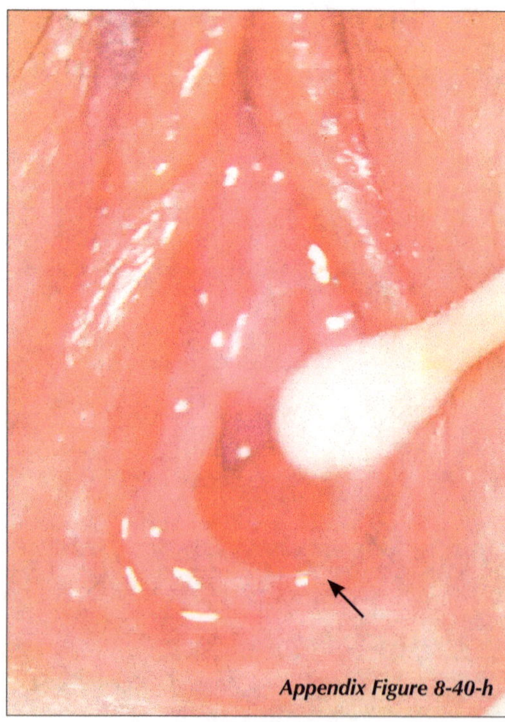

Appendix Figure 8-40-h

Appendix Figure 8-40-g. *At 1 year post-assault, the child has entered puberty, and the hymen is thicker and more pale. There are no visible scars in the fossa or the posterior fourchette. The hymen is folded at the site of the previous tear shown between 5 o'clock and 6 o'clock.*

Appendix Figure 8-40-h. *A swab is used to spread the hymenal fold. The site of the laceration is still evident (arrow).*

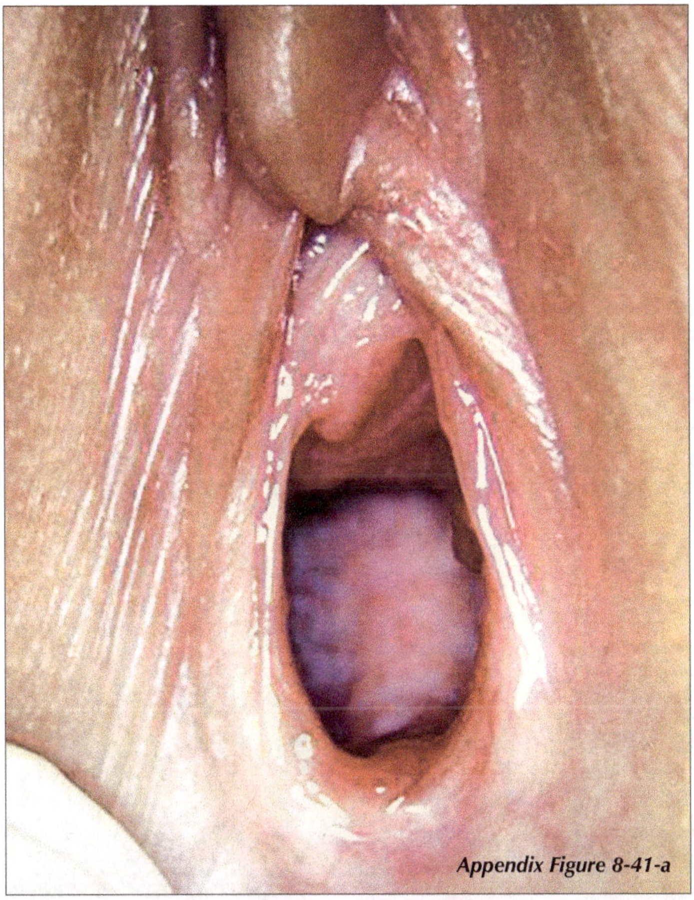

Appendix Figure 8-41-a

Appendix Figure 8-41-a. *This 7-year-old girl was referred for having "no hymen." She denied any history of accidental trauma or abuse, and the child's mother had no explanation for the near absence of her daughter's hymen.*

Appendix Figure 8-41-b. *Using labial traction, it can be seen that only minute remnants of a hymen remain.*

Appendix Figure 8-41-c. *In the prone knee-chest position, it is still not possible to identify any hymenal tissue between 9 o'clock and 4 o'clock. The cause for this disruption was never determined.*

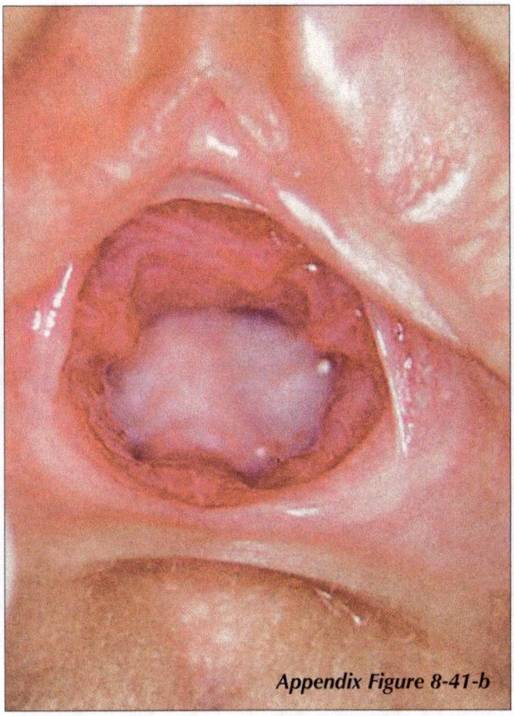

Appendix Figure 8-41-b

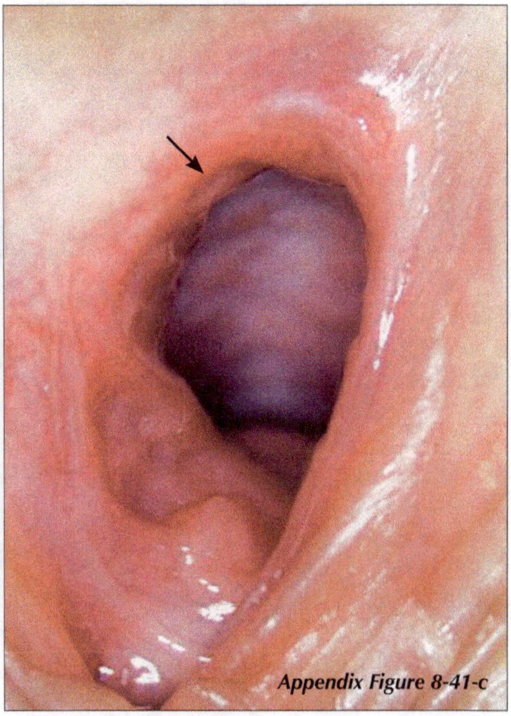

Appendix Figure 8-41-c

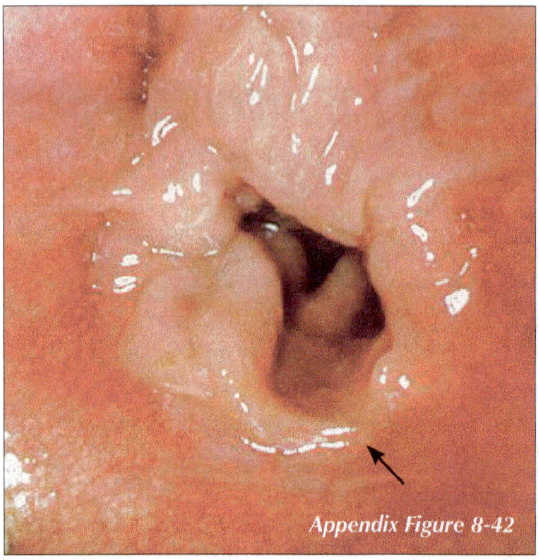

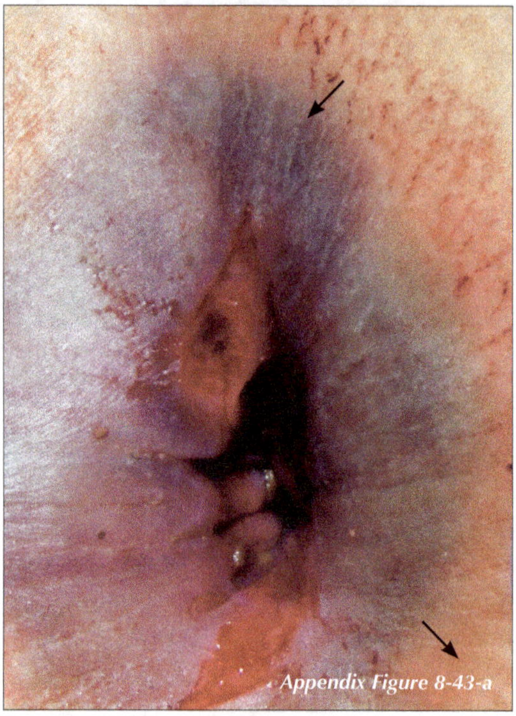

Appendix Figure 8-42. *This 16-year-old girl has been consensually sexually active for 1 year. There is a transection in the hymen at 5 o'clock.*

Appendix Figure 8-43-a. *This 7-year-old boy asked his mother, "Is my bottom still supposed to be hurting?" When asked for details, he disclosed that a 14-year-old male cousin had put his penis in the boy's bottom. The cousin told him it would only hurt for a little while. On examination, there is extensive bruising all around the anus and 2 deep anal lacerations at 6 o'clock and 11 o'clock.*

Appendix Figure 8-43-b. *Ten days after the assault, the bruising has resolved. There is a white scar at the site of the larger laceration (11 o'clock).*

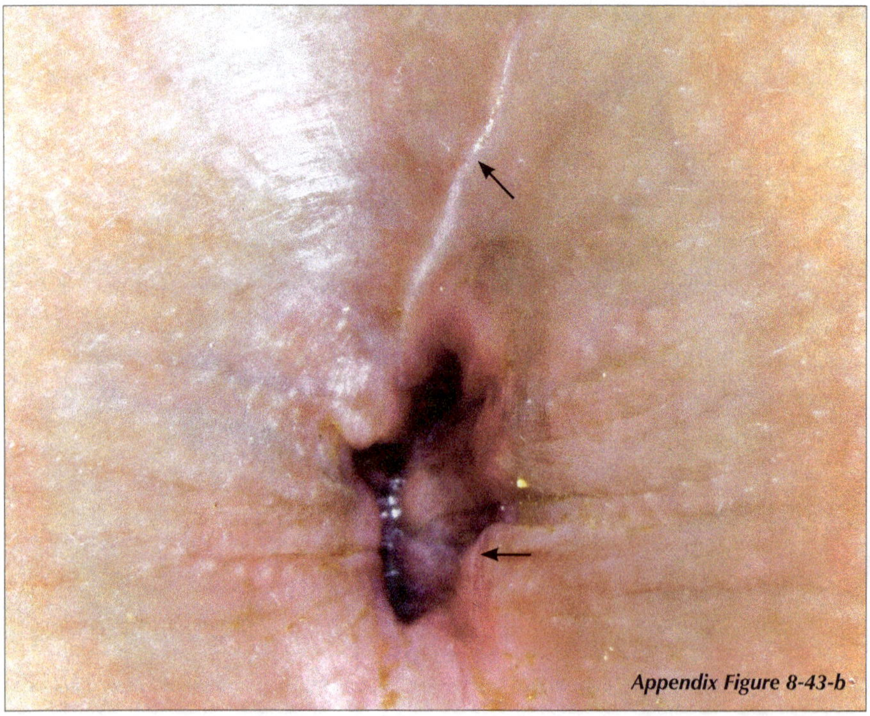

References

1. Adams JA, Harper K, Knudson S. A proposed system for the classification of anogenital findings in children with suspected sexual abuse. *Adolesc Pediatr Gynecol.* 1992;5(2):73-75.
2. McCann J, Voris J, Simon M, Wells R. Perianal findings in prepubertal children selected for nonabuse: a descriptive study. *Child Abuse Negl.* 1989;13(2):179-193.
3. McCann J, Wells R, Simon M, Voris J. Genital findings in prepubertal girls selected for nonabuse: a descriptive study. *Pediatrics.* 1990;86(3):428-439.
4. Berenson A, Heger A, Andrews S. Appearance of the hymen in newborns. *Pediatrics.* 1991;87(4):458-465.
5. American Academy of Pediatrics Committee on Child Abuse and Neglect. Guidelines for the evaluation of sexual abuse of children. *Pediatrics.* 1991;87(2):254-260.
6. Berenson AB, Heger AH, Hayes JM, Bailey RK, Emans SJ. Appearance of the hymen in prepubertal girls. *Pediatrics.* 1992;89(3):387-394.
7. Berenson AB. Appearance of the hymen at birth and one year of age: a longitudinal study. *Pediatrics.* 1993;91(4):820-825.
8. Berenson AB. A longitudinal study of hymenal morphology in the first 3 years of life. *Pediatrics.* 1995;95(4):490-496.
9. Berenson AB, Grady JJ. A longitudinal study of hymenal development from 3 to 9 years of age. *J Pediatr.* 2002;140(5):600-607.
10. Myhre AK, Berntzen K, Bratlid D. Genital anatomy in non-abused preschool girls. *Acta Paediatr.* 2003;92(12):1453-1462.
11. McCann J, Voris J, Simon M. Genital injuries resulting from sexual abuse: a longitudinal study. *Pediatrics.* 1992;89(2):307-317.
12. McCann J, Voris J. Perianal injuries resulting from sexual abuse: a longitudinal study. *Pediatrics.* 1993;91(2):390-397.
13. Heppenstall-Heger A, McConnell G, Ticson L, Guerra L, Lister J, Zaragoza T. Healing patterns in anogenital injuries: a longitudinal study of injuries associated with sexual abuse, accidental injuries, or genital surgery in the preadolescent child. *Pediatrics.* 2003;112(4):829-837.
14. Adams JA. Approach to the interpretation of medical and laboratory findings in suspected child sexual abuse: a 2005 revision. *The APSAC Advisor.* 2005;17:7-13.
15. Adams JA, Kaplan RA, Starling SP, et al. Guidelines for medical care for children who may have been sexually abused. *J Pediatr Adolesc Gynecol.* 2007;20(3):163-172.
16. Adams JA, Kellogg ND, Farst KJ, et al. Updated guidelines for the medical assessment and care of children who may have been sexually abused. *J Pediatr Adolesc Gynecol.* 2016;29(2):81-87.
17. Adams JA, Farst KJ, Kellogg ND. Interpretation of medical findings in suspected child sexual abuse: an update for 2018. *J Pediatr Adolesc Gynecol.* 2018;31(3):225-231.
18. Berenson AB, Chacko MR, Wiemann CM, Mishaw CO, Friedrich WN, Grady JJ. A case-control study of anatomic changes resulting from sexual abuse. *Am J Obstet Gynecol.* 2000;182(4):820-831; discussion 831-834.

19. Adams JA, Botash AS, Kellogg N. Differences in hymenal morphology between adolescent girls with and without a history of consensual sexual intercourse. *Arch Pediatr Adolesc Med.* 2004;158(3):280-285.

20. Heger AH, Ticson L, Guerra L, et al. Appearance of the genitalia in girls selected for nonabuse: review of hymenal morphology and nonspecific findings. *J Pediatr Adolesc Gynecol.* 2002;15(1):27-35.

21. Bacopoulou F, Karakitsos P, Kottaridi C, et al. Genital HPV in children and adolescents: does sexual activity make a difference? *J Pediatr Adolesc Gynecol.* 2016;29(3):228-233.

22. Sehgal VN, Pandhi D, Khurana A. Nonspecific genital ulcers. *Clin Dermatol.* 2014;32(2):259-274.

23. Senusi A, Seoudi N, Bergmeir LA, Fortune F. Genital ulcer severity score and genital health quality of life in Behçet's disease. *Orphanet J Rare Dis.* 2015;10:117.

24. Hupert JS, Gerber MA, Deitch HR, Mortensen JE, Statt MA, Adams Hilliard PJ. Vulvar ulcers in young females: a manifestation of aphthosis. *J Pediatr Adolesc Gynecol.* 2006;19(3):195-204.

25. Delgado-Garcia S, Palacios-Marqués A, Martínez-Escoriza JC, Martín-Bayón TA. Acute genital ulcers. *BMJ Case Rep.* 2014;2014:brc2013202504. doi:10.1136/bcr-2013-202504.

26. Myhre AK, Berntzen K, Bratlid D. Perianal anatomy in non-abused preschool children. *Acta Paediatr.* 2001;90(11):1321-1328.

27. Myhre AK, Adams JA, Kaufhold M, Davis JL, Suresh P, Kuelbs CL. Anal findings in children with and without probable anal penetration: a retrospective study of 1115 children referred for suspected sexual abuse. *Child Abuse Negl.* 2013;37(7):465-474.

28. McCann J, Reay D, Siebert J, Stephens BG, Wirtz S. Postmortem perianal findings in children. *Am J Forensic Med Pathol.* 1996;17(4):289-298.

29. Hobbs CJ, Wright CM. Anal signs of child sexual abuse: a case-control study. *BMC Pediatr.* 2014;14:128.

30. Heger A, Ticson L, Velasquez O, Bernier R. Children referred for possible sexual abuse: medical findings in 2384 children. *Child Abuse Negl.* 2002;26(6-7):645-659.

31. Boos SC. Accidental hymenal injury mimicking sexual trauma. *Pediatrics.* 1999;103(6 pt 1):1287-1290.

32. Herrmann B, Crawford J. Genital injuries in prepubertal girls from inline skating accidents. *Pediatrics.* 2002;110(2 pt 1):e16.

33. Boos SC, Rosas AJ, Boyle C, McCaan J. Anogenital injuries in child pedestrians run over by low-speed motor vehicles: four cases with findings that mimic child sexual abuse. *Pediatrics.* 2003;112(1 pt 1):e77-e84.

34. Gallion HR, Milam LJ, Littrell LL. Genital findings in cases of child sexual abuse: genital vs vaginal penetration. *J Pediatr Adolesc Gynecol.* 2016;29(6):604-611.

35. McCann J, Miyamoto S, Boyle C, Rogers K. Healing of hymenal injuries in prepubertal and adolescent girls: a descriptive study. *Pediatrics.* 2007;119(5):e1094-e1106.

36. McCann J, Miyamoto S, Boyle C, Rogers K. Healing of nonhymenal genital injuries in prepubertal and adolescent girls: a descriptive study. *Pediatrics.* 2007;120(5):1000-1011.

37. Boyle C, McCann J, Miyamoto S, Rogers K. Comparison of examination methods used in the evaluation of prepubertal and pubertal female genitalia: a descriptive study. *Child Abuse Negl.* 2008;32(2):229-243.

38. Kellogg ND, Menard SW, Santos A. Genital anatomy in pregnant adolescents: "normal" does not mean "nothing happened." *Pediatrics.* 2004;113(1 pt 1):e67-e69.

39. Jones JS, Rossman L, Hartman M, Alexander CC. Anogenital injuries in adolescents after consensual sexual intercourse. *Acad Emerg Med.* 2003;10(12):1378-1383.

Chapter 9

Medical Conditions That Mimic Sexual Abuse

Alice Swenson, MD, FAAP
Lori Frasier, MD

Introduction

One of the most common reasons for medical referrals in alleged child abuse cases is to evaluate allegations of sexual abuse. As noted in Chapter 8, physical findings resulting from sexual abuse are exceedingly rare. The child abuse specialist often has special expertise and training in evaluation of a broad variety of anogenital conditions and as such may become the point of referral for these conditions. The referral may be initiated because of a possible history of abuse disclosed by the child, behavioral findings, medical signs, or symptoms. Occasionally a disclosure of abuse accompanies signs or symptoms. The examining clinician must always remain objective in such examinations and not allow the history from the child to overly influence the interpretation of medical findings. The coincidental occurrence of an anogenital condition should not lead the examiner to suggest the condition results from the abuse. Pre-examination bias should especially be guarded against when referrals are exclusively for anogenital complaints by the child or when an observation by a parent or referring medical provider indicates that the child has some finding that may be due to sexual abuse. The differential diagnosis of any anogenital symptom must include a variety of conditions unrelated to sexual abuse because there are many symptoms and diseases that may mimic findings of sexual abuse.

In this chapter, many of the "medical mimics" of child sexual abuse (CSA) that have been both described in the literature and clinically observed are reviewed. Because many patients are referred on the basis of symptoms, the approach of this chapter is symptom based rather than systems based. A differential diagnosis for a variety of symptoms and a diagnostic approach are presented.

Medical Mimics of Child Sexual Abuse

Genital Irritation/Erythema

A common reason a clinician may see a child is to address anogenital redness or erythema discovered or reported by a parent or caregiver. Even in the context of recent abuse allegations, anogenital erythema should not be assumed to be associated with sexual abuse, because it is a nonspecific finding. The clinician should not suggest that such a finding is the direct result of sexual trauma, but instead should explain that the 2 findings are unrelated. The erythema may involve the keratinized epithelium of the vulvar area, perineum, perianal area, penis, or mucosa of the vestibule (anatomically, the area between the labia minora and the periurethral and perihymenal areas, the hymen, and the posterior navicular fossa). The most common causes of genital redness are poor hygiene and contact dermatitis. Also, in prepubertal girls the mucosa of the vestibule may appear erythematous, and what is thought to be an abnormality is a normal appearance caused by the highly vascular nature of these tissues; therefore, what might be thought by the layperson to be an abnormality might in fact be a normal anatomical appearance.

A variety of products can result in a contact irritation of the genital area. These products can be perfume-containing soaps, lotions, bubble baths, toilet paper, and laundry products or any other product that contains irritants. Overzealous cleansing may also cause such irritation. The diagnosis is usually made after clinical observation of erythema. Scaling, crusting, or even blistering can occur. Protected skin folds are usually spared. Edema can be marked if the contact dermatitis involves the penis or the foreskin. The clinical approach to a child with anogenital irritation and redness is first to recommend a regimen of excellent genital hygiene with avoidance of such products. Use of a bland emollient such as zinc oxide or bland occlusive ointment may help to protect the skin as it heals. If skin barrier integrity is lost, overgrowth of bacterial or fungal pathogens may result. These should be treated with appropriate antibiotics or antifungals. A rapid resolution of the condition will reassure the parent and clinician the cause of the child's irritation or redness was related to these products or practices.

Other conditions that mimic chronic genital irritation include psoriasis and seborrheic dermatitis. Psoriasis usually occurs as skin lesions that are sharply demarcated and have fine, silvery scales. Inverse psoriasis is a distinct form of the condition that involves the anogenital area, axillae, and ear canals. Erythema is often the predominant clinical feature, and scaling is minimal, leading to confusion with candidiasis, contact dermatitis, or seborrhea. Skin biopsy is diagnostic and usually recommended only after multiple unsuccessful attempts at topical medications. Treatment of psoriasis is aimed at preventing irritation, with high-potency topical steroids given in short bursts. Evaluation and management of psoriasis is usually in the purview of the pediatric rheumatologist, given the association with other rheumatologic conditions.

Seborrheic dermatitis is a common skin condition that mainly affects the scalp and posterior auricular area but can also be present in the diaper area, leading to a concern of sexual abuse. The condition is usually characterized by greasy, yellow scales. In severe cases, fissures may develop and become secondarily infected. Infantile seborrheic dermatitis generally spontaneously improves by the end of the first year of life.

Anogenital Bruising

Bruising or apparent bruising of the anogenital area may raise concerns for sexual abuse; however, a careful examination may reveal other conditions or a history of accidental trauma. A careful history may reveal a traumatic event such as a straddle-type injury. Given the friability and vascularity of the anogenital tissues, injuries to that area may appear disproportionate to the injury mechanism. Alternatively, venous pooling in the anal area can appear to the layperson to be bruising. Traction on the buttocks for even a few seconds can cause pooling in the venous plexus and appear to be an injury.

Lichen Sclerosus

Descriptions of childhood lichen sclerosus (LS) et atrophicus first appeared in the literature in the 1950s. However, Jenny et al[1,2] noted that LS was being confused with trauma caused by sexual abuse. Since that time, other authors[3,4] have described this condition as one of the most common mimics of anogenital trauma. LS is commonly seen in postmenopausal women as a skin condition of unknown origin. Various causative factors have been suggested. These causes range from infections with Borrelia species to immunological association with certain HLA antigens to familial incidence.[5-7] It is currently commonly understood to be an autoimmune disease.[8] In children, the classic case is seen in a prepubertal child with a history of waxing and waning genital irritation. Children may present with a variety of complaints stemming from the underlying itching and pain. Frequent initial misdiagnoses are common, often for urinary tract infections and yeast infections.[9] Fissuring and stricture in the perianal area have also been reported to cause constipation, a symptom of perianal lichen sclerosus. The skin of the vulva is hypopigmented and atrophic, often in a "figure of 8 pattern" (**Figures 9-1-a**, **b**, and **c**). This pattern may not be as apparent in very fair-skinned individuals. Subcutaneous hemorrhage and hemorrhagic bullae are often the hallmark of LS (**Figure 9-2**). Interestingly, the mucosa, including the hymen, is spared and appears normal.

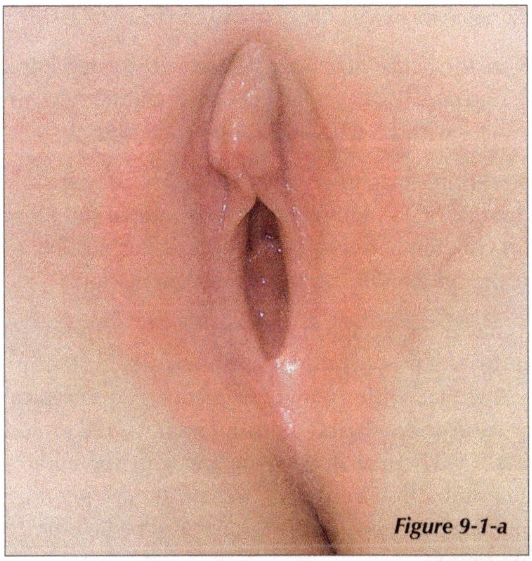

Figure 9-1-a

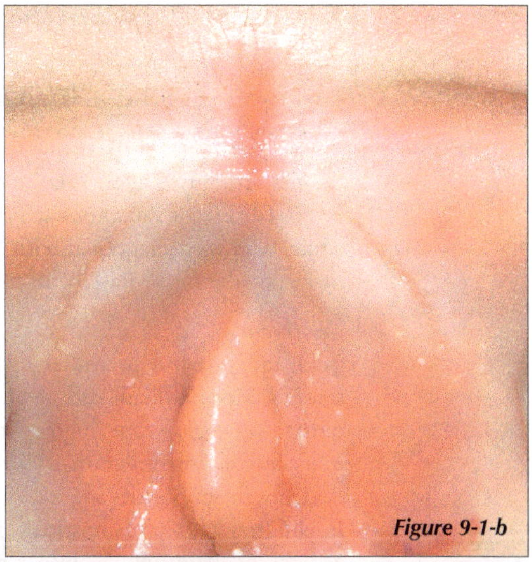

Figure 9-1-b

Figure 9-1-a. *Generalized erythema of the genital mucosa has a variety of causes but often raises a concern about sexual abuse. Removal of irritants and good genital hygiene results in clearing of the skin.*

Figure 9-1-b. *Pale skin anterior to the clitoris in lichen sclerosis et atrophicus. The fissuring is due to friability of the tissue and is a common feature seen in patients with lichen sclerosis.*

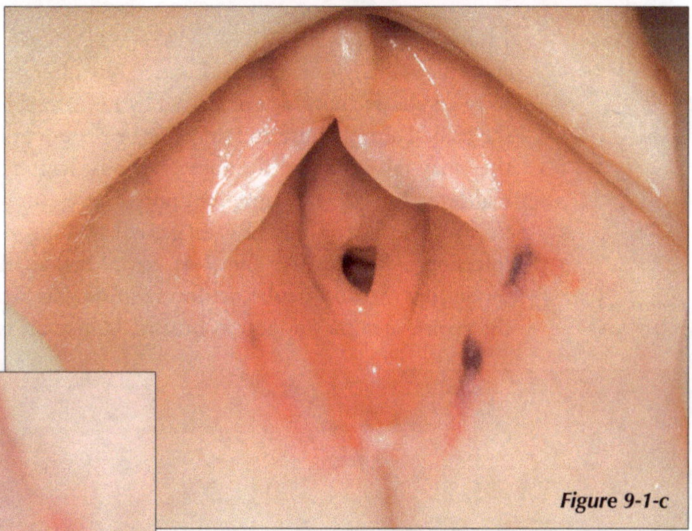

Figure 9-1-c

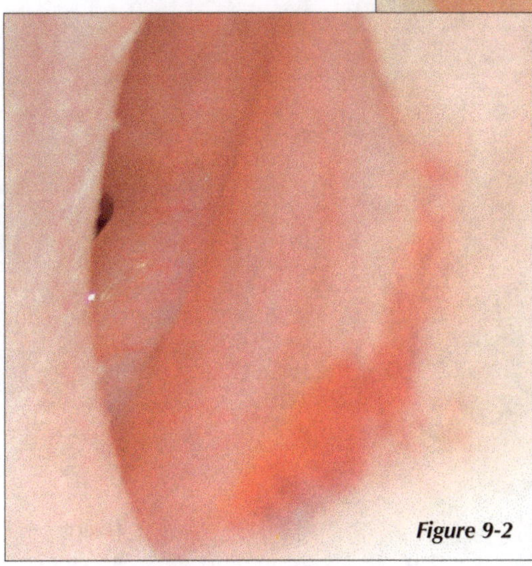

Figure 9-2

Figure 9-1-c. *Typical presentation of lichen sclerosis et atrophicus, with pale atrophic skin and subcutaneous hemorrhage. The mucosa is not involved.*

Figure 9-2. *Another view of the same patient in **Figure 9-1-c**. Subcutaneous hemorrhage can resemble traumatic injury.*

In severe cases of LS, the act of wiping may result in denudation of the atrophic epithelium, with pain and bleeding. On examination, the child appears to have both bruising and ulcerations, raising concerns of trauma or other infections caused by sexual abuse.

Lichen sclerosus is not just a condition of girls. Boys with LS most commonly present with phimosis needing circumcision. Up to 40% of boys undergoing circumcision for phimosis have LS, although some studies estimate the incidence to be closer to 10%.[10]

Some boys who undergo circumcision for lichen sclerosus may go on to develop a subcategory of LS, balanitis xerotica obliterans (BXO), which results in meatal stenosis. This condition occurs in up to 1 in 5 boys with LS who undergo circumcision.[11]

Studies strongly suggest that adults who are diagnosed with LS are at substantially increased risk for squamous cell carcinoma (SCC). However, no longitudinal studies of adults who were diagnosed with LS as children have been done, so it is not possible to make any definitive statements about the risk of SCC in this patient population.

Treatment of LS is aimed at palliation during symptomatic periods. Most cases are mild and respond to the avoidance of irritants, clothing, and activities that cause trauma. More difficult cases have been treated with a variety of agents such as topical estrogens, progesterone, high-potency corticosteroids, immunosuppressants, and topical nonsteroidal anti-inflammatory agents.[12-14] The mainstay of therapy with the bulk of evidence to support its use is ultrapotent topical steroids used over a 3-month period.[15] In children who have constipation or anal stricture, a stool softener may be helpful. In general the condition resolves in adolescence.

Hemangiomas/Vascular Malformations

A vulvar hemangioma that had undergone ulcerative changes and was thought initially to be an abusive burn was described by Levin et al in 1988.[16] Vascular malformations of the genital area are rare and may not be present at birth. When they become apparent, they may raise concern for abuse. Venous, lymphatic, and capillary-lymphatic-venous malformations are the most common. These can manifest in a variety of ways: as cutaneous marks resembling bruises, genital swelling, deformity, bleeding, fluid leakage, or infection[17] (**Figures 9-3** and **9-4**). Sacral hemangiomas can be associated with imperforate anus. Small vascular malformations or strawberry hemangiomas (**Figure 9-4**) on the genital area may appear as bruises. Unlike bruises, these are relatively stable lesions

Figure 9-3. *Clitoral hood vascular lesion and a small anterior fissure as a result of poor hygiene. The child was examined 1 week later; the vascular malformation was stable and the small fissure was resolved.*

Figure 9-4. *Hemangioma.*

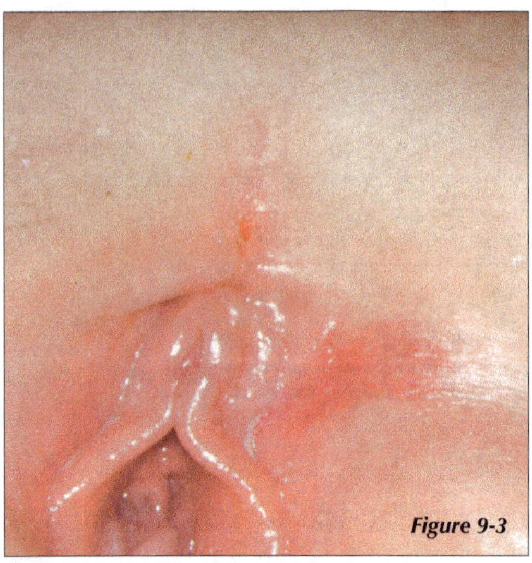

Figure 9-3

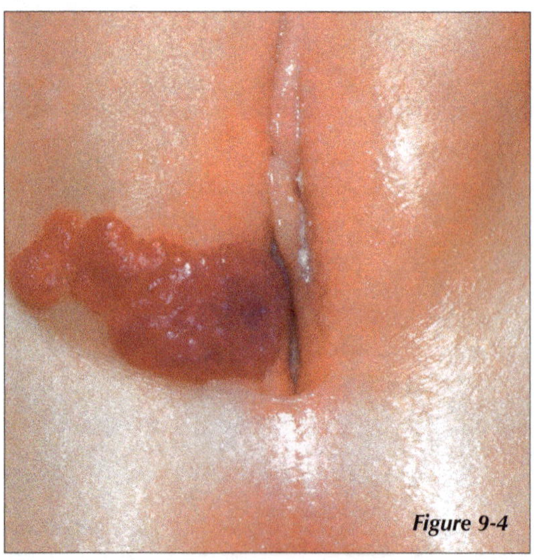

Figure 9-4

that do not change, or the lesions resolve over a relatively short period such as weeks; therefore, reevaluation of the area usually allows the clinician to make a diagnosis of stable vascular lesions, rather than a traumatic bruise or contusion. It is advisable that high-quality photodocumentation be performed in any case that appears to be acute injury. These photos can be compared with those taken at a later date.

Treatment is difficult in some cases and is beyond the scope of this publication.

Purpura as a Mimic of Bruising

Purpura is a common, nonspecific symptom indicative of a pathological condition in which blood leaks into the tissues. Purpuric disorders can be classified according to the pathophysiological processes outlined in **Table 9-1**.

Purpuric lesions can occur in the genital area only, but their manifestation on the genitalia could simply be the first location of a sequence of symptoms that lead to concerns of sexual abuse. More commonly, these conditions have been described as physical abuse mimics. Often, as in Henoch-Schönlein purpura (HSP), if the first symptom appears in the genital area, the extent of the purpura will manifest in a matter of hours to days[18-20] (**Figure 9-5**). Also, the child often has classic accompanying symptoms such as abdominal or joint pain, hematuria, and bloody stools. There is a reported case of a 19-month-old boy who presented to an emergency department with penile and scrotal swelling and apparent bruising and tenderness who eventually developed palpable purpura on the buttocks and was diagnosed with HSP, but only after an extensive workup for child abuse and involvement of law enforcement.[21]

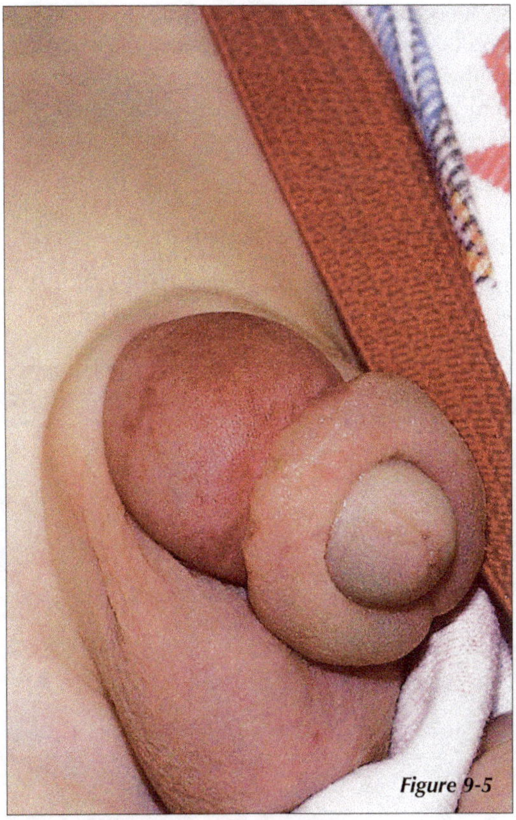

Figure 9-5. *Henoch-Schönlein purpura with involvement of the penis mimicking bruising.*

Table 9-1. Classification of Purpuric Disorders

Classification of Purpuric Disorders
Platelet disorders
— Primary thrombocytopenic purpura such as idiopathic thrombocytopenic purpura
— Secondary thrombocytopenic purpura caused by conditions such as leukemia or aplastic anemias
Vascular disorders
— Vasculitis, as in the case of Henoch-Schönlein purpura
Coagulation disorders
— Disseminated intravascular coagulation resulting from shock or infection; such children are extremely ill
— Hemophilias
— von Willebrand disease

Accidental Genital Injuries

Differentiating an accidental anogenital injury from one due to abuse may be fairly straightforward. The parent—and when possible, the child—often provides a clear history of an impact or penetrating injury to the genital area, followed by bleeding and pain. The injury is often "typical" of a straddle and the child is ambulatory and therefore capable of falling accidentally. Unusual injuries, as discussed within this section, may raise more concern for abuse, either physical or sexual, and may be more difficult to evaluate, particularly if the child is nonverbal.

Most accidental anogenital injuries in girls occur when there is impact between the child's perineum and a hard object such as a bicycle or a metal bar of playground equipment. The soft tissues are compressed between the object and the ischial tuberosities, causing contusions, lacerations, and even injuries reflecting transmitted trauma to different areas. Most straddle injuries are more anterior, external to the hymen, and unilateral (**Figures 9-6** and **9-7**). If there is a history of impalement, a more internal injury such as tearing of perineum or, less commonly, the hymen, may be observed.[22] Unusual injuries have been reported in the literature. In one case a child who fell while waterskiing had a jet of water injected into her vagina, tearing the vaginal wall without injury to the hymen.[23] Other unusual injuries have occurred when a child's pelvic area was crushed by a car rollover.[23] Another accidental perineal injury is described in which a sudden abduction of the legs during rollerblading caused a perineal "split" injury.[24,25]

Merritt's[26] review of genital injuries revealed that the history from the child regarding how the injury occurred remained the most important indicator of whether that injury was accidental or due to sexual abuse. Good photodocumentation with peer review is also helpful in determining the etiological background of injuries. Occasionally, injuries may be repaired surgically before consultation with a child abuse expert. In these cases is important to review the provided clinical description and the history. Photography by the repairing surgeon should be encouraged.

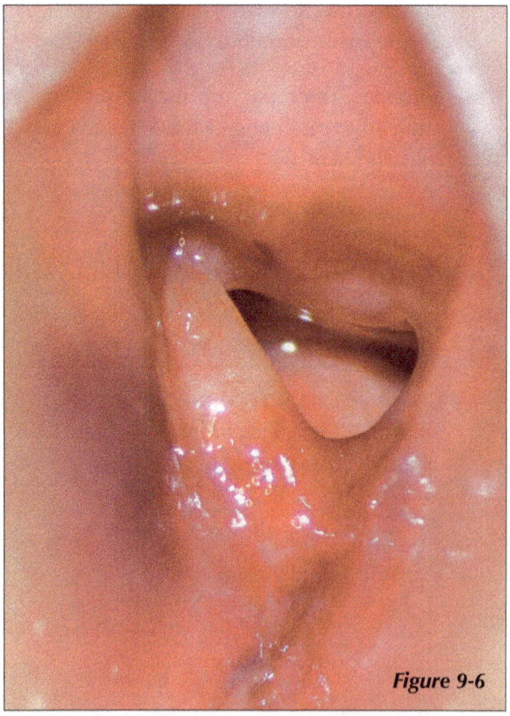

Figure 9-6

Figure 9-6. *Straddle injuries can involve the hymen if there is external to internal injury, as seen in this child who fell astraddle a diving board and has a posterior fourchette injury, external bruise, and hymenal hematoma.*

Figure 9-7. *This child fell astraddle the handle of a child's toy wagon. The hymen is not well visualized but is normal. There is a hematoma in the fossa from the straddle injury.*

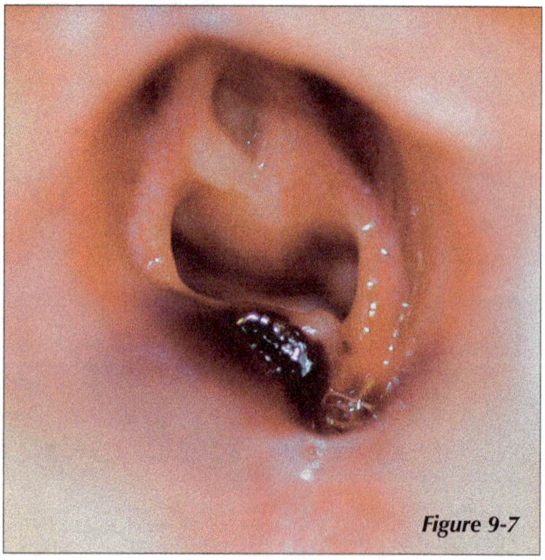

Figure 9-7

A retrospective review of accidental female genital trauma conducted at the Hospital for Sick Children reviewed data for 105 patients aged 1 to 14 years old. The mean patient age was 5.6 years, and the single most common mechanism of injury was straddle injury. Only 5 cases involved the hymen. A total of 22 patients required surgical repair of their injuries.[27]

Skin Discolorations from Dyes, Surgical Adjuncts, and Plants

Although not commonly reported in the literature, marks from dyes (especially those used in colored clothing) can cause discoloration of the skin that resembles a bruise. In addition, this author encountered a patient whose parents had used an aloe vera plant as a diaper rash ointment. This resulted in black streaks on the buttocks that resembled bruises. The clinical test involved wiping the area gently with an alcohol-based wipe, which resulted in removal of the discoloration.

Phytophotodermatitis is a phototoxic dermatitis resulting from contact with psoralen-containing plants such as celery, limes, parsley, figs, eggplant, tomatoes, and carrots. Berloque dermatitis is a variant of phytophotodermatitis and is caused by high concentrations of psoralen-containing fragrances—most commonly, oil of bergamot. The result of exposure to such products and then sunlight may mimic bruises or burns on the skin.

Bleeding

When blood, either bright red or dark, is found in a child's diaper or underwear, it is important to determine the source of the blood. Vaginal bleeding is discussed in a separate section of this chapter. Other sources of bleeding may include the urinary tract, the gastrointestinal tract, or the skin of the anogenital region. All of these must be considered when evaluating a chief complaint of anogenital bleeding.

A careful examination proceeding from external cutaneous structures to more internal structures may lead to a determination of the source of the bleeding and subsequently the appropriate diagnosis. If the origin of blood is not clear, a urinalysis for hematuria, as well as guaiac testing of the stool for occult blood to find the source of the bleeding, should be done. Occasionally, parents may mistake dark-colored stool for blood. Having the parent bring in the child's underwear is often helpful. Frank red blood or slight serosanguineous streaking versus saturation of the underclothing may also guide the clinician in the diagnostic approach.

Skin

Maceration with Irritant Contact

Any product that causes irritation of the skin can result in either localized breakdown due to the dermatitis itself, or it can cause the child to scratch at the area incessantly, causing deep excoriations. Given the friability of the tissues of the anogenital area, bleeding can result and the amount of blood can be quite significant, particularly in prepubertal children. Such products can include lotions, detergents, soaps, perfumes, or even a new brand of diaper. Parents should be carefully questioned about any new product that may have contacted the child's skin in the face of extensive dermatitis or excoriations. Treatment is often accomplished with removal of the offending item and warm soaks (**Figure 9-8**).

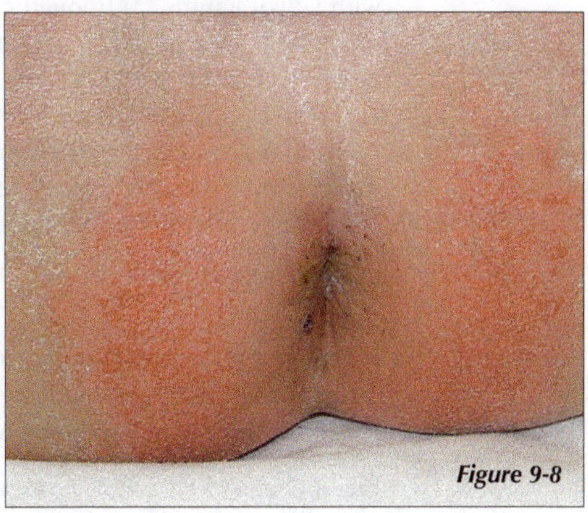

Figure 9-8. *This child presented with blood in his underwear and severe maceration of eczematous skin. This was the cause of the bleeding.*

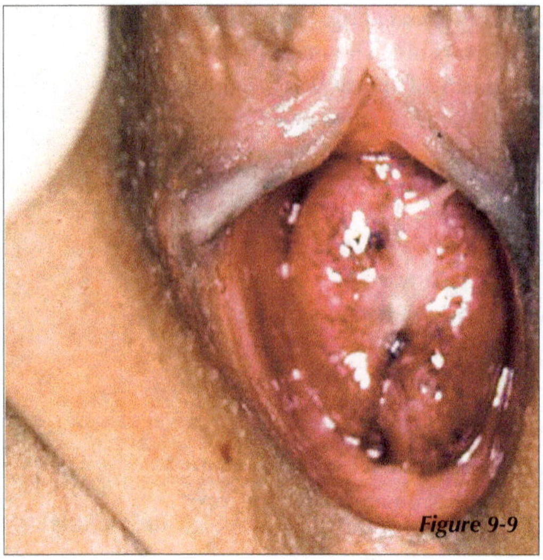

Figure 9-9.
Urethral prolapse.

Urinary Tract

A urinalysis and careful external examination of the periurethral area may reveal the source of bleeding. Urinary tract infections, hematuria from renal origin, and hemorrhagic cystitis may be diagnosed and appropriately treated.

One commonly reported apparent cause of vaginal bleeding is urethral prolapse. A review of the literature spanning 50 years indicates that urethral prolapse has been reported worldwide.[28-34] Urethral prolapse is most often observed as bleeding, initially presumed to be vaginal in origin; furthermore, when examined, the prolapsed, doughnut-shaped urethral tissue is swollen and bleeding and it may obscure the anatomy of the hymen (**Figure 9-9**). It is, therefore, not surprising that genital trauma is immediately considered. Although the incidence is not known, urethral prolapse is rare in all ethnic groups. Anecdotal evidence suggests the condition may be more common in children of African origin. It is rare in Caucasian children, and the reason for this racial disparity is unknown. Various treatments have been proposed, ranging from excision of the prolapsed tissue to conservative approaches of sitz baths and topical estrogens.[35,36] On some occasions the prolapse does not resolve with such treatment, and referral to a pediatric urologist for surgical reduction of the prolapsed tissue may be necessary.

Perivaginal

The perivaginal area—the perineum, posterior commissure and fourchette, labia, and other vulvar structures—may be the source of bleeding. Usually the amount is scant, but it can still be alarming to the caregiver. The clinician should take special care to examine all of the external structures for evidence of bleeding prior to assessing the vaginal area.

Group A β-hemolytic Streptococci

Group A β-hemolytic *Streptococcus* can cause vulvovaginitis in prepubertal girls. It is the most commonly encountered organism on vaginal culture in prepubertal girls with vulvovaginitis.[37] Although such infections may be accompanied by discharge, the mucosa of the perivaginal area is often extremely swollen, beefy in appearance, and bleeding (**Figures 9-10-a** and **b**). Evidence of group A *Streptococcus* dermatitis may be apparent with small satellite lesions consisting of papules, progressing to impetiginous changes. A culture of the perivaginal area is all that is needed to diagnose this condition, which is often quickly responsive to appropriate broad-spectrum oral antibiotics. The child may or may not have evidence of streptococcal pharyngitis.

Vaginal Bleeding

Blood on the child's underwear is often called "vaginal bleeding" by caregivers and referring clinicians. However, only when blood is observed coming from the vagina is this condition considered truly "vaginal" in origin, which necessitates a far different diagnostic approach than blood originating in structures other than the vagina.

Blood observed to originate from above the hymenal opening is true vaginal bleeding. The differential diagnosis is very broad. Without evidence of penetrating trauma (ie, injury to the hymen or the external structures), it would be difficult to speculate that the bleeding resulted from direct vaginal trauma.

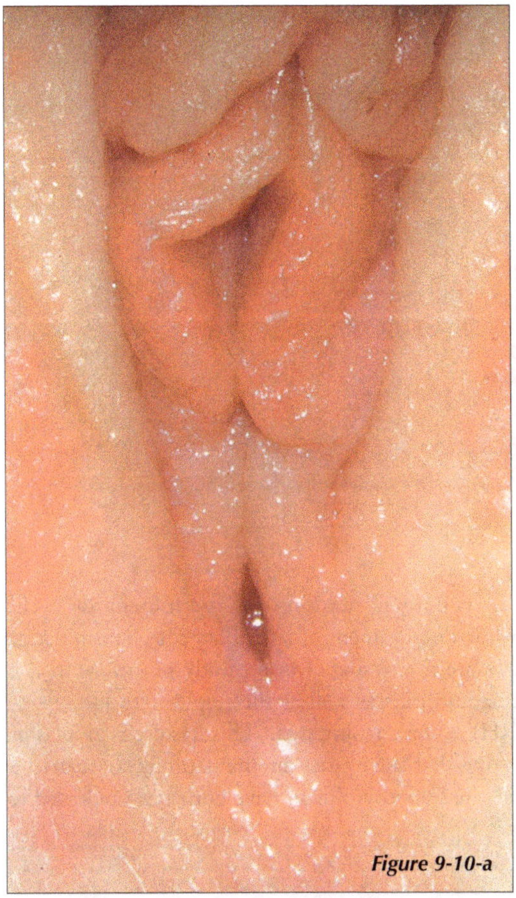

Figure 9-10-a

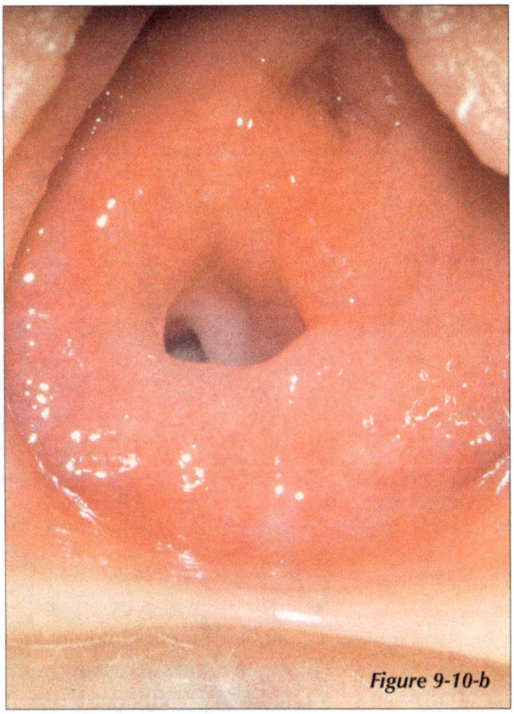

Figure 9-10-b

Figure 9-10-a. *External genital redness in a child with a history of discharge, odor, and slight blood streaking of the underwear.*

Figure 9-10-b. *Extreme erythema of the genital mucosa in the same child as Figure 9-10-a. Both external and mucosal erythema can be a sign of group A* Streptococcus *vulvovaginitis, as seen in this child.*

With signs of sexual development (breast budding, growth acceleration, pubic hair), an endocrine cause becomes the leading diagnosis; in this case, referral to an endocrinologist is recommended, assuming that puberty is unexpected (2-2.5 standard deviations earlier than population norms). Vaginal bleeding without sexual development is rare. In a study by Uli et al,[38] only 3 of 33 cases of prepubertal vaginal bleeding in the absence of sexual development were the result of prepubertal menarche. The majority were vaginitis (30%) or vaginal foreign bodies (30%), with the remainder being benign and malignant vaginal or vulvar tumors. A thorough history and physical examination revealed the need for a comprehensive endocrinological examination in only the minority of cases.

Shigella Vaginitis

A bacterial cause of vulvovaginitis that can result in vaginal bleeding is *Shigella* vaginitis. *Shigella* is a gram-negative bacteria that typically causes enterocolitis (**Figure 9-11**). Vaginal shigellosis may or may not be accompanied by bloody diarrhea or fever.[39] Most *Shigella* infections in the United States are due to *Shigella sonnei* or *Shigella flexneri.*

Endocrine Causes

Newborn Withdrawal Bleeding

Withdrawal bleeding may occur in the female newborn as the result of the discontinuation of maternal estrogens at birth.[40] Mothers should be instructed about the potential for this bleeding, because they might be alarmed when they notice blood in the diapers. This phenomenon generally occurs during the first week of life, peaking at day 5.

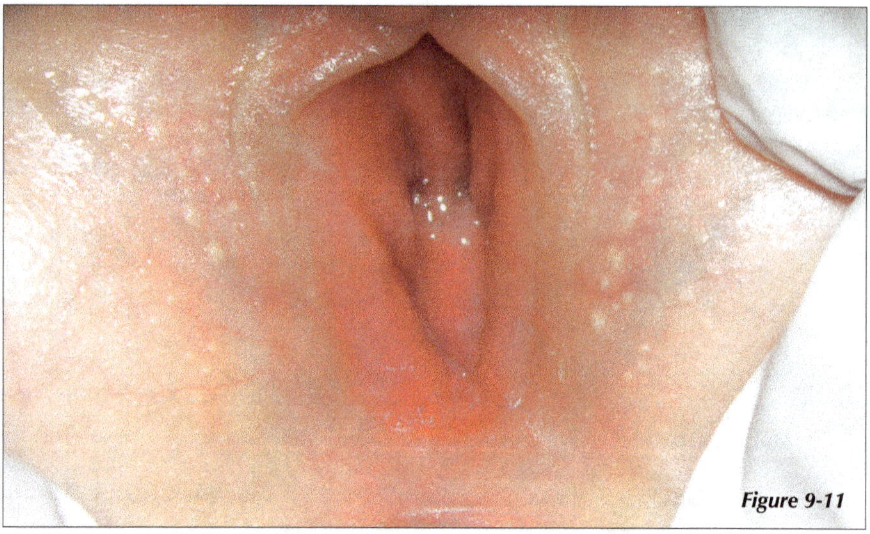

Figure 9-11

Figure 9-11. *This child's vaginal culture grew* Shigella enterocolitica. *She presented with vaginal bleeding and a concern of sexual abuse. There is significant redness and swelling of the mucosa.*

Prepubertal Menarche

Prepubertal menarche is an unusual condition resulting in intermittent or cyclic vaginal bleeding in children without the development of secondary sex characteristics. The vagina and uterus are normal, as are the ovaries. In one study of girls with this condition,[38] prepubertal levels of gonadotropins as well as the response to luteinizing hormone releasing hormone (LHRH) were encountered. This resulted in plasma estradiol levels being elevated, suggesting that the ovaries are prematurely stimulated.[41] Congenital adrenal hypoplasia and severe hypothyroidism have both been reported to cause premenarchal genital bleeding.[38,42]

Precocious Puberty

In the past the definition of ***precocious puberty*** has been the development of breasts or pubic hair before age 8 in girls. This is no longer considered valid in the United States because significant numbers of girls develop breast budding before age 8 years.[43] Recent observations have suggested that, in the United States, a significant percentage of 7- and 8-year-old girls, particularly African-American girls, have breast and pubic hair development.[44] Recent data suggest that a variety of factors, including obesity and race and ethnicity, should be considered when evaluating a girl for precocious puberty. Vaginal bleeding resulting from precocious puberty (premature menarche) is often accompanied by a growth spurt and breast development. In true precocious puberty, menarche is either idiopathic or the result of a variety of cerebral disorders or prolonged exposure to sex steroids from any source (**Table 9-2**). Another form of precocious puberty is termed ***pseudoprecocious puberty*** and is the result of a variety of factors (**Table 9-3**).

Pertinent historical factors for evaluation of precocious puberty include a family history of early development and idiopathic central puberty or previous central nervous system damage. The physical examination should include a careful evaluation for the presence of accelerated growth and advanced skeletal maturation determined radiologically, a skin examination for odor and sweat, and palpation of the thyroid. Laboratory studies may involve testing of levels of serum LH, follicle-stimulating hormone, estradiol, dehydroepiandrosterone sulfate, genetic investigations, and thyrotropin.[45] Imaging modalities include pelvic ultrasound to ascertain whether ovarian cysts are present and to determine uterine size and configuration, bone age assessment, computed tomography, and magnetic resonance imaging of the brain.[45,46]

Table 9-2. Causes of Isosexual Precocious Puberty

Central Precocious Puberty

- Idiopathic
- Cerebral disorders
  - Space-occupying lesions: hypothalamic hamartomas, brain tumors, neurofibromatosis, brain abscess, hydrocephalus, tuberous sclerosis, suprasellar infiltrative lesions (eg, sarcoid, chronic granulomatous disease)
  - Sequelae of cellular damage
  - Meningitis
  - Encephalitis
  - Head trauma
  - Cerebral edema
  - Cranial radiation

Secondary Central Precocious Puberty

- Prolonged exposure to sex steroids for any reason
- Undertreated or late-treated congenital adrenocortical hyperplasia
- Androgen-secreting tumors

Table 9-3. Characteristics of Pseudoprecocious Puberty

- Ovarian tumors
- Adrenal disorders (eg, adrenal carcinoma [estrogen secreting])
- Gonadotropin-independent sexual precocity: recurrent ovarian follicular cysts or McCune-Albright syndrome
- Gonadotropin-producing tumors: tumors that secrete luteinizing hormone (LH) and LH-like substances (eg, human chorionic gonadotropin, estrogen)
- Iatrogenic disorders: prolonged use of estrogen-containing creams or exogen-ous administration or ingestion of estrogens (oral contraceptive pills)
- Primary hypothyroidism

Vaginal Foreign Body

A common cause of vaginal bleeding can be a foreign body in the vagina. The bleeding is accompanied by a foul-smelling purulent discharge. Staphylococcus aureus may grow in pure colonies on culture (**Figure 9-12**). The foreign body may be visible with the child in the frog-leg supine position. The prone knee-chest position is ideal for noninvasively evaluating the length of the vagina. An excellent light source and magnification are helpful. Most vaginal foreign bodies are bits of toilet paper that can flushed out with saline irrigation.[47] Different techniques for visualizing the foreign body include ultrasound and radiography. Foreign bodies have been known to be retained for months, even years. A vaginal examination with the patient under anesthesia is indicated if the following

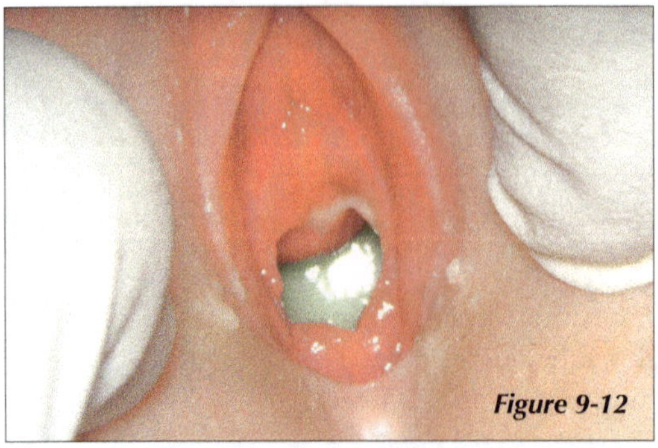

Figure 9-12

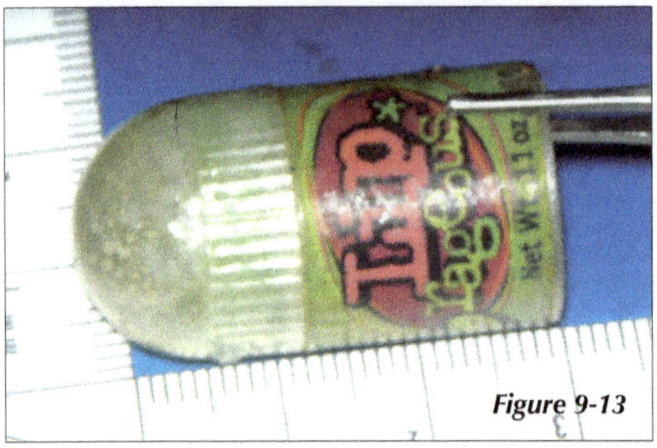

Figure 9-13

sequence of events has been carried out without success in locating a foreign body (**Figure 9-13**): the history and physical examination reveal the presence of intermittent bleeding accompanied by a foul discharge, both suggestive of a foreign body; if no such body is seen during direct visualization of the vagina, flushing the vagina with saline may remove it; a vaginal examination under anesthesia may be indicated if the concern for vaginal foreign body remains high and the child continues to have symptoms.

Neoplasms

Neoplasms of the vagina are rare. Lymphangiomas are congenital lymphovascular neoplasms that tend to bleed spontaneously. They can involve the hymen and the vagina (**Figures 9-14** and **9-15**). Hemangiomas can involve the vagina or the cervix. Some hemangiomas will be fed through large vessels that can be treated through sclerosis. Müllerian papillomas, benign papillomata derived from Müllerian epithelium, are rare. In one 18 month old, the primary symptom was vaginal bleeding.[48,49]

Figure 9-12. *A foul-smelling serosanguinous vaginal discharge can be a sign of a vaginal foreign body. In this case the child had complained for 2 months, and a routine culture met with a hard, resistant green object.*

Figure 9-13. *The top of a lip gloss tube was removed from this child's vagina while she was under anesthesia.*

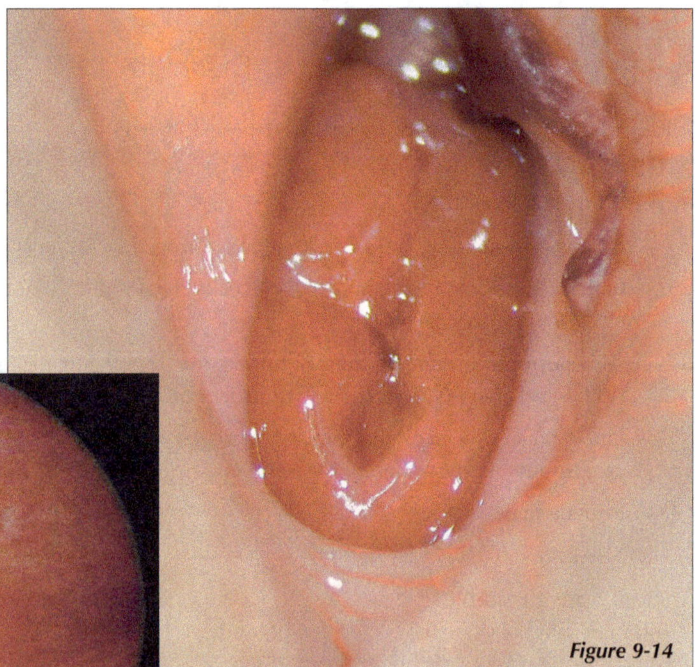

Figure 9-14

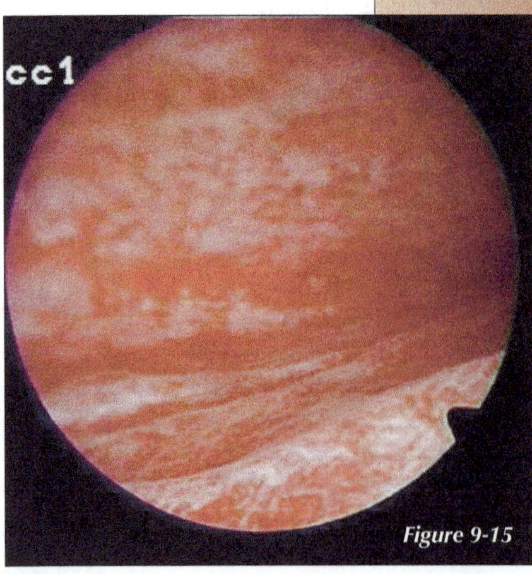

Figure 9-15

Figure 9-14. *This child presented with a beefy red hymen that was negative for bacterial cultures, and the examination findings did not change over several visits. She had intermittent bleeding from the surface of the hymen.*

Figure 9-15. *Photos from vaginoscopy reveal an unusual vascular pattern of the vaginal epithelium; vaginal biopsy revealed a lymphangiomatosis of the vagina.*

Pediatric gynecologic cancers are rare and can be broken down into 3 main types: stromal, ovarian germ cell, and rhabdomyosarcoma. Rhabdomyosarcoma most commonly may be mistaken for sexual abuse.[50]

Sarcoma botryoides, a subtype of embryonal rhabdomyosarcoma, is one of the most common tumors of the pediatric urogenital systems, arising almost exclusively before age 5. This tumor is often misdiagnosed in its early stages because the child has vaginal discharge and bleeding. The diagnosis is usually made when the grapelike clusters extrude through the hymenal opening. The diagnosis of this tumor requires referral to a pediatric center with surgical and oncologic services.[50]

Bleeding of Gastrointestinal Origin

Bleeding from the anus, rectum, or higher gastrointestinal (GI) sources can be confused with blood originating from genital structures. Alternatively, anal or rectal bleeding may raise the specter of sexual abuse. Bleeding from the anus also has a wide-ranging differential diagnosis that includes the entire GI tract.

Fissures

Anal fissures may bleed a surprising amount. The blood may be streaked on the outside of the stool or in the underwear. There may or may not be a history of significant constipation or large, hard stools (**Figure 9-16**). Fissures are exceedingly common, and the only way to determine if a fissure is from sexual abuse is to compare the history, timing, and symptoms in relationship to the examination. Anal tears that involve the sphincters are probably not innocent in origin. Conversely, a small fissure may not be evidence of sexual abuse.

Perianal Bleeding

Group A *Streptococcus* dermatitis can cause a beefy, red, sharply demarcated perianal inflammation that can result in bleeding, pain, and fissuring (**Figure 9-17**). A culture of the area will confirm the diagnosis. Treatment is usually a combination of topical (mupirocin) and oral antistreptococcal antibiotics.[51]

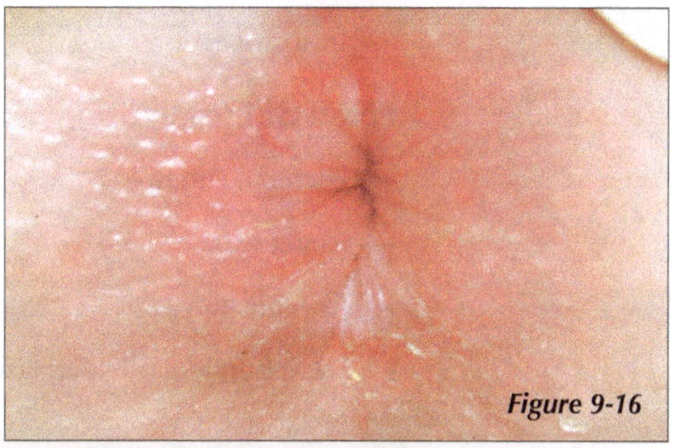

Figure 9-16

Figure 9-16. *Anal fissure. (Image contributed by Joyce Adams, MD.)*

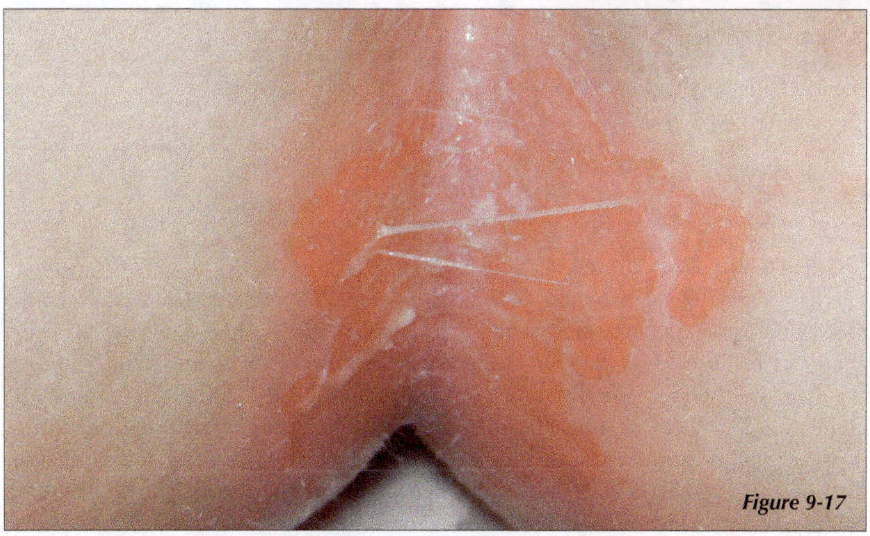

Figure 9-17

Figure 9-17. *Severe perianal maceration. A culture revealed pure group A β-hemolytic Streptococcus.*

Red or maroon blood in the stools is ***hematochezia*** and indicates distal bleeding or massive higher GI bleed above the distal ileum. Moderate blood from above this site tends to cause tarry-appearing stools, or ***melena.*** Diarrhea accompanied by blood suggests an infection or inflammatory bowel disease. Crohn's disease can be accompanied by remarkable anal findings such as fissures, tags, fistulas, pits, scarring, and anal dilatation. Vulvar conditions can also accompany Crohn's disease. There are many case reports of Crohn's disease initially reported as sexual abuse.[52-56] Blood streaked on the stools indicates a distal rectal or anal source such as a fissure or external trauma.

The differential diagnosis of GI bleeding in a child is extensive. **Table 9-4** lists the major causes of GI bleeding by site. It is helpful to keep this differential diagnosis in mind when a child produces blood in the underwear or toilet. Children who may be sexually abused can have coexisting medical conditions.

Table 9-4. Significant Factors in Gastrointestinal Bleeding

Upper GI Bleeding	
— Peptic ulcer/gastritis	— Esophageal varices
— Swallowed blood from epistaxis	— Esophagitis
— Mallory-Weiss syndrome	
Midbowel	
— Intussusception	— Meckel's diverticulum
Lower GI Bleeding	
— Bacterial enteritis	— Foreign body
— Anal fissure	— Hemolytic uremic syndrome
— Colonic polyps	— Inflammatory bowel disease
— Lymphonodular hyperplasia	— Hemorrhoids
— Henoch-Schönlein purpura	
All Locations	
— Hemangioma, arteriovenous malformation	— Coagulopathy

Data from Behrman et al.[58]

Discharge

Discharge may be vaginal, anal, or genital in origin. Prepubertal children evaluated for vaginal discharge are often brought to clinicians because of concerns of sexual abuse. In reality, only a very small percentage of children who are sexually abused are diagnosed with a sexually transmitted infection (STI).[57] On rare occasions the evaluation of a scant to moderate discharge reveals sexually transmitted organisms. A variety of organisms cause discharge in prepubertal girls, and the evaluation of discharge should include an evaluation for common non-sexually transmitted pathogens, and if indicated, tests for STIs.

During a clinical examination, a scant vaginal discharge may be found to be normal (physiologic leukorrhea) or caused by a variety of non-sexually transmitted pathogens. Smegma, the accumulation of exfoliated skin cells and bacteria, is white and curdled in appearance and is usually found in the folds between the labia. Some children may have what appears on the underwear to be discharge when they fail to empty their bladder completely and small reflux of urine into the vagina results in some drainage. Any bacteria found normally in the respiratory tract can be found in the genital area. Nonspecific vaginitis is a condition of poor hygiene or exposure to irritants. On culture a nonspecific vaginitis generally grows mixed normal flora. Nonspecific vaginitis generally responds to a program of topical bland emollients, excellent hygiene, and avoidance of irritants (eg, bubble bath, perfumed soaps, detergents).

A heavy growth of a single organism suggests a possible infection with that organism and may require antibiotic treatment. Yeast infections caused by *Candida albicans* are uncommon in toilet-trained prepubertal children. Children who have just completed a course of broad-spectrum antibiotics, who have diabetes mellitus, or who are immunocompromised are exceptions. Clinicians tend to overtreat children with antifungal creams when children appear for diagnosis of nearly any condition resulting in genital redness, irritation, or itching, presuming it to be *Candida*.

Nonvenereal Pathogens

Many commonly occurring nonvenereal organisms can cause vaginitis. **Table 9-5** lists the common bacterial organisms. In a child with vaginal discharge, STIs are often

Table 9-5. Nonvenereal Pathogens Causing Vulvitis/Vulvovaginitis/Vaginitis

Bacterial	
— Group A *Streptococcus*	— *Neisseria meningitidis*
— Group B *Streptococcus*	— *Staphylococcus aureus*
— *Haemophilus influenzae*	— *Staphylococcus epidermidis*
— *Streptococcus pneumoniae*	— *Gardnerella vaginalis*
Gram-negative Enteric Pathogens	
— *Escherichia coli*	— *Pseudomonas* spp.
— *Streptococcus faecalis*	— *Salmonella* spp.
— *Klebsiella* spp.	— *Shigella* spp.
— *Proteus* spp.	
Gram-negative Anaerobes	
— *Peptococcus* spp.	— *Bacteroides* spp.
— *Peptostreptococcus* spp.	
Viral	
— Rubella (measles)	— Kawasaki disease
— Epstein-Barr virus (infectious mononucleosis)	— Nonspecific viral infections
Fungal	
— *Candida albicans*	— Tinea corporis
Parasitic	
— Pinworms (*Enterobius vermicularis*)	

a major concern. However, STIs are found rarely in sexually abused children; therefore, in addition to cultures for *Chlamydia* and gonorrhea, routine cultures should be performed to identify these common nonvenereal pathogens.

Papules, Macules, and Nodules

Papules and Nodules

Lesions that appear to be genital warts, such as papules and macules in the genital area, raise the specter of sexual abuse. Recent evidence suggests that although human papillomavirus can be transmitted via sexual abuse, vertical and fomite transmission also exist.[57-59]

Molluscum Contagiosum

Molluscum contagiosum is a DNA poxvirus for which humans are the only known reservoir. There appears to be bimodal distribution in childhood and then in young adulthood. Mollusca appear as pearly papules on an erythematous base with a central umbilication (**Figure 9-18**). The lesions can appear clustered in the anogenital area, and the localization of the outbreak in this area is often what raises the red flag of sexual abuse. When the child is carefully examined, as are siblings or close playmates, extragenital mollusca are often found. There may be some risk that the lesions are transmitted sexually; however, mollusca are so common and so easily transmitted from person to person that innocent transmission is most likely the cause.

Perianal Pseudoverrucous Papules and Nodules

Perianal pseudoverrucous papules and nodules (PPPN) is an underreported benign cutaneous condition of flat-topped papules and nodules (**Figure 9-19**). It is a variant of Jacquet's dermatitis (called also ***erosive dermatitis***, ***diaper dermatitis***, or colloquially as ***diaper rash***). Jacquet's dermatitis is a chronic ulcerative condition of the diaper area first described in 1886.[60] It was reported in children who had undergone surgery for Hirschsprung's disease and whose skin was exposed to chronic fecal soiling. Described in peristomal areas, it is also observed in children with urinary or fecal incontinence. The condition clears with removal of the irritant.[61-63]

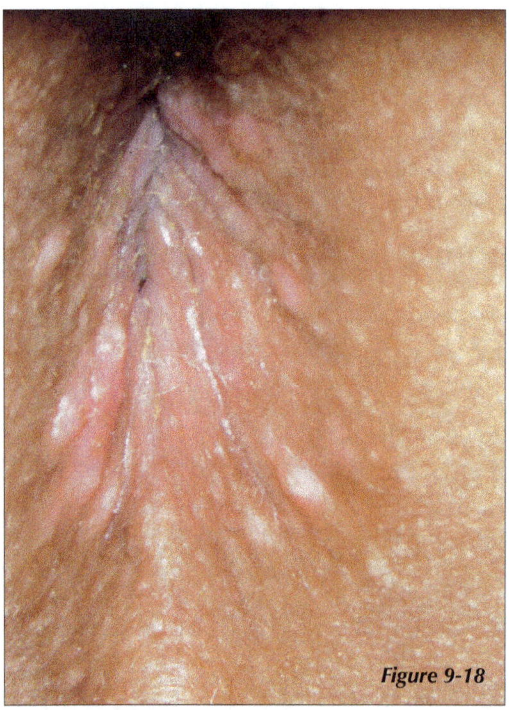

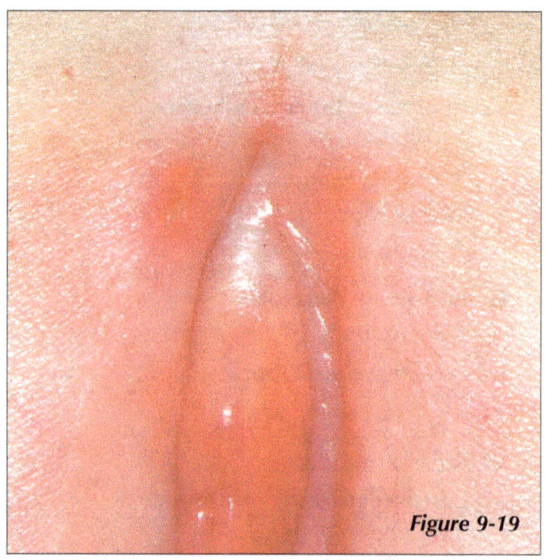

Figure 9-18. *Perianal molluscum contagiosum that can mimic genital warts and raise the suspicion of sexual abuse.*

Figure 9-19. *Pseudoverrucous papules and nodules. Small nodules near the clitoris of this child raised a concern of genital herpes. On careful examination the lesions were nodular and not painful. They cleared with removal of the irritant.*

A variety of rare conditions have been reported to be confused with genital warts, which, in turn raise the concern of sexual abuse. The differential diagnosis of papular and nodular lesions of the anogenital area is broad. **Table 9-6** lists conditions that have been reported or observed in this context.

Table 9-6. Differential Diagnosis of Papules and Nodules
— Benign pigmented apocrine vulvar hamartomas[64]
— Langerhans cell histiocytosis[65]
— Heck disease: focal epithelial hyperplasia[66]
— Epidermal nevus[67]
— Inflammatory linear epidermal nevus Crohn's disease[55]
— Lymphangioma circumscriptum[68]
— Vulvar syringomas[69]
— Bowenoid papulosis
— Xanthogranulomas
— Tuberous sclerosis

Vesicles and Ulcers

Vesicles and ulcerations of the genital area suggest infections such as herpesvirus and therefore hoist the specter of sexual abuse. However, acquiring herpes simplex virus (HSV) from sexual abuse is one of the lowest risks among all STIs. It is not screened for, and therefore only patients with overt symptoms such as vesicles come to the attention of the medical community. See Chapter 10 for a review of HSV as an STI.

Several non-HSV infections can cause vesicles or ulcerations of the genital area. None are known to have any risk for being sexually transmitted. Genital ulcerations caused by Epstein-Barr virus (EBV) have been described infrequently. In studies reviewing 26 cases, the average age is reported as 14.5 years, and sexual contact is rare.[70-72] EBV serologic testing may be helpful, but one must keep in mind that the results are not positive unless testing occurs several days after the development of lesions. Polymerase chain reaction tests of the lesions have yielded positive, confirmatory results of EBV in one study and may be helpful in diagnosis.[72] Another class of herpesviruses, varicella-zoster virus, can cause lesions of the genital area in children. An early occurrence of chickenpox or a later occurrence of shingles in a sacral dermatome may look very much like HSV. Coxsackievirus, first described in 1955, is known to cause oral and cutaneous lesions in children and can also can cause genital lesions.[73] Deitch and colleagues[71] described 9 patients who developed vulvar ulcerations and denied sexual abuse or activity. All were negative for HSV. Six of the patients had systemic symptoms suggestive of a nonspecific viral illness. In a child with other symptoms suggestive of a viral illness and without a history of sexual contact, the clinician must consider genital ulcers as an uncommon occurrence of nonspecific, systemic viral illnesses such as influenza.

Other conditions that have been reported to cause genital ulcerations include localized vulvar pemphigoid in a young girl.[74] Juvenile bullous pemphigoid manifests as localized grouped or single vesicles on the genitals, face, neck, palms, and soles. At least 2 cases that were confused with sexual abuse are reported in the literature.[74,75] The diagnosis of localized genital pemphigoid requires a high index of suspicion, and confirmation depends on biopsy results.

Behçet's disease is a rare systemic condition associated with oral aphthae, genital ulcers, skin lesions, arthritis, and GI involvement. Neuropsychiatric symptoms and the presence of HLA-B51 are also associated with this rare cause of progressive, destructive, painful genital ulcers.[76]

Stevens-Johnson syndrome, or erythema multiforme major, occurs as a reaction to a variety of drugs, mycoplasmas, viruses, or other triggers. The result is a severe vesiculobullous reaction of the mucous membranes that can include the genitalia. In severe cases, vaginal stenosis can result from scarring after involvement of the distal vaginal mucosa.[77-79] Drug reactions can cause genital ulcers (**Figures 9-20** and **9-21**). Usually, exposure to a sulfa-containing antibiotic results in a stereotypic reaction that can be duplicated on reexposure to the drug.

In evaluating lesions of the genital area, a careful history of irritants and potential allergic contact irritants should be sought. Nickel, for example, can be extremely sensitizing. One classic case of allergic contact was that of a child using a bed-wetting alarm, where the contact was nickel. The child was removed from the home and placed in foster care because of the concern that the localized vesicles on the genitals were herpes simplex.[80] This case report demonstrates the potential harm to a child and family when there is a misdiagnosis of sexual abuse.

Conclusion

It is challenging to evaluate any child who has injuries or illness suggestive of sexual abuse. When children or adolescents have anogenital signs or symptoms, a differential diagnosis must be developed. This diagnosis should encompass a variety of acquired and congenital conditions. The co-occurrence of an unusual anogenital condition in the context of a sexual abuse allegation may be coincidental to the allegations. Such conditions should not be considered as evidence of abuse, as normal examination results should not be thought of as definitive evidence of nonabuse. Children who are referred for genital involvement may have other conditions that can mimic the appearance of sexual abuse or an STI. High-quality photodocumentation and review of cases by experienced clinicians, including dermatologists, gynecologists, urologists, and infectious disease specialists, can be critical in coming to a correct diagnosis.

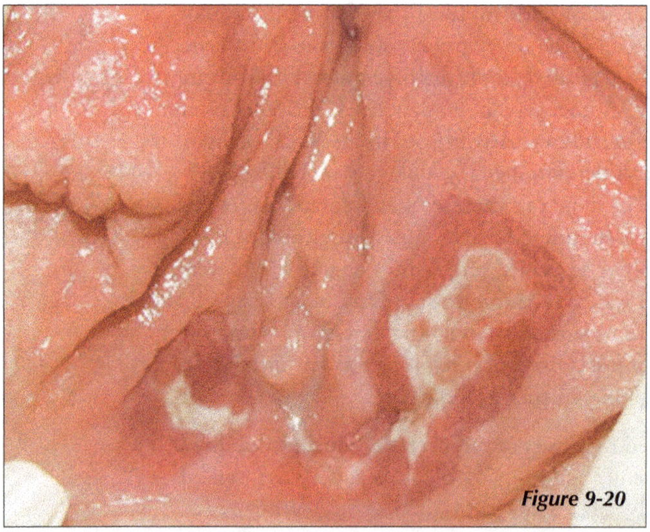

Figure 9-20

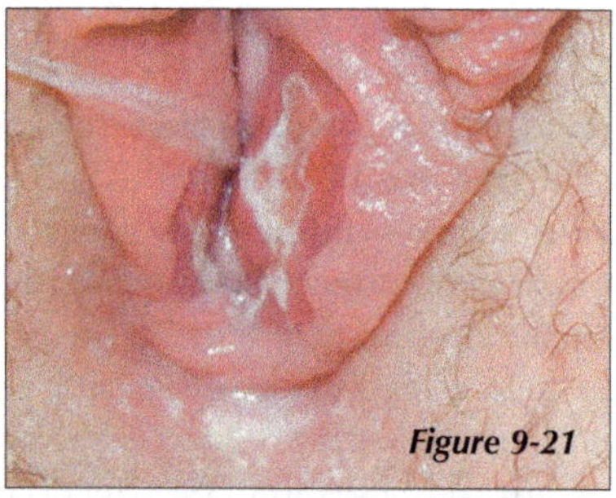

Figure 9-21

Figures 9-20 and 21. *Fixed drug eruption. These severe, shallow, painful genital ulcers in an adolescent were initially thought to be caused by herpes simplex virus. However, HSV culture and polymerase chain reaction testing were negative. The patient was on a sulfa-containing antibiotic for a urinary tract infection. The ulcers cleared with discontinuation of the antibiotic and were felt to be drug reaction.*

References

1. Jenny C, Kirby P, Fuquay D. Genital lichen sclerosus mistaken for child sexual abuse. *Pediatrics*. 1989;83(4):597-599.
2. Ditkowsky SP, Falk AB, Baker N, Schaffner M. Lichen sclerosis et atrophicus in childhood. *AMA J Dis Child*. 1956;91(1):52-54.
3. Al-Khenaizan S, Almuneef M, Kentab O. Lichen sclerosus mistaken for child sexual abuse. *Int J Dermatol*. 2005;44(4):317-320.
4. Loening-Baucke V. Lichen sclerosus et atrophicus in children. *Am J Dis Child*. 1991;145(9):1058-1061.
5. Hagedorn M. Genital vulvar lichen sclerosis in 2 siblings [in German]. *Z Hautkr*. 1989;64(9):810, 813-814.
6. Breier F, Khanakah G, Stanek G, et al. Isolation and polymerase chain reaction typing of Borrelia afzelii from a skin lesion in a seronegative patient with generalized ulcerating bullous lichen sclerosus et atrophicus. *Br J Dermatol*. 2001;144(2):387-392.
7. Buechner SA, Winkelmann RK, Lautenschlager S, Gilli L, Rufli T. Localized scleroderma associated with Borrelia burgdorferi infection: clinical, histologic, and immunohistochemical observations. *J Am Acad Dermatol*. 1993;29(2 pt 1):190-196.
8. Tong LX, Sun GS, Teng JM. Pediatric lichen sclerosus: a review of the epidemiology and treatment options. *Pediatr Dermatol*. 2015;32(5):593-599.
9. Bercaw-Pratt JL, Boardman LA, Simms-Cendan JS; North American Society for Pediatric and Adolescent Gynecology. Clinical recommendation: pediatric lichen sclerosus. *J Pediatr Adolesc Gynecol*. 2014;27(2):111-116.
10. Fistarol SK, Itin PH. Diagnosis and treatment of lichen sclerosus: an update. *Am J Clin Dermatol*. 2013;14(1):27-47.
11. Homer L, Buchanan KJ, Nasr B, Losty PD, Corbett HJ. Meatal stenosis in boys following circumcision for lichen sclerosus (balanitis xerotica obliterans). *J Urol*. 2014;192(6):1784-1788.
12. Beattie PE, Dawe RS, Ferguson J, Ibbotson SH. UVA1 phototherapy for genital lichen sclerosus. *Clin Exp Dermatol*. 2006;31(3):343-347.
13. Wright JE. The treatment of childhood phimosis with topical steroid. *Aust N Z J Surg*. 1994;64(5):327-328.
14. Serrano G, Millán F, Fortea JM, Grau M, Aliaga A. Topical progesterone as treatment of choice in genital lichen sclerosis et atrophicus in children. *Pediatr Dermatol*. 1993;10(2):201.
15. Mashayekhi S, Flohr C, Lewis FM. The treatment of vulval lichen sclerosus in prepubertal girls: a critically appraised topic. *Br J Dermatol*. 2017;176(2):307-316.
16. Levin AV, Selbst SM. Vulvar hemangioma simulating child abuse. *Clin Pediatr (Phila)*. 1988;27(4):213-215.
17. Vogel AM, Alesbury JM, Burrows PE, Fishman SJ. Vascular anomalies of the female external genitalia. *J Pediatr Surg*. 2006;41(5):993-999.
18. Brown J, Melinkovich P. Schönlein-Henoch purpura misdiagnosed as suspected child abuse: a case report and literature review. *JAMA*. 1986;256(5):617-618.
19. Daly KC, Siegel RM. Henoch-Schönlein purpura in a child at risk of abuse. *Arch Pediatr Adolesc Med*. 1998;152(1):96-98.
20. Harley JR. Disorders of coagulation misdiagnosed as nonaccidental bruising. *Pediatr Emerg Care*. 1997;13(5):347-349.

21. Balevic S, Taylor M, Amaya M. Penile and scrotal swelling mimicking child abuse. *Clin Pediatr (Phila).* 2013;52(10):988-990.

22. Rothämel T, Bürger D, Debertin AS, Kleemann WJ. Vaginorectal impalement injury in a 2-year-old child—caused by sexual abuse or an accident? *Forensic Sci Int.* 2001;119(3):330-333.

23. Perlman SE, Hertweck SP, Wolfe WM. Water-ski douche injury in a premenarcheal female. *Pediatrics.* 1995;96(4 pt 1):782-783.

24. Boos SC, Rosas AJ, Boyle C, McCann J. Anogenital injuries in child pedestrians run over by low-speed motor vehicles: four cases with findings that mimic child sexual abuse. *Pediatrics.* 2003;112(1 pt 1):e77-84.

25. Herrmann B, Crawford J. Genital injuries in prepubertal girls from inline skating accidents. *Pediatrics.* 2002;110(2 pt 1):e16.

26. Merritt DF. Evaluation of vaginal bleeding in the preadolescent child. *Semin Pediatr Surg.* 1998;7(1):35-42.

27. Spitzer RF, Kives S, Caccia N, Ornstein M, Goia C, Allen LM. Retrospective review of unintentional female genital trauma at a pediatric referral center. *Pediatr Emerg Care.* 2008;24(12):831-835.

28. Johnson CF. Prolapse of the urethra: confusion of clinical and anatomic characteristics with sexual abuse. *Pediatrics.* 1991;87(5):722-725.

29. Shetty AK, Coffman K, Harmon E. Urethral prolapse. *J Pediatr.* 1998;133(4):552.

30. Templeman C, Hertweck P, Perlman S, Nakajima S. Urethral prolapse in a 7 year old girl. *Aust N Z J Obstet Gynaecol.* 2000;40(4):480.

31. Valerie E, Gilchrist BF, Frischer J, Scriven R, Klotz DH, Ramenofsky ML. Diagnosis and treatment of urethral prolapse in children. *Urology.* 1999;54(6):1082-1084.

32. Rudin JE, Geldt VG, Alecseev EB. Prolapse of urethral mucosa in white female children: experience with 58 cases. *J Pediatr Surg.* 1997;32(3):423-425.

33. Esposito JM. Circular prolapse of the urethra in children: a cause of vaginal bleeding. *Obstet Gynecol.* 1968;31(3):363-367.

34. Neuwirth RS. Urethral prolapse—a cause of vaginal bleeding in young girls: report of 5 cases. *Obstet Gynecol.* 1963;22:290-292.

35. Falandry L. Prolapse of the urethra in black girls: personal experience in 11 cases [in French]. *Med Trop (Mars).* 1994;54(2):152-156.

36. Richardson DA, Hajj SN, Herbst AL. Medical treatment of urethral prolapse in children. *Obstet Gynecol.* 1982;59(1):69-74.

37. Yilmaz AE, Celik N, Soylu G, Donmez A, Yuksel C. Comparison of clinical and microbiological features of vulvovaginitis in prepubertal and pubertal girls. *J Formos Med Assoc.* 2012;111(7):392-396.

38. Uli N, Chin D, David R, et al. Menstrual bleeding in a female infant with congenital adrenal hyperplasia: altered maturation of the hypothalamic-pituitary-ovarian axis. *J Clin Endocrinol Metab.* 1997;82(10):3298-3302.

39. Baiulescu M, Hannon PR, Marcinak JF, Janda WM, Schreckenberger PC. Chronic vulvovaginitis caused by antibiotic-resistant Shigella flexneri in a prepubertal child. *Pediatr Infect Dis J.* 2002;21(2):170-172.

40. Huber A. The frequency of physiologic vaginal bleeding of newborn infants [in German]. *Zentralbl Gynakol.* 1976;98(16):1017-1020.

41. Blanco-Garcia M, Evain-Brion D, Roger M, Job JC. Isolated menses in prepubertal girls. *Pediatrics*. 1985;76(1):43-47.

42. Campaner AB, Scapinelli A, Machado RO, Dos Santos RE, Beznos GW, Aoki T. Primary hypothyroidism presenting as ovarian tumor and precocious puberty in a prepubertal girl. *Gynecol Endocrinol*. 2006;22(7):395-398.

43. Slyper AH. The pubertal timing controversy in the USA, and a review of possible causative factors for the advance in timing of onset of puberty. *Clin Endocrinol (Oxf)*. 2006;65(1):1-8.

44. Herman-Giddens ME, Slora EJ, Wasserman RC, et al. Secondary sexual characteristics and menses in young girls seen in office practice: a study from the Pediatric Research in Office Settings network. *Pediatrics*. 1997;99(4):505-512.

45. Wei C, Davis N, Honour J, Crowne E. The investigation of children and adolescents with abnormalities of pubertal timing. *Ann Clin Biochem*. 2017;52(1):20-32.

46. Emans JS, Laufer MR, Goldstein DP. *Pediatric and Adolescent Gynecology*. 4th ed. Philedelphia, PA: Lippincott Williams & Wilkins; 1998.

47. Smith YR, Berman DR, Quint EH. Premenarchal vaginal discharge: findings of procedures to rule out foreign bodies. *J Pediatr Adolesc Gynecol*. 2002;15(4):227-230.

48. Lane BR, Ross JH, Hart WR, Kay R. Müllerian papilloma of the cervix in a child with multiple renal cysts. *Urology*. 2005;65(2):388.

49. Lüttges JE, Lübke M. Recurrent benign Müllerian papilloma of the vagina: immunohistological findings and histogenesis. *Arch Gynecol Obstet*. 1994;255(3):157-160.

50. Pommert L, Bradley W. Pediatric gynecologic cancers. *Curr Oncol Rep*. 2017;19(7):44.

51. Herbst R. Perineal streptococcal dermatitis/disease: recognition and management. *Am J Clin Dermatol*. 2003;4(8):555-560.

52. Bourrat E, Faure C, Vignon-Pennamen MD, Rybojad M, Morel P, Navarro J. Anitis, vulvar edema and macrocheilitis disclosing Crohn disease in a child: value of metronidazole [in French]. *Ann Dermatol Venereol*. 1997;124(9):626-628.

53. Porzionato A, Alaggio R, Aprile A. Perianal and vulvar Crohn's disease presenting as suspected abuse. *Forensic Sci Int*. 2005;155(1):24-27.

54. Sellman SP, Hupertz VF, Reece RM. Crohn's disease presenting as suspected abuse. *Pediatrics*. 1996;97(2):272-274.

55. Stratakis CA, Graham W, DiPalma J, Leibowitz I. Misdiagnosis of perianal manifestations of Crohn's disease: two cases and a review of the literature. *Clin Pediatr (Phila)*. 1994;33(10):631-633.

56. Wardinsky TD, Vizcarrondo FE, Cruz BK. The mistaken diagnosis of child abuse: a three-year USAF Medical Center analysis and literature review. *Mil Med*. 1995;160(1):15-20.

57. Girardet RG, Lahoti S, Howard LA, et al. Epidemiology of sexually transmitted infections in suspected child victims of sexual assault. *Pediatrics*. 2009;124(1):79-86.

58. Behrman R, Kliegman R, Jenson H. *Nelson Textbook of Pediatrics*. 16th ed. Philedelphia, PA: Saunders; 2000.

59. Hornor G. Ano-genital warts in children: sexual abuse or not? *J Pediatr Health Care*. 2004;18(4):165-170.

60. Siegfried EC, Frasier L. The spectrum of anogenital disease in children. *Curr Probl Dermatol*. 1997;9(2):33-80.

61. Goldberg NS, Esterly NB, Rothman KF, et al. Perianal pseudoverrucous papules and nodules in children. *Arch Dermatol.* 1992;128(2):240-242.
62. Rodríguez Cano L, García-Patos Briones V, Pedragosa Jové R, Castells Rodellas A. Perianal pseudoverrucous papules and nodules after surgery for Hirschsprung disease. *J Pediatr.* 1994;125(6 Pt 1):914-916.
63. Rodriguez-Poblador J, González-Castro U, Herranz-Martínez S, Luelmo-Aguilar J. Jacquet erosive diaper dermatitis after surgery for Hirschsprung disease. *Pediatr Dermatol.* 1998;15(1):46-47.
64. Stephens-Groff SM, Hansen RC, Bangert J. Benign pigmented apocrine vulvar hamartomas. *Pediatr Dermatol.* 1993;10(2):123-124.
65. Papa CA, Pride HB, Tyler WB, Turkewitz D. Langerhans cell histiocytosis mimicking child abuse. *J Am Acad Dermatol.* 1997;37(6):1002-1004.
66. Cohen PR, Hebert AA, Adler-Storthz K. Focal epithelial hyperplasia: heck disease. *Pediatr Dermatol.* 1993;10(3):245-251.
67. Mahto M, Ashworth J, Vickers DM. A case of linear epidermal naevus presenting as genital warts—a cautionary tale. *Int J STD AIDS.* 2005;16(3):267-269.
68. Darmstadt GL. Perianal lymphangioma circumscriptum mistaken for genital warts. *Pediatrics.* 1996;98(3 pt 1):461-463.
69. Tay YK, Tham SN, Teo R. Localized vulvar syringomas—an unusual cause of pruritus vulvae. *Dermatology.* 1996;192(1):62-63.
70. Cheng SX, Chapman MS, Margesson LJ, Birenbaum D. Genital ulcers caused by Epstein-Barr virus. *J Am Acad Dermatol.* 2004;51(5):824-826.
71. Deitch HR, Huppert J, Adams Hillard PJ. Unusual vulvar ulcerations in young adolescent females. *J Pediatr Adolesc Gynecol.* 2004;17(1):13-16.
72. Halvorsen JA, Brevig T, Aas T, Skar AG, Slevolden EM, Moi H. Genital ulcers as initial manifestation of Epstein-Barr virus infection: two new cases and a review of the literature. *Acta Derm Venereol.* 2006;86(5):439-442.
73. Mitchell SC, Dempster G. The finding of genital lesions in a case of Coxsackie virus infection. *Can Med Assoc J.* 1955;72(2):117-119.
74. Levine V, Sanchez M, Nestor M. Localized vulvar pemphigoid in a child misdiagnosed as sexual abuse. *Arch Dermatol.* 1992;128(6):804-806.
75. Hoque SR, Patel M, Farrell AM. Childhood cicatricial pemphigoid confined to the vulva. *Clin Exp Dermatol.* 2006;31(1):63-64.
76. Pivetti-Pezzi P, Accorinti M, Abdulaziz MA, La Cava M, Torella M, Riso D. Behçet's disease in children. *Jpn J Ophthalmol.* 1995;39(3):309-314.
77. Graham-Brown RA, Cochrane GW, Swinhoe JR, Sarkany I, Epsztejn LJ. Vaginal stenosis due to bullous erythema multiforme (Stevens-Johnson syndrome): case report. *Br J Obstet Gynaecol.* 1981;88(11):1156-1157.
78. Marquette GP, Su B, Woodruff JD. Introital adenosis associated with Stevens-Johnson syndrome. *Obstet Gynecol.* 1985;66(1):143-145.
79. Murphy MI, Brant WE. Hematocolpos caused by genital bullous lesions in a patient with Stevens-Johnson syndrome. *J Clin Ultrasound.* 1998;26(1):52-54.
80. Hanks JW, Venters WJ. Nickel allergy from a bed-wetting alarm confused with herpes genitalis and child abuse. *Pediatrics.* 1992;90(3):458-460.

Chapter 10

SEXUALLY TRANSMITTED INFECTIONS

Nancy D. Kellogg, MD
Lora Spiller, MD
Michelle I. Amaya, MD, MPH

INTRODUCTION

The identification of sexually transmitted infections (STIs) in suspected victims of sexual abuse presents clinical and diagnostic challenges. Each STI may present with varying or no clinical features, and in the case of human papillomavirus (HPV), the incubation period may extend for months. Once a clinician has decided to test for an STI, a number of diagnostic tests are available, each with varying sensitivity and specificity rates as well as site-specific restrictions. Even when an STI is identified in a child, the determination that the infection was sexually transmitted can be problematic (**Table 10-1**). In order to accurately interpret and treat an STI in a child or adolescent, clinicians must be knowledgeable about indications for STI testing, appropriate tests to use, and possible modes of transmission.

Table 10-1. Implications of Commonly Encountered STIs for the Diagnosis and Reporting of Sexual Abuse of Infants and Prepubertal Children

STI CONFIRMED	SEXUAL ABUSE	SUGGESTED ACTION
Gonorrhea*	Diagnostic†	Report‡
Syphilis*	Diagnostic	Report
HIV infection§	Diagnostic	Report
C. trachomatis infection*	Diagnostic†	Report
T. vaginalis infection	Highly suspicious	Report
C. acuminata infection* (anogenital warts)	Suspicious	Report
Herpes simplex (genital location)	Suspicious	Report¦
Bacterial vaginosis	Inconclusive	Medical follow-up

* *If not perinatally acquired and rare nonsexual vertical transmission is excluded.*

† *Although the culture technique is the "gold standard," current studies are investigating the use of nucleic acid amplification tests as an alternative diagnostic method in children.*

‡ *To the agency mandated in the community to receive reports of suspected sexual abuse.*

§ *If not acquired perinatally or by transfusion.*

¦ *Unless there is a clear history of autoinoculation.*

Reproduced with permission from Journal Pediatrics, Vol. 116, Pages 506-512, Copyright © 2005 by the AAP.

Interpreting the presence of an STI within the context of sexual abuse or assault also presents challenges for the clinician who works with investigative agencies. The clinician must become knowledgeable about sensitivities and specificities for various testing modalities, in addition to positive predictive values when such tests are used in low- and high-prevalence populations. Investigative agencies are most interested in testing that is considered the legally acceptable standard, with little or no possibility of false positive results. The clinician, on the other hand, must consider the low sensitivities of some "gold standards" and may wish to use a test that optimizes detection of the STI. In some situations, such as a sexually active adolescent who is also sexually assaulted, the presence of an STI will have no forensic significance but is significant as a public health issue; therefore, using the most sensitive test in this high-prevalence population is optimal. Confirming an STI in a sexually active adolescent also enables treatment of presumably infected sexual contacts. The sexual abuse or assault examination is often the first time a sexually active adolescent has ever been screened for STIs and the first opportunity for clinicians to impact this problem on a public health level.

The medical evaluation of a child or adolescent for sexual abuse or assault may include testing and treating for STIs. The medical history and examination findings should guide the clinician in deciding which sites (ie, oral, genital/vaginal/urine, anal) should be tested for STIs.[1] Additionally, the clinician should consider testing more sites if there is a suspicion that the child's disclosure is incomplete or partial and alter testing sites (eg, obtain urine instead of vaginal swab) if the child does not tolerate the examination. The Centers for Disease Control and Prevention[2] (CDC) and the American Academy of Pediatrics Committee on Child Abuse and Neglect[2,3] have recommended that adolescents be tested for gonorrhea and *Chlamydia* using nucleic acid amplification tests (NAATs). Urine and vaginal specimens from prepubertal girls can also be tested with NAATs. NAATs are acceptable for testing extragenital sites in adolescents,[4] but culture is still recommended for extragenital sites in prepubertal children and all sites in prepubertal boys.[2] However, culture is less sensitive than any NAAT, and *Chlamydia* culture is no longer readily available for clinical use in many hospitals.[5] Disadvantages to using NAATs include the lack of information about antibiotic sensitivity. Retesting for cure in areas where resistant strains are endemic is one alternative to confirm successful treatment. Confirmatory testing of positive NAAT results may be required in prepubertal children. The CDC has indicated that when collected from an adolescent or adult, a positive *Chlamydia* result no longer necessitates routine additional testing, but retesting should still be considered for positive gonorrhea results due to cross-reactivity with other *Neisseria* species. Additionally, consultation with an expert is recommended when using NAATs in situations where the result has legal implications.[6] Additional recommended tests include vaginal swabs for *T. vaginalis* culture[7] or NAAT and serum samples for *Treponema pallidum*, human immunodeficiency virus (HIV), and hepatitis B virus and hepatitis C virus. (**Table 10-2**).[4] Testing for hepatitis C in adolescents should be considered based on risk factors (eg, intravenous drug use).[4] Even when such recommendations are employed, the prevalence of STIs in prepubertal children evaluated for sexual abuse is low. In one multicenter study[8] of 536 boys and girls aged 13 years and younger who were examined for STIs as part of the medical evaluation for sexual abuse, a *Chlamydia* and/or gonorrhea NAAT or culture was positive in about 3% of girls tested, *Trichomonas vaginalis* identified on wet mount was found in 5.9%, one child had serologic evidence of syphilis, and none had a positive HIV serologic test. Five of 12 girls cultured for herpes virus were positive for type 2. No boys in this study had a positive HIV serologic test, however, not all children had serologic testing performed.

Table 10-2. Suggested Testing Schedule for Sexually Transmitted Infections*

STI	Initial†	2 Weeks	6 Weeks	12 Weeks	6 Months
Gonorrhea	X	X			
Chlamydia	X	X			
Trichomonas	X	X			
Syphilis	X		X		
Hepatitis‡	X		X	X	
HIV	X		X		
Human papillomavirus§	X			X	

* *Schedule is based on examination conducted within 5 days of sexual assault. If abuse is chronic, or last abusive sexual contact occurred several weeks prior to examination, testing schedule should be established based on timing of last sexual contact.*

† *Not all these tests are appropriate for every patient; testing should be tailored based on type of sexual contact, age of child, symptomatology, and patient or parent requests.*

‡ *Hepatitis B surface antigen, surface antibody and core antibody for adolescents, and hepatitis C antibody if risk factor(s) (eg, intravenous drug use) present.*[4]

§ *The diagnosis of HPV is made clinically, but due to the prolonged incubation period of this disease, follow-up examinations 6 months to 1 year from the last abusive sexual contact should be considered. If patient has received at least 1 dose of HPV vaccine, follow-up may not be needed.*

Considerations for Sexually Transmitted Infection Testing

Testing for STIs in children and adolescents can be uncomfortable, intrusive, and traumatic. Obtaining blood for syphilis, hepatitis, and HIV testing is certainly uncomfortable. Additionally, repeat testing for syphilis, HIV, hepatitis B and hepatitis C is recommended in some patients 3-6 months past the last abusive sexual contact. Vaginal sampling for gonorrhea and *Chlamydia* cultures involves the insertion of a cotton-tipped applicator past the hymenal ring into the vaginal vault; gentle scraping is required to harvest cells for culture because *C. trachomatis* is an obligate intracellular organism. Smaller Dacron® swabs may be less traumatic because they are easier to pass into the vagina without touching the more sensitive hymen. Additionally, urine samples can be submitted for NAA testing in prepubertal children and older patients who experience difficulty tolerating examination. In post-pubertal patients, cervical samples can be obtained in those who have had a previous speculum examination. Vaginal samples are also acceptable and may be more comfortable for the patient, with comparable sensitivity rates to cervical specimens for *Chlamydia*.[9] Rectal samples for gonorrhea and *Chlamydia* are obtained with cotton-tipped or Dacron® swabs inserted into the rectum up to a few centimeters. Swabs can be moistened with nonbacteriostatic saline, which may improve comfort for the patient. Oral samples involve swabbing the tonsillar pillars and may produce a gag reflex. Once the testing is complete, *Chlamydia* samples are refrigerated and gonorrhea samples are incubated if there is a delay in transport to the laboratory. NAATs generally do not require special handling or refrigeration if transported to the lab within 24 hours.

Several factors should be considered in deciding who needs STI testing, which STIs to test for, and what sites should be tested. In addition to the medical history and any examination findings that suggest infection or trauma, the clinician should consider the patient's age, health concerns, confirmed presence of an STI, and risk factors relating to the sex offender in deciding their approach to STI testing. Criteria for testing include (1) history of penetration or evidence of recent or healed penetrative injury to oropharynx, genitals, or anus; (2) abuse by a stranger; (3) an abuser known to be infected with an STI or at high risk for an STI; (4) a sibling or another relative in the household with an STI; (5) a high STI rate in community; (6) signs or symptoms of STIs; or (7) a patient already diagnosed with at least 1 STI.[4] It is recommended, however, that adolescents be screened for all STIs regardless of disclosure,[10] due to high prevalence (up to 22.9%)[4,6,11] and a tendency for some STIs to be asymptomatic.

Proposed criteria for testing are sometimes based on forensic rather than medical indications. The rationale for this approach is that identification of an STI in sexually active adolescents is forensically insignificant and may, in fact, make the victim appear "promiscuous" to a jury. In addition, prophylactic antibiotic treatment with azithromycin, ceftriaxone, and metronidazole costs approximately $165.00, which is generally less expensive than the cost of STI testing. However, the prevalence of STIs in the adolescent population is high, and many infected individuals are asymptomatic, undetected, and untreated. Because of the risks of ascending infection and poor compliance with follow-up examinations, prophylaxis after an acute assault is generally recommended in adolescents in addition to testing. If infected adolescents are treated but not tested, their infected partners will likely be undetected and untreated. Testing and treating adolescent survivors of sexual assault, regardless of past sexual activity is recommended.[4]

NEISSERIA GONORRHOEAE AND *CHLAMYDIA TRACHOMATIS*

Because symptomatology, indications for testing, and coinfection are similar or common for *N. gonorrhoeae* and *C. trachomatis*, these STIs will be discussed jointly. Among sexually abused children, the reported rates of gonorrhea or *Chlamydia* infection range from 3% to 20%, with higher prevalence among adolescents.[12,13] Currently, *C. trachomatis* is more common than *N. gonorrhoeae* in the adult population so a similar trend is anticipated among children and adolescents sexually victimized by adults. Pediatric and adult populations infected with these STIs may be asymptomatic although symptoms such as vaginal discharge and vaginitis may be more commonly seen among prepubertal females infected with gonorrhea (**Figures 10-1**, **10-2**, and **10-3**).[14] Genital and anal *Chlamydia* infections are often asymptomatic; however, some infected patients report discharge, dysuria, abdominal pain, and rectal pain.[15] Genital *Chlamydia* and gonorrhea infections in adolescents may also progress to pelvic inflammatory disease and infertility. Pelvic inflammatory disease is not commonly seen among prepubertal children with *Chlamydia* or gonorrhea.[2,16] The incubation period for chlamydial disease is variable but usually takes at least 1 week. Neonatal chlamydial conjunctivitis typically develops 5 to 12 days after birth, but may occur up to 30 days after birth. The incubation period for gonorrhea is usually 2 to 7 days.[2,16]

The selection of sampling sites depends primarily on the patient's history and clinical signs. Because oral gonorrhea infections may be asymptomatic, it is recommended that testing of the oropharynx be conducted when the history or examination suggests contact between the patient's mouth and another individual's genitals. Through contiguous spread, patients sometimes present with conjunctivitis. Testing for oral or pharyngeal *Chlamydia* infection is usually not recommended because the yield is low, perinatally acquired infection has been reported to persist past age 2 years,[17] and some laboratories

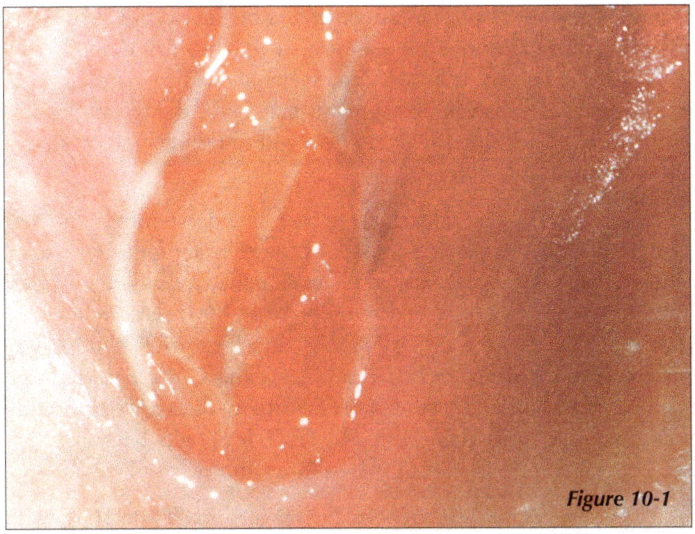

Figure 10-1. *The yellow vaginal discharge present is consistent with* Neisseria gonorrhoea, *which grew in the vaginal culture of a 4-year-old Hispanic child.*

Figure 10-2. *Photo of a 3-year-old girl with yellow-green vaginal discharge and history that "Daddy hurt my pee pee." Culture was positive for* N. gonorrhoea *including confirmatory testing.*

Figure 10-3. *Photo of same child as seen in Figure 10-2, examined 2 weeks after treatment for gonorrhea. This photo shows a hymen with no signs of injury and an opening that was estimated to be 2 to 3 mm wide. Gonorrhea causes a vulvovaginitis in prepubertal girls; penetration beyond the hymen is not necessary to transmit the infection.*

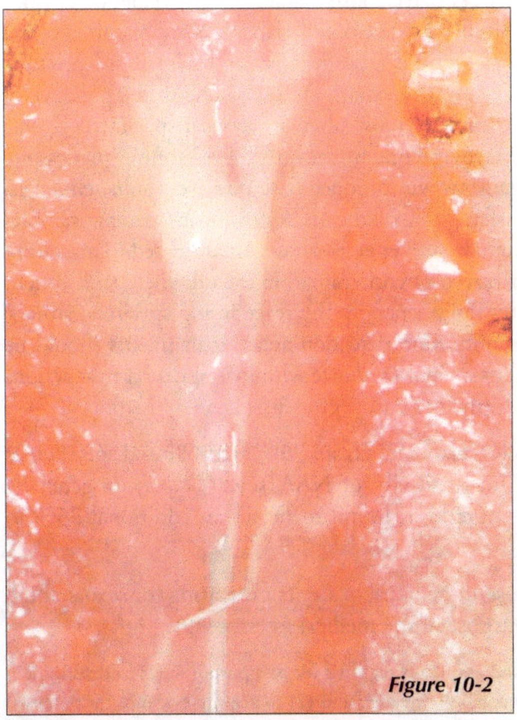

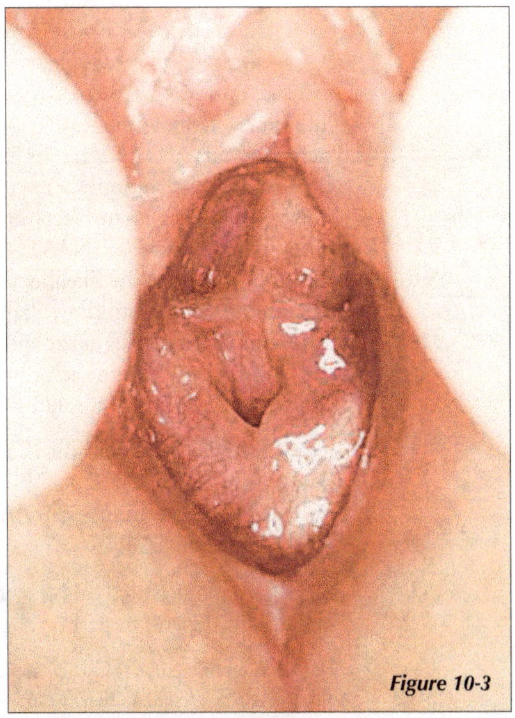

utilizing cultures do not distinguish between *C. trachomatis* and *C. pneumonia*.[2] However, in one study[18] 6% of patients tested for oral *Chlamydia* and gonorrhea with a NAAT had a positive result, and more than half that tested positive did not provide a history of genital-oral contact. Decisions regarding testing for gonorrhea and *Chlamydia* should not be based on examination findings alone because many patients with these infections are asymptomatic. The patient's comfort, especially during an assessment for sexual abuse or assault, is of paramount importance, and the clinician may opt to alter sampling sites to reduce trauma.

If a gonorrhea culture is done, a positive result must be validated with 2 confirmatory tests (eg, carbohydrate degradation, enzyme substrate tests) or by alternative independent methods. These tests will differentiate *N. gonorrhoeae* from other *Neisseria* species.

The isolation of *C. trachomatis* by culture can be confirmed by microscopic identification of inclusions by staining with fluorescein-conjugated monoclonal antibody specific for *C. trachomatis*. Although there is little risk of bacterial cross-contamination in *Chlamydia* cultures, oral and rectal bacteria overgrowth may make the test impossible to interpret. In addition, menstrual blood may interfere with interpretation of vaginal swabs submitted for *Chlamydia* cell culture.

Other detection techniques for these organisms have been tested extensively in adult populations and to some extent in pediatric populations, some with promising results. These techniques include enzyme immunoassay, direct fluorescent antibody, nucleic acid hybridization (or probe) tests, and NAATs. Examples of NAATs include polymerase chain reaction, transcription mediated assay (APTIMA), and Becton-Dickinson assay probe. Of particular note is the distinction between NAATs and DNA hybridization, often confused because both detect DNA sequences. Sensitivity rates are significantly lower with DNA hybridization tests than with NAATs.[16] It should be noted that antibiotic susceptibility tests can only be done from culture samples.

The sensitivity of NAATs for *N. gonorrhoeae* is reported to range from 89% to 100% with specificities of 99% to 100%.[19-21] NAATs detect both viable and nonviable organisms. Therefore, a test may be positive due to the presence of nonviable DNA remaining several weeks after effective treatment. Although both false negative and false positive results are uncommon with these assays, false negative results can occur due to the presence of inhibitors of the amplification process found most often in cervical specimens.[22] One source of false positive results is carryover contamination during sample processing. Because carryover of only a few organisms will produce false positive results, clinicians must ensure that any objects or surfaces that come in contact with patient samples other than culture or NAAT materials are effectively decontaminated. Laboratory measures to reduce the likelihood of carryover contamination include the establishment of a unidirectional workflow that physically separates the reagent and specimen storage area, sample processing area, and amplification/detection area.[23] Instruments should be decontaminated prior to each run of assays in accordance with manufacturer instructions and weekly swipe tests should be performed to ensure effective decontamination.

The sensitivity of NAATs for *C. trachomatis* ranges from 99% to 100% and specificities range from 98% to 100%.[20,21,24] The sensitivity of NAATs for *Chlamydia* generally exceeds culture techniques: NAATs have been found to detect an additional 25% to 30% of infected adults.[25]

Decisions about which STI test to use in pediatric patients presenting for sexual abuse evaluations depend in part on the purpose of the medical assessment[26]:

> Examination of victims (of sexual abuse and assault) is required for two purposes: (1) to determine if an infection is present so that it can be successfully treated; and (2) to acquire evidence for potential use in a legal investigation. Testing to satisfy the first purpose requires a method that is highly sensitive, whereas satisfying the second purpose requires a method that is highly specific. Because of the health and legal implications of test results, the additional time, labor, and cost of performing tests that are sensitive and highly specific are justified.

The latter statement is true if the forensic implications of the test, which require minimizing false positive results, are more important than detection and treatment of the disease, which require minimizing false negative results. If there is other compelling evidence of abuse, the risk of attributing a false positive NAAT to sexual abuse is small. The child's history is the most important evidence and is the only evidence in the majority of child sexual abuse cases. Screening a general population of children for gonorrhea or *Chlamydia* with NAATs and interpreting a positive result as conclusive evidence of sexual abuse in the absence of a clear history or other compelling evidence is misleading and inappropriate. In legal proceedings, the physician may be asked to explain why he or she used NAATs in situations where the culture is still considered to be the "gold standard," and how he or she interprets a positive test. Although all medical evaluations of suspected victims of child and adolescent sexual abuse involve diagnosis and treatment of the physical and emotional consequences of abuse, few also involve testimony. For example, in San Antonio, Texas, fewer than 5% of child sexual abuse cases that include a medical evaluation result in a criminal trial. The risks and relative costs of treating a false positive result by NAAT are small. The cost is generally less than $100 for outpatient antibiotic therapy. The risks of antibiotic treatment for *N. gonorrhoeae* with Ceftriaxone include diarrhea (2.7%); pain, induration, and tenderness at injection site (1%); headache or dizziness (<1%); nausea and vomiting (<1%); and rash (1.7%). The side effects of Azithromycin for treatment of *C. trachomatis* include diarrhea/loose stools (7%), nausea (5%), abdominal pain (5%), vomiting (2%), and dyspepsia (1%).[27] The benefits of treating additional victims who are identified as infected or possibly infected with *Chlamydia* or gonorrhea (as detected by NAATs) include a reduction in the probability of pelvic inflammatory disease, infertility, and ectopic pregnancy. Treatment can also provide reassurance to the victim that the sequelae of abuse are effectively addressed and treated.

An initial positive NAAT test for gonorrhea or *Chlamydia* in a victim of acute assault may reflect perpetrator secretions rather than victim infection.[4,18] Additionally, positive tests from both vaginal and anal sites may represent contiguous spread of infection or multiple deposition sites of infective assailant secretions.[4,18] Even when a positive result may represent infected assailant secretions rather than patient infection, prophylactic antibiotic treatment and follow-up assessment to ensure that the patient is appropriately evaluated for all STIs and that potential infections are eradicated is indicated.

Once gonorrhea or *Chlamydia* infection is reliably identified with the appropriate test, the probability of sexual transmission is addressed. Gonorrhea and *Chlamydia* are transmitted by sexual contact unless there is evidence of perinatal transmission or "clearly, reasonably and independently documented but rare nonsexual transmission."[1] Overall, possible modes of transmission include the following:

1. *Vertical transmission from mother to infant during birth*: Congenital *Chlamydia* infections involving genital and nongenital sites have been documented in rare cases up to almost 3 years after birth.
2. *Horizontal transmission through sexual contact.*
3. *Close nonsexual contact between individuals*: There is limited research available to support the transmission of these diseases through close nonsexual contact between individuals and even less (aside from anecdotal reports) to support transmission between individuals and fomites. *Chlamydia* is an obligate intracellular organism and does not survive on inanimate surfaces. Gonorrhea survives under strict growth requirements, such as a specific carbon dioxide concentration.

The treatment of gonorrhea and *Chlamydia* includes providing prophylaxis and treating the identified disease. CDC recommendations for prophylactic treatment of adolescents older than 12 years of age is azithromycin (1 gram orally in a single dose) or doxycycline (100 mg orally twice daily for 7 days) for *C. trachomatis* and ceftriaxone (250 mg IM in a single dose) for *N. gonorrhoeae*.[2]

The recommended treatment of *C. trachomatis* for children aged 6 months to 12 years is erythromycin or azythromycin.[2,16] The recommendation for infants younger than 6 months of age is erythromycin base or ethylsuccinate 50 mg/kg/day orally, divided into 4 doses daily for 14 days. Treatment with erythromycin is approximately 80%

effective, so follow-up assessment is recommended to determine whether retreatment is necessary. Infants treated with erythromycin who are younger than age 6 weeks have an increased risk of infantile hypertrophic pyloric stenosis. Azithromycin 20 mg/kg/day orally given as a single dose daily for 3 days may be effective; however, data are limited and reassessment post-treatment is recommended. When needed, a test of cure should be done at least 3 weeks after treatment is completed because NAATs (if used) will detect viable and nonviable organisms for up to 3 weeks. Children heavier than 45 kg or older than 12 years of age may receive a single 1-gram oral dose of azithromycin. Doxycycline 100 mg orally twice daily for 7 days is a recommended alternative, but it should not be given to pregnant adolescents or children younger than age 8 years.[2,16]

In adults, a minority of untreated *Chlamydia* infections (up to 30%) may resolve spontaneously without treatment. Additionally, treatment for other infections, such as benzathine penicillin for syphilis may also eradicate *Chlamydia* infections.

The recommended treatment of gonococcal infections is intramuscular ceftriaxone in adolescents with uncomplicated infection.[2,16] The prevalence of quinolone-resistant *N. gonorrhoeae* (QRNG) is high in Europe, Asia, the Middle East, and the Pacific (including California and Hawaii) and is increasing in the United States. It is also more common among men who have sex with men (MSM). In April 2007, the CDC recommended removal of quinolones as an option for treatment of *N. gonorrhoeae* in the United States.[28] Gonococcal infections of the pharynx are more difficult to eradicate than anogenital infections, though a single intramuscular dose of ceftriaxone remains the treatment of choice.[29]

If NAAT results are not available or *Chlamydia* testing is negative with a test other than NAAT, patients treated for gonorrhea should also be treated for *Chlamydia*. Recommendations apply for pharyngeal gonorrhea infection because of risk of coinfection of a genital site (see **Table 10-3**).[2]

When utilizing cultures and some NAATs to detect gonorrhea, cross-contamination with other species is possible. These species include *Neisseria meningitidis*, *Neisseria lactamica*, *Neisseria cinerea*, *Neisseria sicca*, *Neisseria subflava biovar perflava*, *Neisseria*

Table 10-3. Treatment Recommendations for Gonorrheal and Chlamydial Infections

Infections	Children < 8 years and < 45 kg	Children < 8 years and > 45 kg	Children/Adolescents ≥ Age 8 years and ≥ 45 kg
C. trachomatis (uncomplicated anogenital or oral infection or prophylaxis in adolescents)	Erythromycin base orally 50 mg/kg/day divided into 4 doses for 14 days (retest) *OR* Azithromycin 20 mg/kg orally daily for 3 days*	Azithromycin 1 gm orally (single dose)	Azithromycin 1 gm orally as a single dose *OR* Doxycycline 100 mg orally twice daily for 7 days
N. gonorrhoeae (uncomplicated anogenital or oral infection or prophylaxis in adolescents)	Ceftriaxone 125 mg IM (single dose)	Ceftriaxone 25-50 mg/kg IV or IM in single dose (up to125 mg IM)	Ceftriaxone 250 mg IM (single dose)

**Azithromycin 20 mg/kg/day for 3 days may be considered as an alternative if EES unavailable or too costly.*

mucosa, *Neisseria flavescens*, *Neisseria polysaccharea*, *Branhamella catarrhalis*, and *Kingella denitrificans*.[30] If the diagnostic tests and interpretation are appropriately conducted to minimize false positive results, a positive test for gonorrhea or *Chlamydia* is reliable and other infectious causes can be excluded from the differential diagnosis.

Human Papillomavirus

Condyloma acuminata (venereal warts) is frequently diagnosed in sexually abused children (**Figures 10-4**, **10-5**, **10-6**, and **10-7**). In adults, transmission of this disease is predominantly sexual, and the prevalence of genital human papillomavirus (HPV) infections in adults age 18 to 59 years is approximately 45% in men and 40% in women.[31] Some are infected with multiple HPV types. How HPV is transmitted to children is controversial and has remained so despite ongoing active research in this area for the last 30 years. In the most recent *Guidelines for the Medical Assessment and Care of Children Who May Have Been Sexually Abused*,[1] genital or anal condyloma acuminatum in the absence of other indicators of abuse is considered a finding with no expert consensus on interpretation with respect to sexual contact. Lesions that first appear in a child older than 5 years are considered more likely to have been transmitted through sexual contact.[32]

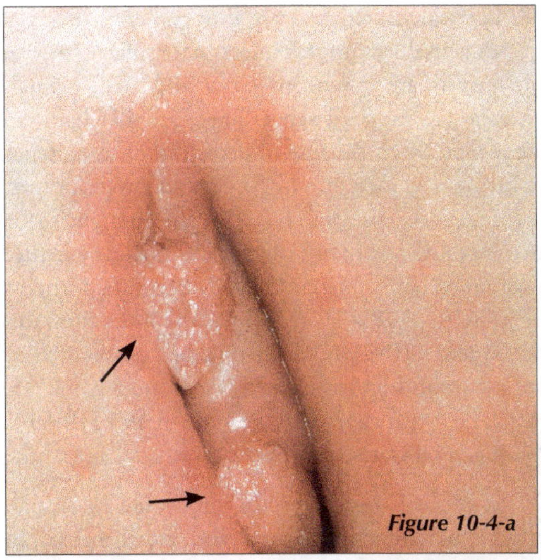

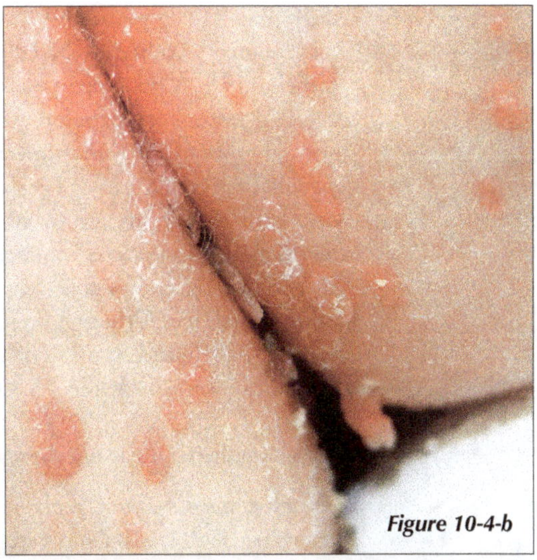

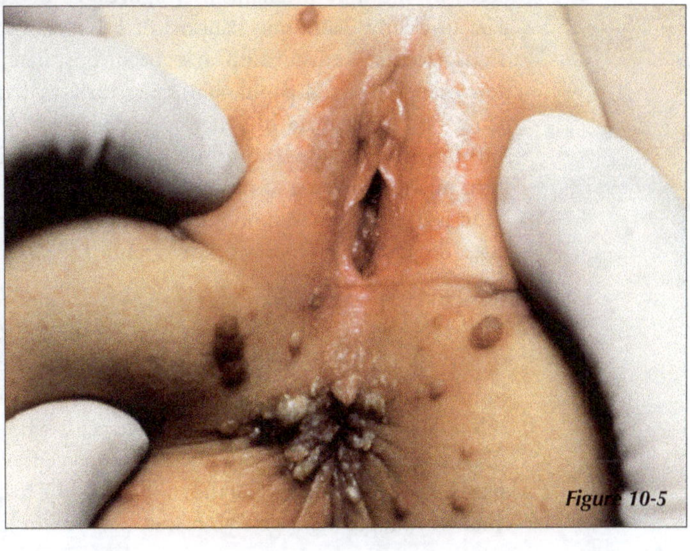

Figure 10-4-a. *Three-year-old child in the supine position. There are 2 cauliflower-like, warty clusters of condyloma acuminata (HPV). One is on the periurethral area and the other on the posterior hymen. There are several isolated warts on the labia majora.*

Figure 10-4-b. *Flat and sessile warts visible on the buttocks of the child. G. vaginalis and group B streptococcus were cultured from the vagina (35mm).*

Figure 10-5. *Condyloma acuminata is evident in the perianal area (35mm).*

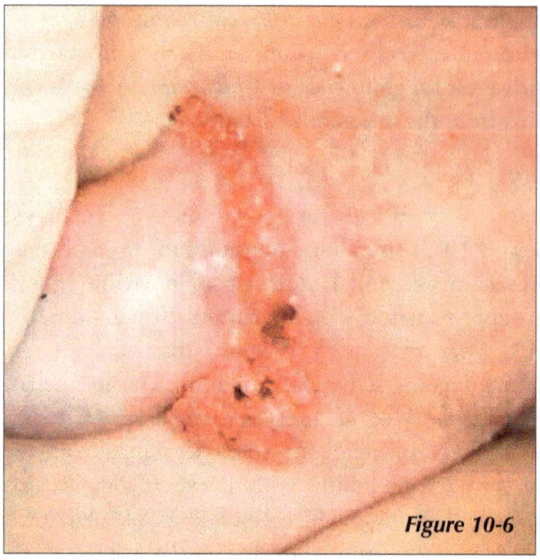

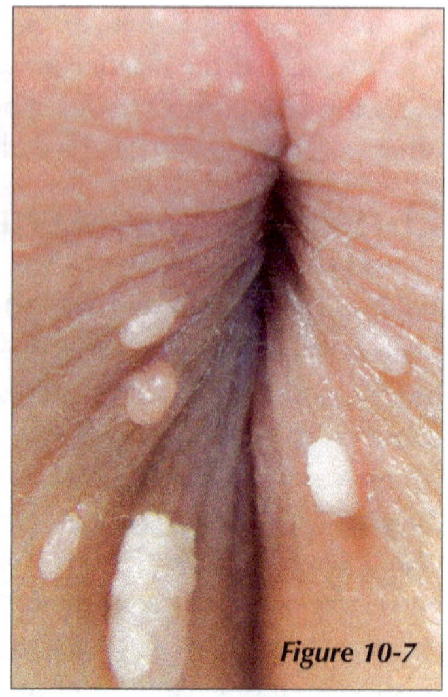

Figure 10-6. Condyloma at the base of the penis in a 3-year-old boy. Child did not give a disclosure of abuse.

Figure 10-7. Condyloma in the anal area of a 4-year-old girl who gave no disclosure of sexual abuse. Mother had a history of an abnormal Pap smear several years prior.

More than 100 types of HPVs have been identified and are grouped into mucosal and cutaneous subtypes based on their predilection to infect particular types of epithelium.[2,16] Most often, nongenital warts are cutaneous types and anal, genital, oral, and respiratory papillomas/dysplasias are mucosal types. There are 40 identified mucosal types of HPV that infect the genital tract. Because of detection of some types in genital cancers, mucosal HPVs are further grouped into high-risk and low-risk types. Most HPV infections (up to 90% of infections within 2 years)[33-35] are thought to be cleared by the immune system before they cause any harm, though it is unclear whether infected persons completely clear infection or HPV infection simply becomes dormant and undetectable. Although there are more than 18 high-risk types, the most common are HPV-16 (found in 50% of cancers) and HPV-18, which together cause 70% of cervical cancers worldwide.[16,36] Other common high-risk genital types are 31, 33, 35, 39, 45, 51, 52, 56, 58, 59, 68, and 82. Low-risk types include HPV-6 and HPV-11, which together cause more than 90% of genital warts.[37]

Though transmission of genital HPV in adults is believed to be almost always sexual, mechanisms of transmission in children remain controversial and are theorized to occur by multiple mechanisms (**Figures 10-8**, **10-9**, **10-10**, and **10-11**). Sufficient data to clearly define mechanisms of HPV transmission in children are still lacking. Transplacental transmission has been postulated due to rare reports of infants developing laryngeal papillomatosis as early as 1 day of age,[38] presence of nongenital condyloma acuminata in a newborn delivered by Cesarean section (C-section) with intact membranes,[39] identification of HPV in amniotic fluid and umbilical cord blood from infants delivered to mothers with HPV infection,[40,41] and identification of HPV-16 in peripheral blood mononuclear cells.[42] These reports involve very few numbers of cases, despite the high prevalence of adult HPV.

Vertical and postnatal transmission has been studied by assessing frequency of positive HPV DNA in oral or genital swabs in infants and children.[43-47] Chatterjee et al[46] found 16% (5 of 31) newborn buccal smears to be positive for HPV DNA (types 6,11,16,18). Summersgill et al[45] collected oral squamous cells from swabs or oral saline solution from 268 healthy infants, children, and adolescents who were 20 years old or younger. HPV DNA was detected in 6% of subjects. Five percent of the adolescents (more than 12 years of age) were positive, none of the children aged 7 to 12 years were positive, and 9% of the children younger than age 7 years were positive. In Japan, 45% of healthy 3 year olds and

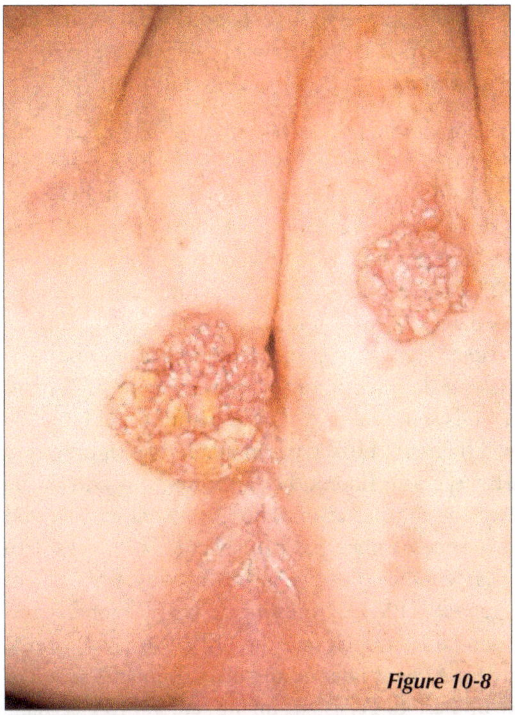
Figure 10-8

Figure 10-8. *Giant, pedunculated condyloma in an 8-month-old female. Both parents had genital warts at the time of the baby's birth. The source of the baby's HPV could have been from either parent. No other STDs were found in the infant.*

Figure 10-9. *Anal condyloma in a 2-month-old breastfed infant. This child was removed from the parents because the physician who examined the baby said that the warts could only have been spread by sexual contact. Further history revealed that mother had a past history of genital warts but currently had no lesions. The mode of transmission in this infant was most likely not sexual.*

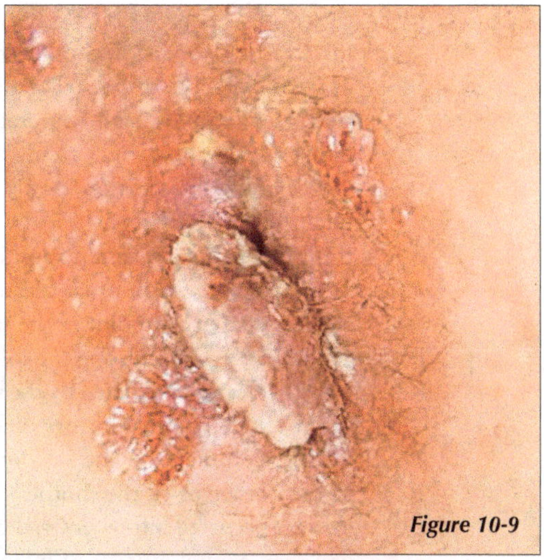
Figure 10-9

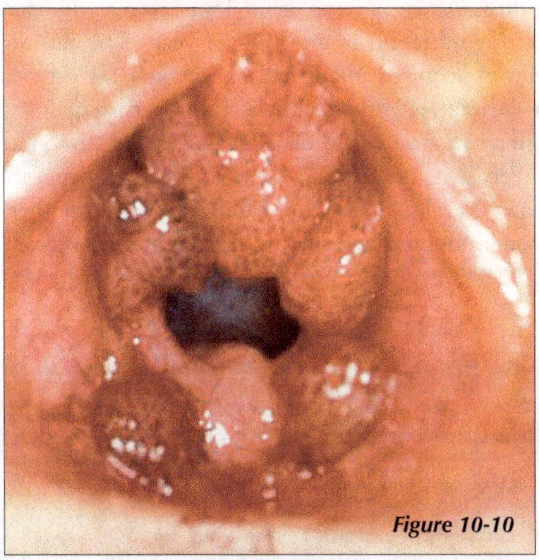
Figure 10-10

Figure 10-10. *This 6-year-old girl gave a history of penile-genital contact by her stepfather. She was brought for an examination because of genital bleeding, which was determined to have been caused by condyloma. In this case, transmission was likely sexual.*

Figure 10-11. *This 3-year-old child has anal warts, noticed first at 12 months. The child's mother had noted 1 small wart for several years. Recently, the warts appeared to spread, and she brought him for an examination. The child denied any abuse. Several others in the family had warts on their hands. These warts were not biopsied but were treated with topical medication and resolved.*

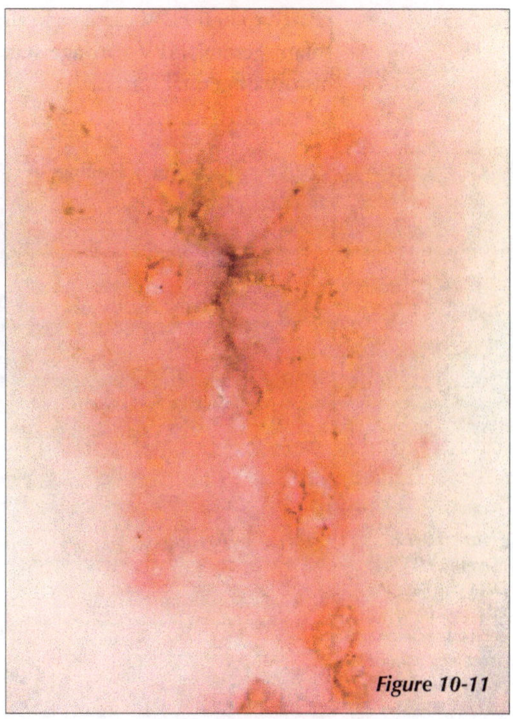
Figure 10-11

50% of healthy 5 year olds attending the same nursery school had HPV DNA detected on oral buccal swabs, especially HPV-16, HPV-1, HPV-2, and HPV-75.[44] These studies raise an unanswered question: Is this colonization, infection, or contamination?

Finnish researchers addressed this question with a prospective study of 324 infants and their parents over 36 months, assessing oral and genital swabs for 12 high-risk HPV DNA types.[43] Although these researchers did not report concordance of mother/baby HPV DNA or whether subjects had any visible warts or condyloma, they described acquisition, clearance, and persistence of high-risk HPV DNA detected in infant oral and genital specimens (**Figure 10-12**). Patterns were very similar for oral and genital mucosa. At delivery, HPV DNA was detected in 14% of infant oral swabs. Of these infants, 10% (1.4% of total) had persistent HPV carriage at 36 months of age and 11% cleared the HPV. No HPV DNA was ever detected in oral specimens from 37% of all infants. New (or acquisition of) HPV DNA in oral mucosa was demonstrated in 42% of the infants. Persistent oral carriage of high-risk HPV types in infants was significantly associated with (1) high-risk oral HPV types in the mother at 36 months and in the father at 24 months, (2) young age of the mother at initiation of sexual activity and use of oral contraception, and (3) presence of maternal hand warts. With regard to infant genital specimens, 15% were HPV DNA–positive at birth. Only 1.5% (5) of these infants had persistent positive genital HPV DNA testing at age 36 months, and 14% of infants with initial positive genital testing cleared the HPV. No genital HPV was detected at any point in the study for 47% of infants, and 36% of infants acquired genital HPV DNA during the follow-up period. Persistent infant genital HPV carriage was significantly predicted by the mother's history of recent genital warts at over 20 years of age and a maternal history of smoking initiation at age 18 to 21 years. The authors did not comment on the relationship of acquired infant oral and genital HPV types to each other or to the mother's or father's HPV types. Importantly, persistent HPV carriage occurred infrequently, though persistent carriage of HPV was more common in oral than genital mucosa of infants. Persistent oral carriage of HPV in infants appears related to oral HPV carriage in the parents and to presence of hand warts in the mother. Infant genital HPV carriage was uncommon and appeared related to mother's recent history of genital warts.

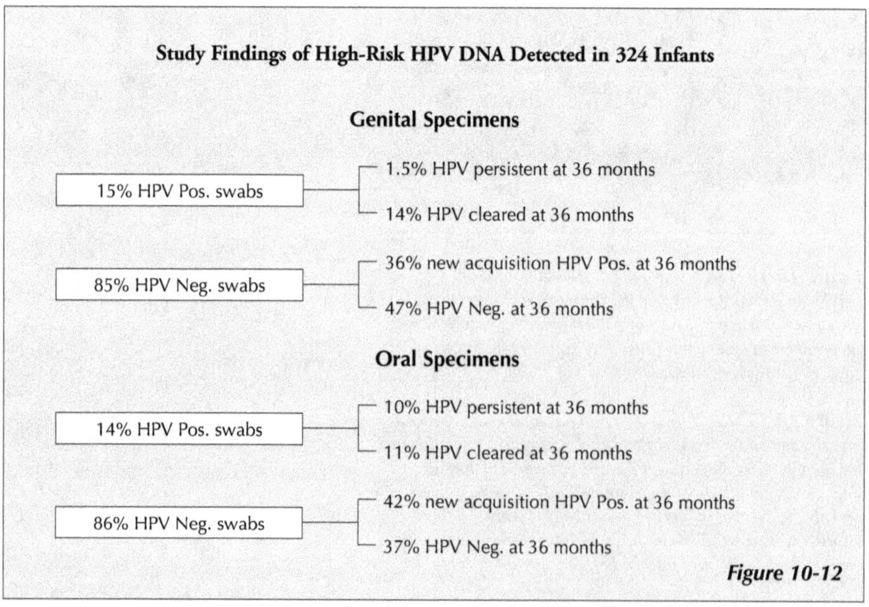

Figure 10-12. *High-risk HPV DNA detected in infant oral and genital specimens, describing acquisition, clearance, and persistence.*

Another study of buccal samples from 267 children aged 3 to 11 years showed much higher prevalence of HPV DNA in children when using type-specific PCR testing (HPV-16, a high-risk mucosal type).[47] Prevalence of HPV-16 was 52% compared to 17% by generic PCR. All controls and 20 tested fomite surfaces in the school environment tested HPV-negative. This author also summarized serologic studies demonstrating presence of antibodies by EIA to HPV-16 in 4% to 14% of children aged 1 to 13 years as well as detection of IgM antibody to HPV-16 among 50% of children aged 1 to 10 years presented as evidence for recent or persistent HPV-16 infection in children. This study did not differentiate vertical transmission from early childhood acquisition. A follow-up study by the same group tested for persistence of oral HPV-16 in 20 children aged 4 to 9 years, comparing them to a negative control group.[48] The time interval tested was 30 months. Of the HPV-16–positive group, 40% were subsequently negative, and 63% of the negative control group had become HPV-16–positive. The authors concluded that (asymptomatic) oral HPV-16 DNA in children is likely transient. It is possible that the high rates may reflect false positive PCR results.[49]

The high rates of infant HPV DNA detection in some of the above studies and lack of comparison to parent HPV DNA rates are in contrast to 2 large prospective longitudinal studies of infant and parent HPV DNA.[50,51] Both studies describe women with relatively high rates of genital/cervical HPV DNA (Smith et al 29%; Watts et al 41% cervical and 74% with cervical, vulvovaginal, and history of condyloma or abnormal Pap smear). Infants had very low rates of oral or genital HPV (Smith et al 1.6%; Watts et al 1.5% genital, 1.2% anal, none oral or nasopharyngeal). Furthermore, the infants with HPV DNA were not concordant with their mother's HPV DNA types. Results from both of these studies support the conclusion that vertical transmission of HPV infection is rare.

An unanswered question is whether presence of HPV DNA represents true infection. Respiratory papillomatosis (RP) is interesting to study because it clearly represents infection, not colonization or carriage. Frequently, RP is presumed to occur through vertical transmission because most of the affected children with this disorder have HPV-6 or HPV-11 and obstetric delivery of women with genital HPV by C-section may be associated with lower rates of infant laryngeal infection,[52] although C-section to prevent transmission of HPV to the newborn is currently not indicated.[2] Vertical transmission as explanation for all or even most cases of respiratory papillomas has been challenged because the disease also develops in older children and adults. There are no reported cases of respiratory or laryngeal papillomas in siblings, marital partners, or family members.[40] Sinclair et al[53] highlight the bimodal age distribution for peak diagnosis of RP (between ages 2 and 5 years in children and between ages 20 and 30 years in adults). They also point out the paucity of studies that consider acquisition of RP from child sexual abuse, despite adult RP being attributed to oral-genital contact. Wiatrak et al[40] have published a 10-year longitudinal prospective study of 74 children with recurrent respiratory papillomatosis followed from time of diagnosis. In this series, the mean age of diagnosis was 4 years old, with the youngest child diagnosed at age 4 months and the oldest at age 12 years. No type of screening for sexual abuse was described.

Horizontal transmission and autoinoculation are additional proposed modes of transmitting HPV to children's genitals. It is unknown how commonly this occurs; however, HPV types 2, 3, 27, and 57 have been shown to be present in pediatric anogenital warts.[49,54] Because these 4 types are commonly seen in cutaneous warts, it is speculated that children may transfer HPV to their genitals when scratching, toileting, et cetera. Additionally, horizontal transmission is theorized to occur from an adult caregiver when assisting with diaper changes or toileting, or during sexual abuse of the child, as many disclosures of sexual abuse involve fondling and digital penetrative acts. HPV DNA has been found in finger brush samples of adults with genital HPV disease. It is unknown whether this transient hand carriage is adequate to allow transmission without abraded skin.[54]

Attempts to demonstrate fomite transmission of HPV from floors, toys, humid surfaces of bathhouses, et cetera have not yielded any positive HPV DNA samples.[47,49] Fomite transmission is speculated to be a cause of plantar warts; however, demonstration of fomite transmission has not been reported.

Evaluation of a child, especially an older child (>5 years of age) who presents with genital or oral warts should include consideration of sexual abuse. A complete medical evaluation is recommended, including a child forensic interview, and caretaker interview to assess maternal history of condyloma or abnormal Pap smears, and history of cutaneous warts affecting the child or family members. Although vertical transmission does not appear to be common, absence of a clear maternal history does not preclude it. Physical examination of the entire child including the oral cavity should be performed and testing for other STIs should be considered. Consensus is currently lacking on when to report these cases to child protective services (CPS). Routine reporting to CPS has been suggested for children over age 4 years presenting with anogenital warts, with referral to CPS for younger children guided by overall history, forensic interview, and clinical findings.[53]

Other methods of transmission including nonsexual horizontal transmission and autoinoculation are possible. Fomite transmission is unlikely though described.[53] Blood transfusion is a theoretical risk with limited, inconclusive data.[42] Host factors also influence viral transmission, persistent carriage of HPV, and rate of HPV disease. Patients with immunosuppression—either from immunodeficiency, HIV infection, or iatrogenic immunosuppression—have higher rates of HPV disease. Patients with mucosal breaks [ie, ulcerative diseases including herpes simplex virus (HSV)] may also be at increased risk of HPV disease; however, data are lacking to support skin disorders such as eczema as a factor increasing infection rate with HPV.

The diagnosis of condyloma acuminata (venereal warts) is primarily clinical. During clinical examination, application of acetic acid (ie, TCA or BCA used for treatment) to a suspicious skin lesion may elicit a characteristic "white frosting" of HPV infected tissue. Although the application of acetic acid is not a specific test for HPV, the white frosting effect is not expected to occur in HPV-uninfected lesions. Application of acetic acid can be quite painful[55] and is not advised for patients undergoing a sexual abuse evaluation. Other diagnostic tests include histologic examination and detection of HPV DNA in biopsied material. HPV DNA can be detected with dot blot hybridization, DNA blotting, and modifications of PCR.[56] While costly and labor-intensive, the DNA blot is considered the "gold standard."[57] Although genital HPV subtypes have been detected in oral mucosal scrapings of asymptomatic prepubertal children,[58] subtyping of HPV appears to have no diagnostic or therapeutic value when performed on asymptomatic patients. HPV colonization can occur via sexual and nonsexual transmission. Subtyping of HPV in patients with clinically apparent lesions does not assist physicians in determining whether such lesions are sexually transmitted. A biopsy should be considered if the diagnosis is uncertain, lesions do not respond or appear to worsen during standard treatment, the patient is immunocompromised, or if the warts appear atypical.[2] Histopathologic detection of HPV in cervical scrapings or biopsies of suspicious lesions depends on the identification of koilocytosis. False negatives are problematic with inexperienced personnel.[57] In a study of several sexually active adolescent girls, non-sexually active adolescent girls, and prepubertal girls presenting for gynecological care or complaints, vaginal samples were positive for HPV in 37.9% of patients, including 34.5% of prepubertal girls.[59] The relationship between a positive vaginal sample, clinical disease, and sexual transmission remain to be clarified. Currently, HPV researchers have found the presence of cutaneous HPV DNA and antibodies to the same HPV type are not significantly correlated, thus concluding "the biologic meaning of seropositivity as a marker of cutaneous HPV infection" is as yet uninterpretable.[60] HPV serologic tests are not available commercially, and the usefulness of this test for clinical or forensic purposes in child abuse pediatrics is unknown, unstudied, and should not be used at this time.

The quadrivalent HPV vaccine (Gardasil®, Merck) was FDA approved in June 2006 to prevent cervical cancer and lesions caused by HPV-6, HPV-11, HPV-16, and HPV-18. International studies confirm the vaccine is nearly 100% effective at preventing HPV-16 and HPV-18 infection. Within 6 years of this vaccine's introduction, there has been a 64% decrease in the prevalence of quadrivalent HPV types among females aged 14 to 19 years.[61] The CDC recommends routine vaccination of girls 11 to 12 years old, with catch-up vaccination for young women who missed routine vaccination between ages 13 to 26 years. Girls as young as 9 years old may be vaccinated at the discretion of health care providers. Clinicians should consider providing this vaccine to sexually abused or assaulted children (older than 9 years) and adolescents who are unvaccinated or incompletely vaccinated. If the series is initiated before the patient's 15th birthday, a two-dose schedule is recommended, with vaccines given at 0 and 6 to 12 months.[62]

A number of treatments for condyloma acuminata are available; however, no definitive evidence exists to support best efficacy of any single treatment. Treatment efficacy varies among patients. The effect of treatment on limiting HPV transmission is unknown, so treatment should be considered only for patients with visible lesions. Regardless of treatment, lesions may spontaneously resolve, and are likely to recur. Because most lesions are small in number and asymptomatic, it is likely best to first observe without therapy for several months to establish whether lesions spontaneously resolve. Decision to treat may be influenced by development of symptoms including pruritus, pain, or bleeding or by increasing number or size of warts. Ablative surgery should be reserved for extensive lesions, particularly those interfering with urogenital function (eg, obstructive, painful). Most warts respond to a course of treatment (or spontaneously involute) within 3 months. Complications are rare but include post-treatment pigmentation change, depressed or hypertrophic scars, chronic pain syndromes (vulvodynia, analdynia, hyperesthesias, painful defecation, or fistulas), and limited reports of severe systemic side effects from interferon and podophyllin treatments exist.[2] Patient-applied therapies are likely to have optimal response with supervision and follow-up to assist compliance and efficacy and to monitor for side effects (see **Table 10-4**). Podofilox 0.5% solution or gel is a safe, easy-to-use antimitotic drug. Most patients experience mild to moderate local pain or irritation with treatment. Imiquimod is a topical immune enhancer that stimulates interferon and other cytokines. Treatment is usually associated with mild to moderate redness and irritation. Referral may be made to dermatologists or gynecologists for provider-administered treatments. Side effects may be minimized by limiting treatment cycles to 3 months and allowing sufficient time to heal between therapy regimens. Trichloroacetic acid (TCA) or Bichloroacetic acid (BCA) 80% to 90% may be applied weekly if necessary in the office setting. A small amount is applied only to the warts and allowed to dry (lesions will whiten). Excess acid should be removed by powdering the treated area with talc, baking soda, or liquid soap preparations. Podophyllin resin 10% to 25% may be applied in the office weekly as needed. Toxicity may be associated with systemic absorption; therefore, only a small amount should be used (maximum 0.5 mL) and application should be limited to small area less than 10 cm^2 per session. Other modalities are cryotherapy, surgical removal (eg, excision, curettage, electrosurgery), carbon dioxide laser surgery, or injection of intralesional interferon.[2] Differential diagnosis of external warts includes molluscum contagiosum, linear epidermal nevus, syphilis (condyloma lata), skin tags, and pearly penile papules (benign).

Table 10-4. Treatment Modalities for Anogenital Warts

Treatment Modalities	
Anal Warts	Cryotherapy (liquid nitrogen) OR TCA/BCA 80% to 90% applied to warts OR Surgical removal (if on rectal mucosa)
Vaginal Warts	Cryotherapy (liquid nitrogen—do not use cryoprobe) OR TCA/BCA 80% to 90% applied to warts
Urethral Meatus Warts	Cryotherapy (liquid nitrogen) OR Podophyllin 10% to 25% in compound tincture of benzoin OR Podofilox* 0.5% solution or gel OR Imiquimod* 5% cream
External Genital Warts (Patient-Applied)	Podofilox 0.5% solution or gel: twice a day x 3 days (then 4 days no treatment); may repeat up to 4 cycles. Max 0.5 ml/day to max area 10 cm^2 OR Imiquimod 5% cream: 3 times a week once daily at bedtime, up to 16 weeks. Wash treated area 6 to 10 hours after application
External Genital Warts (Provider-Applied)	Cryotherapy (liquid nitrogen or cryoprobe) every 1 to 2 weeks OR Podophyllin resin 10% to 25% in compound tincture of benzoin OR TCA/BCA 80% to 90% applied to warts OR Surgery (excision, curettage, electrocautery, carbon dioxide laser) OR Intralesional interferon (injection)

** Limited data.*

TRICHOMONAS VAGINALIS

Infection with *T. vaginalis* is another STI that can occur in sexually abused children and adolescents (**Figure 10-13**). In the United States, it is considered the second most common STI, and the most common curable STI.[63] However, it is not a reportable sexually transmitted disease in the United States. Epidemiologically, *Trichomonas* is considered a marker for high-risk sexual behavior in adults and is commonly associated with other STIs, especially gonorrhea. In women, bacterial vaginosis (BV) commonly occurs concurrently with *Trichomonas*, and *Trichomonas* infection has been found to be an important cofactor that amplifies HIV transmission.[16,63,64] Its incubation period ranges from 4 to 28 days (averaging 1 week).[16,63]

Figure 10-13. *Appearance of* Trichomonas vaginalis *on wet preparation examination.*

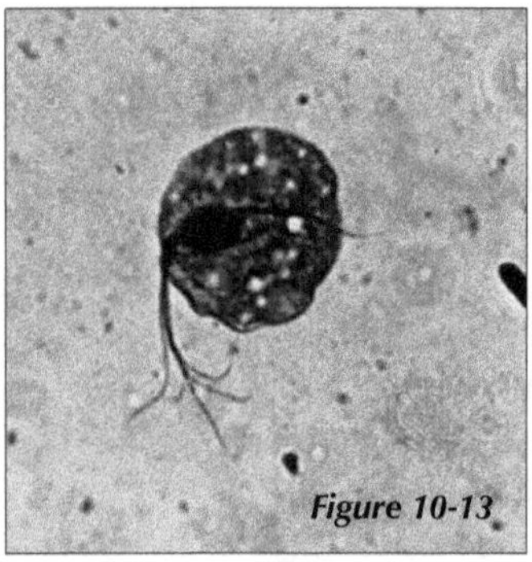

Trichomoniasis is asymptomatic in most infected men (90%) and in half of infected women. The organism is a flagellated protozoan slightly larger than a white blood cell. Typical symptoms in women, when present, include frothy pale yellow to gray-green vaginal discharge, odor, pruritus, and irritation (vaginal redness and edema, "strawberry" cervix). Dysuria and lower abdominal pain are also common. The urethra is infected in most cases. Males may develop urethritis, epididymitis, or prostatitis, albeit uncommonly. Reinfection by infected partners is common.[63,65]

The diagnosis is typically made by microscopic examination of vaginal secretions. Male urine, prostatic secretions, or semen may be tested.

Vaginal smear (wet prep) examination has a low sensitivity rate (13% to 80%),[2,16,63,66-69] in part because nonmotile trichomonads closely resemble white blood cells and can be overlooked. Hence, detection relies heavily on the microscopic expertise of the examiner, appropriate preparation of the vaginal smear to preserve motility of the trichomonads, and inspection of the vaginal smear slide within 10 to 20 minutes of sample collection. Alternative detection techniques for *Trichomonas* include culture, latex agglutination, direct fluorescent antibody, and PCR. Culture has a low cost: approximately $2.50 per test (excluding laboratory and pathologist fees). There are 3 culture media available: Diamond's media, Kupferberg's Trichosel media, and InPouch™ TV. In a study that compared the sensitivity of these 3 media, the InPouch™ TV test was significantly more sensitive than either the Diamond's or Trichosel media and detected approximately twice as many infected patients at 48 hours.[70] Tests with better clinical utility than vaginal smear and culture are nonamplified molecular tests and NAATs, which are more expensive than culture.[71] NAATs performed on vaginal specimens have a sensitivity greater than 76% and specificity greater than 96% for detection of *Trichomonas* and are recommended by the CDC for adult and adolescent survivors of sexual assault.[4] In contrast to culture, false positives may occur with these tests, especially in low prevalence populations.[2] Direct fluorescent antibody (DFA) has been demonstrated to be more sensitive than vaginal smear but less sensitive than culture or PCR.[69] In the same study, cultures utilizing Trichosel media detected 46 positive results whereas PCR detected 61 positive results. However, PCR is expensive and laborious compared to all other detection techniques for *T. vaginalis*.[2,16]

Metronidazole is the treatment of choice for trichomoniasis. Adolescent dose is 2 grams orally in a single dose or, alternatively, tinidazole 2 grams orally in a single dose. Patients unable to tolerate the single dose (eg, because of nausea) or with treatment failure may take metronidazole 500 mg orally twice a day for 7 days.[2] Recommended treatment for children weighing less than 45 kg is oral metronidazole 15 mg/kg per day divided (maximum 2 grams/day) into 3 doses per day for a total of 7 days.[16] Low-grade resistance to metronidazole has been described in vitro but has not yet become clinically important.[2,72] Although metronidazole can be offered as prophylaxis following an acute sexual assault, clinicians may opt to have the patient delay treatment for a few days due to side effects of nausea, especially if taken with post-coital contraception medications.

Differential diagnosis of *T. vaginalis* includes other infectious and non-infectious causes of vaginitis. Additionally, *T. vaginalis* must be reliably distinguished from other human *Trichomonas* species, *Trichomonas tenax* and *Pentatrichomonas hominis* (ie, *Trichomonas hominis*), which are nonpathogenic and occur infrequently. *T. tenax* is found in oral gingival and tracheobronchial secretions. *P. hominis* is found in the gastrointestinal tract, therefore stool contamination of vaginal or urethral specimens makes identification of *T. vaginalis* more difficult. *Trichomonas* species have strict habitat restriction meaning *T. tenax* and *P. hominis* are not viable in the vagina or urethra and cannot be sexually transmitted. Consequently, the diagnosis of infection with *T. vaginalis* is best made from vaginal or urethral samples. In young patients, bagged urine samples may be contaminated with *Pentatrichomonas*. The decision to test for *T. vaginalis* cannot be based on the presence of patient symptoms or signs as most males and many females are asymptomatic.[2,16,63] Testing criteria for *T. vaginalis* should complement testing criteria for *N. gonorrhoeoa* and *C. trachomatis*, and include a patient history for vaginal-penile contact.

Duration of *Trichomonas* infection is not well described; however, one study using mathematical models to study epidemiology of *Trichomonas* estimated average duration of *Trichomonas* infection in women to be 3 to 5 years and in men to be 4 months.[73]

Data are lacking on duration of infection in neonates, however newborn infection is considered to be self-limited and treatment unnecessary.[16,63] Few papers describe neonatal or prepubertal infection and duration of infection in these ages. One 1974 study of 984 newborn subjects describes 0.6% to 5% of infants of *Trichomonas*-positive mothers to have evidence of infection, with infection persisting until treatment (oldest infant 8 weeks of age).[74] The authors postulate that the hyperestrogenic acidic environment of the neonatal vagina allows *Trichomonas* infection to develop (nonetheless rarely described in this population). Once the estrogenic environment subsides and vaginal pH neutralizes (around 6 to 8 weeks of life), conditions are less favorable for *Trichomonas*. Other papers describe case reports of neonatal nasal or respiratory infection.[64,75,76] Vertical transmission is thus possible, though uncommon. Persistence of neonatal infection is not well documented but is thought to be rare outside of the neonatal period. Although fomite transmission is also theoretically possible as *Trichomonas* has been shown to be viable for several hours in urine and washcloths, transmission has not been reported and is likely to be infrequent given the strong association of *Trichomonas* infections with other STIs.[63,74,77,78] Presence of *Trichomonas* infection in an adolescent or child outside of the neonatal period is, therefore, most likely to be sexually transmitted. Reporting to social services, investigation, and evaluation of the child for other STIs is indicated.

Herpes Simplex Viruses

There are 2 types of herpes simplex viruses and both cause genital herpes infections in children and adults. Herpes simplex type 2 (HSV-2) accounts for the majority of genital herpes infections.[79,80] Orolabial HSV-2 occurs much less frequently than genital infections, measured by studies of HSV shedding using daily swabs for PCR testing. In these adult studies, oral HSV-2 shedding was not associated with any visible oral lesions, though was usually associated with HSV-2 genital lesions or genital shedding.[79,81,82] The majority of people (>85%) with HSV-2 specific antibodies do not report symptoms of genital herpes,[79,80] yet persons infected with HSV-2 have been shown to have asymptomatic HSV-2 shedding by PCR on 20% to 25% of all days. Furthermore, people who are HSV-2 seropositive without symptomatic genital herpes have been shown to be equally likely to shed HSV as those with symptomatic genital herpes.[83] Therefore, most HSV-2 transmission occurs from asymptomatic infected persons. This fact is important to consider when evaluating a child who presents with genital herpes caused by HSV-2, as the infected perpetrator would generally be expected to lack a history of symptomatic genital or oral HSV-2 while being HSV-2 seropositive (**Figure 10-14**).

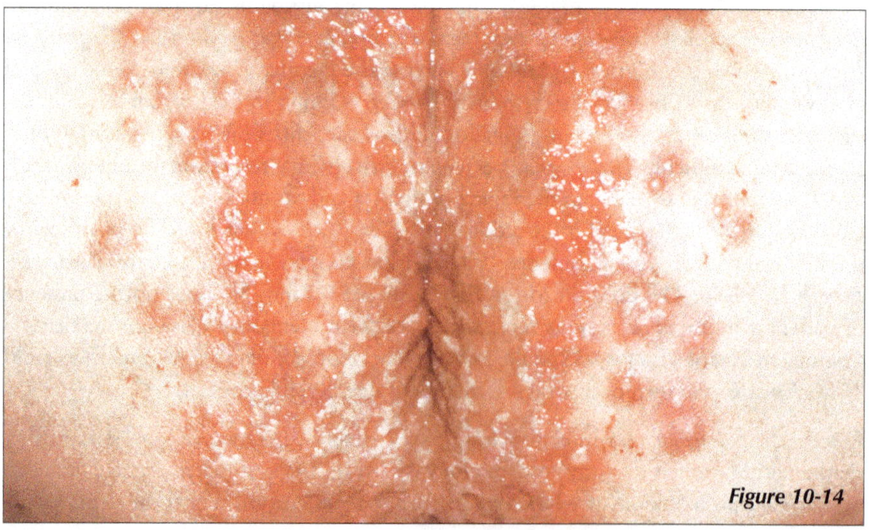
Figure 10-14

Figure 10-14.
This 3 year old has extensive herpes simplex type 2 (HSV-2) around her anus and on her perineum and labia majora (35mm).

Herpes simplex type 1 (HSV-1) is frequently transmitted in childhood by nonsexual contacts, most often via infectious saliva. Seroprevalence is approximately 20% in children younger than age 5 years and then increases linearly to age 70 years.[79,84] Genital HSV-1 infections have been reported more frequently in the United States and Europe during the last 20 years. Nearly half of all first episodes of genital herpes in Canada and the United Kingdom are HSV-1 infections.[83] Genital herpes infections with HSV-1 are associated with receptive oral sex[85] and are less infectious compared to HSV-2, as recurrences are much less frequent and rates of asymptomatic genital shedding are much lower for both men and women.[83,86]

Examples of nonsexual transmission of HSV-1 include herpes gladiatorum (transmission during sports activities with close skin-to-skin contact like wrestling) and more commonly from patients with herpes labialis to health care personnel, especially dentists.[87,88] The risk of transmission from health care personnel with HSV infection is theoretically possible but highly unlikely,[16,63] with the exception of personnel with herpetic whitlow. There are a very limited number of studies or case reports describing nosocomial (nonsexual) transmission. Most of these papers describe possible but unproven cases involving very few patients. There are no data on whether HSV transmission can occur by an uninfected person via hand contamination with infected secretions. Data are also lacking on nonsexual transmission by persons with genital lesions (eg, while changing diapers). In 1982, Turner et al[89] studied 9 adults with herpes labialis and with viral culture found that 7 (78%) demonstrated HSV-1 viral shedding from the mouth, and 6 (67%) had HSV-1 virus isolated from their hands. The study also demonstrated that HSV-1 survives poorly outside of the body (2 to 4 hours on skin, cloth, or plastic).

Autoinoculation is defined as self-infection of another body site and thus another dorsal root ganglion. Transmission by autoinoculation of HSV-1 is known to occur, as exemplified by cases of herpetic whitlow (ie, HSV-1 infection of the hand and one or more fingers) transmitted by patients with herpes labialis to themselves.[90,91] Most people with ocular HSV have herpes labialis. Although ocular infection may occur by direct infection of the conjunctivae with infected saliva (via autoinoculation or from someone else), mouse studies have shown that the virus can spread through the nervous system (among branches of the trigeminal ganglion).[83,86] Cases are rarely reported however. A few cases of HSV-2 autoinoculation have been reported. Gill et al[92] describe 79 patients with HSV hand infections, including HSV-2. All the included children younger than age 10 years had HSV-1 lesions associated with gingivostomatitis. Of the adult cases, 7 of 49 occurred in health professionals (15%). All of the 20 hand infections with HSV-2 occurred in adults over age 20 years with genital herpes.

Herpes infections may present clinically in children in several ways. Most primary infections are asymptomatic, except in neonates where asymptomatic infection is not known to occur.[16,63] In most symptomatic cases, the virus produces a painful vesiculopustular lesion; however, HSV may also cause subtle and even painless ulcers.[93] Lesions may occur on the face and orolabially. Genital herpes infection in children may present with dramatic dysuria and urinary retention, genital discharge (urethral, vaginal), or skin inflammation and irritation (vulvar irritation, perianal, scrotal, or vulvar fissures). Adenopathy is commonly associated. Systemic symptoms are more common with primary infections and include fever, headache, nausea, vomiting, and myalgia. After primary infection, HSV becomes latent, persisting most frequently in the trigeminal (herpes labialis) or sacral ganglia (genital herpes). Reactivation is most often asymptomatic. Symptomatic herpes labialis usually recurs on the vermillion border of the lips but may also recur on the face, nares, or conjunctiva. Genital herpes vesicular lesions recur on the penis, scrotum, vulva, cervix, thighs, buttocks, perianal regions, or lower back.[16,63] HSV infections may be complicated by meningitis, encephalitis, ascending myelitis, Bell's palsy, neuralgias, and post infectious encephalomyelitis. The incubation period for newborn disease is usually up to 4 weeks. Beyond the neonatal period, incubation is 2 to 14 days. (See **Figures 10-15** through **10-20** for examples of HSV-1 and HSV-2.)

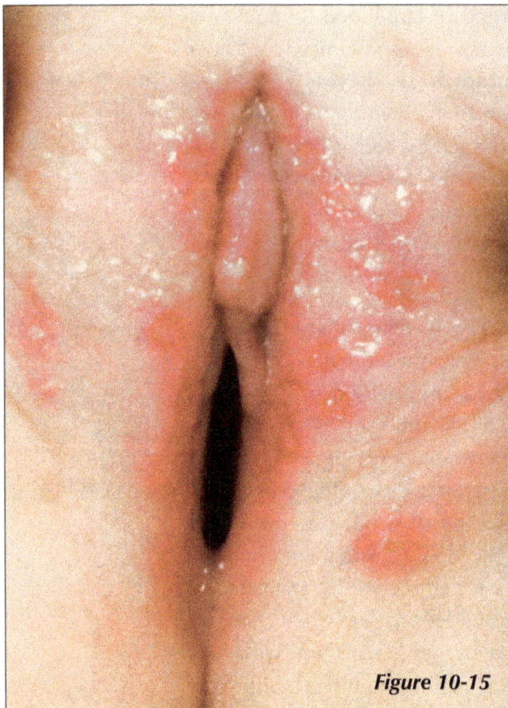

Figure 10-15

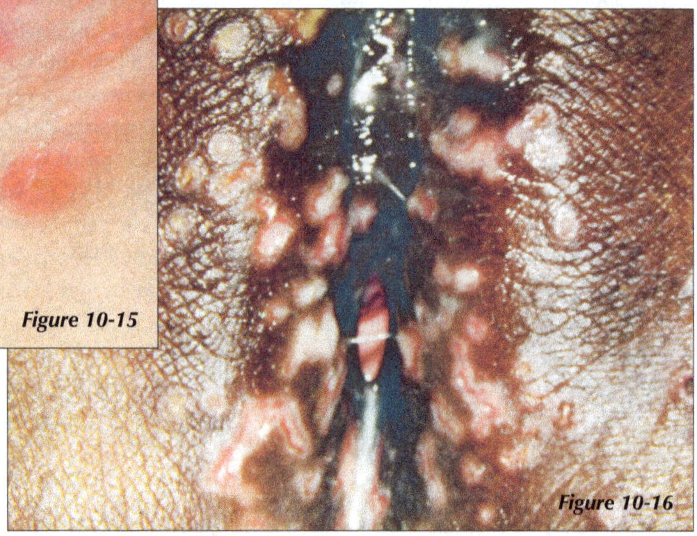

Figure 10-16

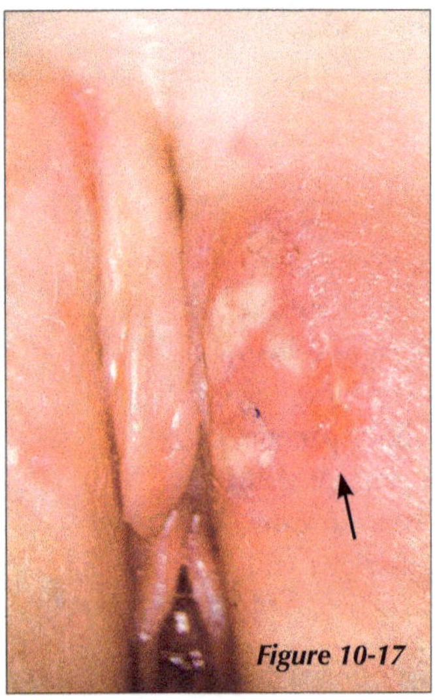

Figure 10-17

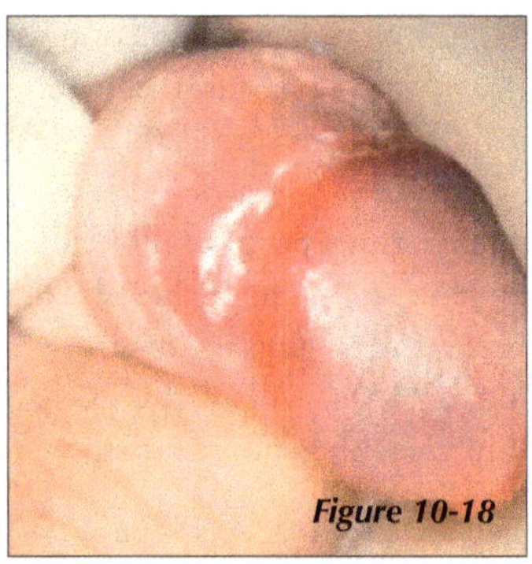

Figure 10-18

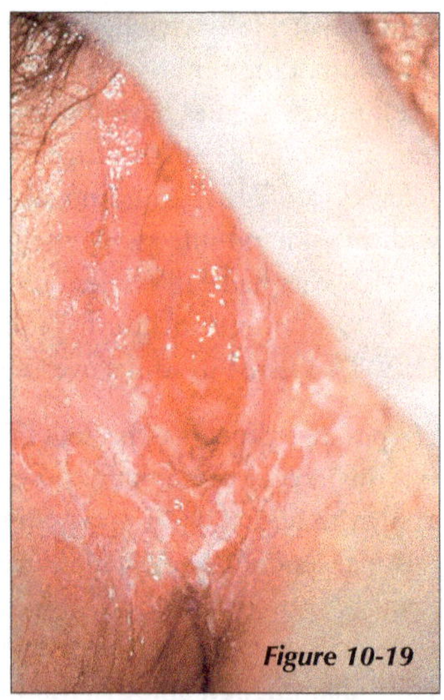

Figure 10-19

Figure 10-15. *This photo shows vesicles on the medial aspect of the labia majora and around the introitus (35mm) of a 6-year-old female.*

Figure 10-16. *Painful sores in genital area in a 4-year-old girl with severe eczema. The child denied sexual contact. Lesions were positive for herpes simplex type 1 (HSV-1). Antibodies were negative for HSV-2 but positive for HSV-1. No one in the family had a history of "cold sores." Mode of transmission was indeterminate.*

Figure 10-17. *A 6-year-old girl with sores on labia. She gave a history of oral-genital contact by her mother's boyfriend, who did have a history of cold sores. These lesions cultured positive for HSV-1.*

Figure 10-18. *This 3-year-old boy complained of pain in his genital area. He gave no disclosure of abuse. The culture of the penile lesion was positive for HSV-1. The mode of transmission was indeterminate.*

Figure 10-19. *In this 14-year-old patient, the sores appeared 1 week after being sexually assaulted by a stranger. The lesions were positive for HSV-2.*

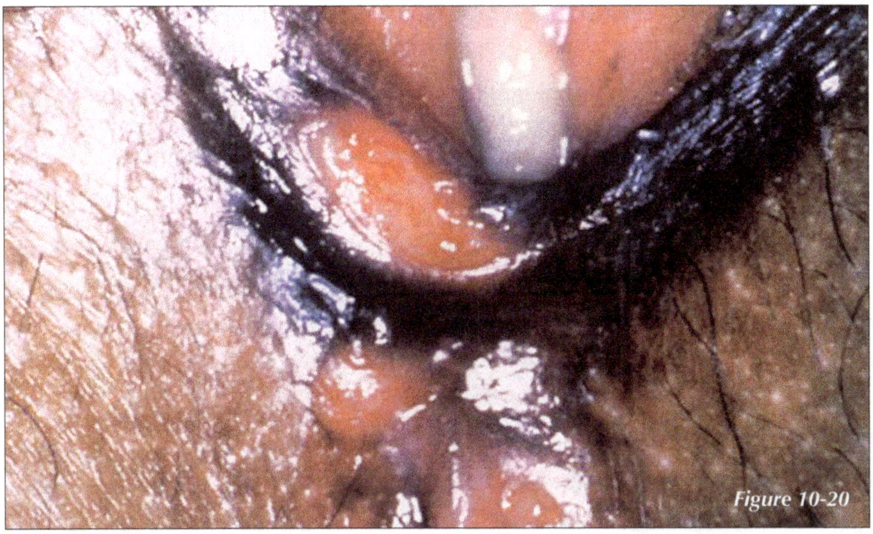

Figure 10-20. *This 16-year-old adolescent girl had a history of genital herpes, first appearing following consensual sexual activity at age 15 years. She was seen for possible sexual abuse due to the presence of these lesions, which were positive for HSV-2. This likely represents a recurrence of her original infection.*

Differential diagnoses of herpes ulcers in children depend somewhat on oral versus genital location. They include (1) infectious causes [eg, coxsackievirus, Epstein-Barr virus, cytomegaloviruses, varicella, syphilis (though ulcers are typically non-painful), tuberculosis ulcers (especially oral), beta-hemolytic streptococcus, chancroid (*Haemophilus ducreyi*), fungal (ie, mucormycosis), and granuloma inguinale (outside the United States)]; (2) malignancy; (3) trauma; or (4) autoimmune or other (eg, Behçet's disease, aphthous stomatitis, drug-related eruption, and Jacquet's diaper dermatitis). Chancroid is an uncommon infection that is only known to be transmitted sexually. Its incubation period typically spans 3 to 10 days, which presents with painful genital ulcer(s) and tender suppurative inguinal adenopathy. Culture (about 80% sensitive) requires special media, which is not widely available, and PCR, which is available in some clinical laboratories. As of yet, there is no FDA-approved test available in the United States.[2] Chancroid is treated with azithromycin or ceftriaxone.

Any vesicular, excoriated, or ulcerative lesions should be cultured for HSV, and a bacterial culture should also be submitted. HSV PCR may be performed from the same swab specimen placed in appropriate liquid viral media. The HSV cell culture becomes less sensitive as viral shedding decreases, typically when lesions are no longer vesicular. Because PCR is highly sensitive and specific, it may be used when suspicious lesions are ulcerative or excoriated. Rapid diagnostic tests such as direct fluorescent antibody staining or enzyme immunoassay detection techniques and histologic identification of multinucleated giant cells and eosinophilic intranuclear inclusions are less sensitive and not recommended.[16]

Obtaining serologic HSV titers for diagnosis of acute disease or for subtyping of HSV-1 and HSV-2 is problematic and not recommended by the CDC.[2] Because many victims of sexual abuse or assault do not present clinically during the acute phase of the disease, an acute elevation in titers may be missed. If titers are elevated, and clinical presentation is delayed, acute primary disease or recurrent disease are both possible explanations.[16,63] Type-specific assays for HSV-1 and HSV-2 that are not based on detection of glycoprotein G2 (diagnostic for HSV-2) and glycoprotein G1 (diagnostic for HSV-1) do not accurately distinguish HSV-1 from HSV-2, despite the claims of manufacturers and laboratories.[2] FDA-approved, gG-based type-specific assays include the following: POCkit™HSV-2 (Diagnology), HerpeSelect™-1 ELISA IgG or HerpeSelect™-2 ELISA IgG (Focus Technology, Inc.), and HerpeSelect™ 1 and 2 Immunoblot IgG (Focus Technology). One study of 61 patients 1 to 14 years of age reports specificity rates of 97% for HSV-1 and 100% for HSV-2 with the HerpeSelect ELISA (Focus Technologies).[94] The study by

Ramos et al[95] of 150 children shows better specificity (less false positives) of the Biokit HSV-2 Rapid Test compared to the HerpeSelect ELISA (Focus Technologies).

As with any antibody test, the statistical odds of a false positive are higher in low prevalence populations, such as sexually abused children. Although data regarding the use of anti-HSV gG testing in children is limited (but promising), certain laboratory measures may reduce the likelihood of false positive results. Laboratories should be able to reproduce a positive result in at least 2 separate runs, determine that the absorbance reading was at least 3 times higher than the positive cutoff value, and conduct confirmatory testing with enzyme-linked immunosorbent assay (ELISA) or immunoblot (Western blot) for samples detecting the presence of anti-HSV gG.

The distinction between HSV-1 and HSV-2 in children and adolescents evaluated for sexual abuse is important for diagnosis and management. HSV-2 is predominantly a sexually transmitted disease, while HSV-1 may be sexually transmitted or non-sexually transmitted. HSV-2 is more likely to recur in genital regions than HSV-1. It is common for children and adults, especially from lower socioeconomic groups, to have HSV-1 antibodies and no history of clinical disease.[2,16] Fomite transmission has not been documented. Data are lacking regarding sexual transmission of herpes in children[96]; however, sexual abuse includes oral, genital, and digital touching, which are all mechanisms of transmitting herpes viruses. Diagnosis of genital herpes infection in children should be investigated for possible sexual abuse and children with genital herpes should be tested for other STIs including syphilis and HIV. History of neonatal herpes infection should be obtained and is unlikely to be missed, because asymptomatic cases are not reported.

Treatment of primary or first clinical episodes of herpes is most effective when initiated within 3 to 6 days of the onset of lesions. Treatment of recurrent disease is effective if initiated within 24 hours of the appearance of lesions. Valacyclovir and famciclovir have not been FDA approved for children younger than 12 years of age (see **Table 10-5** for dosing recommendations).[2,16]

Table 10-5. Treatment Regimens for Primary and Recurrent Herpes Simplex Outbreaks

Oral Dosing	Adolescent	Child < 45 kg (Not Neonate)
FIRST CLINICAL EPISODE		
Acyclovir	400 mg 3 times daily for 7 to 10 days	80 mg/kg daily in 3 to 4 divided doses for 10 days
Valacyclovir	1 gm twice daily for 10 days	
Famciclovir	250 mg 3 times daily for 7 to 10 days	
RECURRENT EPISODE		
Acyclovir	400 mg 3 times daily for 5 days; OR 800 mg twice daily for 5 days; OR 800 mg 3 times daily for 2 days	40 to 80 mg/kg daily in 3 divided doses for 5 days
Valacyclovir	500 mg twice daily for 3 days; OR 1 g daily for 5 days	
Famciclovir	125 mg twice daily for 5 days; OR 1 g twice daily for 1 day	

Syphilis (*Treponema pallidum*)

Syphilis has been described in infants since 1497. Its causative organism, *Treponema pallidum*, was discovered in 1905. Humans are the only natural host of this thin, mobile spirochete, which has very limited survival outside an infected host.[97] In 2000, rates of primary, secondary, and congenital syphilis were the lowest they have ever been since onset of surveillance in 1941 (approximately 2 per 100 000). Since 2000, rates of congenital syphilis have remained fairly low (8 cases per 100 000 live births in 2005). Lack of prenatal care is the most important contributor to increased rates of vertical transmission. Vertical transmission rates remain very high for 4 years after maternal infection (70% to 100%).[98] Due to a lack of available prenatal health services, rates of congenital syphilis in Russia increased 26 fold between 1991 and 1999.[97]

Rates of primary and secondary syphilis have been gradually increasing since 2000, with rates highest among African American men (15.7 cases/100 000 population) and Hispanic men (5.5/100 000), as compared to the rate in women (0.8/100 000 population).[99] Disease is more commonly found in sub-Saharan Africa, South and Southeast Asia, and South America. In the United States, syphilis remains an uncommon complication of child sexual abuse, found in fewer than 1% of children screened.[98,100-102] There is some thought that this may be due to limited testing, limited recognition of physical manifestations of classic disease in children, and the availability of antibiotics for routine childhood illnesses that may partially treat congenital syphilis and alter appearance of late clinical manifestations.[98]

Congenital syphilis may present early (first 2 years of life) or late. Congenital syphilis results from transplacental infection of the developing fetus. Perinatal transmission through infant contact with maternal primary or secondary genital lesions during delivery is possible, but is reported to be extremely uncommon.[101] Symptoms most commonly include mucocutaneous symptoms within the first month of life (as many as 70%), hepatomegaly with or without splenomegaly (70%), leukocytosis, and most importantly, bone involvement seen on radiographs (60% to 80%). Bony findings appear early, typically with multiple symmetric lesions (especially of the femur and humerus). They are often painful and consist of periostitis, cortical demineralization, and osteochondritis. Other presenting symptoms include intrauterine growth retardation and failure to thrive, generalized lymphadenopathy, syphilitic profuse and sometimes bloody rhinitis ("snuffles") which may occur as late as age 3 months, anemia and thrombocytopenia, pneumonia alba (ie, fibrosing pneumonitis), nephrotic syndrome, neurosyphilis, and ocular involvement (eg, chorioretinitis, glaucoma, uveitis).[97,102] Late findings of congenital syphilis occur in approximately 40% of untreated survivors and include perforation of the hard palate, Hutchinson teeth (ie, peg-shaped, notched central incisors), sensorineural hearing loss, blindness (eg, interstitial keratitis, secondary glaucoma, corneal scarring), and bony deformities [eg, saddle nose deformity, frontal bossing, anterior "saber" bowing of shins, thickening of the clavicle, Clutton joints (symmetric, painless sterile joint effusions, usually of the knees)].[94,102] Description of clinical presentation is provided here to assist in differentiation from acquired syphilis, as acquired syphilis in children is considered to be sexually transmitted except in rare circumstances. Even though the rash of secondary syphilis has been shown to contain viable treponemes, close physical contact with mucosal surfaces is necessary for transmission and transmission from secondary syphilis is rarely described.[78,97,101,103] Children presenting with symptoms of primary syphilis after age 6 months or secondary syphilis after age 15 months should be presumed to be victims of sexual abuse (even if there is no disclosure) and should be evaluated comprehensively for other STIs and abnormal physical findings, be reported to protective services, and undergo forensic interviewing. All infants and children diagnosed with syphilis should be tested for HIV.[2] Medical providers evaluating children older than 1 month should conduct a cerebrospinal fluid (CSF) examination for neurosyphilis, obtain long bone films, and review infant birth and maternal prenatal and delivery medical records to assess for evidence of congenital syphilis.[2]

Acquired syphilis in children may be detected when asymptomatic children (latent phase) undergo serologic screening. Primary syphilis may present as marked nontender adenopathy (especially inguinal). A chancre (not always seen by the patient or on examination) appears at the primary inoculation site 10 to 90 days (average 21 days) after contact and may be vaginal, labial, cervical, penile, scrotal, anal, rectal, oral, or occur on any extragenital site where there has been a break in the epidermal barrier. The chancre is typically a solitary, erythematous papule that rapidly erodes, leaving a painless, smooth, yellow-red ulcer with regular margins (**Figures 10-21** and **10-22**). It contains viable treponemes and may be crusted or there may be a serous and highly infectious discharge, but purulent discharge is uncommon.[103] Lesions heal in 3 to 12 weeks when untreated. Secondary syphilis presents with generalized involvement of skin and mucous membranes and constitutional symptoms. Constitutional symptoms are variable and sometimes vague. They most commonly include malaise, anorexia, headache, and a low-grade fever with generalized lymphadenopathy. The rash (or secondary eruption) usually appears 6 to 8 weeks after the chancre, and in most cases the chancre has resolved. The rash is a polymorphous maculopapular rash typically extending to the palms and soles. Scaling may be prominent, especially on hands and feet. Moist areas may develop coalescing small fleshy plaques (ie, condyloma lata) that can be confused with condyloma acuminata (ie, HPV). Mucous patches may occur on any mucous membrane, most often oropharynx and rectum, and appear as painless, gray-white erosions.[16,103] Neurosyphilis is present in approximately 30% of patients with secondary syphilis. Skin and mucous membrane lesions contain treponemes and are contagious with significant direct contact. Iritis, uveitis, arthritis, and nephrotic syndrome may all occur as part of secondary syphilis, likely secondary to immune complex formation.[97] Primary and secondary syphilis lesions will resolve without treatment, though the infection persists in a latent form. Secondary syphilis signs can recur during the first year after infection (ie, early latency) but not later.[97]

Figure 10-21. *This 12-year-old male has a syphilitic chancre visible on the upper lip (35mm).*

Figure 10-22. *A syphilis primary chancre on the penis of a 14-year-old male.*

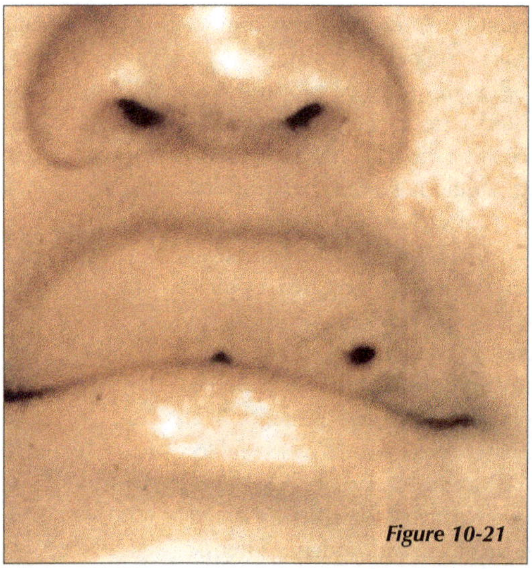
Figure 10-21

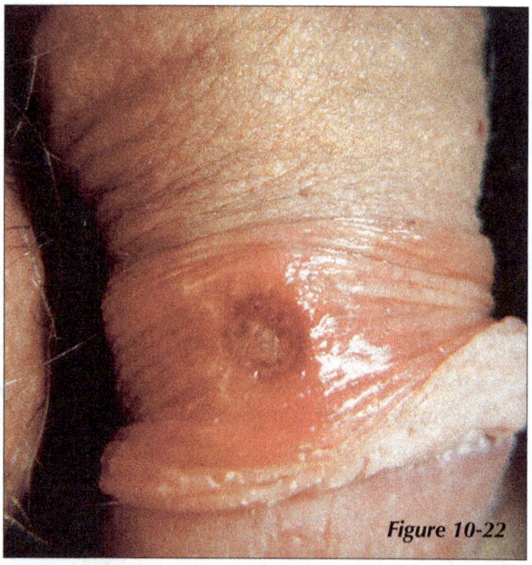
Figure 10-22

Differential diagnosis of primary syphilis includes herpes simplex, trauma, Behçet's disease, Jacquet's diaper dermatitis, furuncle or impetigo, and other ulcerative lesions (**Figure 10-23**). Syphilitic chancres are usually painless. Differential diagnosis of secondary syphilis includes pitiriasis rosea, psoriasis, tinea versicolor, drug reactions, nummular eczema, and nonspecific viral exanthems.[97,103]

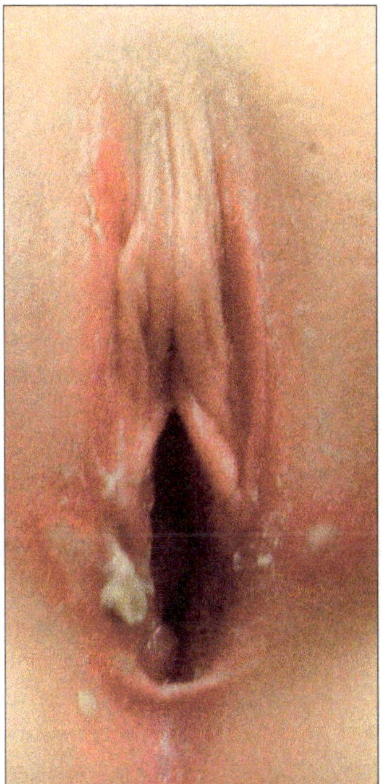
Figure 10-23

Figure 10-23. *Painful vulvar ulcers on a 10-year-old girl, with no disclosure of abuse. The child and other family members were recently diagnosed with influenza A infection. Cultures for herpes were negative and blood test for syphilis was negative.*

Definitive diagnosis of acute syphilis infection is made with darkfield microscopy or direct fluorescent antibody (DFA) testing exudate or tissue obtained from a primary or secondary mucocutaneous lesion.[2] This is especially important when skin lesions are present, as serologic tests are usually negative during the first 7 to 10 days of infection.[103] In the absence of a lesion, serologic testing is recommended. Like HIV screening, syphilis screening is a two-step protocol consisting of a highly sensitive but less specific test, then confirmed with a highly specific test. Nontreponemal tests, such as rapid plasma reagin (ie, RPR, the more sensitive of nontreponemal tests)[97] or Venereal Disease Research Laboratory (VDRL) detects nonspecific anticardiolipin antibodies and must be confirmed with a test that detects specific antitreponemal antibodies. Specific treponemal tests include *Treponema pallidum* particle agglutination (TP-PA), fluorescent treponemal antibody absorbed (FTA-ABS), *Treponema pallidum* hemagglutination test (MHA-TP), which has been replaced by the TP-PA test, and ELISA. The FTA-ABS is the most sensitive of these tests (detecting 85% of patients with primary syphilis and 100% of patients with secondary syphilis) but is more difficult to perform.[97] Nontreponemal tests, such as RPR and VDRL, usually become negative (months to years) after successful treatment but may remain positive for life at a persistently low titer, a condition termed serofast. Nontreponemal tests should be reported quantitatively (as a titer). Serial testing using the same test type can give information about disease activity, but importantly, RPR and VDRL titers are not comparable. In contrast, the specific treponemal tests (ie, TP-PA, FTA-ABS) do not give an index of disease activity. Most patients who have a reactive treponemal test will have reactive tests throughout their lives, regardless of disease activity[2]; therefore, a reactive test indicates the patient has had syphilis sometime in life but is not helpful in determining the time during which infectious contact occurred.

Newer approaches to screening and diagnosing syphilis involve an initial screen with a treponemal-specific test such as an enzyme immunoassay (EIA), which is more specific and as sensitive as an RPR test.[2,104] Rapid tests on finger-stick specimens (Abbott Determine TP) are available and have shown sensitivity of 88%, and specificity comparable to TP-PA.[105] Other significant advantages relate to laboratory processing. For example, ELISAs are less labor intensive and less dependent on technician interpretation. If an initial screen for antitreponemal antibodies is positive, an RPR is done to differentiate active from previously treated disease.

Syphilis treatment recommendations are based on the child's stage of syphilis infection. Congenital syphilis and neurosyphilis require the most aggressive and prolonged treatment; therefore, the workup of any child with suspected syphilis or positive serologies must exclude congenital or central nervous systems (CNS) involvement. Neurosyphilis in children should be treated with aqueous crystalline penicillin G (200 000 to 300 000 U/kg per day, given every 4 to 6 hours intravenously for 10 to 14 days) not to exceed the adolescent and adult dose of 18 to 24 million U per day, administered as 3 to 4 million U IV every 4 hours for 10 to 14 days. Some infectious disease experts recommend

3 additional weekly intramuscular injections of benzathine penicillin G (children 50 000 U/kg per dose; adolescents or adults 2.4 million U per dose). Early congenital syphilis is treated with aqueous penicillin G 100 000 to 15 000 U/kg per day given as 50 000 U/kg per dose IV every 12 hours during the first 7 days of life and then every 8 hours to complete a total of 10 days of treatment. Daily IM procaine penicillin G (50 000 U/kg/dose) may be given as an alternate treatment for 10 days. Late congenital syphilis treatment is aqueous penicillin G 200 000 to 300 000 U/kg per day IV for 10 days.[2]

Human Immunodeficiency Virus

Although the majority of children infected with human immunodeficiency virus (HIV) (>90%) acquired infection from their mothers in the perinatal period, transmission to children also occurs sexually.[106] In 1998, Lindegren et al[106] analyzed national HIV/AIDS surveillance data retrospectively and found 26 of 9136 children with HIV/AIDS had acquired HIV through sexual abuse. Of these sexually abused children, 18 (69%) were reported in the 3-year period 1993-1996 after the CDC revised the pediatric HIV/AIDS case report form to collect standardized information about sexual contact with a male or female. The authors concluded that these cases were likely underestimated because sexual abuse was and remains underrecognized and underreported to child protection services as well as HIV/AIDS surveillance systems. There are few other studies of HIV incidence in sexually abused children. Diagnosis of sexually transmitted HIV in young children requires exclusion of perinatal transmission through review of maternal records of HIV testing and infant birth records.

HIV is transmitted through body secretions and unfixed tissues, especially blood and secretions containing blood. Saliva, urine, feces and diarrhea, and vomit are highly unlikely to transmit HIV unless mixed with blood. Receptive anal intercourse is the most likely route of sexual transmission, with a risk of 0.5% to 3% per episode. Receptive vaginal intercourse carries a risk of 0.1% to 0.2% per episode. Insertive vaginal intercourse with an infected recipient carries the lowest known sexual transmission risk of 0.03% to 0.09% per episode.[107] Oral sex is estimated to convey a lower risk per episode (though increasingly recognized as the sole reported risk factor in a subset of cases).[2] Sexual intercourse combined with trauma, and therefore, contact with bloody secretions, increases transmissibility; thus, forced insertive anal or vaginal intercourse carries a higher risk than consensual or oral contact. Risk is also related to the stage of the infected person. Periods of highest level viremia are at the two extremes of disease: during the weeks following acute infection (when risk may be 1000 times higher) and at the end-stages of untreated AIDS.[108,109] Efficacy of transmission is increased with concurrent genital infections (especially ulcerative STDs), syphilis, and BV. The local prevalence of HIV is important in estimating the risk of transmitting HIV to a sexually abused child or adolescent. Risk is highest for perpetrators with known HIV infection. For those with unknown HIV status, risk is higher when the alleged perpetrator has a history of intravenous (IV) drug use, crack cocaine drug use, promiscuity, incarceration, infection with other STIs, or is a man who has sex with other men.[2]

Testing for HIV should be voluntary and conducted with the patient's knowledge (or assent from his or her legally authorized representative). Testing should be offered as part of routine care for patients aged 13 to 64 years[110] and as part of the initial evaluation of sexually assaulted adolescents.[4] In most states, public health statutes allow for evaluation and treatment of minors for STIs without parental knowledge, allowing adolescents aged 13 and older to give consent for STI testing, including for HIV; however, not every state has explicitly included HIV testing as not requiring parental consent.[110] In 2014, the CDC recommended another testing algorithm for HIV.[111] The initial screening test is a fourth generation HIV-1/2 antigen/antibody combination immunoassay followed by an HIV-1/HIV-2 antibody differentiation immunoassay for positive initial screens. If the result of the HIV-1/HIV-2 antibody differentiation test is nonreactive or indeterminate, testing of the specimen is reflexed to an HIV-1 nucleic acid test. This new testing algorithm allows for earlier detection of HIV infections and the ability to accurately classify HIV-1 and HIV-2 infections. In situations where exposure is within hours or results are indeterminate, repeat testing can be done in 2 to 4 weeks.

The former ELISA test for HIV antibodies confirmed with a Western blot assay or an immunofluorescence assay (IFA) is no longer recommended. Rapid test results are available as soon as 20 minutes (eg, Oraquick) or within 1 hour.[112] Negative antibody tests cannot exclude recent infection and should be repeated in 3 months if clinical suspicion warrants further testing.

Sexual abuse victims may present with a history of symptoms that may suggest acute retroviral syndrome. These influenza-like symptoms (eg, fever, malaise, lymphadenopathy, rash) frequently occur in the first 4 to 6 weeks following HIV infection, before the ELISA antibody test becomes positive.[113] Therefore, standard serologic testing will fail to detect these very early cases and direct testing for virus, rather than antibody, is required, typically using PCR-based testing for HIV RNA (ie, "viral load") or testing for the HIV marker, p24 antigen. Infants with perinatal exposure to HIV may have positive ELISA testing in the absence of HIV infection due to presence of maternal antibodies in the infant for up to 18 months. Infant infection may be determined using HIV DNA PCR serial testing consisting of 3 total determinations: once after age 1 month and one other testing between ages 2 and 4 months in conjunction with evaluation by a pediatric HIV expert. PCR testing is most accurate with HIV DNA PCR assays (a negative RNA PCR may occur in HIV-infected patients), especially in children younger than age 18 months.[2] Testing of the alleged perpetrator is recommended when obtainable (voluntary or by court order).

Questions are frequently raised about the HIV exposure risk following child sexual abuse and sexual assault, and the utility of HIV postexposure prophylaxis (PEP). Medical providers may seek to offer treatment with any hope of benefit to sexually traumatized children, particularly for this eventually fatal disease. Current recommendations for HIV prophylaxis are based on very limited data. To date, there are no randomized controlled trials of PEP for nonoccupational exposure (sexual) or occupational exposure. The 1997 case-control study published in the *New England Journal of Medicine* assessing outcomes of occupational exposure in health care settings after percutaneous needle stick with HIV-infected blood is the most compelling existing report of PEP effectiveness.[108,114] In this retrospective analysis, zidovudine alone appeared to reduce the risk of transmission by greater than 60%. Despite study limitations, these results are believable because risk reduction is in the same range as perinatal transmission prevention with zidovudine alone. Although uncontrolled and far from definitive, there is also a growing experience with offering PEP following nonoccupational sexual exposures in adults.[115] Based on these studies; animal models; the demonstrated effectiveness of perinatal prophylaxis; and the great strides in making antiretroviral regimens more potent, tolerable, and convenient, PEP in acute child and adolescent sexual abuse cases might be effective in preventing HIV transmission.[2,116] Medical providers making the decision to recommend PEP must, therefore, take into consideration risk of infection, likelihood of efficacy of prophylaxis, medication side effects, and likelihood of adherence to medications and medical follow-up.

The most recent guidelines from the CDC recommend a 28-day course of PEP using a 3-drug regimen (tenofovir-emtricitabine and raltegravir) only for those persons seeking care within 72 hours of a substantial exposure to blood, genital secretions, or other potentially infectious body secretions of a known HIV-infected person.[2,108,116] Patients initiating PEP should have baseline HIV and lab testing (ie, CBC, serum chemistry), be able to receive the first dose of PEP as soon as possible after the decision is made to treat, and agree to close medical follow-up in 3 to 5 days. Baseline HIV and lab testing assesses for HIV infection prior to the current exposure and gives a baseline for monitoring antiretroviral toxicities. The sooner PEP is administered after HIV exposure, the more likely it is to interrupt transmission. Use of an FDA-approved rapid HIV test is preferred if available (results within an hour), as patients who test HIV-positive should be excluded from PEP. It is generally not recommended to provide HIV PEP in cases when therapy will not be initiated until more than 72 hours after the exposure. In sexual assault cases where the alleged perpetrator has unknown HIV status, the CDC recommends that clinicians evaluate the risks and benefits of PEP and individualize recommendations on a case-by-case basis.[4] In these cases, it is important to gather as much information about the potential HIV risk factors of the alleged perpetrator(s). When the alleged perpetrator is known to be HIV infected, exploring his or her detailed treatment history in collaboration with an experienced HIV clinician is critically important for planning an appropriately individualized PEP regimen based on prior drug exposures and documented antiretroviral resistance.

Prior to initiation of PEP, clinicians should explain to patients that the agents used for PEP have unproven benefit and documented toxicities in these circumstances. Patients should also understand the importance of adherence to recommended dosing in order to receive maximum potential benefit and to reduce the risk of selecting for drug-resistant HIV strains. If PEP is given, clinicians should consult with a specialist in HIV treatment, provide a 3 to 5 day starter pack of the recommended antiretroviral regimen, and have patients return to assess tolerance of medication and to make a better assessment of HIV risk.[2,108] If it is possible to test the alleged perpetrator, PCR testing is preferred because of the possibility the perpetrator has acute infection and had not yet seroconverted. If the perpetrator's HIV PCR test is negative, the patient's antiretroviral treatment should be stopped.

Treatment regimens may consist of 2 or 3 antiretrovirals (2 nucleoside analogue reverse transcriptase inhibitors plus either a protease inhibitor or a non-nucleoside reverse transcriptase inhibitor). Two-drug therapy is used most commonly in developing countries, while 3-drug therapy is used in areas with available HAART treatment and increased risk for primary transmission of a resistant HIV strain.[2,16,116] Commonly used regimens in children and adolescents include tenofovir-emtricitabine and raltegravir.[4,117]

Several studies have demonstrated poor adherence of sexual assault survivors to PEP protocols.[116,118] Olshen et al[119] reported 13 of 110 adolescents who had been sexually assaulted and offered HIV PEP completed their 28-day PEP course (12%). Only 37 of these adolescents returned for a follow-up examination, and half of them (46%) developed an adverse reaction to the PEP medicines. Medication adherence may be improved with fewer doses and fewer pills per dose, counseling about importance of adherence and potential side effects, use of supportive medicines like antiemetics to treat side effects, and access to help and encouragement by phone or office visit.[116]

Hepatitis A, B, and C

Serologic testing in children and adolescents evaluated for sexual abuse or assault may include HIV; RPR; and tests for hepatitis A, B, and C. Although hepatitis A is usually transmitted by fecal-oral contact, it can be transmitted during sexual activity.[2] The diagnosis of acute hepatitis A is based on the presence of serum IgM antibody to hepatitis A virus (HAV). Total anti-HAV does not differentiate individuals with acute disease, past disease, or hepatitis A immunization.

Among adolescents and adults, sexual activity is the most common mode of transmission for hepatitis B infections[2]; other modes of transmission include mucous membrane contact and intravenous contact with infected needles or syringes. The presence of IgM antibody to hepatitis B core antigen confirms the diagnosis of acute infection. The presence of hepatitis B surface antigen can indicate acute or chronic infection. In uninfected, immunized individuals, only the antibody to hepatitis B surface antigen will be positive. Because the duration of vaccine-induced immunity to hepatitis B is unknown and may wane, baseline hepatitis B testing is recommended for adolescents.[4]

Hepatitis C is primarily transmitted by percutaneous exposure to blood products and by sexual activity. Screening victims of sexual abuse or assault should include serum antibody to hepatitis C virus (HCV). Antibody assays include an initial enzyme immunoassay (EIA) and positive results are confirmed by a recombinant immunoblot assay (RIBA).[16,63] An alternative diagnostic test for hepatitis C is serum HCV RNA. Risk factors including multiple sexual partners, other STIs, and intravenous drug use should be considered in deciding whether to screen for hepatitis C.

The clinician may opt to screen for hepatitis A, B, and C whenever risk factors for HIV are detected, or when the assailant is known to have hepatitis or liver disease. Risk factors in the assailant include but are not limited to the following: stranger to victim, multiple sexual partners, drug use, history of incarceration, and other health risk markers, such as membership in a gang. In cases where children or adolescents are victims of acute sexual assault, it is prudent to ascertain whether they have been fully immunized against hepatitis B (3 doses). If the patient is unimmunized, an initial dose of hepatitis B vaccine should be given, preferably within 24 hours of exposure, with the remainder of the vaccine doses given at appropriate intervals. For patients whose hepatitis B status is unknown and cannot be ascertained within 24 hours of the exposure, practitioners may opt to send a blood specimen for hepatitis B immune status and give the first vaccine dose. Additional doses at follow-up visits would be given only if the test showed the patient to be nonimmune. Hepatitis B immune globulin (HBIG) should be given in those cases where the perpetrator is known to be hepatitis B surface antigen positive.[16]

Bacterial Vaginosis

Bacterial vaginosis (BV) is a clinical syndrome characterized by malodorous vaginal discharge caused by replacement of normal *Lactobacillus* species in the vagina with overgrowth of anaerobic bacteria, *Gardnerella vaginalis*, and *Mycoplasma hominis*. It is described as the most prevalent adult and adolescent vaginal infection worldwide,[16,120] but there are limited studies of prevalence in prepubertal children. The incubation period is unknown. The disease state of BV is associated with multiple sexual partners, a new sex partner, lack of vaginal lactobacilli, and douching. Douching itself is also associated with sexual activity.[120] As many as 50% of women with clinical BV are asymptomatic. Diagnosis of BV requires presence of three of the following clinical findings[2,16]:

— Homogeneous thin white discharge that smoothly coats the vaginal walls

— "Clue cells" on microscopic examination (vaginal smear) making up at least 20% of vaginal epithelial cells (clue cells are vaginal epithelial cells covered with bacteria so that they appear granular and ragged) (**Figures 10-24-a** and **b**)

— Vaginal fluid pH > 4.5

— Positive amine test or whiff test (fishy odor of vaginal discharge before or after addition of 10% potassium hydroxide)

Culture is not recommended because it is not specific.

Figure 10-24-a. *Microscopic appearance of "clue cells," vaginal epithelial cells, using saline wet mount preparation. Provided with permission from Seattle STD/HIV Prevention Training Center.*

Figure 10-24-b. *Microscopic appearance of normal vaginal epithelial cells using saline wet mount preparation. Provided with permission from Seattle STD/HIV Prevention Training Center.*

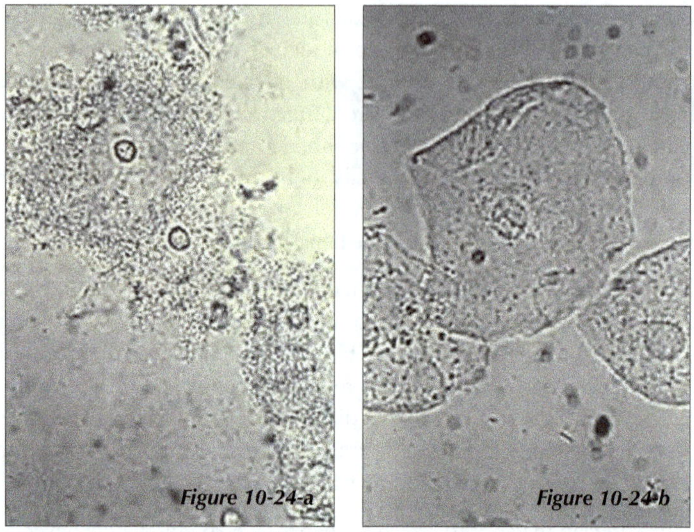

The mechanism of transmission of BV remains unclear. Although women who have never been sexually active are rarely affected, it is still unclear whether BV results from a sexually transmitted pathogen.[2] Part of the confusion stems from the fact that diagnosis of BV cannot be based on isolation of *G. vaginalis*, as this organism is present in as many as 50% of women without BV, and may also be present in asymptomatic females who are sexually inexperienced.[16,121-123] In a 2005 study by Schwebke and Desmond,[120] the authors followed 94 sexually active women without BV aged 18 years or older for development of BV. Their male partners were also studied. Their data support sexual transmission of BV. Multivariate analysis showed that incident BV was most significantly associated with exposure to a new sexual partner. Use of condoms with occasional partners was also found to be protective. The authors reviewed studies citing evidence for and against sexual transmission of BV and concluded that "while the etiology of BV remains unproven, evidence continues to accumulate in favor of sexual transmission." Evidence for sexual transmission was cited from several studies. Gardner and Dukes[124] induced bacterial vaginosis in a woman by introducing vaginal secretions from an infected woman into the subject's vagina. Schwebke and Desmond also cite studies reporting increased rates of BV and trichomonas associated with increased number of sexual partners, not frequency of intercourse[125]; up to 90% of male partners of women with BV having *G. vaginalis* and other BV bacteria[124]; balanoposthitis in sexually active males caused by BV organisms[126,127]; and isolating BV organisms (especially *G. vaginalis*) from semen of asymptomatic males.[128] Evidence cited against sexual transmission includes 2 types of studies. The Bump and Buesching[121] study reports similar rates of *G. vaginalis* and BV in sexually active versus self-reported sexually inexperienced adolescents. The "virginal" group of 14 to 17 year old girls was defined by self-report and included one girl with chlamydial cervicitis. Additionally virginal designation excluded only sexual intercourse, with no mention of excluded external rubbing, oral, rectal, or digital touching. There are also a group of studies of male partners that fail to show reduction in BV recurrence rates among women whose male sexual partners were treated with a single 2-gram dose of metronidazole.[129,130] Schwebke and Desmond point out that those studies are several decades old, do not include a measure of compliance with treatment, and that single-dose therapy has been shown to be marginally effective in infected females and is likely to be poorly effective in infected males. Wahl et al[131] demonstrated *G. vaginalis* could not be found in urethra, glans, or rectal cultures of asymptomatic non-abused prepubertal boys, while reporting a case of a 3-year-old male with symptomatic balanitis with culture positive for *G. vaginalis*. These authors concluded that while significance of *G. vaginalis* as an STI in prepubertal boys is currently unknown, isolation in a symptomatic boy raises questions of sexual abuse, as would isolation in a prepubertal girl with symptoms of BV. Although studies to date do not conclusively support sexual transmission of BV or a diagnosis of sexual abuse in a prepubertal child with bacterial vaginosis, the child with BV should be tested for other sexually transmitted pathogens (*N. gonorrhoeae*, *C. trachomatis*, *T. vaginalis*). Forensic interview and medical examination are recommended.

Treatment for children (< 45 kg) with BV is metronidazole, 15 mg/kg per day orally, in 2 divided doses for 7 days (maximum 1 gram/day). Adolescents may be treated with metronidazole, 2 grams, orally in a single dose. Alternate regimens are metronidazole gel, 0.75% intravaginally daily for 5 days, or clindamycin cream, 2% intravaginally at bedtime for 7 days. The clindamycin cream is oil based and may weaken condoms and diaphragms, and may be less efficacious than metronidazole.[2,16]

Differential diagnosis of bacterial vaginosis includes other causes of vaginal discharge. Other infectious causes include *N. gonorrhoeae*, *C. trachomatis*, *T. vaginalis*, and *Shigella* species (or other enteric bacteria). Candidiasis, pin worms, and group A streptococcus would be less likely causes, as pain or pruritus are much more prevalent with these infections than in BV. Noninfectious causes include foreign body and nonspecific vaginitis (due to constipation, bubble baths, poor hygiene, et cetera).

Testing the Suspect

When an STI is identified in a child or adolescent victim of sexual abuse or assault, investigators frequently ask whether testing the suspect for disease would provide important information for criminal investigation. Most of the time, testing a suspect for STIs is uninformative, confusing, or even damaging to the prosecution of the suspect. In general, most sexual offenders are males, and males are more difficult to test for STIs than females. Many diseases can resolve without treatment, so a negative test does not preclude prior disease. For example, most venereal HPV lesions resolve within 3 to 5 years without treatment.[132] If the suspect is treated for an STI or for another infection that eradicates an existing STI, then the suspect will be disease-free at the time of testing. Serologic tests for syphilis, hepatitis A, hepatitis B, hepatitis C, and gG-based type-specific assays for HSV-1 and HSV-2 can confirm the presence of past disease in the suspect. Treponemal-specific tests should be performed because non-treponemal tests may become non-reactive with treatment. The presence of total anti-HAV titers, in the absence of HAV immunization, confirms past infection with hepatitis A. The presence of antibody to hepatitis B surface antigen indicates resolved infection or immunity following immunization. The presence of hepatitis B surface antigen would confirm active or chronic disease[16] in a suspect. The presence of antibody to hepatitis C virus confirms disease and is positive in 80% of infected patients 15 weeks after exposure. In the acute phase (up to 15 weeks after exposure) anti-HCV is sometimes negative.[16] Screening for HIV should be performed using a fourth generation HIV-1/HIV-2 antibody differentiation immunoassay. With this dilemma, the bottom line for medical providers remains what is best medical care for the patient.

References

1. Adams JA, Kellogg ND, Farst KJ, et al. Updated guidelines for the medical assessment and care of children who may have been sexually abused. *J Pediatr Adolesc Gynecol.* 2016;29(2):81-87.

2. Workowski KA, Bolan GA. Sexually transmitted diseases treatment guidelines, 2015. *MMWR Recomm Rep.* 2015;64(RR-03):1-137.

3. Jenny C, Crawford-Jakubiak JE; Committee on Child Abuse and Neglect, American Academy of Pediatrics. The evaluation of children in the primary care setting when sexual abuse is suspected. *Pediatrics.* 2013;132(2):e558-e567.

4. Seña AC, Hsu KK, Kellogg N, et al. Sexual assault and sexually transmitted infections in adults, adolescents, and children. *Clin Infect Dis.* 2015;61(suppl 8):S856-S864.

5. Black CM, Driebe EM, Howard LA, et al. Multicenter study of nucleic acid amplification tests for detection of *Chlamydia trachomatis* and *Neisseria gonorrhoeae* in children being evaluated for sexual abuse. *Pediatr Infect Dis J.* 2009;28(7):608-613.

6. Papp JR, Schachter J, Gaydos CA, Van Der Pol B. Recommendations for the laboratory-based detection of *Chlamydia trachomatis* and *Neisseria gonorrhoeae*—2014. *MMWR Recomm Rep.* 2014;63(RR-02):1-19.

7. Gallion HR, Dupree LJ, Scott TA, Arnold DH. Diagnosis of *Trichomonas vaginalis* in female children and adolescents evaluated for possible sexual abuse: a comparison of the InPouch TV culture method and wet mount microscopy. *J Pediatr Adolesc Gynecol.* 2009;22(5):300-305.

8. Girardet RG, Lahoti S, Howard LA, et al. Epidemiology of sexually transmitted infections in suspected child victims of sexual assault. *Pediatrics.* 2009;124(1):79-86.

9. Falk L, Coble BI, Mjörnberg PA, Fredlund H. Sampling for *Chlamydia trachomatis* infection: a comparison of vaginal, first-catch urine, combined vaginal and first-catch urine and endocervical sampling. *Int J STD AIDS.* 2010;21(4):283-287.

10. Williams HN, Letson MM, Tscholl JJ. Sexually transmitted infections in child abuse. *Clin Pediatr Emerg Med.* 2016;17(4):264-273.

11. Jo S, Shin J, Song KJ, Kim JJ, Hwang KR, Bhally H. Prevalence and correlated factors of sexually transmitted diseases—*Chlamydia, Neisseria, cytomegalovirus*—in female rape victims. *J Sex Med.* 2011;8(8):2317-2326.

12. Ingram DL. *Neisseria gonorrhoeae* in children. *Pediatr Ann.* 1994;23(7):341-345.

13. Siegel RM, Schubert CJ, Myers PA, Shapiro RA. The prevalence of sexually transmitted diseases in children and adolescents evaluated for sexual abuse in Cincinnati: rationale for limited STD testing in prepubertal girls. *Pediatrics.* 1995;96(6):1090-1094.

14. American Academy of Pediatrics, Committee on Child Abuse and Neglect. Gonorrhea in prepubertal children. *Pediatrics.* 1998;101(1 pt 1):134-135.

15. Fuster CD, Neinstein LS. Vaginal *Chlamydia trachomatis* prevalence in sexually abused prepurbertal girls. *Pediatrics.* 1987;79(2):235-238.

16. Kimberlin DW, Brady MT, Jackson MA, Long SS. *Red Book 2015: 2015 Report of the Committee on Infectious Diseases.* 30th ed. Elk Grove Village, IL: American Academy of Pediatrics; 2015.

17. Bell TA, Stamm WE, Wang SP, Kuo CC, Holmes KK, Grayston JT. Chronic *Chlamydia trachomatis* infections in infants. *JAMA.* 1992;267(3):400-402.

18. Kellogg ND, Melville JD, Lukefahr JL, Nienow SM, Russell EL. Genital and extragenital gonorrhea and *Chlamydia* in children and adolescents evaluated for sexual abuse. 2018;34(11):761-766.

19. Buimer M, van Doornum GJ, Ching S, et al. Detection of *Chlamydia trachomatis* and *Neisseria gonorrhoeae* by ligase chain reaction-based assays with clinical specimens from various sites: implications for diagnostic testing and screening. *J Clin Microbiol.* 1996;34(10):2395-2400.

20. Carroll KC, Aldeen WE, Morrison M, Anderson R, Lee D, Mottice S. Evaluation of the Abbott LCx ligase chain reaction assay for detection of *Chlamydia trachomatis* and *Neisseria gonorrhoeae* in urine and genital swab specimens from a sexually transmitted disease clinic population. *J Clin Microbiol.* 1998;36(6):1630-1633.

21. Van Dyck E, Ieven M, Pattyn S, Van Damme L, Laga M. Detection of *Chlamydia trachomatis* and *Neisseria gonorrhoeae* by enzyme immunoassay, culture, and three nucleic acid amplification tests. *J Clin Microbiol.* 2001;39(5):1751-1756.

22. Hammerschlag MR. Use of nucleic acid amplification tests in investigating child sexual abuse. *Sex Transm Infect.* 2001;77(3):153-154.

23. *Chlamydia trachomatis* assay: Abbott LCx Probe System [package insert]. Abbott Park, IL: Abbott Laboratories; 1996.

24. Hook EW 3rd, Smith K, Mullen C, et al. Diagnosis of genitourinary *Chlamydia trachomatis* infections by using the ligase chain reaction on patient-obtained vaginal swabs. *J Clin Microbiol.* 1997;35(8):2133-2135.

25. Black CM. Current methods of laboratory diagnosis of *Chlamydia trachomatis* infections. *Clin Microbiol Rev.* 1997;10(1):160-184.

26. Johnson RE, Newhall WJ, Papp JR, et al. Screening tests to detect *Chlamydia trachomatis* and *Neisseria gonorrhoeae* infections—2002. *MMWR Recomm Rep.* 2002;51(RR-15):1-38; quiz CE1-CE4.

27. *Physicians' Desk Reference.* 60th ed. Montvale, NJ: Medical Economics Company, Inc; 2006.

28. Centers for Disease Control and Prevention. Update to CDC's sexually transmitted diseases treatment guidelines, 2006: fluoroquinolones no longer recommended for treatment of gonococcal infections. *MMWR Morb Mortal Wkly Rep.* 2007;56(14):332-336.

29. Ota KV, Fisman DN, Tamari IE, et al. Incidence and treatment outcomes of pharyngeal *Neisseria gonorrhoeae* and *Chlamydia trachomatis* infections in men who have sex with men: a 13-year retrospective cohort study. *Clin Infect Dis.* 2009;48(9):1237-1243.

30. Whittington WL, Rice RJ, Biddle JW, Knapp JS. Incorrect identification of *Neisseria gonorrhoeae* from infants and children. *Pediatr Infect Dis J.* 1988;7(1):3-10.

31. McQuillan G, Kruszon-Moran D, Markowitz LE, Unger ER, Paulose-Ram R. Prevalence of HPV in adults aged 18-69: United States, 2011-2014. *NCHS Data Brief.* 2017(280):1-8.

32. Hammerschlag MR, Guillén CD. Medical and legal implications of testing for sexually transmitted infections in children. *Clin Microbiol Rev.* 2010;23(3):493-506.

33. Dunne EF, Unger ER, Sternberg M, et al. Prevalence of HPV infection among females in the United States. *JAMA.* 2007;297(8):813-819.

34. Franco EL, Villa LL, Sobrinho JP, et al. Epidemiology of acquisition and clearance of cervical human papillomavirus infection in women from a high-risk area for cervical cancer. *J Infect Dis.* 1999;180(5):1415-1423.

35. Moscicki AB, Shiboski S, Broering J, et al. The natural history of human papillomavirus infection as measured by repeated DNA testing in adolescent and young women. *J Pediatr*. 1998;132(2):277-284.

36. Cohen J. Public health: high hopes and dilemmas for a cervical cancer vaccine. *Science*. 2005;308(5722):618-621.

37. Centers for Disease Control and Prevention. *Human Papillomavirus: HPV Information for Clinicians*. Atlanta, GA: Centers for Disease Control and Prevention; 2006.

38. Derkay CS. Task force on recurrent respiratory papillomas: a preliminary report. *Arch Otolaryngol Head Neck Surg*. 1995;121(12):1386-1391.

39. Rogo KO, Nyansera PN. Congenital condylomata acuminata with meconium staining of amniotic fluid and fetal hydrocephalus: case report. *East Afr Med J*. 1989;66(6):411-413.

40. Wiatrak BJ, Wiatrak DW, Broker TR, Lewis L. Recurrent respiratory papillomatosis: a longitudinal study comparing severity associated with human papilloma viral types 6 and 11 and other risk factors in a large pediatric population. *Laryngoscope*. 2004;114(11 pt 2 suppl 104):1-23.

41. Tang CK, Shermeta DW, Wood C. Congenital condylomata acuminata. *Am J Obstet Gynecol*. 1978;131(8):912-913.

42. Bodaghi S, Wood LV, Roby G, Ryder C, Steinberg SM, Zheng ZM. Could human papillomaviruses be spread through blood? *J Clin Microbiol*. 2005;43(11):5428-5434.

43. Rintala MA, Grénman SE, Järvenkylä ME, Syrjänen KJ, Syrjänen SM. High-risk types of human papillomavirus (HPV) DNA in oral and genital mucosa of infants during their first 3 years of life: experience from the Finnish HPV Family Study. *Clin Infect Dis*. 2005;41(12):1728-1733.

44. Kojima A, Maeda H, Kurahashi N, et al. Human papillomaviruses in the normal oral cavity of children in Japan. *Oral Oncol*. 2003;39(8):821-828.

45. Summersgill KF, Smith EM, Levy BT, Allen JM, Haugen TH, Turek LP. Human papillomavirus in the oral cavities of children and adolescents. *Oral Surg Oral Med Oral Pathol Oral Radiol Endod*. 2001;91(1):62-69.

46. Chatterjee R, Mukhopadhyay D, Murmu N, Mitra PK. Correlation between human papillomavirus DNA detection in maternal cervical smears and buccal swabs of infants. *Indian J Exp Biol*. 1998;36(2):199-202.

47. Rice PS, Mant C, Cason J, et al. High prevalence of human papillomavirus type 16 infection among children. *J Med Virol*. 2000;61(1):70-75.

48. Mant C, Kell B, Rice P, Best JM, Bible JM, Cason J. Buccal exposure to human papillomavirus type 16 is a common yet transitory event of childhood. *J Med Virol*. 2003;71(4):593-598.

49. Syrjänen S, Puranen M. Human papillomavirus infections in children: the potential role of maternal transmission. *Crit Rev Oral Biol Med*. 2000;11(2):259-274.

50. Smith EM, Ritchie JM, Yankowitz J, et al. Human papillomavirus prevalence and types in newborns and parents: concordance and modes of transmission. *Sex Transm Dis*. 2004;31(1):57-62.

51. Watts DH, Koutsky LA, Holmes KK, et al. Low risk of perinatal transmission of human papillomavirus: results from a prospective cohort study. *Am J Obstet Gynecol*. 1998;178(2):365-373.

52. Shah K, Kashima H, Polk BF, Shah F, Abbey H, Abramson A. Rarity of cesarean delivery in cases of juvenile-onset respiratory papillomatosis. *Obstet Gynecol.* 1986;68(6):795-799.

53. Sinclair KA, Woods CR, Kirse DJ, Sinal SH. Anogenital and respiratory tract human papillomavirus infections among children: age, gender, and potential transmission through sexual abuse. *Pediatrics.* 2005;116(4):815-825.

54. Jayasinghe Y, Garland SM. Genital warts in children: what do they mean? *Arch Dis Child.* 2006;91(8):696-700.

55. Sinal SH, Woods CR. Human papillomavirus infections of the genital and respiratory tracts in young children. *Semin Pediatr Infect Dis.* 2005;16(4):306-316.

56. Hammerschlag MR. Sexually transmitted diseases in sexually abused children: medical and legal implications. *Sex Transm Infect.* 1998;74(3):167-174.

57. Muram D, Stewart D. Sexually transmitted diseases. In: Heger A, Emans SJ, Muram D, eds. *Evaluation of the Sexually Abused Child: A Medical Textbook and Photographic Atlas.* 2nd ed. New York, NY: Oxford University Press; 2000:187-224.

58. Jenison SA, Yu XP, Valentine JM, et al. Evidence of prevalent genital-type human papillomavirus infections in adults and children. *J Infect Dis.* 1990;162(1):60-69.

59. Bacopoulou F, Karakitsos P, Kottaridi C, et al. Genital HPV in children and adolescents: does sexual activity make a difference? *J Pediatr Adolesc Gynecol.* 2016;29(3):228-233.

60. Andersson K, Waterboer T, Kirnbauer R, et al. Seroreactivity to cutaneous human papillomaviruses among patients with nonmelanoma skin cancer or benign skin lesions. *Cancer Epidemiol Biomarkers Prev.* 2008;17(1):189-195.

61. Markowitz LE, Liu G, Hariri S, Steinau M, Dunne EF, Unger ER. Prevalence of HPV after introduction of the vaccination program in the United States. *Pediatrics.* 2016;137(3):e20151968.

62. Meites E, Kempe A, Markowitz LE. Use of a 2-Dose schedule for human papillomavirus vaccination: updated recommendations of the advisory committee on immunization practices. *MMWR Morb Mortal Wkly Rep.* 2016;65(49):1405-1408.

63. Schwebke JR, Burgess D. Trichomoniasis. *Clin Microbiol Rev.* 2004;17(4):794-803.

64. Rughooputh S, Greenwell P. *Trichomonas vaginalis*: paradigm of a successful sexually transmitted organism. *Br J Biomed Sci.* 2005;62(4):193-200.

65. Seña AC, Miller WC, Hobbs MM, et al. *Trichomonas vaginalis* infection in male sexual partners: implications for diagnosis, treatment, and prevention. *Clin Infect Dis.* 2007;44(1):13-22.

66. Blake DR, Duggan A, Joffe A. Use of spun urine to enhance detection of *Trichomonas vaginalis* in adolescent women. *Arch Pediatr Adolesc Med.* 1999;153(12):1222-1225.

67. Borchardt KA, al-Haraci S, Maida N. Prevalence of *Trichomonas vaginalis* in a male sexually transmitted disease clinic population by interview, wet mount microscopy, and the InPouch TV test. *Genitourin Med.* 1995;71(6):405-406.

68. Ohlemeyer CL, Hornberger LL, Lynch DA, Swierkosz EM. Diagnosis of *Trichomonas vaginalis* in adolescent females: InPouch TV culture versus wet-mount microscopy. *J Adolesc Health.* 1998;22(3):205-208.

69. van Der Schee C, van Belkum A, Zwijgers L, et al. Improved diagnosis of *Trichomonas vaginalis* infection by PCR using vaginal swabs and urine specimens compared to diagnosis by wet mount microscopy, culture, and fluorescent staining. *J Clin Microbiol.* 1999;37(12):4127-4130.

70. Borchardt KA, Zhang MZ, Shing H, Flink K. A comparison of the sensitivity of the InPouch TV, Diamond's and Trichosel media for detection of Trichomonas vaginalis. *Genitourin Med.* 1997;73(4):297-298.

71. Hobbs MM, Seña AC. Modern diagnosis of Trichomonas vaginalis infection. *Sex Transm Infect.* 2013;89(6):434-438.

72. Schwebke JR, Barrientes FJ. Prevalence of *Trichomonas vaginalis* isolates with resistance to metronidazole and tinidazole. *Antimicrob Agents Chemother.* 2006;50(12):4209-4210.

73. Bowden FJ, Garnett GP. *Trichomonas vaginalis* epidemiology: parameterising and analysing a model of treatment interventions. *Sex Transm Infect.* 2000;76(4):248-256.

74. al-Salihi FL, Curran JP, Wang J. Neonatal *Trichomonas vaginalis*: report of three cases and review of the literature. *Pediatrics.* 1974;53(2):196-200.

75. Szarka K, Temesvári P, Kerekes A, Tege A, Repkény A. Neonatal pneumonia caused by *Trichomonas vaginalis. Acta Microbiol Immunol Hung.* 2002;49(1):15-19.

76. Temesvári P, Kerekes A. Newborn with suppurative nasal discharge and respiratory distress. *Pediatr Infect Dis J.* 2004;23(3):282-283.

77. Emans SJH, Laufer MR, Goldstein DP, Goldstein DP. *Pediatric and Adolescent Gynecology.* 5th ed. Philadelphia, PA: Lippincott Williams & Wilkins; 2005.

78. Neinstein LS, Goldenring J, Carpenter S. Nonsexual transmission of sexually transmitted diseases: an infrequent occurrence. *Pediatrics.* 1984;74(1):67-76.

79. Corey L, Handsfield HH. Genital herpes and public health: addressing a global problem. *JAMA.* 2000;283(6):791-794.

80. Xu F, Sternberg MR, Kottiri BJ, et al. Trends in herpes simplex virus type 1 and type 2 seroprevalence in the United States. *JAMA.* 2006;296(8):964-973.

81. Kim HN, Meier A, Huang ML, et al. Oral herpes simplex virus type 2 reactivation in HIV-positive and -negative men. *J Infect Dis.* 2006;194(4):420-427.

82. Wald A, Ericsson M, Krantz E, Selke S, Corey L. Oral shedding of herpes simplex virus type 2. *Sex Transm Infect.* 2004;80(4):272-276.

83. Sacks SL, Griffiths PD, Corey L, et al. HSV shedding. *Antiviral Res.* 2004;63(suppl 1):S19-S26.

84. Johnson RE, Nahmias AJ, Magder LS, Lee FK, Brooks CA, Snowden CB. A seroepidemiologic survey of the prevalence of herpes simplex virus type 2 infection in the United States. *N Engl J Med.* 1989;321(1):7-12.

85. Lafferty WE, Downey L, Celum C, Wald A. Herpes simplex virus type 1 as a cause of genital herpes: impact on surveillance and prevention. *J Infect Dis.* 2000;181(4):1454-1457.

86. Wald A, Zeh J, Selke S, Ashley RL, Corey L. Virologic characteristics of subclinical and symptomatic genital herpes infections. *N Engl J Med.* 1995;333(12):770-775.

87. Adams G, Stover BH, Keenlyside RA, et al. Nosocomial herpetic infections in a pediatric intensive care unit. *Am J Epidemiol.* 1981;113(2):126-132.

88. Rowe NH, Heine CS, Kowalski CJ. Herpetic whitlow: an occupational disease of practicing dentists. *J Am Dent Assoc.* 1982;105(3):471-473.

89. Turner R, Shehab Z, Osborne K, Hendley JO. Shedding and survival of herpes simplex virus from 'fever blisters'. *Pediatrics.* 1982;70(4):547-549.

90. Cengizlier R, Uysal G, Güven A, Tülek N. Herpetic finger infection. *Cutis.* 2002;69(4):291-292.

91. Novick NL. Autoinoculation herpes of the hand in a child with recurrent herpes labialis. *Am J Med.* 1985;79(1):139-142.

92. Gill MJ, Arlette J, Buchan K. Herpes simplex virus infection of the hand: a profile of 79 cases. *Am J Med.* 1988;84(1):89-93.

93. Cowan FM, Copas A, Johnson AM, Ashley R, Corey L, Mindel A. Herpes simplex virus type 1 infection: a sexually transmitted infection of adolescence? *Sex Transm Infect.* 2002;78(5):346-348.

94. Leach CT, Ashley RL, Baillargeon J, Jenson HB. Performance of two commercial glycoprotein G-based enzyme immunoassays for detecting antibodies to herpes simplex viruses 1 and 2 in children and young adolescents. *Clin Diagn Lab Immunol.* 2002;9(5):1124-1125.

95. Ramos S, Lukefahr JL, Morrow RA, Stanberry LR, Rosenthal SL. Prevalence of herpes simplex virus types 1 and 2 among children and adolescents attending a sexual abuse clinic. *Pediatr Infect Dis J.* 2006;25(10):902-905.

96. Reading R, Rannan-Eliya Y. Evidence for sexual transmission of genital herpes in children. *Arch Dis Child.* 2007;92(7):608-613.

97. Woods CR. Syphilis in children: congenital and acquired. *Semin Pediatr Infect Dis.* 2005;16(4):245-257.

98. Christian CW, Lavelle J, Bell LM. Preschoolers with syphilis. *Pediatrics.* 1999;103(1):E4.

99. US Department of Health and Human Services, Centers for Disease Control and Prevention, Division of STD Prevention. *Sexually Transmitted Disease Surveillance 2005 Supplement: Syphilis Surveillance Report.* Atlanta, GA: Centers for Disease Control and Prevention; 2006.

100. Everett V, Ingram D, Flick L, Russell T, Tropez-Sims S, McFadden A. A comparison of sexually transmitted diseases (STDs) found in a total of 696 boys and 2973 girls evaluated for sexual abuse. *Pediatr Res.* 1998;43(4 suppl 2):91.

101. Rawstron SA, Bromberg K, Hammerschlag MR. STD in children: syphilis and gonorrhoea. *Genitourin Med.* 1993;69(1):66-75.

102. Starling SP. Syphilis in infants and young children. *Pediatr Ann.* 1994;23(7):334-340.

103. Ginsburg CM. Acquired syphilis in prepubertal children. *Pediatr Infect Dis.* 1983;2(3):232-234.

104. Egglestone SI, Turner AJ. Serological diagnosis of syphilis: PHLS Syphilis Serology Working Group. *Commun Dis Public Health.* 2000;3(3):158-162.

105. Siedner M, Zapitz V, Ishida M, De La Roca R, Klausner JD. Performance of rapid syphilis tests in venous and fingerstick whole blood specimens. *Sex Transm Dis.* 2004;31(9):557-560.

106. Lindegren ML, Hanson IC, Hammett TA, Beil J, Fleming PL, Ward JW. Sexual abuse of children: intersection with the HIV epidemic. *Pediatrics.* 1998;102(4):E46.

107. Havens PL; American Academy of Pediatrics Committee on on Pediatric AIDS. Postexposure prophylaxis in children and adolescents for nonoccupational exposure to human immunodeficiency virus. *Pediatrics.* 2003;111(6 pt 1):1475-1489.

108. Ellen JM. Human immunodeficiency virus prophylaxis for sexual assault survivors: what we need to know. *Arch Pediatr Adolesc Med.* 2006;160(7):754-755.

109. Pilcher CD, Tien HC, Eron JJ Jr, et al. Brief but efficient: acute HIV infection and the sexual transmission of HIV. *J Infect Dis.* 2004;189(10):1785-1792.

110. Branson BM, Handsfield HH, Lampe MA, et al. Revised recommendations for HIV testing of adults, adolescents, and pregnant women in health-care settings. *MMWR Recomm Rep.* 2006;55(RR-14):1-17; quiz CE11-14.

111. Branson BM, Owen SM, Wesolowski LG, et al. Quick Reference Guide - Laboratory Testing for the Diagnosis of HIV Infection: Updated Recommendations. Centers for Disease Control and Prevention Web site. https://stacks.cdc.gov/view/cdc/23446. Published June 27, 2014. Accessed June 7, 2018.

112. Greenwald JL, Burstein GR, Pincus J, Branson B. A rapid review of rapid HIV antibody tests. *Curr Infect Dis Rep.* 2006;8(2):125-131.

113. Kahn JO, Walker BD. Acute human immunodeficiency virus type 1 infection. *N Engl J Med.* 1998;339(1):33-39.

114. Cardo DM, Culver DH, Ciesielski CA, et al. A case-control study of HIV seroconversion in health care workers after percutaneous exposure: Centers for Disease Control and Prevention Needlestick Surveillance Group. *N Engl J Med.* 1997;337(21):1485-1490.

115. Pinkerton SD, Martin JN, Roland ME, Katz MH, Coates TJ, Kahn JO. Cost-effectiveness of HIV postexposure prophylaxis following sexual or injection drug exposure in 96 metropolitan areas in the United States. *AIDS.* 2004;18(15):2065-2073.

116. Dominguez KL, Smith DK, Thomas V, et al. Updated Guidelines for Antiretroviral Postexposure Prophylaxis After Sexual, Injection Drug Use, or Other Nonoccupational Exposure to HIV—United States, 2016. Centers for Disease Control and Prevention Web site. https://stacks.cdc.gov/view/cdc/38856. Published April 18, 2016. Updated May 23, 2018. Accessed June 7, 2018.

117. Jain S, Mayer KH. Practical guidance for nonoccupational postexposure prophylaxis to prevent HIV infection: an editorial review. *AIDS.* 2014;28(11):1545-1554.

118. Schremmer RD, Swanson D, Kraly K. Human immunodeficiency virus postexposure prophylaxis in child and adolescent victims of sexual assault. *Pediatr Emerg Care.* 2005;21(8):502-506.

119. Olshen E, Hsu K, Woods ER, Harper M, Harnisch B, Samples CL. Use of human immunodeficiency virus postexposure prophylaxis in adolescent sexual assault victims. *Arch Pediatr Adolesc Med.* 2006;160(7):674-680.

120. Schwebke JR, Desmond R. Risk factors for bacterial vaginosis in women at high risk for sexually transmitted diseases. *Sex Transm Dis.* 2005;32(11):654-658.

121. Bump RC, Buesching WJ 3rd. Bacterial vaginosis in virginal and sexually active adolescent females: evidence against exclusive sexual transmission. *Am J Obstet Gynecol.* 1988;158(4):935-939.

122. Bump RC, Sachs LA, Buesching WJ 3rd. Sexually transmissible infectious agents in sexually active and virginal asymptomatic adolescent girls. *Pediatrics.* 1986;77(4):488-494.

123. Morris MC, Rogers PA, Kinghorn GR. Is bacterial vaginosis a sexually transmitted infection? *Sex Transm Infect.* 2001;77(1):63-68.

124. Gardner HL, Dukes CD. *Haemophilus vaginalis* vaginitis: a newly defined specific infection previously classified non-specific vaginitis. *Am J Obstet Gynecol.* 1955;69(5):962-976.

125. Barbone F, Austin H, Louv WC, Alexander WJ. A follow-up study of methods of contraception, sexual activity, and rates of trichomoniasis, candidiasis, and bacterial vaginosis. *Am J Obstet Gynecol.* 1990;163(2):510-514.

126. Kinghorn GR, Jones BM, Chowdhury FH, Geary I. Balanoposthitis associated with *Gardnerella vaginalis* infection in men. *Br J Vener Dis.* 1982;58(2):127-129.

127. Masfari AN, Kinghorn GR, Duerden BI. Anaerobes in genitourinary infections in men. *Br J Vener Dis.* 1983;59(4):255-259.

128. Hillier SL, Rabe LK, Muller CH, Zarutskie P, Kuzan FB, Stenchever MA. Relationship of bacteriologic characteristics to semen indices in men attending an infertility clinic. *Obstet Gynecol.* 1990;75(5):800-804.

129. Moi H, Erkkola R, Jerve F, et al. Should male consorts of women with bacterial vaginosis be treated? *Genitourin Med.* 1989;65(4):263-268.

130. Swedberg J, Steiner JF, Deiss F, Steiner S, Driggers DA. Comparison of single-dose vs one-week course of metronidazole for symptomatic bacterial vaginosis. *JAMA.* 1985;254(8):1046-1049.

131. Wahl NG, Castilla MA, Lewis-Abney K. Prevalence of *Gardnerella vaginalis* in prepubertal males. *Arch Pediatr Adolesc Med.* 1998;152(11):1095-1099.

132. Powell LC, Jr. Condyloma acuminatum: recent advances in development, carcinogenesis, and treatment. *Clin Obstet Gynecol.* 1978;21(4):1061-1079.

Chapter 11

Collection and Testing of DNA Evidence

Marcella F. Scott, MSPH

Introduction

The role of the forensic biologist in a child sexual abuse case is to examine items of evidence for the presence of body fluid stains, hair, or other DNA-containing cellular material. The DNA analysis of this evidence can establish associations between victim, suspect, and crime scene. The quality of DNA testing results begins with the collection of evidence. In cases of sexual abuse, evidence deposited on the victim's body will be lost over time due to biological degradation and everyday actions like bathing, showering, drinking, eating, urinating, and defecating. Therefore, evidence collection must be completed as promptly as possible in order to minimize loss. Additionally, the potential that tangential individuals will deposit biological material increases with time. Even skin cells or sweat from caregivers and first responders can interfere with detection and interpretation of DNA left behind by a perpetrator. Evidence collection from the prepubescent victim's body should occur up to 72 hours post-assault.[1] For adolescent victims, considerations should be made to extend that examination time.[2] The adolescent victim's physical development and physiological characteristics may be similar to an adult's. Examinations up to 120 hours post-assault are recommended for adult victims.[3] In cases involving unusual circumstances such as prolonged incapacitation or captivity, collecting evidence from the body beyond recommended time frames may produce foreign DNA results; however, additional items of evidence, such as clothing worn by the victim at the time of or immediately after the assault, can be collected beyond those time frames. The scene of the assault should also be processed for evidence collection, especially in cases involving a delayed report.

Advances in DNA analysis have led to more sensitive techniques and processing for the detection of male-specific DNA. These methods are also more sensitive than the conventional body fluid testing that has been in use since the mid-1950s, late 1960s, and late 1990s.[4,5] Body fluids such as semen, saliva, and blood have always been excellent sources of DNA, but now, samples collected from skin-to-skin contact (eg, fingernail swabbings or scrapings, body swabs from locations where the victim was grabbed or restrained) can yield a foreign DNA profile.

Short tandem repeat (STR) DNA is characterized by short sequences of nucleotides, typically 2 to 7 bases, which repeat a varying number of times among individuals. The highly polymorphic nature of STRs makes them useful for distinguishing one individual from another. The testing of STR markers in the human genome has been the standard forensic DNA technique since 1997, when the Federal Bureau of Investigation (FBI) established via the DNA Identification Act of 1994 a core of 13 STR loci for use in the Combined DNA Index System (CODIS), a nationwide database of DNA profiles used to identify potential suspects.[6] STR markers on the Y chromosome (ie, Y-STRs) have also been identified. Only males possess the Y chromosome; however, in the absence of mutation, all patrilineal relatives will have the same Y-STR DNA profile. STR testing for Y-STR loci can isolate and detect male DNA masked by large quantities of female DNA, which may occur in a given sexual assault involving a female and a male.[7]

For cases involving an assailant whose STR-DNA profile is not included in CODIS, another genetic tool can be used to assist in identifying some of the assailant's physical characteristics. Single nucleotide polymorphisms (SNPs) are differences in the genome that occur at a single base. The testing of SNP markers has led to the identification of phenotypic traits for eye color, hair color, and skin color.[9] SNPs have also been used to estimate ancestry.[10] Mainstream use of SNP analysis by forensic laboratories is still under development; however, phenotypic and ancestry testing have been commercially available for forensic casework since late 2014.[11] This analysis provides physical characteristics for the DNA donor that can be used to aid the investigation.

Routine STR-DNA testing often results in mixed DNA profiles of victims and other donors, potentially even perpetrators. Probabilistic genotyping software is available to assist in the interpretation of mixed DNA results and can also generate likelihood ratios for any DNA associations made.[12,13]

Evidence Collection

When collecting evidence from a victim's body, it should be borne in mind that any and all technological advances and forensic biological tools are rendered useless by improper evidence collection. The sexual assault evidence kit (SAK) is the basic tool for the collection of evidence from the victim's body. It is collected by a specially trained medical professional as part of the forensic medical examination. There are various terms used to describe these kits: rape kit, victim physical evidence recovery kit, and sexual assault evidence kit. The contents of the SAK may vary by jurisdiction. **Figure 11-1** shows an example of an SAK. The *National Best Practices for Sexual Assault Kits*[3] recommends the creation of national minimum standards for the SAK. The forensic medical provider should collaborate with local crime laboratory personnel to establish standardized items to collect in an SAK. **Table 11-1** and **Table 11-2** lists items typically found in an SAK.

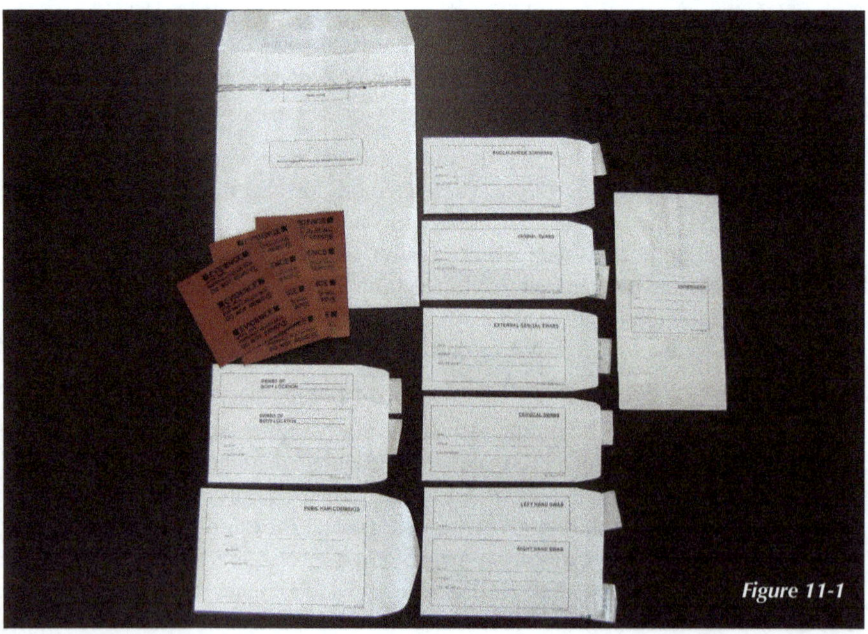

Figure 11-1. *A sexual assault evidence collection kit.*

Table 11-1. Items Commonly Found in a Sexual Assault Evidence Kit (Female Victim)

Sample	Adolescent	Prepubescent	Specimen Details
Vaginal swabs	Collect	Only if injury requires sedation	Use 2 dry swabs, covering surfaces, packaged together.
Cervical swabs	Collect	Only if injury requires sedation	Use 2 dry swabs, covering surfaces, packaged together.
External genitalia swabs	Collect	Collect—avoid insertion into the introitus	Use 2 slightly moistened swabs, covering surfaces, packaged together.
Anal/perianal swabs	Collect	Collect	Use 2 slightly moistened swabs, covering surfaces, packaged together.
Oral swabs	Collect	Collect	Use 2 dry swabs along gums, teeth, and cheeks. Body jewelry or dental appliances can be swabbed if they cannot be collected.
Skin swabs (possible semen; possible saliva: breast/chest, neck)	Collect	Collect	Use 2 slightly moistened swabs per area. Package each area separately.
Fingernail samples/clippings	Collect	Collect	Use 1 slightly moistened swab per hand and swab under the fingernails. Scrapings or clippings may also be collected per hand. Package each hand separately.
Buccal reference swabs	Collect	Collect	Use 2 dry swabs, covering the surface, package together. Collected after the oral swab and following a rinsing of the mouth. This will be used as the victim's known DNA source.
Underwear	Collect	Collect	Package in the kit
Pubic hair combing	Collect	Collect	Comb the pubic hair over the collection paper to capture any loose hairs or debris. If the victim doesn't have pubic hair then look for loose hairs to pick, and two slightly moistened swabs may be collected from the mons pubis.

Data from US Department of Justice, Office on Violence Against Women[1]*; US Department of Justice, Office on Violence Against Women*[2]*; US Department of Justice, Office of Justice Programs, National Institute of Justice.*[3]

Table 11-2. Items Commonly Found in a Sexual Assault Evidence Kit (Male Victim)

Sample	Adolescent	Prepubescent	Specimen Details
Anal/perianal swabs	Collect	Collect	Use 2 slightly moistened swabs, covering surfaces, packaged together.
Oral swabs	Collect	Collect	Use 2 dry swabs along gums, teeth and cheeks. Body jewelry or dental appliances can be swabbed if they cannot be collected.
Skin swabs (possible semen; possible saliva: chest, neck)	Collect	Collect	Use 2 slightly moistened swabs per area. Package each area separately.
Fingernail samples/clippings	Collect	Collect	Use 1 slightly moistened swab per hand and swab under the fingernails. Scrapings or clippings may also be collected per hand. Package each hand separately.
Buccal reference swabs	Collect	Collect	Use 2 dry swabs, covering the surface, package together. Collected after the oral swab and following a rinsing of the mouth. This will be the used as the victim's known DNA source.
Underwear	Collect	Collect	Package in the kit
Pubic hair combing	Collect	Collect	Comb the pubic hair over the collection paper to capture any loose hairs or debris. If the victim doesn't have pubic hair then look for loose hairs to pick, and 2 slightly moistened swabs may be collected from the mons pubis.
Penile and scrotum swabs	Collect	Collect	Use 2 slightly moistened swabs, covering the surface, package together. Swab the shaft, glans, under the foreskin, and scrotum, avoid the urethra.

Data from US Department of Justice, Office on Violence Against Women[1]; US Department of Justice, Office on Violence Against Women[2]; US Department of Justice, Office of Justice Programs, National Institute of Justice.[3]

Samples collected should be guided by the case history. If this information is incomplete or absent, samples should be collected from areas that may yield foreign DNA, including the neck, breast, and external genitalia. Swabs should also be collected from body areas commonly contacted during sexual assault (eg, vagina or penis, anus, oral cavity). Sample collection should be concentrated on only 1 or 2 swabs to ensure concentration of possible samples for testing, as spreading the foreign donor's biological material across multiple swabs lessens the likelihood of detection in typical crime laboratory workflows. The 2 swabs should be collected simultaneously or using the same technique in order to secure homogenous samples.[3] Collecting a single moistened swab followed by a dry swab has been shown to produce a heterogeneous sample.[14] This technique requires identification of the "wet" and "dry" samples to ensure that the laboratory analyzes the sample containing the greatest amount of DNA. Homogenous samples obviate the need to specify swab sampling order and allow the laboratory to test either swab with an analogous outcome. Additionally, the literature demonstrates that the single moistened swab technique produces results comparable to the double swab method.[15] Using too much water to moisten a swab can also dilute the sample and hinder collection of material onto the swab.

An alternate light source (ALS) (**Figure 11-2**) can aid in the identification of dried secretions on the victim's body. Flavins are found in various tissues in the body. They possess photochemical sensitivity and fluoresce under ultraviolet light. Semen contains high concentrations of flavins. Semen stains can be detected at the blue ~455nm range, using an orange filter (typically a visor or goggles) to visualize. **Figures 11-3** are a semen stain on cloth under normal lighting and with an ALS. The ALS can also be used to identify possible saliva stains.[4]

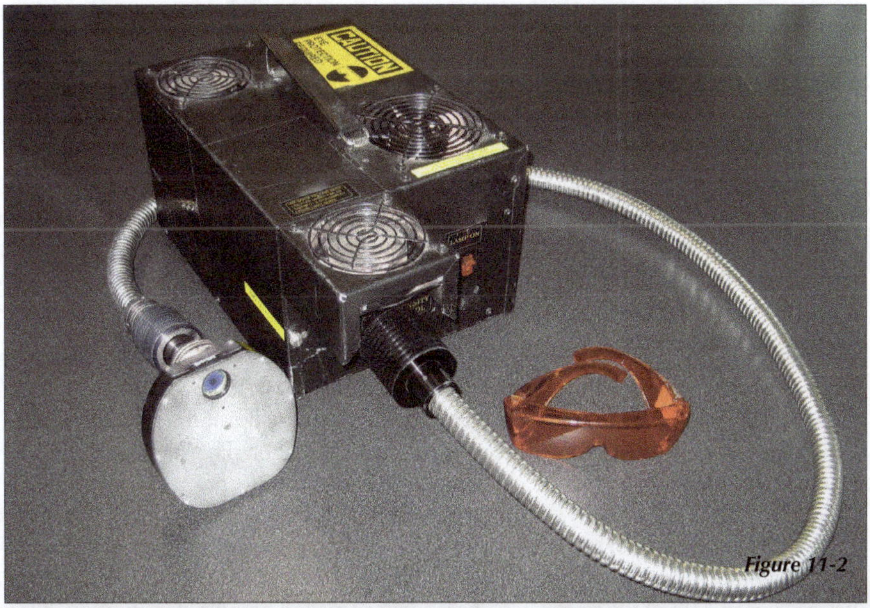

Figure 11-2. *An alternate light source (ALS) used to visualize stains.*

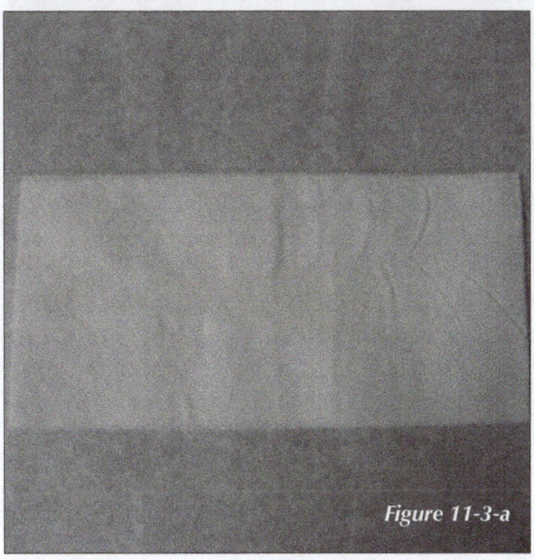

Figure 11-3-a. *A semen stain on material under normal lighting.*

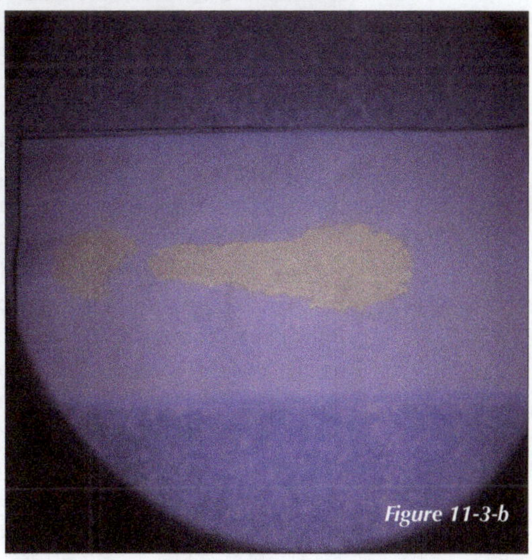

Figure 11-3-b. *The same semen stain on material under an ALS at 455nm.*

The clothing worn by the victim during and immediately following assault should be collected. Valuable evidence can be identified on the clothing items worn at the time of the sexual assault. In cases of child sexual abuse, probative evidence is often found on the victim's clothing.[16] If a patient is wearing the same garments worn during or immediately following assault at the time of examination, each item of clothing should be collected and packaged in its own paper bag, separate from the SAK. If the clothing worn during or after assault is not available during the examination, law enforcement may collect it separately. If clothing worn during or immediately after assault has been laundered, it should still be collected, as semen stains can persist even after laundering.[17] However, special considerations are warranted in the event of a cohabitant being the alleged abuser, as semen donors' DNA can be transferred in the laundry. A study by Noël et al[18] demonstrated the presence of DNA from all family members on the underwear of children living in the home. Presumptive (acid phosphatase) and confirmatory testing (prostate-specific antigen) for semen were negative, and swabbings of the underwear yielded no transferred DNA. All transferred DNA was identified on cuttings.

Additional items that may be collected in the SAK and during examination include the following. Feminine products, like tampons and pads used during or immediately after assault should be collected. If secretions are found in the victim's head hair, they can be swabbed using the technique previously described. Condoms found inside the victim's body or left at the scene must be collected. All items containing biological evidence should be dried and packaged in breathable materials, including paper envelopes, bags, or cardboard boxes. Plastic packaging such as baggies or specimen containers should be avoided. A sterile gauze square can be placed in an envelope with a used condom if needed. Once dried, the ideal storage conditions are in a temperature- and humidity-controlled environment away from any direct sunlight. This will minimize the risk of bacteria and mold growth on the evidence. Bacteria and mold degrade DNA and can prevent a result from being obtained.[19]

The following items are no longer routinely collected in SAKs: vaginal, anal, or oral smears; pulled head or pubic hair; and dental flossing.[3] Smears may not be routinely examined by a crime laboratory due to the laborious process of the examination. Preparation of a slide by the medical professional collecting a kit may waste evidence better preserved on a swab for laboratory analysis. If the SAK requires examination for the presence of spermatozoa, the collected swabs are used for this analysis. Additionally, the hospital wet mount examination of vaginal smears for spermatozoa has been shown to be ineffective, only identifying spermatozoa in 41% of the cases where the laboratory made a positive identification, likely due to the differential staining technique used in the forensic laboratory.[20] The results of the wet mount examination have no impact on how the laboratory processes swabs.

In the past, pulled head and pubic hairs would be collected from the victim as a hair reference sample, used for comparison in morphological hair analysis. The examination involves the visual and microscopic comparison of hair found in pubic and head hair combings or picked from the victim's body in an attempt to locate hair different from the victim's. The 2009 National Academy of Sciences report on forensic science, *Strengthening Forensic Science in the United States: A Path Forward*, described hair analysis as "highly unreliable."[24] Hair analysis is a type of forensic examination that is now coupled with DNA testing and used as a screening tool for mitochondrial DNA analysis.[25] If a case warrants hair analysis, reference samples from the victim can be collected at a later time. Hairs pulled from deceased, decomposing victims may be a suitable reference standard when buccal swabs or blood are not available. Although hair comparisons have been deemed unreliable, the examination of hairs found at a crime scene to determine if they are suitable for STR-DNA analysis (actively growing root or adhering follicular tissue) is still conducted in the absence of other probative samples. The ubiquitous nature of hairs in the environment makes hair evidence prone to question and circumstance. An obvious pubic hair (for example, from the genital examination of a child) should be collected within any SAK. As with semen and saliva transfer among the clothing and bedding of cohabitants or individuals known to one another, the presence of hair can be somewhat meaningless.

Dental flossing has, in the past, been used for the collection of spermatozoa following oral assault. Persistence of seminal constituents after deposition is diminished in the mouth, as compared with other areas of the body. The literature currently recommends against the use of dental floss in evidence collection, due to risk for disease introduction through gum disruption.[3] In a 2014 study consisting of 87 samples, 38% demonstrated spermatozoa on both floss and swabs, and 29% were negative for both sample types.[26] However, 25% of the floss samples were negative when the swab was positive for spermatozoa, and conversely, 8% of the swabs were negative when the floss samples were positive. The collection of both swabs and flossing did increase the chance of obtaining a positive result. However, the results do support the recommendation to only use swabs when collecting samples from the oral cavity following an oral assault.

Touch DNA Samples

Increased sensitivity of DNA analysis methods has allowed for the detection of the DNA in cells transferred from an individual touching an item with their bare skin. The average person will shed approximately 400 000 skin cells a day, although the outermost cornified epithelial layer no longer contains nuclei. Prolonged contact or friction will cause increased sloughing of living skin cells. This DNA originates from the epithelial cells themselves, rather than from body fluid. Sweat also carries epithelial cells, although far less than saliva. This type of evidence is referred to as "touch DNA evidence." The amount of cells left from handling an object depends on a number of factors. Initial studies of the detection of DNA from touch evidence suggested that individuals could be categorized as "good sloughers" and "non-sloughers."[27,28] However, this simplified categorization of individuals into 2 types could not be reproduced, as individuals varied in the amount of cells they shed from sample to sample. Length of time between handwashing was the largest factor that impacted individuals' ability to shed skin cells. The longer an individual goes between handwashing, the more cells they tend to shed when touching or handling an item. Differences have also been observed between dominant and nondominant hands, with the dominant hand tending to shed more cells when handwashing is limited.[29] Ultimately, an individual's ability to shed cells is complex and depends on handwashing habits, length of contact, and contacted surface.

The single moistened swab technique is the appropriate procedure to collect touch DNA evidence.[15] The case scenario is key to determining whether touch DNA samples should be collected. Offenders in juvenile sexual assaults are most often family members (34.2%) and acquaintances (58.7%).[8] Family members often have skin-to-skin contact through normal activities like holding hands, carrying, assisting a child with dressing or bathing, and diaper changing. Acquaintances may or may not engage in these types of skin-to-skin contact. In 2008, Graham and Rutty[15] conducted a study to assess the level of background DNA an adult might have on the skin of his or her neck. (See **Table 11-3** for a summary of the DNA results from collected samples.) In this study, a single swab was collected from 5 different areas of the neck on 24 participants, totaling 120 samples. Of the 120 samples collected, 23% demonstrated alleles from a nondonor. Of the samples that demonstrated nondonor alleles, 79% (22 samples) detected 5 alleles or less. The nondonor alleles were observed in 13% of the samples from the front of the neck and 9% from the back of the neck. Potential sources of the nondonor DNA include primary transfer through skin contact and oral projection of saliva particles or secondary transfer from shared items. Individuals who were living with a partner during sample collections demonstrated higher levels of nondonor DNA.

Table 11-3. The Detection of Background DNA from Adults' Necks

Number of Subjects	Sex	Neck Area (24 samples per location)				
		Front Right	Front Center	Front Left	Back Left	Back Right
15	F	5* – 6† (7)‡	4 – 3 (4)	6 – 3 (13)	3 – 3 (9)	2 – 0
19	M	5 – 3 (14)	7 – 2 (6)	4 – 2 (13)	3 – 4 (3)	3 – 2 (3)

**Number of samples producing a complete DNA profile from the DNA donor (study participant)*
†Number of samples demonstrating nondonor alleles
‡Maximum number of alleles detected for the nondonor (out of 22 total alleles)
Data from Graham EAM, Rutty GN.[15]

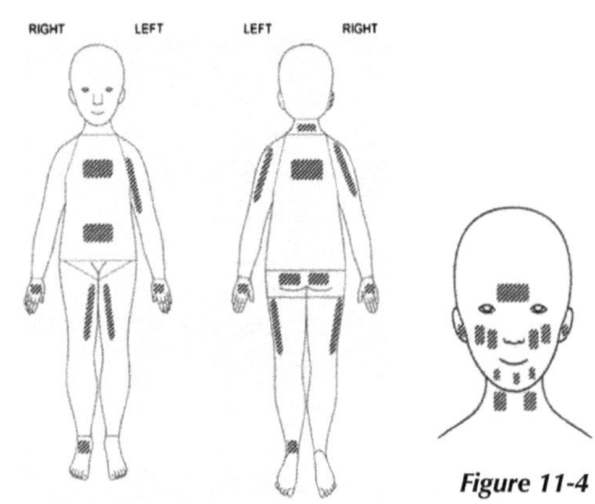

Figure 11-4

Figure 11-4. *Areas swabbed from a child's face (12 sites) and body (20 sites). Reprinted from Graham EAM, Watkins WJ, Dunstan F, et al.30 https://creativecommons.org/licenses/by/4.0/.*

The contact between adults may differ from contact between adults and children. The level of background DNA on children aged 0 to 5 has been researched and can aid in the assessment of the collection of touch DNA evidence. In a study of 47 children, samples were collected from 12 sites on the face and neck and 20 sites elsewhere on the body using a single swab (**Figure 11-4**), totaling 944 samples from 32 sites.[30] Nondonor DNA was detected in 35% of the samples, with 90% of these samples demonstrating 5 or fewer foreign alleles.Of all sampled sites, the front of the hands and the cheeks demonstrated the most nondonor DNA. The biological source of the nondonor DNA was not assessed.

Overall, the frequency of background DNA is low but still present. Collection of touch DNA evidence should be based on case details, including type of assault and the identity of the alleged perpetrator. In cases in which a child's genitals were fondled or digital assault occurred, a swab of the area should be collected. It is also conceivable that a perpetrator would use saliva as a lubricant in penetrating a child, which would result in transfer of his or her DNA.

Contamination Prevention

Throughout the process of collection, the examiner must take precautions to prevent the contamination of evidence. DNA contamination is the unintentional introduction of exogenous DNA to a sample.[31] The use of personal protective equipment (PPE) is critical to contamination prevention. PPE serves two purposes: (1) protecting the examiner from exposure to potentially infectious disease, and (2) protecting the evidence from the introduction of exogenous DNA. PPE includes gloves, laboratory coats, face masks, and hair covers. DNA from the examiner, case coordinator, law enforcement officer, or family members could be transferred onto the victim's body during the examination. Limiting who is in the room during the examination not only protects the victim's privacy, it also limits the number of possible sources of contamination. The examiner should wear gloves throughout the entire evidence collection process and should be aware of items in the room that are touched with gloved hands. In order to prevent transfer of DNA from area to area, gloves should be changed when they may have been contaminated or when touching different areas of the victim's body.[1]

As previously described, oral projection of saliva can introduce DNA onto a sample or the body. The examiner should be mindful of this when explaining procedures during the examination. A face mask covering the nose and mouth can prevent this type of contamination. The process of packaging evidence following the examination can be a source of contamination. Following the steps described above during sample packaging may ensure the integrity of evidence.

All evidence must be properly labelled and sealed, protecting it from loss, contamination, or deleterious change. Care should be taken to carefully identify the location on the body from which samples are collected. Documentation of the examination and the assault must be collected. Forensic examination documentation can be included in the kit or provided to the laboratory during evidence submission by law enforcement.[1] Documentation valuable to the forensic laboratory includes:

— Dates and times of assault and examination

— Post-assault activities like bathing, washing, or changing clothes

— Type(s) of assault (eg, penile-vaginal, digital-vaginal, penile-anal, digital-anal, penile-oral)

— Body surfaces sampled for saliva, semen, or epithelial cells (touch DNA)

— For adolescents, consensual contact within 5 days prior to assault and the approximate timeline and type of contact

Once the evidence is collected, the chain of custody begins. Chain of custody documents and tracks the movement of evidence from person to person and location to location. Chain of custody documentation can be handwritten or electronic. The key aspect of the record is that the whereabouts of the evidence are known at all times from time and place of collection to disposal or entry at court. A law enforcement agency will retrieve the sealed evidence from the collection site and maintain the chain of custody.[32]

Serological Laboratory Analysis

Law enforcement will transfer evidence to a crime laboratory for analysis. The crime laboratory may be a publicly funded facility operating at the federal, state, county, or city level, or it may be a private facility. At all facilities the chain of custody will be maintained throughout evidence processing procedures. The evidence (eg, SAK, clothing) submitted to the crime laboratory will be based on that facility's case acceptance procedures. Some laboratories restrict the initial submission to the SAK.[33-35] If testing of the SAK does not establish a biological link to the suspect, additional evidence like clothing and bedding can be submitted. Once the evidence is accepted into the laboratory it will be transferred to the forensic biology section for analysis. Historically, items of evidence submitted in a sexual assault case would initially be tested for body fluid stains such as semen, saliva, and blood. Components of these body fluids are forensically significant (**Table 11-4**). These testing methods involve rudimentary techniques, with little advancement over time. Basic testing principles begin with a presumptive test and, if the presumptive test is positive, a confirmatory test. The characteristics of effective presumptive and confirmatory tests can be seen in **Table 11-5**. A presumptive test should be relatively easy to use and very sensitive. The specificity of the test allows for a narrowing-down of possible sources of the positive reaction but does not identify a substance to the exclusion of all others. A confirmatory test will positively identify a substance. It should be sensitive to the level of the DNA testing methods being employed if it is being used as a screening tool. Both tests should be stable and able to be reproduced.[4] The selection of which presumptive and confirmatory tests are used is based on the laboratory's validated methods.

Table 11-4. The Forensically Significant Components of Body Fluids

Body Fluid	Component	Forensic Use
Semen	Flavins	— ALS (location of stains)
	Acid phosphatase	— Presumptive serology testing
	PSA (P30)	— Presumptive/confirmatory* serology testing
	Spermatozoa	— Confirmatory serology testing — Autosomal DNA testing — Y chromosome DNA testing
Saliva	α-Amylase	— Presumptive serology testing
	Buccal cells	— Autosomal DNA testing — Y chromosome DNA testing
Blood	Red blood cells (hemoglobin)	— Presumptive serology testing — Confirmatory serology testing
	Serum proteins	— Confirmatory serology testing
	White blood cells	— Autosomal DNA testing — Y chromosome DNA testing

**Confirmatory when coupled with other testing*

Table 11-5. Characteristics of Effective Presumptive and Confirmatory Tests

Presumptive Test	Confirmatory Test
— High sensitivity	— Moderate sensitivity
— Low specificity	— High specificity
— Ease of use	— Reproducible
— Nondestructive to evidence	— Legal and scientific acceptance
— Reproducible	
— Legal and scientific acceptance	

Data from Gaensslen RE, ed.[4]

Accredited laboratories must perform validation studies on all tests before they are used on evidence. The conception of new or novel methods requires a developmental validation. The developmental validation is the collection of data to establish the conditions and limitations of the new method.[36] The steps taken to validate a method include determining the new method's sensitivity, robustness, and reproducibility. It will include conducting the test on reference materials and mock evidence, comparing the new method's results to prior testing methods, and assessing factors impacting the new method's results.[37] Internal validation is performed when a laboratory wants to implement an existing method. It includes performing the method using established protocols to confirm that expected results are obtained. On completion of the validation, all laboratory members must undergo training and competency testing using the new method.

Semen

The laboratory will have written protocols for all testing methods used. The serological testing for the presence of semen will begin with a presumptive test. Semen is a heterogeneous mixture of fluid and cells produced by the male reproductive organs. It contains spermatozoa and secretions from the prostate, seminal vesicles, and bulbourethral (Cowper's) glands. The forensically significant constituents of semen persist inside the body for varying lengths of time (**Table 11-6**). Detection of acid phosphatase is a common presumptive test for semen. Acid phosphatase is a component of semen produced by the prostate. Acid phosphatase hydrolyzes phosphate esters at an acidic pH. It is this chemical property that is exploited in the presumptive test. The chemicals used to conduct this test are ortho-dianisidine, sodium acetate, glacial acetic acid, α-naphthyl phosphate disodium salt, and water. In the presence of acid phosphatase the α-naphthyl phosphate will be hydrolyzed into sodium phosphate and α-naphthol. The α-naphthol then couples with the ortho-dianisidine (Brentamine Fast Blue B), producing a purple azo dye (**Figure 11-5**). The deep purple color is indicative of acid phosphatase. Levels of acid phosphatase are 20 to 400 times higher in semen than in other body fluid or tissue sources. Positive reactions are characterized by the deep purple color occurring in less than 30 seconds. Compounds containing amines and phenols can produce a false positive reaction. Oftentimes this reaction will not produce the same color as the seminal acid phosphatase.[4] A positive presumptive test will require additional testing to confirm the presence of the semen. A confirmatory test for the presence of semen is the microscopic identification of spermatozoa. Differential histological stains like kernechtrot and picroindigocarmine dye (KPIC) are used. The kernechtrot stains nuclear material red and picroindigocarmine dye stains all cellular material green. The spermatozoa will have red heads with a very light red to clear acrosomal cap and, if present, a pinkish-green midpiece and green tail (**Figure 11-6-a**).[21] The vaginal epithelial cells will have light red nuclei and green cytoplasm. The sperm heads are approximately 3.5 μm, with the tail being 10 times longer.[22] The diameter of vaginal epithelial cells are approximately ten times larger. The examination is conducted using a compound light microscope. Spermatozoa were first observed microscopically in 1677, and the use of histological stains employed since the nineteenth century.[4] Advancements in this area have involved the use of immunofluorescent stains, which are specific to spermatozoa. A monoclonal mouse anti-human sperm antibody will have a fluorescent label attached. The antibody will bind with a protein in the human spermatozoa head. Using a fluorescent microscope with appropriate filters for the dyes, the spermatozoa heads will fluoresce while the background is blacked out.[23] **Figure 11-6-b** shows sperm visualized using a fluorescent tag. Laser microdissection of individual sperm cells from a slide has been perfected, but STR-DNA testing still requires numerous spermatozoa (20 copies or ~60pg of the DNA at minimum) to yield a profile suitable for comparison.[38] All of the microscopic techniques are laborious and do not lead to the individualization of the semen.

Table 11-6. Persistence of Seminal Components Inside the Body

Body Orifice	Spermatozoa	Acid Phosphatase	Prostate Specific Antigen (P30)A
Vagina (postpubescent)	3 to 7.5 days	1 to 3 days	1 to 2 days
Anal	46 hours	--	--
Oral	6 hours	--	--

Data from Hochmeister MN, Budowle B, Rudin O, et al[5]; Davies A, Wilson E[41]; Willott GM, Allard JE.[42]

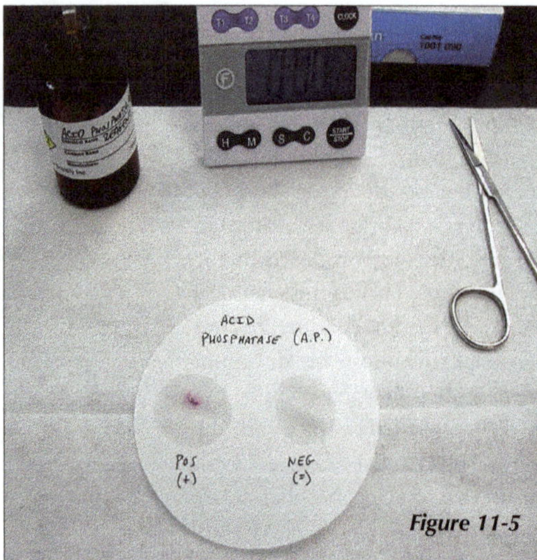

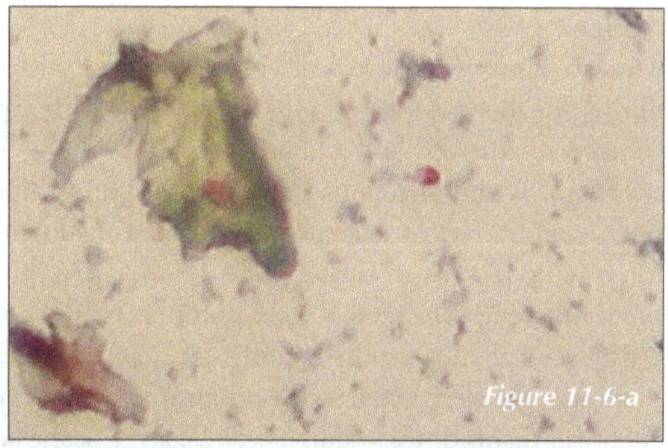

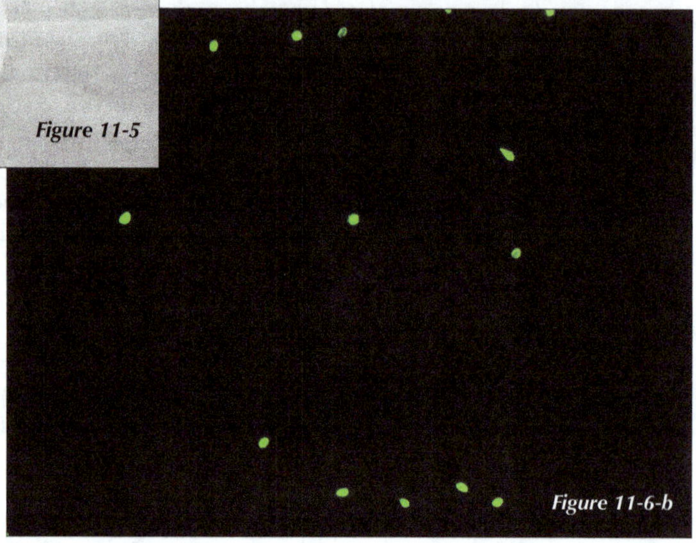

Figure 11-5. *A positive and negative test for acid phosphatase.*

Figure 11-6-a. *A spermatozoa head stained with KPIC.*

Figure 11-6-b. *Spermatozoa visualized with a fluorescent tag.*

Semen may be azoospermic (containing no mature spermatozoa), aspermic (containing no testicular elements), or oligospermic (containing less than the normal amount of spermatozoa).[22] A male may also be vasectomized. Another test exists to detect the presence of semen without spermatozoa. It tests for the presence of prostate-specific antigen (PSA), also known as P30. This glycoprotein is produced in the prostate and was once thought only to be found in semen, postejaculation urine, and the blood of males with prostate cancer. Further research has found PSA in breast milk and other body fluids, though in much lower concentrations than semen.[39] The detection of PSA is based on antigen-antibody reactions. Electrophoretic test methods for the detection of PSA can be performed; however, the rapid and simple immunochromatographic membrane test card can be used. A line in both the T (test) and C (control) zones indicates a positive test (**Figure 11-7**).[5] Due to the presence of PSA in other body fluids, a positive presumptive test for acid phosphatase followed by a positive PSA test result could confirm the presence of semen, depending on the manufacturer of the PSA membrane.[40]

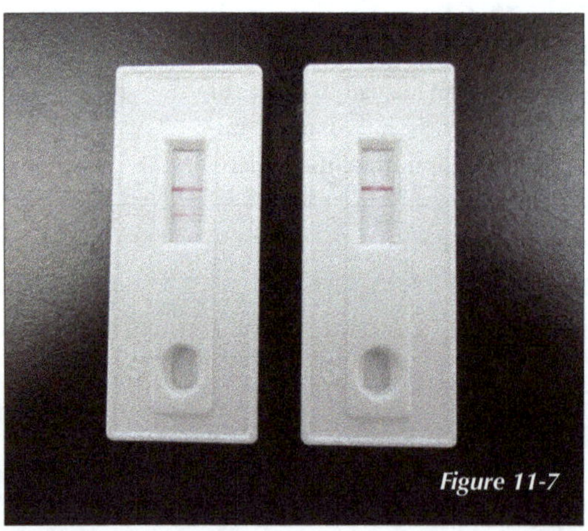

Figure 11-7. *Positive and negative test strip for the presence of prostate-specific antigen (PSA).*

Saliva

Evidence in a sexual assault case can also be tested for the presence of saliva. Saliva is a thin colorless fluid secreted by 3 pairs of glands in the mouth. Saliva can transfer cells from an individual's mouth to surfaces with which it comes into contact. If a perpetrator places his or her mouth on a victim's body or uses saliva as a lubricant, saliva and DNA can be transferred. Unlike semen, there is no serological confirmatory test for the presence of saliva. Saliva lacks a sufficient amount of unique substances for identification. It is primarily made up of water and contains thiocyanate, nitrite, alkaline phosphatase, and α-amylase. The composition of saliva varies between individuals. There are presumptive tests for saliva that test for the presence of α-amylase. Amylases are found in other body fluids, some omnivores (eg, rodents, pigs), and plant sources.[4] Salivary α-amylase is also known as ptyalin. Its purpose is to hydrolyze starches into maltose and dextrin.[43]

The radial diffusion test can be used for the detection of α-amylase. First, an agarose gel is prepared containing starch. The possible saliva sample is added to a well in the gel and incubated for 12 to 24 hours. Following incubation, iodine is added to the gel. The iodine will bind to the starch molecules and the gel will display a dark blue color. If the starch has been hydrolyzed, the iodine cannot bind and the gel will remain clear. Clearing around the sample well indicates a positive reaction (**Figure 11-8**). The size of the circle can indicate the amount of α-amylase in the sample. A negative reaction would be no clearing with only a blue color present (**Figure 11-9**).[44] A similar method wherein the item of evidence is placed in contact with a larger starch-impregnated gel can be used to identify possible saliva stains on articles of clothing.

The Phadebas® test is another method that has been used as a presumptive test for saliva. The test is conducted in a culture tube. It employs a water-insoluble, cross-linked blue starch polymer, which incubates with the possible saliva sample. If α-amylase is present, the polymer will hydrolyze, releasing the blue starch. The appearance of blue color in the tube indicates a positive reaction. The amount of α-amylase activity can be quantified using a spectrometer at 620 nm. A colorless solution indicates a negative reaction.

Immunochromatographic membrane test cards can also be used to test for the presence of α-amylase, functioning like the test card for semen detection. If α-amylase is present it will bind to a dye-labeled mobile antibody and migrate through the card to an immobile antibody. An antibody-antigen-antibody complex is formed, and the

Figure 11-8. Positive results for α-amylase shown by the clearing around each well.

Figure 11-9. Negative results for α-amylase, displaying no clearing of the gel.

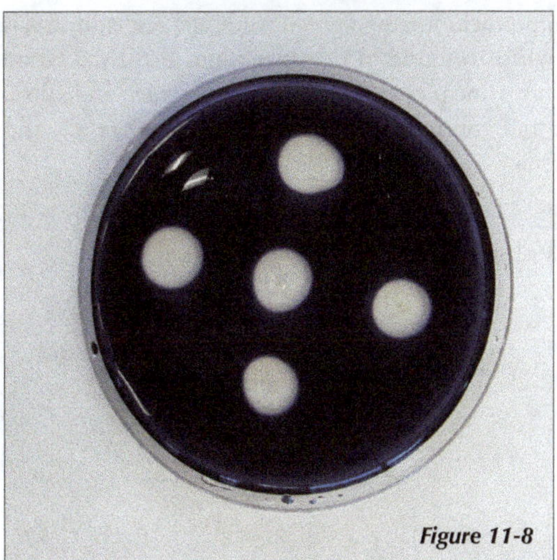

Figure 11-8

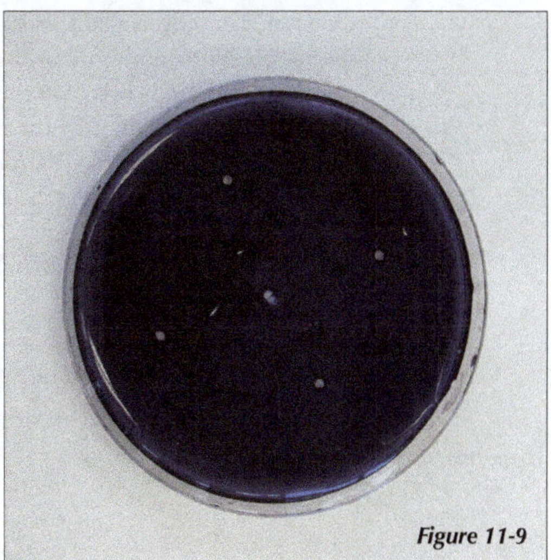

Figure 11-9

accumulation of the dye will be visualized as a line. The unbound, dye-labeled antibody will migrate through the card to a control zone where it will bind to an immobile anti-immunoglobulin antibody and a line will form. This is an internal control that indicates the test card performed as expected. The presences of lines in the test and control zones indicates a positive result.[45]

All of the testing methods described in this section will indicate the presence of amylase, which is found in saliva, other body fluids, and other biological and commercial substances. Fecal matter contains high levels of α-amylase produced in the pancreas. Therefore, it should be noted that a positive result only indicates the *possible* presence of saliva.

Blood and Hair

The presence of blood in a sexual assault case could be due to injury or menstruation. In cases involving female adolescents, serological testing for the presence of blood on swabs from the body or the underwear cannot distinguish between menstrual and nonmenstrual blood. The presence of blood in a prepubescent child's genital swabs or underwear could corroborate assault. Both presumptive and confirmatory tests exist for testing blood. The development of serological blood tests dates back to the nineteenth century. Many presumptive methods for detecting blood are catalytic tests that exploit the peroxidase-like activity of hemoglobin. Hemoglobin and many of its derivatives will catalyze the oxidation of substances in the presence of hydrogen peroxide.[4] The basic formula for the chemical reaction can be seen in **Figure 11-10**. The phenolphthalin test was first developed in 1901 and 1903 by scientists Kastle and Meyer, respectively. This test is also known as the Kastle-Meyer test and is still in use.[46,47] Phenolphthalein is a pink substance in an alkaline solution. In its reduced state, phenolphthalin, it is colorless. When blood is present at a detectable level, the hemoglobin will catalyze hydrogen peroxide breakdown, and the colorless reduced phenolphthalin will be oxidized, resulting in the pink phenolphthalein. An immediate pink color indicates a positive reaction. No color change indicates a negative reaction. As with most colorimetric assays, the timeframe of the color change is relevant, because the substances sought in the detection only catalyze the reactions that would naturally occur given sufficient time. There are some false positives like chemical oxidants and metal catalysts; however, adding the test solutions in a multistep approach can aid in the identification of chemical oxidants. These substances will drive the redox reaction without the addition of hydrogen peroxide.[4] Confirmatory tests for blood can be immunological. One test currently available is an immunochromatographic membrane test card that is specific for human glycophorin A, which is found in the membrane of the red blood cell. This test card is based on the same principles as the test cards for semen and saliva. The appearance of lines in the test and control zones indicates a positive result, and a line only in the control zone indicates a negative result.[48]

The Basic Peroxidase-Mediated Oxidation-Reduction Formula

$$\underset{\text{(Reduced)}}{AH_2} + H_2O_2 \xrightarrow{\text{Peroxidase}} \underset{\text{(Oxidized)}}{A} + 2H_2O$$

Figure 11-10

Figure 11-10. *The basic peroxidase-mediated oxidation reduction formula.*

Pubic hair combings and hair recovered from the genitals of prepubescent children can be examined to assess suitability for DNA testing. The hair will be evaluated to determine if it is human and its phase of growth. There are 3 growth phases of hair: anagen, catagen, and telogen. The anagen phase is the active growth phase (**Figure 11-11**). Hair in this phase is more likely to be left behind if forcibly pulled. Telogen hairs are in the resting phase. These are hairs that are naturally shed from the body in an ongoing fashion. A telogen hair has a club-shaped root (**Figure 11-12**). When a hair is transitioning from the growth phase to the resting phase, it is in the catagen phase.[49] Nuclear DNA is found in the hair root and mitochondrial DNA in the hair shaft. Nuclear DNA remnants may also be found in the hair shafts. The roots of hair in anagen and catagen phases often contain a sufficient amount of nuclear DNA for detection and typing. These hairs are suitable for DNA testing. Hair roots in the telogen phase may or may not be suitable for nuclear DNA testing. It will depend on how much adhering cellular material is associated with the root. A study of 3 forms of telogen hairs found that the types of cells found on these roots were non-nucleated epithelial cells and nucleated epithelial cells, along with keratinized remnant follicle and trichilemmal keratin. One form of a telogen hair is a root without tissue associated with it, as seen in **Figure 11-12**. This form would not be suitable for nuclear DNA testing. Another is an enlarged club with a germinal nipple attached at the end. The enlarged club is made up of keratinized remnant follicle, which is non-nucleated, and trichilemmal keratin. The germinal nipple consists of trichilemmal keratin, and nuclear material is not present. The third is a club with tissue adhering above or below the root. The tissue is most often seen above the club and consists of both nucleated and non-nucleated epidermal cells. This form of telogen root would be suitable for nuclear DNA testing.[50]

A study to assess if telogen hair, regardless of form, contained a sufficient amount of nuclear DNA to obtain results demonstrated that 66.9% of 510 hairs tested from 60 individuals contained 0.1ng to greater than 0.55ng of nuclear DNA.[51] This DNA was found to be degraded, due to the keratinization process. Degraded DNA is characterized by shortening of the DNA strand. Due to the level of degradation, only partial DNA results were obtained for the majority of the tested samples. Nine hairs quantified with a high concentration of DNA (0.025ng/ul) when extracted. The DNA testing of these hairs produced partial results at 9 of 12 loci tested. Overall, very low amounts of nuclear DNA were obtained from telogen hairs. More recent research has identified remnants of incomplete removal from hair corneocytes as the source of the nuclear DNA. The use of in-situ labeling of DNA fragments using DNA-specific dye Hoechst 33258 has shown that the number of nuclear fragments found in the hair shaft varies greatly between individuals. The number of fragments detected is also directly related to the amount of DNA quantified and detected.[52] This research suggests a new tool to assess a telogen hair for potential nuclear DNA analysis. However, the degradation of the nuclear DNA in the remnant will always limit the results obtained. Telogen hairs without cellular material may be recommended for mitochondrial DNA testing.

Figure 11-11. *A human anagen hair.*

Figure 11-12. *A human hair root in the telogen phase.*

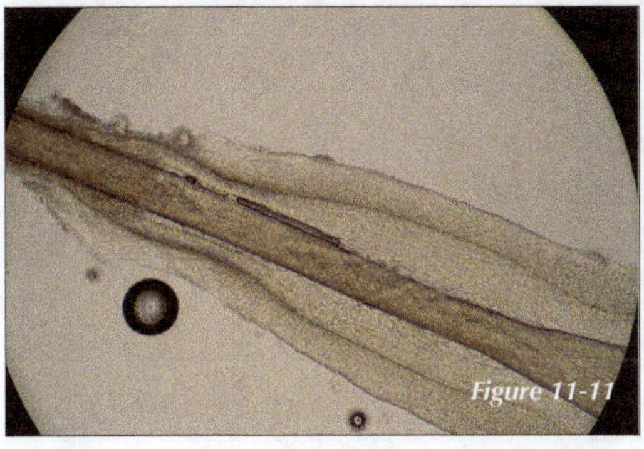

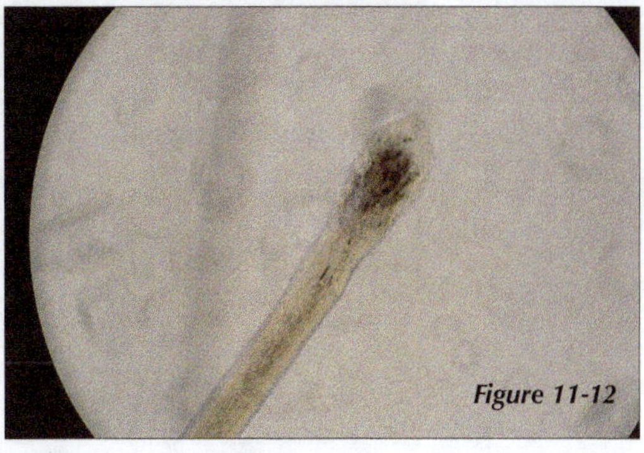

Evidence Testing Triage

The first items tested in any sexual assault case include swabs from the body and underwear. Serological analysis of the swabs will often be based on type of swab and case information provided. Swabs from the genitals should be screened for semen and possibly saliva. Internal orifice swabs that are presumptively tested and negative for semen should still undergo a microscopic examination. As listed in **Table 11-6**, spermatozoa persist much longer in the body than acid phosphatase. The presence of spermatozoa, even in the absence of a positive presumptive test confirms the presence of semen. Other body swabs may be screened or directly sampled for DNA testing. In the laboratory, an ALS is used as an aid in locating possible semen stains on clothing and bedding. Stains located using the ALS would undergo presumptive testing and, if positive, confirmatory testing. Semen stains that have been deposited outside of the body might not incur degradation of the proteins of interest (acid phosphatase and PSA) as would occur inside of the body. In order to conduct these tests, a small cutting is taken from the swab or material. Clothing items or other textiles with numerous stains can also be screened using a mapping technique verses testing individual stains.[53]

The serological testing process can be laborious and consume valuable quantities of potential DNA evidence. The confirmation of a body fluid may be helpful in a case of child sexual assault, as consensual sexual encounters are not a reasonable explanation for its presence. However, identifying the person who is the source of the body fluid will aid in the investigation, arrest, and prosecution of the crime. The results of serological testing cannot be used to identify an individual. The determination whether to conduct serological testing will be based on a laboratory's standard operating procedures.

Untested Sexual Assault Kits

In 2011, the National Institute of Justice published a report regarding untested SAKs that were being discovered across the Nation and how to go about testing them.[54] Subjecting samples from an SAK to targeted testing known as direct to DNA is one approach to increase testing efficiency and promote high-throughput processing. The standardized SAK sample type, a swab, lends itself to this approach.[55] This procedure screens SAK samples for the presence of male DNA and only forwards for additional testing those demonstrating a sufficient amount. It is effective in cases where the victim is female and the suspect is male. This is the case in the majority of the sexual assaults for both juveniles and adults. For all juveniles, 82% of reported assaults involved female victims and 94% involved male offenders (**Table 11-7**).[8] The direct-to-DNA process alleviates the need to screen the items in the SAK for any body fluids. The samples are screened by quantitation. If needed for prosecution or investigation, testing for the

Table 11-7. Juvenile Victim and Offender Genders for Reported Assaults

Victim Age	Female Victim	Male Offender
Victim: < 6 years old	69%	88%
Victim: 6 to 12 years old	75%	94%
Victim: 12 to 17 years old	91%	97%
Overall	82%	96%

Data from Snyder HN.[8]

presence of semen can be conducted at a later time, if samples remain. For the small number of remaining cases involving male victims, or when the suspect is a female, some samples such as penile, breast, and neck swabs can be processed using a direct-to-DNA approach with samples not being screened during quantitation. Other items in the SAK, like anal swabs and underwear, may undergo serological testing.

Forensic DNA Testing Procedure

The DNA molecule and the information it holds has been used as a forensic tool in the United States since the late 1980s.[56,57] Since that time, many advancements and improvements have been made in forensic DNA processes. DNA testing is used to identify individuals who may have left a body fluid or cellular material at a crime scene. The DNA molecule is the basic information carrier for all living things. The structure of the molecule is a double helix composed of sugar and phosphate backbones with nitrogenous bases forming hydrogen bonds in the center, joining the 2 strands. Each nucleotide consists of 1 of 4 nitrogenous bases—adenine (A), thymine (T), guanine (G), or cytosine (C)—bound to a sugar-phosphate molecule. Complementary base-pairing dictates that A binds with T and G with C. The sequence of the nucleotides determines the species of the living thing as well as unique characteristics. Human beings have approximately 3 billion pairs of bases, and only 0.1% of the bases are different from one another. DNA is bundled into structures known as chromosomes. There are 22 pairs of autosomal chromosomes and a single pair of sex-determining chromosomes (X,X or X,Y). A person inherits his DNA from his parents, receiving one set of chromosomes from the mother and the other set from the father. Only identical twins share the same genetic information which would result in the same STR-DNA profile. One copy of the DNA is found in the cell's nucleus.[58] Semen, saliva, epithelial cells, hair, and blood may be the source of DNA in sexual assault cases.

DNA Extraction

DNA testing is a multi-step process. The first step is to extract the DNA from the dried stain. There are many methods for extracting DNA. The first method used in forensic science and still in use today is an organic extraction using phenol/chloroform/isoamyl alcohol (PCI). The process begins with adding stain extraction buffer [tris(hydroxymethyl) aminomethane, sodium chloride, sodium dodecyl sulfate, and ethylenediaminetetraacetic acid] and proteinase K. The chemicals will lyse the cells, denaturing proteins and releasing the DNA into the solution. The PCI is used to isolate and purify the DNA. The result of this extraction protocol is double-stranded DNA in a buffered solution. The PCI extraction technique is laborious and the chemical is a health hazard that requires the method to be performed in a safety hood.[59] A simpler extraction method was developed and uses Chelex 100® chelating resin. The Chelex suspension is added to the sample, incubated, and then boiled. The high temperature disrupts the cell membrane and denatures the DNA. The resin will chelate metal ions, required as cofactors for nucleases, which can degrade the DNA.[60] In addition to exogenous nucleases, the cell itself contains nucleases in the cytoplasm, which could damage the DNA if activated. This method is easy to perform and rapid, but the resulting pH of the solution is a harsh environment, and potential PCR inhibitors, dirt, and cellular debris all remain in solution with the freed DNA. The DNA is in a single-stranded form following this technique.

The need to perform extractions of larger numbers of samples containing smaller quantities of DNA has led to the development of automated extraction procedures. Vendors have developed instruments that can extract and purify small amounts of DNA with little examiner interaction. The automated instruments use paramagnetic, silica-coated beads to bind the DNA and wash away inhibitors and cellular debris. The DNA is then eluted from the beads into a buffer for further processing.[61,62] The endpoint is a more purified and thus protected DNA sample in solution. **Figure 11-13** is one instrument available for automated DNA extraction. Manual methods using this same technology preceded their automation and may still be used in some laboratories.

The samples from an SAK may contain spermatozoa and epithelial cells from the victim and offender. Mixed DNA profiles can be difficult to interpret. There are several techniques to separate spermatozoa DNA from epithelial cell DNA. These include differential lysis; selective degradation; and less commonly, laser microdissection, membrane filtration and microdevices, and flow cytometry. Laser microdissection removes and collects spermatozoa from mixed samples. This is a physical separation of the cells by visualizing them on a microscope slide and then dissecting them from the surrounding material.[63] Membrane filtration uses the differences in the cells' size and shape to separate the different cell types.[64] Flow cytometry is another physical separation process that uses specific membrane proteins to mark and sort cells. Most forensic laboratories use differential lysis. The differential process uses chemicals to lyse the epithelial cells' membranes, remove that DNA, and use stronger chemicals to lyse the spermatozoa cells' membranes.[65,66] The sample undergoes a series of centrifugation and wash steps in an effort to separate cell types. The last technique, selective degradation, is similar to differential lysis; however, following the removal of the epithelial cell DNA sample, the enzyme DNase is used to remove any DNA not contained in the spermatozoa heads. The DNase is then deactivated and spermatozoa lysis can occur. This procedure eliminates additional centrifugation and washes steps required in the differential lysis process.[67] All of these techniques require numerous manipulations by the examiner. The differential lysis technique has been automated, resulting in reduced examiner processing time and more consistent results. The instrument performs the separation and lysis portions of the protocol by automating pipetting and centrifugation.[68] Following extraction, the samples are ready for quantification.

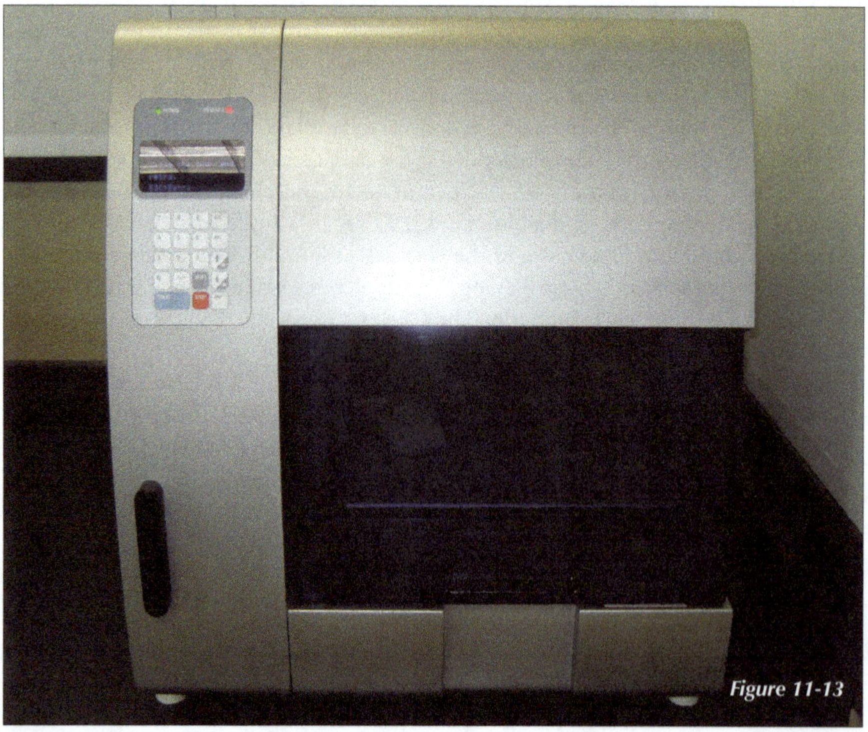

Figure 11-13. *An automated DNA extraction instrument.*

Polymerase Chain Reaction/Amplification

Polymerase chain reaction (PCR) was developed in 1985, and its inventor received the Nobel Prize in Chemistry in 1993. The simple temperature-driven steps of the PCR are an in-vitro DNA replication process. The template DNA along with the following components are required for the PCR to occur: deoxynucleotide triphosphates (dNTPs), which are used to build the new strand; a thermostable DNA polymerase, which uses the dNTPs to synthesize DNA; 3' (reverse) and 5' (forward) primers, which identify where the synthesis will begin; and buffers, salts, and chemicals, which maintain the optimum environment for replication to occur. The PCR consists of 3 steps to complete 1 cycle:

1. The sample is heated to nearly 100° C, denaturing the double-stranded DNA.
2. The temperature is lowered, allowing the primers to anneal to the single-stranded DNA.
3. A slight temperature increase occurs, which promotes the addition of the dNTPs by the DNA polymerase, synthesizing the DNA strand.

These 3 steps are repeated for 28 to 34 cycles, depending on the protocol being used. The number of strands of DNA will increase exponentially with each cycle (**Figure 11-14**). The primers will isolate and replicate specific loci of interest on the DNA molecule. Current forensic STR-DNA testing techniques use the primers to visualize the DNA. A fluorescent dye is bound to the forward primer. This process is optimized to function with a specific quantity of input template DNA.[69] The amplified product from the PCR is detected once the cycles have been completed, unless utilizing real-time detection. PCR is the basis of multiple steps in the DNA analysis process.

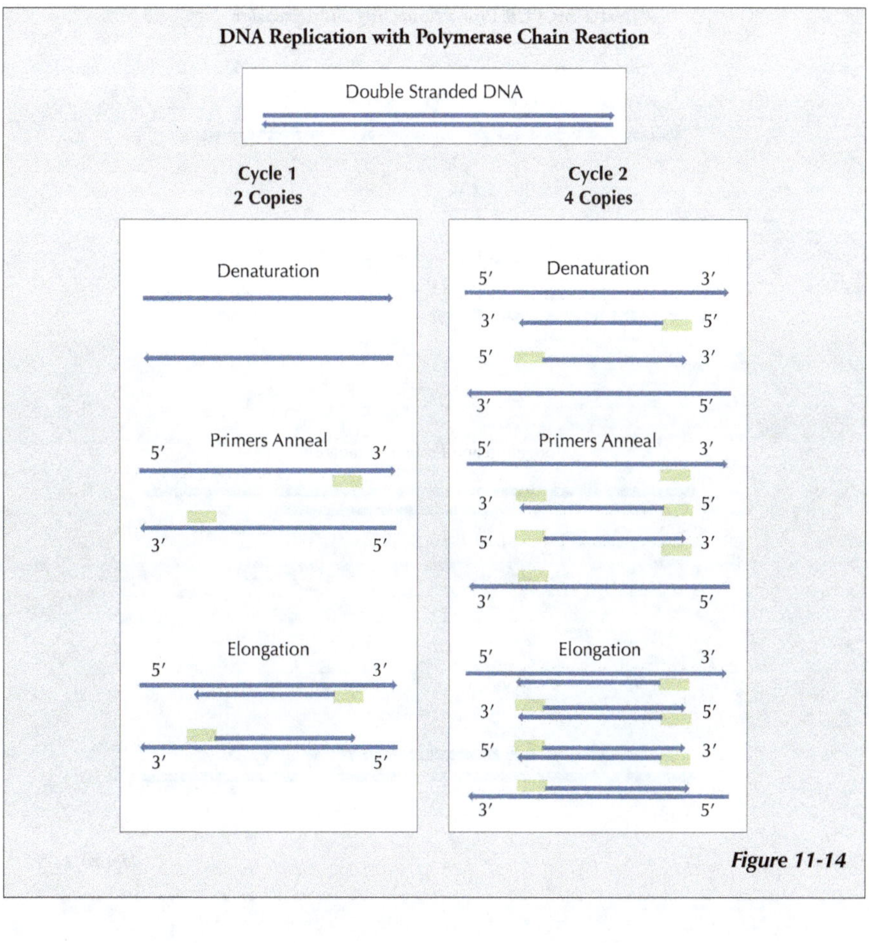

Figure 11-14. DNA replication with the polymerase chain reaction.

DNA Quantification

Quantitation of human DNA samples is necessary to optimize the amplification process. Quantitative real-time polymerase chain reaction (qPCR) is the most commonly used quantitation process. The basis of this technique is PCR. During qPCR, the quantity of DNA being synthesized during each cycle is captured in real time. Commercially available assays have been designed for the simultaneous detection of targets used to predict total human and human male-specific DNA amounts in samples.[70,71] The assays either capture the increase or decrease in fluorescence as the amplified product accumulates. The method employing an increase in fluorescence uses a probe with a fluorophore attached to the 5' end and a quencher dye at the 3' end. The presence of the quencher dye prevents fluorescence. During the annealing step of the PCR, the probe will attach within the region being copied along with the primers. As the DNA is synthesized during elongation, the DNA polymerase cleaves the probe, causing the fluorophore and quencher to separate (**Figure 11-15**). Once separated, the fluorophore's signal is detected. As the number of degraded probes increases, fluorescence intensifies.[71] The assay detecting the loss of signal uses the same quencher-fluorophore mechanism. The fluorophore is attached to a modified nucleotide during elongation. The quencher is bound to the complementary modified nucleotide. As the cycles proceed and elongation occurs, the modified nucleotides are incorporated into the new DNA strands. Once the double-stranded DNA is formed, the fluorescent signal will be quenched. During each cycle the amount of free fluorophore-labeled nucleotides will decrease.[70]

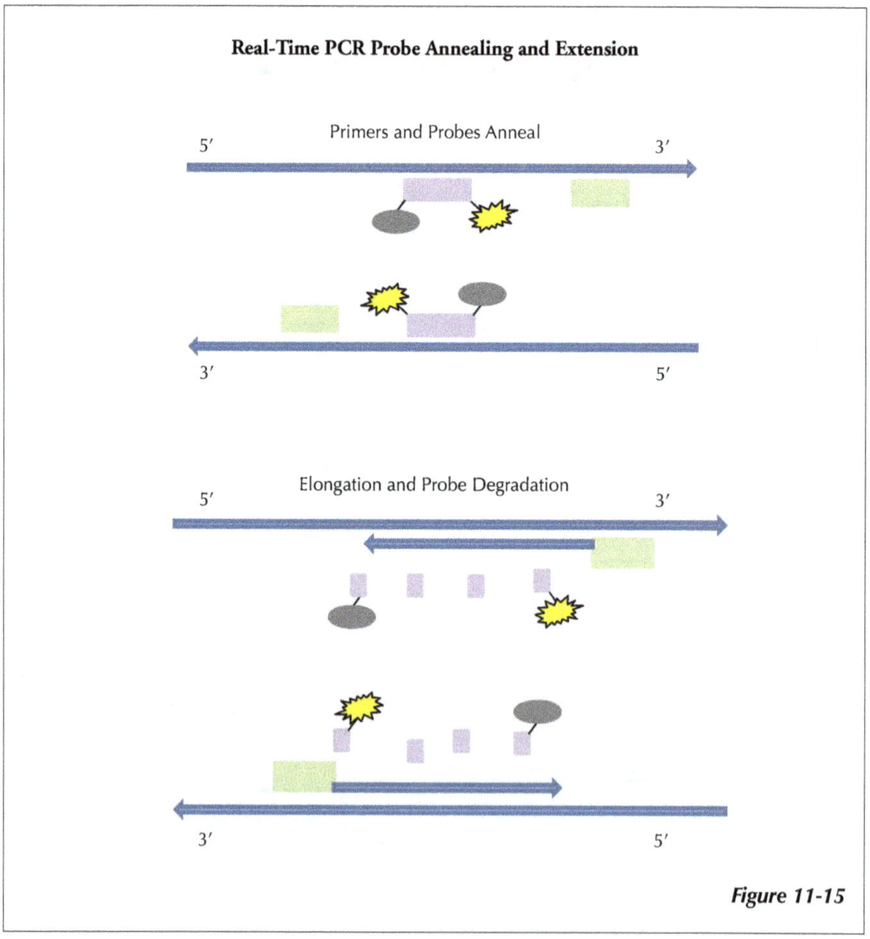

Figure 11-15. *Real-time PCR probe annealing and extension.*

Interpretation of Quantitation Results

The results of the qPCR is an estimation of the total amount of human DNA and the total human male-specific DNA in a sample in nanograms per microliter. The results can be used to create a ratio of the total human DNA to male DNA in the sample, or the ratio of female DNA to male DNA present. These results can then be used to evaluate SAK samples. **Table 11-8** shows possible quantitation results for SAK samples. There are 2 types of assaults represented: (1) a vaginal assault and (2) a vaginal-oral assault. The samples processed when following a direct-to-DNA protocol (female victim and male offender) require any sample that may potentially contain semen be extracted using some type of differential process. The Quality Assurance Standards for Forensic

Table 11-8. Examples of qPCR Results for SAK Samples

Penile-Vaginal Assault	[Auto] ng/ul	[Y] ng/ul	Male:Female
Vaginal swabs (sperm fraction)	0.0623	0.0050	1:11.46
Vaginal swabs (epithelial fraction)	7.3635	0.0000	
External genital swabs (sperm fraction)	0.0188	0.0112	
External genital swabs (epithelial fraction)	2.3179	0.0000	
Underwear (sperm fraction)	0.0160	0.0125	
Underwear (epithelial fraction)	0.3233	0.0001	1:3232
Reagent blank (sperm fraction)	0.0000	0.0000	
Reagent blank (epithelial fraction)	0.0000	0.0000	
Breast swabs	1.0325	0.0099	1:103.3
Neck swabs	0.9921	0.0085	1:115.1
Reagent blank	0.0000	0.0000	
Oral Assault			
Vaginal swabs (sperm fraction)	0.0015	0.0001	1:14
Vaginal swabs (epithelial fraction)	0.9874	0.0003	1:3290.3
External genital swabs (sperm fraction)	0.0028	0.0000	
External genital swabs (epithelial fraction)	0.2742	0.0058	1:46.2
Underwear (sperm fraction)	0.0670	0.0000	
Underwear (epithelial fraction)	4.4003	0.3066	1:13.4
Reagent blank (sperm fraction)	0.0001	0.0000	
Reagent blank (epithelial fraction)	0.0000	0.0000	
Breast swabs	1.0235	0.0226	1:44.2
Neck swabs	0.0054	0.0015	1:2.58
Reagent blank	0.0000	0.0000	

DNA testing laboratories, as issued by the Director of the FBI, requires an accredited laboratory possess and follow a technique for the differential extraction of samples suspected of containing semen.[72] Body orifices would be treated in this manner even when no penile penetration has been reported, because juveniles may not articulate exactly what occurred or may have been incapacitated with alcohol or drugs. Samples collected that may not represent semen may be tested using a nondifferential procedure. This would include samples of possible saliva or touch DNA. The quantitation results can then be evaluated to determine if any samples will proceed with additional testing. The laboratory will identify through validation studies cut-off values and ratios for anticipating interpretable results from the male donor.

The qPCR results for the SAK collected in the example penile-vaginal assault theoretically indicate male DNA in all of the spermatozoa cell portions of the differential extractions, as well as the breast and neck swabs, and a trace amount in the underwear epithelial cell portion. The ratio of female to male DNA is extremely high for the underwear sample and the breast and neck swabs. Due to the ratio, these samples would not undergo further processing at this time. The amplification PCR process which follows is a competition of sorts, wherein the DNA from a donor present at a given amount versus a lesser donor would win and ultimately mask the presence of the lesser donor. The vaginal, cervical, and underwear spermatozoa cell fractions all demonstrate results consistent with a sufficient amount of male DNA and very little to no female DNA. A laboratory may proceed with the testing of all of these samples or select a portion of the positive samples to continue testing depending on the circumstances surrounding the case. If there were multiple offenders or an unknown number of offenders, then more samples may be processed. If an adolescent of consenting age had a consensual encounter within 5 days before the assault, this may be considered when determining which samples to process. The paperwork associated with the SAK should contain information that will assist the laboratory in making analysis triage determinations.

For the oral assault example, the results indicate that all of the spermatozoa cell fractions contained no male DNA except the vaginal swabs, which contained a trace amount. The epithelial cell fraction of the vaginal swabs also contained a minimal amount of male DNA, along with an extremely high ratio of female DNA to male DNA. All of these samples would be dropped for further testing. The epithelial cell fractions, where DNA would typically be found in an oral assault, and the breast and neck swabs demonstrate male DNA. The ratios for some of these samples are elevated. Similar to the previous example, those positive samples would be evaluated based on the specifics surrounding the case, like number of perpetrators and post-assault activities. Laboratories will establish triaging protocols for assessing the quantitation results for samples in the SAK when using a direct-to-DNA approach. This protocol will be used to determine which samples will progress to the next step of the DNA process.[55]

Autosomal Short Tandem Repeat Multiplex

The next step in the DNA process following quantitation is amplification using PCR. The purpose of this PCR is to replicate the specific loci used to obtain a DNA profile. Attempts will be made to obtain a DNA profile from the evidence that can be compared to the DNA profile from the known reference samples from the victim and suspect. The qPCR results (in ng/µl) will be used to determine the volume of an extracted sample to add to the reaction. PCR has an optimum range of input template DNA. This amount will be based on the developmental and internal validation studies but will generally be between 0.5 to 1.5 ng.

Short tandem repeats (STRs) are the standard type of DNA loci examined in forensic biology. STRs are small fragments of DNA consisting of 2-7 base pairs. The fragments then repeat in tandem a varying number of times between individuals. The number of times the fragment repeats will be the allele designation for the locus and is expressed as a number. Most of the STR loci used in forensic DNA testing are tetranucleotides (4 base fragments). The small sizes of the STR loci make them amendable to multiplexing and use on degraded DNA.[7,69] In the United States, a core of 20 STR loci has been established, which includes the original 13 CODIS core loci (**Table 11-9**). There are a number of commercially available amplification kits that contain the minimum core loci, along with some others (**Table 11-10**).[6,73,74] These test kits allow for the simultaneous amplification of all core loci. The PCR process occurs in a thermal cycler (**Figure 11-16**). This instrument will rapidly heat and cool the samples driving the PCR process. As previously described, the forward primer used in the reaction is labeled with a fluorophore. In order to easily visualize and analyze the results for all of the loci, multiple fluorophores are used in each test kit. Following the PCR, samples will be placed on a capillary electrophoresis instrument.

Table 11-9. The CODIS Core Loci (Effective January 1, 2017)

— CSF1PO*	— D3S1358*	— D16S539*	— D2S1338
— FGA*	— D5S818*	— D18S51*	— D10S1248
— THO1*	— D7S820*	— D21S11*	— D12S391
— TPOX*	— D8S1179*	— D1S1656	— D19S433
— VWA*	— D13S317*	— D2S441	— D22S1045

**CODIS Core Loci October 1998 to December 31, 2016. Data from Federal Bureau of Investigations.*[74]

Table 11-10. Commercially Available Amplification Kits Containing the 20 CODIS Core Loci

— AB GlobalFiler™ Express

— AB GlobalFiler™

— Promega PowerPlex® Fusion

— Promega PowerPlex® Fusion 6C

— QIAGEN Investigator 24plex QS

— QIAGEN Investigator 24plex GO!

Data from Federal Bureau of Investigation.[74]

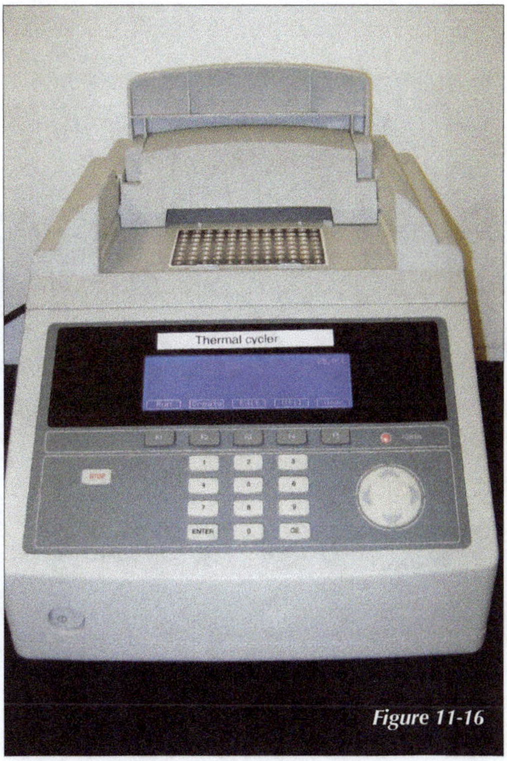

Figure 11-16. *A thermal cycler used to perform the polymerase chain reaction.*

DNA Detection

Capillary electrophoresis is the separation of particles by size using an electrical charge inside of a capillary that contains some type of medium. The DNA fragments will be denatured following PCR and have a negative charge. As the DNA molecules move through the capillary, the different fragments (amplicons) are separated by size (**Figure 11-17**). Fragments of similar size representing different loci will have different fluorescent dyes attached. There is a detection window in the capillary, and as the fragments move past the window, a laser will excite the dye, resulting in a fluorescent signal captured by the instrument and converted into a digital image called an electropherogram. The electropherogram displays the DNA profile (**Figure 11-18-a**). The fragments of DNA are represented by peaks on the plot. The height of a peak is loosely proportional to the amount of DNA in the sample in terms of relative florescence units (RFU).[69] For each locus, an individual will normally have either a single peak (homozygote), with each chromosome having the same allele, or two peaks (heterozygote), with each chromosome having a different allele. The sister alleles in the heterozygous profile will have similar peak heights. During validation studies, a laboratory will establish a minimum analytical threshold.[72] This threshold represents a cut-off for interpreting a peak as DNA versus being potential background noise or unreliable signal. A stochastic threshold may also be established. This threshold is higher than the analytical threshold and is the cut-off for interpreting a single DNA peak as a homozygote genotype versus a heterozygous result, from which the sister allele is missing. Mixtures are identified by more than 2 peaks at multiple loci and loci with 2 alleles that are not balanced (**Figure 11-18-b**).[75] Amelogenin is a gender marker included with the core loci. DNA from a male will have two peaks—an X and Y—and a female will only have a single peak representing the XX. DNA profiles are generated for the samples from the SAK and the known reference samples (buccal swabs).

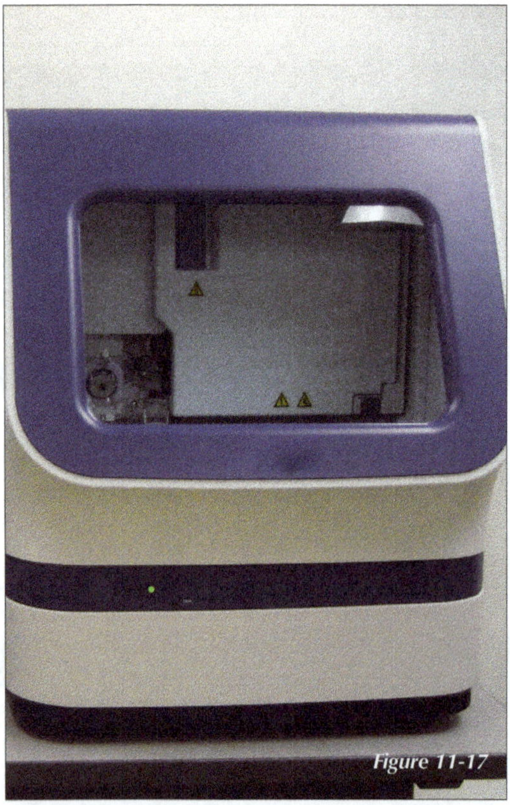

Figure 11-17. *A capillary electrophoresis instrument.*

DNA Conclusions

Following the interpretation of DNA results and the determination of the profiles, comparisons are made. The following conclusions are possible when making comparisons: match/inclusion, exclusion, or no determination/inconclusive. The term "match" is sometimes used for single DNA donor samples. It indicates the DNA profile on the evidence is the same as the profile of the known reference. "Inclusion" can be used for comparison to single-source or mixed samples. The term used when there is a positive association will be based on a laboratory's protocols. An "exclusion" means the individual's DNA profile could not be the source of the results. The term "no determination"/"inconclusive" can be used for comparisons of known reference profiles to mixed DNA profiles.

If the results for the sample are incomplete or there is DNA from too many donors, it may not be possible to draw a conclusion.[58,75] The samples in an SAK will often contain DNA from more than 1 individual because the samples have been collected from an individual's body. The victim, offender, and when applicable, the consensual partner are typical sources of DNA. It can be challenging to

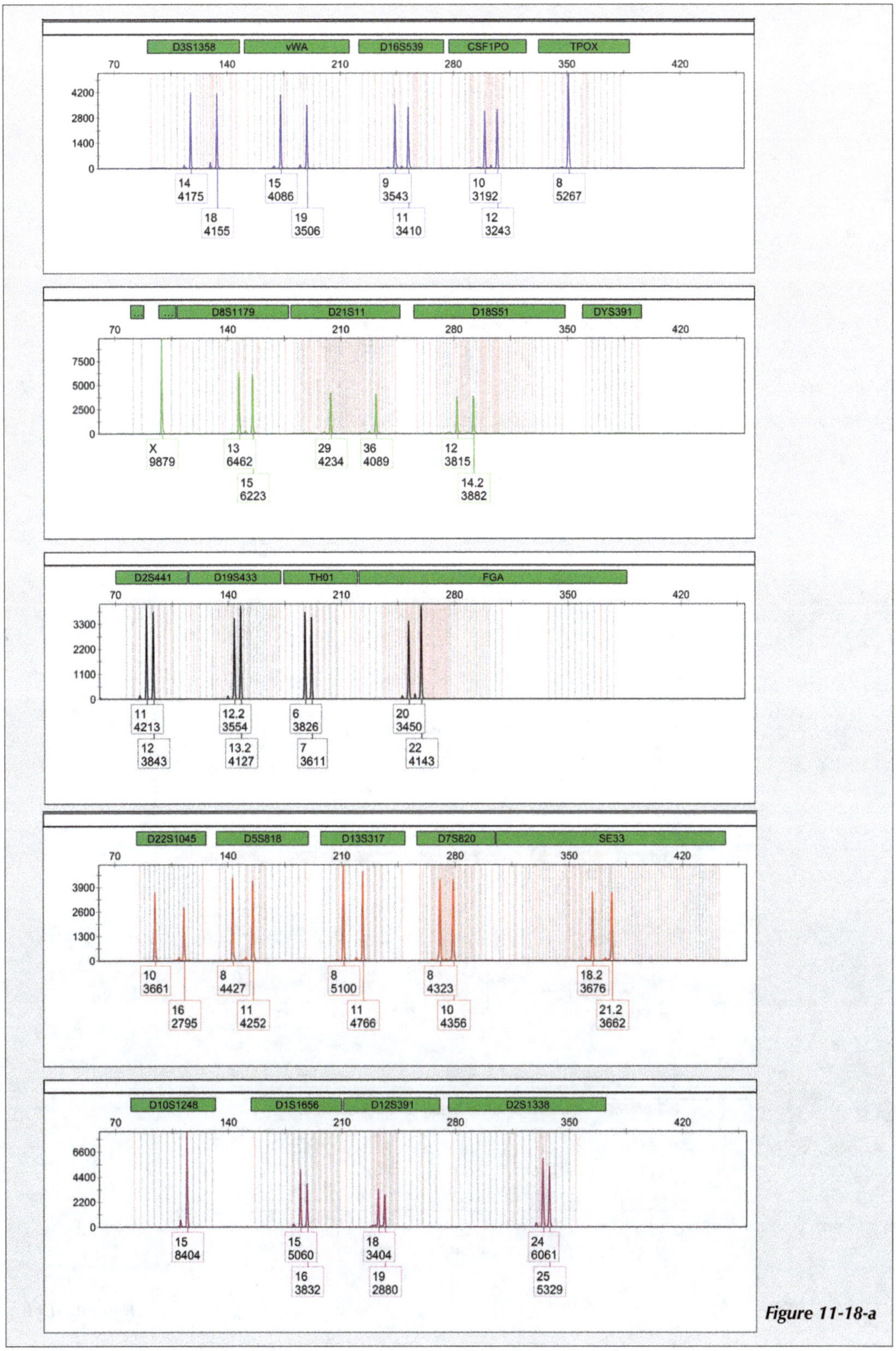

Figure 11-18-a. *An electropherogram for a single DNA donor.*

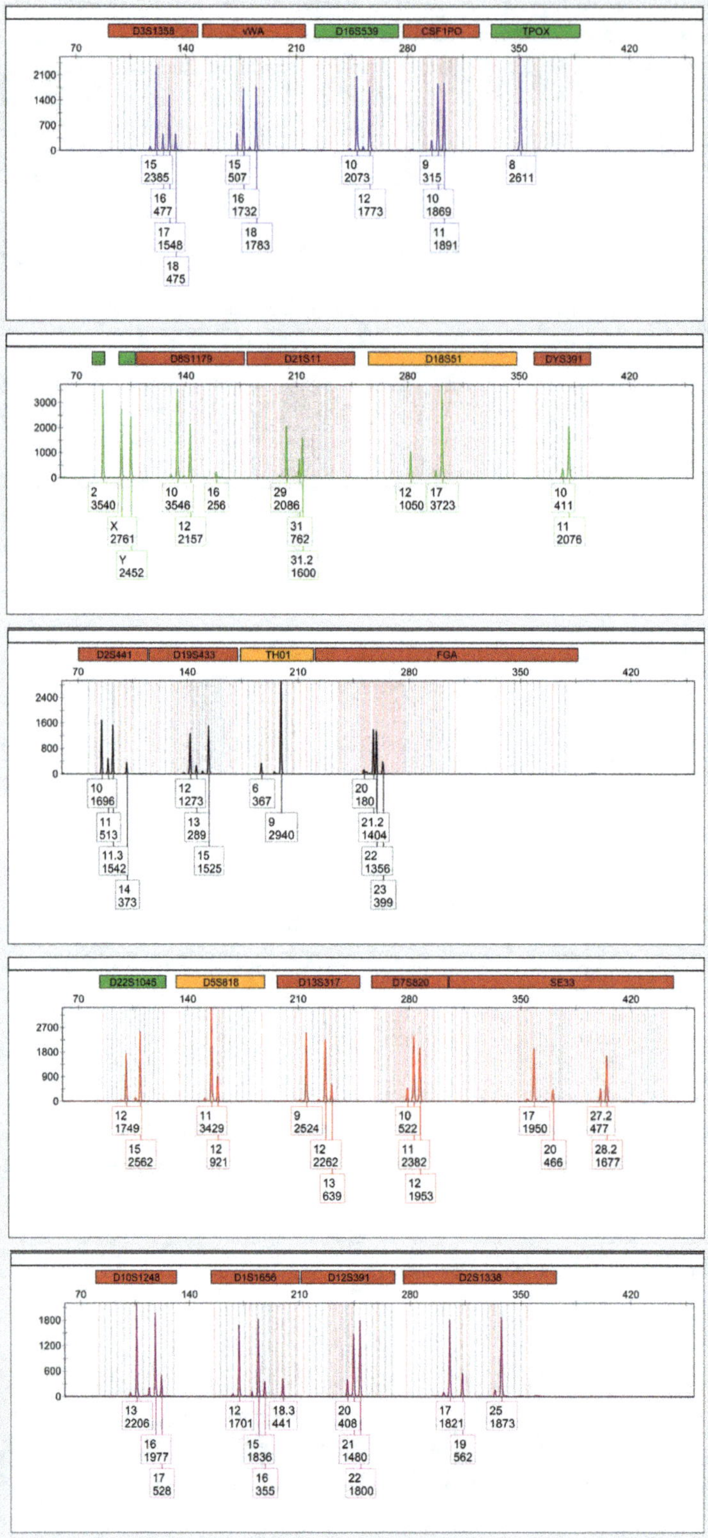

Figure 11-18-b

Figure 11-18-b. An electropherogram from a mixture of 2 DNA donors.

interpret mixtures; however, using DNA profiles from individuals who are expected to have DNA present can aid in identifying DNA foreign to that person.[75] Additionally, use of probabilistic genotyping software to aid in the interpretation of mixtures is gaining widespread use in the United States, with many laboratories in the process of implementing this type of software on evidence.[76] This software use biological modeling, statistical theory, and computer algorithms to determine which genotypes will best fit the data. It can also calculate likelihood ratios for the comparison of known references to the DNA results.[12,13] A statistical weight must be reported with positive associations, which can be a likelihood ratio, random match probability, or combined probability of inclusion or exclusion. A likelihood ratio will compare 2 propositions to see which is more likely (**Figure 11-19**). The numerator can be referred to as the "prosecution" hypothesis and the denominator would be the "defense" hypothesis. A number greater than 1 would favor the "prosecution" hypothesis. The larger the value the more the hypothesis is favored. A number less than 1 would favor the "defense" hypothesis.

The random match probability (RMP) is most often used for single-source DNA profiles. It represents the frequency of occurrence of the DNA profile in the general population, or the probability of selecting an unrelated individual at random from the population and that individual matching the DNA profile. A modified RMP can be used for mixture when the number of DNA donors is known. The combined probability of inclusion (CPI) is used for mixed DNA profiles. It is the probability of selecting an unrelated individual at random from the population and having his or her DNA profile included in the mixture. It includes the probabilities for all the possible genotypes represented in the mixed DNA profile. The probability of exclusion is the probability that a randomly selected unrelated individual would be excluded from the mixture.[75] A foreign DNA profile obtained from the body swabs of a sexual assault victim establishes a positive association between those individuals. As part of the case analysis, the DNA profile belonging to the putative perpetrator would be entered into CODIS.

Combined DNA Index System

The Combined DNA Index System (CODIS) is computer software created in 1990 at the direction of the Federal Bureau of Investigation. It consists of DNA profiles from forensic casework samples, qualifying offenders, missing persons, unidentified persons or remains, relatives of missing persons, and profiles defined by each state's laws. The software compares DNA profiles to one another to see if any match based on the level of stringency for the search. The purpose of CODIS is to provide investigative leads through matches made between cases and offenders and between cases and other cases. A match in CODIS is called a "hit." Each state's laws will indicate which samples will be stored in CODIS. There are 30 states that store profiles from arrestees and all states collect samples from convicted offenders. As of September 2017, CODIS had produced 392 684 DNA hits assisting in more than 377 507 investigations. CODIS is comprised of 3 levels. The eligibility criteria for a specimen can be different at each level. The Local DNA Index System (LDIS) and State DNA Index System (SDIS) criteria can be defined by the individual and state laboratories, respectively. The LDIS exists in individual, caseworking crime laboratories. Profiles from cases thought to belong to a putative perpetrator are entered into the system. Then on a routine basis, the profiles in all of the LDIS laboratories are uploaded to the state level. The SDIS laboratory also processes qualifying offender samples for the

The Likelihood Ratio Equation for DNA Association Assessment

$$LR = \frac{Pr(E|H_p)}{Pr(E|H_d)}$$

Figure 11-19

Figure 11-19. *The likelihood ratio equation for DNA association assessment (ie, probability of the evidence given the prosecution's hypothesis divided by probability of the evidence given the defense's hypothesis).*

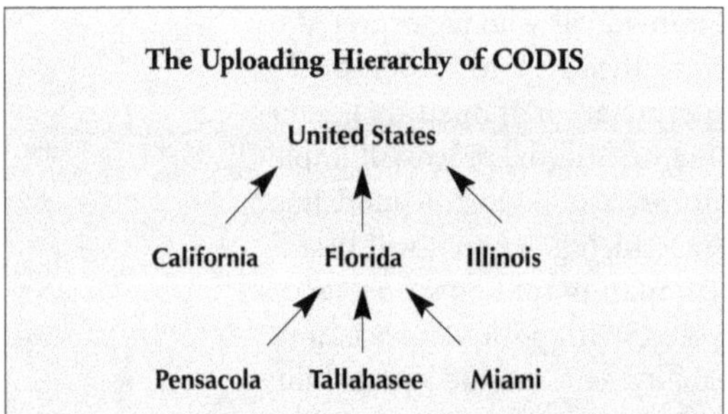

Figure 11-20

Figure 11-20. *The uploading hierarchy of CODIS from LDIS to SDIS to NDIS.*

state. Finally, the SDIS laboratory will upload the state's qualifying offenders and casework profiles to the National DNA Index System (NDIS), which is maintained by the FBI (**Figure 11-20**). DNA results at less than the 20 core loci may prevent a profile from being uploaded to NDIS. Uploads and searches will generally occur on a weekly basis or more frequently. Hits made at any level will result in all involved laboratories receiving an electronic notification. This information is then passed onto law enforcement agencies.[77,78] CODIS is most useful to cases in which the suspect is unknown. If a foreign DNA profile is identified on any samples from the SAK, it will be entered into CODIS. The average CODIS hit rate for untested SAK evidence in New Orleans, Los Angeles, and Detroit has been reported to be approximately 13.8%, 18%, 28.5%, respectively.[79-81]

Y Chromosome STR Multiplex

The contributions of the victim's DNA to the SAK samples may preclude a foreign DNA profile being obtained. In cases where spermatozoa is not the source of the male DNA, oral or digital assaults, or if the male is vasectomized, the ratio of female to male DNA may be too high to amplify any male autosomal DNA. In the oral assault example in **Table 11-8**, the breast swab contains a sufficient amount of male DNA to obtain a complete autosomal STR-DNA profile. However, there is 46 times more female DNA in that sample than male DNA; therefore, the autosomal STR results of this sample will show only minor alleles for the male contributor. Another type of DNA test can be used for samples with a high ratio of female to male DNA. This test examines STR loci on the Y chromosome. Only males have a Y chromosome; therefore, the competition with the victim's DNA to amplify STRs no longer exists. There are several drawbacks to Y-STR testing when compared to autosomal STR testing (**Table 11-11**). The results of Y-STR testing are not unique; therefore, CODIS cannot be used to identify a suspect, as with autosomal STRs. However, it can be used in CODIS, in conjunction with autosomal STRs, to identify unknown remains and missing persons as well as in paternity cases involving a male child with a missing father and an available paternal male relative.[82] The Y chromosome is passed on from a father to all of his sons, just like he inherited

Table 11-11. Comparison of Autosomal STRs, Y-STRs, and Mitochondrial DNA Testing Methods

Autosomal STRs	Y-STRs	Mitochondrial DNA
CODIS searchable	Limited CODIS	Limited CODIS
Inherited from both parents	Inherited from father only	Inherited from mother only
Unique among individuals, except identical twins	All patrilineal relatives same profile	All matrilineal relatives same profile
RMP/ LR statistics	Counting statistics	Continuing statistics
1 copy per cell	1 copy per cell	Multiple copies per cell

Data from Butler JM.[69]

the same Y chromosome from his father. If a child sexual abuse case involves patrilineal relatives then Y-STR testing cannot assist in identifying the donor of the foreign DNA. Y-STR testing requires a known reference from the offender to make a direct comparison. The statistical technique used to assign significance to a positive Y-STR association is called the counting method. This technique is performed by counting how many times the Y-STR profile was observed in a database of Y-STR profiles. The weight of the association is completely dependent on the size of the database.[69]

Digital assault of a female victim by a male offender could result in the transfer of epithelial cells from the offender to the victim. Recent research suggests it may be possible to detect that male DNA using Y-STR testing. In a controlled study involving a small sample of adult volunteers (8 couples) swabs were collected at 1, 6, 12, 24, or 72 hours after 5 minutes of digital penetration. A total of 60 swabs were collected. A partial or complete Y-STR DNA profile was obtained for at least 1 sample from each couple (see **Table 11-12**). A subset of samples underwent quantitation prior to amplification (personal communication), but this data was not included in publication. All but 2 samples indicated quantities that would not reach the target DNA amount of 1.0 ng with the maximum volume added (17.5 µl) or no male quantitation results (personal communication).[83] This limited study suggests the possibility of obtaining Y-STR results when only digital penetration has occurred. Current optimized testing procedures to screen samples for male DNA would result in the majority of these samples being dropped without additional processing. However, considerations may need to be made when the case scenario suggests a digital assault with a collection of vaginal swabs at less than 72 hours. This study should also encourage collection of genital swabs in cases in which only digital assault is reported. Additional research is needed in this area, especially data that includes casework samples.

Table 11-12. Y-STR Results (Number of Alleles Detected) Following 5 Minutes of Digital Penetration

Subject Pairs	Collection Times (Hours)				
	1	6	12	24	72
1	Partial (19)	Partial (6)	Partial (4)	Partial (10)	Partial (19)
2	Partial (19)	Complete	Partial (8)	Partial (5)	Partial (16)
3	Partial (8)	Partial (1)	Partial (6)	NR	Partial (7)
4	Partial (11)	Partial (6)	Partial (15)	Partial (10)	Partial (3)
5	Complete	Partial (5)	NC	NC	NC
6	NC	NC	Partial (7)	NC	NC
7	Complete	Complete	Partial (18)	Partial (22)	NR
8	Complete	NC	NC	NC	NC

Complete profiles have 23 alleles.
NR = No Results
NC = Not Collected
Data from Sween KR, Quarino LA, Kishbaugh JM.[83]

Mitochondrial DNA Testing

Mitochondrial DNA testing is another method that may be useful in a child sexual abuse case. This technique has similar drawbacks to Y-STR testing (**Table 11-11**). Children only inherit their mitochondrial DNA (mtDNA) from their mothers. All maternal relatives will have the same mitochondrial DNA; therefore, it is not unique. It is used in CODIS to aid in the identification of unknown remains and missing persons, but cannot be used to identify a suspect. The statistics used to provide weight to a positive association are also calculated by the counting method. Mixtures can be difficult to interpret because the DNA is being sequenced for detection.[84] It is also highly susceptible to contamination by exogenous DNA. Benefits of mtDNA testing include sensitivity (there can be thousands of mtDNA copies in a single cell), capacity to test degraded samples, and capacity to test shed hairs and hairs without roots.[69] In child sexual abuse cases involving family members or acquaintances, shed hairs removed from the outer clothing of the victim would not provide a meaningful association. These hairs can be picked up from common household items or the laundry. If a hair is located in the genital area of a prepubescent child, an intimate association may explain its presence. Pubic hair combings from adolescent victims can also produce foreign hairs and establish intimate contact.

Emerging Techniques

Many laboratories are moving away from conducting the old serological tests for body fluid stains because they are time intensive and consume samples, and at present, new testing methods that use messenger RNA (mRNA) are being developed to confirm the presence of body fluid. Messenger RNA is single-stranded RNA that is transcribed from the DNA in the nucleus. Its purpose is to carry the code for proteins from the nucleus to the ribosomes where mRNA is translated into amino acids, which then form proteins. Tissue-specific mRNA have been isolated and can be used to identify blood, semen, saliva, vaginal secretions, and menstrual blood.[69] There are a number of commercially available extraction systems designed to coextract DNA and mRNA, simplifying the first step in the DNA process and conserving samples.[85] The detection methods used include qPCR, PCR, and capillary electrophoresis. Current research is developing a non–PCR-based method of identifying mRNA that can be rapidly completed and could potentially be portable. This technique would use molecular beacons (MBs). MBs are molecular probes that contain a quencher and fluorophore on either end. The design results in a hairpin shape, with fluorescence quenched. In the presence of the target RNA, the structure would unfold and a signal would be generated. The signal would be captured using a fluorospectrometer. The results of this research are promising, but more work is needed to create a multiplex system for this technique.[86] None of these testing methods is widely used in forensic casework laboratories at this time.

Forensic DNA phenotyping is another new tool, which is currently only commercially available. This technique predicts physical characteristics and ancestry and is designed to provide an investigative lead when traditional DNA tools like CODIS cannot produce a match. It could be used in cases involving a stranger or an unknown offender. This technique would require a sample with only a single DNA donor present or a mixture of only 2 individuals when a major donor and a minor donor can be observed. The quantity of DNA required is comparable to STR-DNA testing. The technology behind this process is massive parallel sequencing of hundreds of thousands of single-nucleotide polymorphisms (SNPs) (ie, variations in a single nucleotide). There are millions of SNPs throughout an individual's genome. SNPs associated with eye color, hair color, skin pigmentation, freckling, face morphology, and biogeographic ancestry have been identified and characterized. Once SNPs have been typed, the results are analyzed using prediction algorithms to provide a genetic composite of the individual.[9,69,87,88] The use of SNPs for phenotyping and distinguishing between individuals will continue to advance. With the expansion of the CODIS core loci on January 1, 2017, it is unlikely that SNPs will replace STRs as the forensic standard anytime soon.[74]

Once laboratory analysis is complete, a report will be generated. For accredited laboratories, the report will include the items being tested and the results for all tests performed. It will also contain interpretations and conclusions made by the author of the report. Any samples entered into the CODIS will be identified in the report and the disposition of the evidence will also be included. The evidence submitted to a state laboratory by local municipalities will be returned to that local police agency. Chain of custody will be complete and the evidence can then be stored for potential future prosecution.[37]

Further Research

The timing of post-assault evidence collection has been the subject of 2 notable studies. In 2000, Christian et al[89] conducted a retrospective study of the detection of body fluids using serological techniques in prepubescent victims. They concluded that swabbing the prepubescent child after 24 hours was unnecessary because it failed to produce any positive results. However, this study failed to evaluate any DNA testing that may have been performed. In 2011, Thackeray et al[16] conducted another retrospective study emphasizing the frequency of obtaining positive DNA results from samples collected from the body. This study concluded that evidence will be missed in rare cases if sampling isn't performed beyond 24 hours.

The expansion of the CODIS core loci in 2017 resulted in the development of new amplification kits that are more sensitive and robust than what was in use in 2011. Instrumentation for the extraction and detection of the DNA has also improved since that time. Studies suggest that detection of male offenders' DNA with Y-STR testing may be possible in cases of digital assault in adults and adolescents. In 2015, Speck and Ballantyne[90] reported the detection of Y-STR results in postcoital samples collected from adults at 4, 7, and 9 days. DNA left behind from skin-to-skin contact can now be detected. All of this suggests the need for a large scale prospective study of child sexual abuse cases in which samples are collected up to 72 hours post-assault, based on the circumstance of each case. All collected samples should then undergo autosomal STR testing and, potentially, Y-STR testing. Effective recommendations can only be made after this type of study.

Conclusion

The proper and complete collection of evidence in child sexual abuse cases has a direct impact on laboratory results. Recent recommendations for SAK evidence collection promote the use of standardized kits and practices and discontinuation of antiquated techniques. Collection of body swabs based on the circumstances of a given case can also improve the chances of obtaining probative DNA data. In a vast majority of cases, offenders are known to their victims, and sample collection should take that into consideration. In addition to semen and blood, saliva, skin cells, hair, and vaginal and nasal secretions are sources of detectable DNA. Serological testing of SAKs is being phased out for more efficient and sensitive methods. The use of automated instruments has improved consistency while increasing throughput. SAK samples from cases involving a female victim and male offender, which represent the majority of cases, can be screened for the presence of male DNA during quantitation. Those results will impact further testing. Cases involving digital assault only may be considered for Y-STR testing, although more research is needed. Once DNA profiles are developed from SAK samples, they will be compared to known reference samples from the victim and offender. Eligible DNA profiles developed from evidence samples from the perpetrator of a crime will be entered into the CODIS database, which may result in new investigative leads for law enforcement. DNA testing methods like Y-STR and mtDNA provide additional tools for evidence assessment, as do newer techniques such as mRNA body fluid confirmation and phenotypic profiling. All completed laboratory analysis will be documented in a report authored by the examiner. The report is then provided to law enforcement and the evidence is re-sealed and returned to the law enforcement agency or the evidence vault to await its potential use in judicial proceedings.

References

1. US Department of Justice, Office on Violence Against Women. A national protocol for sexual abuse medical forensic examinations: pediatric. https://www.justice.gov/ovw/file/846856/download. Published April 2016. Accessed December 28, 2018.

2. US Department of Justice, Office on Violence Against Women. A national protocol for sexual assault medical forensic examinations: adults/adolescents: second edition. https://www.ncjrs.gov/pdffiles1/ovw/241903.pdf. Published April 2013. Accessed December 28, 2018.

3. US Department of Justice, Office of Justice Programs, National Institute of Justice. National best practices for sexual assault kits: a multidisciplinary approach. https://www.ncjrs.gov/pdffiles1/nij/250384.pdf. Accessed December 28, 2018.

4. Gaensslen RE. *Sourcebook in Forensic Serology, Immunology, and Biochemistry*. Washington, DC: US Department of Justice, National Institute of Justice; 1983.

5. Hochmeister MN, Budowle B, Rudin O, et al. Evaluation of prostate-specific antigen (PSA) membrane test assays for the forensic identification of seminal fluid. *J Forensic Sci*. 1999;44(5):1057-1060.

6. Hares DR. Expanding the CODIS core loci in the United States. *Forensic Sci Int Genet*. 2012;6(1):e52-e54.

7. Butler JM. Genetics and genomics of core short tandem repeat loci used in human identity testing. *J Forensic Sci*. 2006;51(2):253-465.

8. Snyder HN. *Sexual Assault of Young Children as Reported to Law Enforcement: Victim, Incident, and Offender Characteristics*. Washington, DC: US Department of Justice, Office of Justice Programs; 2000.

9. Valenzuela RK, Henderson MS, Walsh, MH, et al. Predicting phenotype from genotype: normal pigmentation. *J Forensic Sci*. 2010;55(2):315-322.

10. Halder I, Shriver M, Thomas M, Fernandez JR, Frudakis T. A panel of ancestry informative markers for estimating individual biogeographical ancestry and admixture from four continents: utility and applications. *Hum Mutat*. 2008;29(5):648-658.

11. Parabon Nanolabs. Parabon Snapshot™ gives crime solvers a new way to use DNA. https://parabon-nanolabs.com/news-events/2014/12/announcing-parabon-snapshot.html. Published December 17, 2014. Accessed December 28, 2018.

12. Bright JA, Taylor D, McGovern C, et al. Developmental validation of STRmix™, expert software for the interpretation of forensic DNA profiles. *Forensic Sci Int Genet*. 2016;23:226-239.

13. Perlin MW, Legler MM, Spencer CE, el al. Validating TrueAllele® DNA mixture interpretation. *J Forensic Sci*. 2011;56(6):1430-1447.

14. Pang BC, Cheung BK. Double swab technique for collecting touched evidence. *Leg Med (Tokyo)*. 2007;9(4):181-184.

15. Graham EA, Rutty GN. Investigation into "normal" background DNA on adult necks: implications for DNA profiling of manual strangulation victims. *J Forensic Sci*. 2008;53(5):1074-1082.

16. Thackery JD, Horner G, Benzinger EA, Scribano PV. Forensic evidence collection and DNA identification in acute child sexual assault. *Pediatrics*. 2011;128(2):227-232.

17. Brayley-Morris H, Sorrell A, Revoir AP, Meakin GE, Court DS, Morgan RM. Persistence of DNA from laundered semen stains: implications for child sex trafficking cases. *Forensic Sci Int Genet*. 2015;19:165-171.

18. Noël S, Lagacé K, Rogic A, et al. DNA transfer during laundering may yield complete genetic profiles. *Forensic Sci Int Genet*. 2016;23:240-247.

19. Technical Working Group on Biological Evidence Preservation. The biological evidence preservation handbook: best practices for evidence handlers. https://nvlpubs.nist.gov/nistpubs/ir/2013/NIST.IR.7928.pdf. Accessed December 28, 2018.

20. Cavness S, Choudhury A, Sensabaugh G. Hospital wet mount examination for the presence of sperm in sexual assault cases is of questionable value. *J Forensic Sci*. 2014;59(3):729-734.

21. National Institute of Justice. DNA analyst training: laboratory training manual: protocol 2.05: semen stain identification: Kernechtrot Picoindigocarmine Stain (KPIC) (identification). https://static.training.nij.gov/lab-manual/Linked%20Documents/Protocols/pdi_lab_pro_2.05.pdf. Accessed December 28, 2018.

22. Baechtel FS. Identification and individualization of semen statins. In: Saferstein R, ed. *Forensic Science Handbook*. Vol 2. Englewood Cliffs, NJ: Prentice Hall; 1988:347-392.

23. Miller KW, Old J, Fischer BR, Schweers B, Stipinaite S, Reich K. Developmental validation of the SPERM HY-LITER™ kit for the identification of human spermatozoa in forensic samples. *J Forensic Sci*. 2011;56(4):853-865.

24. Committee on Identifying the Needs of the Forensic Sciences Community. *Strengthening Forensic Science in the United States: A Path Forward*. Washington, DC: National Academies Press; 2009.

25. Federal Bureau of Investigation. FBI/DOJ microscopic hair comparison analysis review. Federal Bureau of Investigation Web site. https://www.fbi.gov/services/laboratory/scientific-analysis/fbidoj-microscopic-hair-comparison-analysis-review. Accessed October 3, 2018.

26. Roberts KA, Johnson DJ, Cruz S, Simpson H, Safer A. A comparison of the effectiveness of swabbing and flossing as a means of recovering spermatozoa from the oral cavity. *J Forensic Sci*. 2014;59(4):909-918.

27. Wickenheiser RA. Trace DNA: a review, discussion of theory, and application of the transfer of trace quantities of DNA through skin contact. *J Forensic Sci*. 2002;47(3):442-450.

28. Lowe A, Murray C, Whitaker J, Tully G, Gill P. The propensity of individuals to deposit DNA and secondary transfer of low level DNA from individuals to insert surfaces. *Forensic Sci Int*. 2002;129(1):25-34.

29. Phipps M, Petricevic S. The tendency of individuals to transfer DNA to handled items. *Forensic Sci Int.* 2007;168(2-3):162-168.

30. Graham EA, Watkins WJ, Dunstan F, et al. Defining background DNA levels found on the skin of children aged 0-5 years. *Int J Leg Med.* 2014;128(2):251-258.

31. Scientific Working Group on DNA Analysis Methods. Contamination prevention and detection guidelines for forensic DNA laboratories. https://docs.wixstatic.com/ugd/4344b0_c4d4dbba84f1400a98eaa2e48f2bf291.pdf. Approved January 12, 2017. Accessed December 28, 2018.

32. Office of Justice Programs. SART toolkit: chain of custody. National Criminal Justice Reference Service Web site. https://ovc.ncjrs.gov/sartkit/develop/issues-coc.html. Accessed October 1, 2107.

33. Florida Department of Law Enforcement. Crime laboratory evidence submission manual. http://www.flaccreditation.org/docs/resources/2013evidencesubmissionmanuel.pdf. Published 2013. Accessed December 28, 2018.

34. North Carolina Department of Justice. Policy and procedure for evidence submission. https://www.ncdoj.gov/getdoc/0d2d2d94-2519-46a8-88f1-2989ef651433/Evidence-Guide-10-16-2013-(1).aspx. Effective October 15, 2018. Accessed December 28, 2018.

35. Virginia Department of Forensic Science. Evidence handling & laboratory capabilities guide: forensic biology. https://www.dfs.virginia.gov/wp-content/uploads/2017/02/Forensic-Biology-2015-07.pdf. Updated August 17, 2015. Accessed December 28, 2018.

36. Scientific Working Group on DNA Analysis Methods. SWGDAM guidelines for the collection and serological examination of biological evidence. http://media.wix.com/ugd/4344b0_bce915901bb14b9cb36049df6a8441e2.pdf. Approved January 1, 2015. Accessed December 28, 2018.

37. International Organization for Standardization. *General Requirements for the Competence of Testing and Calibration Laboratories.* 2nd ed. Geneva, Switzerland: International Organization for Standardization; 2005.

38. Sanders CT, Reisenbigler EK, Peterson DA. Laser microdissection separation of pure spermatozoa populations from mixed cell samples for forensic DNA analysis. https://www.ncjrs.gov/pdffiles1/nij/grants/217268.pdf. Published February 2007. Accessed December 28, 2018.

39. Yu H, Diamandis EP. Prostate-specific antigen in milk of lactating women. *Clin Chem.* 1995;41(1):54-58.

40. Bitner SE. False positives observed on the Seratec® PSA SemiQuant Cassette Test with condom lubricants. *J Forensic Sci.* 2012;57(6):1545-1548.

41. Davies A, Wilson E. The persistence of seminal constituents in the human vagina. *Forensic Sci.* 1974;3(1):45-55.

42. Willott GM, Allard JE. Spermatozoa: their persistence after sexual intercourse. *Forensic Sci Int.* 1982;19(2):135-154.

43. Nelson DF, Kirk PL. The identification of saliva. *J Forensic Med.* 1963;10(1):14-21.

44. National Institute of Justice. DNA analyst training: laboratory training manual: protocol 2.09: saliva stain indication: radial gel diffusion test. https://static.training.nij.gov/lab-manual/Linked%20Documents/Protocols/pdi_lab_pro_2.09.pdf. Accessed December 28, 2018.

45. Pang BC, Cheung BK. Applicability of two commercially available kits for forensic identification of saliva stains. *J Forensic Sci.* 2008;53(5):1117-1122.

46. New York City Office of the Chief Medical Examiner. Forensic biology serology procedures manual: Kastle-Meyer (KM) presumptive testing for blood. https://www1.nyc.gov/assets/ocme/downloads/pdf/technical-manuals/serology-procedures-manual/kastle-meyer-km-presumptive-testing-for-blood.pdf. Effective April 24, 2017. Accessed December 28, 2018.

47. North Carolina Department of Justice. Procedure for blood analysis. https://www.ncdoj.gov/getdoc/0dbd274a-3855-4eec-96d6-c4813878b212/Procedure-for-Blood-Analysis.aspx. Effective April 6, 2016. Accessed December 28, 2018.

48. Rapid stain identification of human blood (RSID™-Blood): technical information and protocol sheet for dual buffer system. Independent Forensics Web site. https://ifi-test.com/documents/BLOOD-Dual-Buffer-with-SpinEZE-042016.pdf. Published April 2016. Accessed December 28, 2018.

49. Deedrick DW. Hair, fibers, crime, and evidence, part 1: hair evidence. *Forensic Sci Commun.* 2000;2(3). https://archives.fbi.gov/archives/about-us/lab/forensic-science-communications/fsc/july2000/deedric1.htm. Accessed December 28, 2018.

50. Linch CA. The ultrastructure of tissue attached to telogen hair roots. *J Forensic Sci.* 2008;53(6):1363-1366.

51. Opel KL, Fleishaker EL, Nicklas JA, Buel E, McCord BR. Evaluation and quantitation of nuclear DNA from human telogen hairs. *J Forensic Sci.* 2008;53(4):853-857.

52. Szabo S, Jaeger K, Fischer H, Tschachler E, Parson W, Eckhart L. In situ labeling of DNA reveals interindividual variation of nuclear DNA breakdown in hair and may be useful to predict success of forensic genotyping of hair. *Int J Legal Med.* 2012;126(1):63-70.

53. National Institute of Justice. DNA analyst training: laboratory training manual: protocol 2.04: semen stain identification: acid phosphatase mapping (indication). https://static.training.nij.gov/lab-manual/Linked%20Documents/Protocols/pdi_lab_pro_2.04.pdf. Accessed December 28, 2018.

54. US Department of Justice, Office of Justice Programs, National Institute of Justice. The road ahead: unanalyzed evidence in sexual assault cases. https://www.ncjrs.gov/pdffiles1/nij/233279.pdf. Published May 2011. Accessed December 28, 2018.

55. Scientific Working Group on DNA Analysis Methods. Recommendations for the efficient DNA processing of sexual assault evidence kits. https://docs.wixstatic.com/ugd/4344b0_4daf2bb5512b4e2582f895c4a133a0ed.pdf. Published December 5, 2016. Accessed December 28, 2018.

56. Baechtel FS. A primer on the methods used in the typing of DNA. *Crime Laboratory Digest.* 1988;15(suppl 1):3-9.

57. Eubanks WG. Expenses associated with DNA typing methods. *Crime Laboratory Digest.* 1988;15(suppl 1):10-11.

58. National Human Genome Research Institute. Fact sheets on science, research, ethics and the Institute. National Human Genome Research Institute Web site. https://www.genome.gov/10000202/fact-sheets/. Updated November 9, 2015. Accessed October 3, 2018.

59. Comey CT, Koon BW, Presley KW, et al. DNA extraction strategies for amplified fragment length polymorphism analysis. *J Forensic Sci.* 1994;39(5):1254-1269.

60. Walsh PS, Metzger DA, Higuchi R. Chelex-100 as a medium for simple extraction of DNA for PCR-based typing from forensic material. *Biotechniques.* 1991;10(4):506-513.

61. Montpetit SA, Fitch IT, O'Donnell PT. A simple automated instrument for DNA extraction in forensic casework. *J Forensic Sci.* 2005;50(3):555-563.

62. Liu JY, Zhong C, Holt A, et al. AutoMate Express™ forensic DNA extraction system for the extraction of genomic DNA from biological samples. *J Forensic Sci.* 2012;57(4):1022-1030.

63. Sanders CT, Sanchez N, Ballantyne J, Peterson DA. Laser microdissection separation of pure spermatozoa from epithelial cells for short tandem repeat analysis. *J Forensic Sci.* 2006;51(4):748-757.

64. Chen J, Kobilinsky L, Wolosin D, Shaler R, Baum H. A physical method for separating spermatozoa from epithelial cells in sexual assault evidence. *J Forensic Sci.* 1998;43(1):114-118.

65. Vuichard S, Borer U, Bottinelli M, et al. Differental DNA extraction of challenging simulated sexual-assault samples: a Swiss collaborative study. *Investig Genet.* 2011;2:11.

66. Gill P, Jeffreys AJ, Werrett DJ. Forensic application of DNA "fingerprints". *Nature.* 1985;318(6046):577-579.

67. Campbell R, Pierce SJ, Sharma DB, et al. Comparing standard and selective degradation DNA extraction methods: results from a field experiment with sexual assault kits. *J Forensic Sci.* 2017;62(1):213-222.

68. QIAGEN. *Developmental Validation of QIAcube™ Automated Platform and Differential Wash Protocol for Forensic DNA Testing Laboratories.* Hilden, Germany: QIAGEN, Inc; 2013.

69. Butler JM. *Advanced Topics in Forensic DNA Typing: Methodology.* Waltham, MA: Elsevier; 2012.

70. Krenke BE, Nassif N, Sprecher CJ, Knox C, Schwandt M, Storts DR. Developmental validation of a real-time PCR assay for the simultaneous quantification of total human and male DNA. *Forensic Sci Int Genet.* 2008;3(1):14-21.

71. Horsman KM, Hickey JA, Cotton RW, Landers JP, Maddox LO. Development of a human-specific real-time PCR assay for the simultaneous quantitation of total genomic and male DNA. *J Forensic Sci.* 2006;51(4):758-765.

72. Federal Bureau of Investigation. Quality assurance standards for forensic DNA testing laboratories. https://www.fbi.gov/file-repository/quality-assurance-standards-for-forensic-dna-testing-laboratories.pdf/view. Effective September 1, 2011. Accessed December 28, 2018.

73. Hares DR. Addendum to expanding the CODIS core loci in the United States. *Forensic Sci Int Genet.* 2012;6(5):e135.

74. Federal Bureau of Investigation. Frequently asked questions on CODIS and NDIS. Federal Bureau of Investigation Web site. https://www.fbi.gov/services/laboratory/biometric-analysis/codis/codis-and-ndis-fact-sheet. Accessed October 3, 2018.

75. Scientific Working Group on DNA Analysis Methods. Interpretation guidelines for autosomal STR typing by forensic DNA testing laboratories. https://docs.wixstatic.com/ugd/4344b0_50e2749756a242528e6285a5bb478f4c.pdf. Published January 12, 2017. Accessed December 28, 2018.

76. STRmix. News. STRmix Web site. https://www.strmix.com/#news. Accessed December 28, 2018.

77. Federal Bureau of Investigation. CODIS: NDIS statistics. Federal Bureau of Investigation Web site. https://www.fbi.gov/services/laboratory/biometric-analysis/codis/ndis-statistics. Accessed October 3, 2018.

78. Federal Bureau of Investigations. National DNA index system (NDIS) operational procedures manual. https://www.fbi.gov/file-repository/ndis-operational-procedures-manual.pdf/view. Effective June 1, 2018. Accessed December 28, 2018.

79. Nelson MS. Analysis of untested sexual assault kits in New Orleans. National Criminal Justice Reference Service Web site. https://www.ncjrs.gov/pdffiles1/nij/242312.pdf. Accessed December 28, 2018.

80. Peterson J, Johnson D, Herz D, Graziano L, Oehler T. Sexual assault kit backlog study. National Criminal Justice Reference Service Web site. https://www.ncjrs.gov/pdffiles1/nij/grants/238500.pdf. Accessed December 28, 2018.

81. Campbell R, Fehler-Cabral G, Pierce SJ, et al. The Detroit sexual assault kit (SAK) action research project (ARP): final report. https://www.ncjrs.gov/pdffiles1/nij/grants/248680.pdf. Published November 9, 2015. Accessed December 28, 2018.

82. Mulero JJ, Chang CW, Calandro LM, et al. Development and validation of the AmpFlSTR Yfiler PCR amplification kit: a male specific, single amplification 17 Y-STR multiplex system. *J Forensic Sci.* 2006;51(1):64-75.

83. Sween KR, Quarino LA, Kishbaugh JM. Detection of male DNA in the vaginal cavity after digital penetration using Y-chromosome short tandem repeats. *J Forensic Nurs.* 2015;11(1):33-40.

84. Scientific Working Group on DNA Analysis Methods. Interpretation guidelines for mitochondrial DNA analysis by forensic DNA testing laboratories. http://media.wix.com/ugd/4344b0_c5e20877c02f403c9ba16770e8d41937.pdf. Approved July 18, 2013. Accessed December 28, 2018.

85. Schweighardt AJ, Tate CM, Scott KA, Harper KA, Robertson JM. Evaluation of commercial kits for dual extraction of DNA and RNA from human body fluids. *J Forensic Sci.* 2015;60(1):157-165.

86. Young ST, Moore JR, Bishop CP. A rapid, confirmatory test for body fluid identification. *J Forensic Sci.* 2018;63(2):511-516.

87. Wiley R, Zeng X, Larue B, Greytak EM, Armentrout S, Budowle B. Blind testing and evaluation of a comprehensive DNA phenotyping system. Promega Web site. https://www.promega.com/-/media/files/products-and-services/genetic-identity/ishi-27-poster-abstracts/89-ellen-greytak.pdf. Published 2016. Accessed October 3, 2018.

88. Breslin K, Muralidharan C, Walsh S. Forensic DNA phenotyping through massive parallel sequencing. Promega Web site. https://www.promega.com/-/media/files/products-and-services/genetic-identity/ishi-27-poster-abstracts/88-krystal-breslin.pdf. Published 2016. Accessed October 3, 2018.

89. Christian CW, Lavelle JM, De Jong AR, Loiselle J, Brenner L, Joffe M. Forensic evidence findings in prepubertal victims of sexual assault. *Pediatrics*. 2000;106(1 pt 1):100-104.

90. Speck P, Ballantyne J. Post-coital DNA recovery study. https://www.ncjrs.gov/pdffiles1/nij/grants/248682.pdf. Published March 2015. Accessed December 28, 2018.

Chapter 12

Child Sexual Abuse Medical Examiners

Randell Alexander, MD, PhD
Nancy Harper, MD, FAAP

Importance of the Sexual Abuse Evaluation

Child abuse medicine is a highly integrated discipline which requires the ability to identify or exclude various types of abuse, and requires knowledge of the social and legal aspects of abuse. A diagnosis of child abuse is multifaceted. Child abuse affects children's health and may affect their social situation as well. After a diagnosis of child abuse, the child and family may have interactions with social services, police, mental health providers, and the legal system. A medical diagnosis of abuse may lead to the incarceration of a family member and disruption of the child's family life. An error may lead to prosecution of an innocent person. Failure to make a correct diagnosis of abuse may leave the child in an unsafe environment at risk for ongoing abuse and potentially place other children at risk. An accurate medical evaluation is, therefore, critical to the well-being of the child and the multidisciplinary assessment of child abuse.

Knowledge and Reliability of Examiners About Sexual Abuse

Child sexual abuse examiners come from a diverse group of medical practitioners and bring with them the views and values of their fields. All examiners, regardless of training and expertise, share a common goal: an accurate assessment and diagnosis capable of meeting the needs of the child while also meeting the requirements of the legal system. Physicians, nurse practitioners (NPs), physician assistants (PAs), and nurses bring different skill levels and training to the comprehensive medical evaluation. Even within the different fields, a great diversity of expertise is found. It is imperative that consistent and accurate knowledge and abilities are developed and maintained by all examiners.

Medical providers who examine children for suspected sexual abuse must be well trained, knowledgeable, and comfortable performing a specialized anogenital examination. They must be astute at diagnosing findings related to abuse and findings that mimic abuse. They should be adept and capable of diagnosing other forms of abuse, and it is desirable if they can diagnose and treat other medical conditions that may be present. Each of the many medical disciplines involved in the medical evaluation of child abuse has different training and skills. As of 2019, no national consensus exists on the appropriate levels of training for medical providers examining children for suspected sexual abuse, but basic concepts about skill levels needed for examining children apply (see the National Children's Alliance 2017 *Standards for Accredited Members*[1]). This important examination should be provided by the most qualified person available; however, a clear idea of what constitutes "medically qualified" for such a diverse group of providers is sometimes not well defined.

The first skill required to conduct the physical examination portion of the evaluation is to be capable of identifying the anatomy itself. This is relatively simple, but few medical personnel are taught this in their training. This indicates a cultural discomfort with examining the genitalia that may have negative consequences for women's and men's health. In 1987, Ladson and colleagues[2] surveyed pediatricians and family practitioners who were asked to identify genital structures on a photograph of female genitalia. Only 59% of the physicians could correctly identify the hymen on the photograph. In a follow-up study published in 2000, Lentsch,[3] using the same photograph, surveyed 166 pediatricians, family practitioners, and emergency medicine physicians. Only 61.7% of physicians correctly identified the hymen. When shown a photograph of a hymen with normal findings, 64% of the physicians believed the photograph depicted abnormal findings and 62% believed the photograph depicted signs of possible sexual abuse, even in the absence of a history concerning for abuse. The authors specifically noted that physicians seeing more than 25 patients per week for sexual abuse allegations were more likely to correctly identify genital structures, highlighting the importance of clinical experience in the diagnostic process. A subsequent study of NPs yielded similar results. Less than 60% of NPs could correctly identify 2 genital structures (the hymen and vaginal opening) on a photograph.[4]

Many authors have studied examiner agreement on physical examination findings. In 1993, Adams and Wells[5] showed 170 colposcopic photographs to examiners who were blinded to the history of the allegation. Examiners with more experience (based on the number of cases an examiner had seen in a month) agreed more with the expert than those examiners with less experience. The less-experienced examiners overstated the findings more often, diagnosing a normal examination as an abnormal one. Similarly, in 1997, Paradise and colleagues[6] measured diagnostic agreement among physicians who identified themselves as skilled in child sexual abuse examinations and compared their opinions with those of an expert panel. The opinions of the physicians with the most experience resembled those of the experts more closely than did the opinions of the less-experienced physicians. In a subsequent study, Paradise and colleagues[7] found that the history could influence the examination findings of less-experienced physicians. Inexperienced physicians asked to evaluate a photograph depicting normal findings accompanied by a normal history diagnosed the examination as normal. However, when later presented with the same photograph coupled with a history of trauma, they would often reinterpret the examination as abnormal, reflecting the history. In 2002, Makoroff and colleagues[8] studied the diagnostic accuracy of emergency medicine physicians. They found that in 79% of the female genital examinations diagnosed as abnormal and indicative of sexual abuse by pediatric emergency medicine physicians, 70% were diagnosed as normal and another 9% as nonspecific when reviewed by physicians trained in child abuse.

Diagnostic acumen in child abuse can be a reflection of the decade during which a physician trained. Child sexual abuse research did not become prevalent until the late 1980s. Physicians trained during or before that time who have not had updated training may be basing their knowledge on obsolete and incorrect information. It may be assumed that more recently trained physicians would be better trained, more comfortable, and more knowledgeable about sexual abuse. Dubow et al[9] tested this assumption in 2005 by surveying all the pediatric chief residents in the United States to determine their ability to recognize prepubertal female anatomy. They found that 30% incorrectly identified the hymen on a photograph. These chief residents indicated that the child sexual abuse training in their residencies varied widely. Half felt their training was inadequate; however, the authors did not correlate the amount of training with the residents' scores. A 2006 national study of residents' child abuse training, knowledge, and comfort found that only 13% of residents could identify 3 genital structures (the hymen, labia minora, and urethra) on a photograph.[10] Residents in that study also reported they were uncomfortable performing an anogenital examination. As seen in earlier studies, increased training and increased patient exposure led to higher comfort levels and higher knowledge scores in these residents.

Less is known about the diagnostic accuracy for boys with physical examination findings indicative of sexual abuse. Research on the ability of practitioners to determine the significance of anal findings is lacking. Although medical practitioners may be skilled at diaper rashes and other common skin conditions, some structural variants (eg, failure of midline fusion), certain medical conditions (eg, prolapsed urethra), or identification of sexually transmitted infections (STIs) may continue to test their skills.

The conclusion that must be drawn from the summary of the literature to date is that the majority of medical providers remain inadequately trained to examine children for sexual abuse. Although research has identified pediatricians as the best trained and most experienced in examinations, many still are not well trained. Many examiners are unfamiliar with prepubertal genital anatomy and the range of anatomic findings that can be considered normal. An untrained or undertrained medical provider should not provide an expert opinion in a case of child sexual abuse. Inexperienced examiners tend to overstate positive examination findings, which can lead to inappropriate legal consequences in the investigation of potential child abuse.

A national call to action to identify the requisite knowledge and skills of the trained examiner and to improve the education and qualifications of medical providers in the evaluation and referral of child sexual abuse is needed. This should begin with basic training about genital anatomy in medical training. Perhaps no one should graduate if they cannot identify 6 or 7 key genital structures for girls, for example. Although the diagnosis of abnormalities indicating sexual abuse is much more complicated, a good start is made in understanding what is normally seen. This also means that as part of comprehensive physical examinations, examiners should be taught that they should also examine the genitalia routinely, in accordance with the recommendations of the American Association of Pediatricians (AAP) and others.[11-13]

Purpose of the Medical Evaluation for Sexual Abuse

Collection of Evidence and Protection of the Child

The medical evaluation consists most importantly of the history, but it also encompasses the physical examination and possibly the collection of forensic evidence. Purposes of a physical examination for sexual abuse should be clearly delineated in order to determine the qualifications for the examiner. Although collection of evidence necessary for a legal proceeding may be one goal of the examination, issues related to the child's well-being and safety are of primary importance.

The health care provider must help ensure the safety and well-being of the child. An appropriate diagnosis can assist in the adjudication of a civil or criminal court case and the protection of the child. Assessment of the child for developmental, emotional, or behavioral concerns may reveal the need for further evaluation and treatment. In addition, the child and family may benefit psychologically from reassurance that the child's examination findings are normal. Referrals for appropriate mental health counseling, if not in place, can be initiated by the medical provider.

Medical providers and the system within which they work should be able to fully diagnose, document, and address medical conditions resulting from abuse and other medical conditions that may also be present. When an abnormal genital finding is present, often the family can be assured that it will heal and can be advised of any further medical treatment that may be necessary. An examiner must differentiate medical findings indicative of abuse from those that may be explained by other medical conditions or accidental injuries. Conditions such as urethral prolapse, lichen sclerosis, or genital hemangiomas may be mistaken for abuse by an inexperienced examiner.[14] Accidental mechanisms such as straddle injuries also may be mistaken for abuse and must be diagnosed and appropriately treated.

Untrained examiners may make 2 types of diagnostic errors. First, physical findings may be misinterpreted; for example, an examiner may see a case of lichen sclerosis and misdiagnose it as sexual trauma. Another diagnostic error occurs when examiners overlook findings that may be diagnostic. Providers who cannot identify a hymen on a photograph will not be able to identify injury to a hymen.

The provider must also be able to diagnose, document, and address health conditions unrelated to abuse. Many children have limited contact with health care providers after infancy and may not have had recent contact. At the time of their examinations they may have unmet health needs. Children arrive in child sexual abuse clinics with serious untreated heart conditions, undiagnosed diabetes and other endocrine disorders, and dermatologic problems needing immediate referrals. The provider should be able to assess the health needs of the child and make referrals as necessary. Linkage to a tertiary care center or specialized medical assessment facility allows isolated examiners and those with less training in general pediatric diagnosis to properly care for these children.

History Taking

Usually the most important aspect of the child sexual abuse evaluation is the history. A health care provider may be the first professional a child has contact with after a disclosure of sexual abuse. Some children may share a special bond with a health care provider and may disclose information to the provider that they might not share with investigators. Although all health care providers learn diagnostic history taking in their general training, obtaining a specialized medical history from a child for suspected sexual abuse requires specific skills and knowledge not normally possessed by an untrained provider. The provider must have the ability to gather a history that is both forensically sensitive and medically relevant. Untrained examiners may mistakenly ask leading questions or misinterpret a child's statements. Formal training in obtaining such histories in suspected child sexual abuse cases is recommended.[15,16]

A child does not live in isolation; therefore, inquiry about the histories of the caregivers is often important. Referral for treatment also may be important for others in the family, especially because a caregiver needs to support the child as well. Sexual abuse is prevalent, and a specific case may bring out concerns that transcend the specific patients themselves. The history provided by the child and family should be documented in direct quotations whenever possible. An accurate history and diagnosis must be accompanied by detailed documentation. A health care provider must document the history, physical examination findings, and interpretation of the examination accurately and in detail. This type of documentation can be learned from extensive training and from mentors. Comfort with this level of documentation usually develops over time.

Photodocumentation

Another aspect of documentation in child abuse cases is photodocumentation. Examination findings should be captured photographically for peer review, second opinion consultation, and potential use within the court system. An examiner should remain open to the scrutiny involved in peer review of photographs. The ability to obtain still or video images is mandatory. Photographic systems vary widely. Although photographic technique can be learned in a training session, ongoing experience with the equipment is necessary to adequately obtain high-quality documentation of examination findings. The examiner must have policies in place for secure storage and distribution of the images.

Collaboration Between Health Professionals

A health care provider must interact effectively within a multidisciplinary team. The examiner will be a member of a team that may consist of law enforcement, child protective services, prosecutors, and mental health providers. Accurate and timely information must be conveyed to other professionals to assist in the protection of the child and/or the adjudication of a criminal proceeding. The provider should be willing to share information and cooperate with various agencies to provide the best outcome for a child. Often the health care provider will provide court testimony regarding the medical findings. As with many of the skills necessary for child abuse evaluations, the more experience an examiner has testifying in court, the more comfortable the process becomes. The multidisciplinary team is discussed in more detail in Chapter 13.

Children who are victims of sexual abuse may also be victims of physical abuse and neglect. Although physicians, NPs, and PAs typically are trained to evaluate and treat all aspects of the medical care of a child, most nurses who are trained as sexual assault examiners are trained only to evaluate acute sexual assault. Such providers will need written procedures for medical intervention when there are physical injuries present, when a child needs a referral for emergency medical care, or when the children may need a second comprehensive examination by a more qualified provider. Second examinations or follow-up examinations in children and adolescents are recommended with some criteria suggested, such as when there is an acute injury identified on initial examination, when the findings on initial examination are uncertain, when additional testing or reassessment for STIs is indicated, and most importantly when the initial examiner is less experienced (eg, has conducted fewer than 100 evaluations of children or adolescents).[17,18]

In some cases, nonmedical investigators make decisions about which children should receive a medical evaluation. However, it is important that all children suspected of being victims of sexual abuse receive medical evaluations. At some point during the development of new programs, parameters should be set for selecting the most appropriate type of evaluation needed to provide the level of care that is in the best interest of the child. It is important to define on a case-by-case basis the type of physical examination needed for a child who may have been sexually abused. The purpose of a pediatric examination may be limited (eg, an acute illness, a distinct problem, or for the purpose of this chapter, a report of suspected sexual abuse). The child sexual abuse examination may, at times, be described as an examination for the collection of forensic medical evidence, best performed within 24 hours but commonly performed within 72 hours after an alleged abuse event (a disclosure of abuse).[19-21] As DNA techniques evolve, it is important to reevaluate the best timing for evidence collection.

Children who disclose abuse beyond the time frame compatible with a forensic evaluation require at least an examination focused on medical history and a physical examination of the oral, anal, and genital areas. In addition, most children are best served by a more comprehensive pediatric medical evaluation, which may be conducted by a licensed physician, certified and licensed advanced practice nurse, or licensed physician assistant. A comprehensive medical evaluation can be defined as a thorough medical history, a complete physical examination, an assessment of behavior and development, a diagnosis, and a treatment plan. If the child has an established medical home, the evaluation is part of the child's primary care. If the child does not have a primary care provider, the comprehensive evaluation can be performed at the time of the sexual abuse evaluation, or later, and should be performed by a provider with training in and knowledge of child development, normal prepubertal and pubertal anatomy, interpretation of physical findings, and differential diagnoses with abuse and other medical conditions considered. Careful consideration of differential diagnoses is important, especially among children with physical or behavioral symptoms but no clear disclosure of abuse. Although many physicians and nurses have most of the requisite skills, not all have more than a basic understanding of child abuse, forensic interviewing, and physical examination for abuse. Collaboration with or referral to a physician, physician assistant, or advanced practice nurse specializing or experienced in child abuse pediatrics is helpful in those situations.

The purpose of the medical evaluation should be in the best interest of the child. The evaluation should follow a best practice model with findings that are evidence based.[13] Determining who should be allowed to do what to whom should be based on the knowledge, education, training, and experience of the examiner. In fairness to the child, the child's family, and the systems depending on medical findings (or lack of findings), examinations beyond forensic evidence collection are optimally performed by health care professionals who have specific education and training in the field of child sexual abuse medicine, a knowledge of child physical and emotional development, and training in other appropriate pediatric care areas. Training in child sexual abuse evaluations should include a component of closely supervised experience performing and interpreting examinations.

Three broad areas of preparation should be evaluated before deciding who is best able to provide medical evaluations for sexually abused children. These areas are (1) education, training, certification, and licensing; (2) supervision, ongoing continuing education, and case review experience; (3) sufficient experience to maintain skills, and (4) ongoing peer review of findings and opinions after examinations.[22] Not all physicians and nurses have the necessary education and training to be skilled in child sexual abuse examination techniques, interpretation of findings, laboratory testing, diagnosis, and management. Consequently, to guarantee best practice models for the medical care of possibly sexually abused children, both doctors and nurses must meet certain advanced skill levels through education, continuing education, supervised experience, and peer review of opinions and findings before working independently.

Peer review is a process of continually presenting findings and opinions before a group of health care professionals of varying skill levels for the purpose of confirmation of findings, discovery of new ideas, and discussion of controversial issues. All health care professionals who engage in child sexual abuse evaluations should avail themselves of opportunities for peer review.

All examinations must be free from personal bias. Examiners must resist the lure of "making the case" for investigators or prosecutors by overinterpreting a normal or nonspecific finding.

Who Examines Children for Sexual Abuse?

Many different medical disciplines are involved in the evaluation of child sexual abuse. The examiner may be a physician, nurse practitioner, physician assistant, or sexual assault nurse examiner (SANE). A telemedicine nurse may assist at a remote site. The training and experiences of each of these groups varies (**Table 12-1**).

Table 12-1. Comparison of Different Medical Providers With the Sexual Abuse Evaluation

Examiner	Scope of Service	Diagnose and Treat Other Medical Conditions	Child Needs Additional Medical Examination	Review
Child abuse pediatrician and other pediatricians trained in child abuse	Diagnose and treat all forms of abuse	Yes	No	Peer review sufficient
General pediatricians, other physicians, general NPs or PAs	Vary in ability to diagnose and treat all forms of abuse	Yes	Maybe	Peer, or possibly part of an organized system with an advanced consultant
Trained NP	Diagnose and treat all forms of abuse	Yes	No	Peer, or possibly part of an organized system of hierarchal review
Trained PA	Diagnose and treat all forms of abuse	Yes	No	Peer, or possibly part of an organized system of hierarchal review
Trained RN (SANE)	History, physical evidence collection, and photodocumentation Identify physical findings of concern	No	Yes	Should be part of an organized system of hierarchal review
Telemedicine nurse	Assist in examinations and evidence collection	No	No	Should be included in peer review

There is no national standard for training medical students or residents in child abuse. Physicians often have little, if any, exposure to abuse training in their residencies. Even programs that offer educational rotations and education in sexual abuse may not offer acute sexual assault training to students and residents. Pediatricians receive the most training on abuse-related topics, but they are still undertrained.[9,13] Other physicians such as gynecologists, emergency medicine, and family medicine physicians who may see child sexual abuse victims may receive little, if any, training in sexual assault and abuse of children.

The American Board of Pediatrics (ABP) established the subspecialty of child abuse pediatrics in 2006 and the first certifying examination was given in 2009. Before the availability of fellowship training, physicians were largely self-trained, and their expertise was dependent on their years of experience in the field. Although many physicians will elect to continue to evaluate child abuse without subspecialty certification, all eligible pediatricians who wish to become board certified will be required to complete an approved 3-year fellowship and then apply to the ABP to sit for the child abuse pediatrics certifying examination. The curricula across the training programs is reasonably standardized based on the Accreditation Council for Graduate Medical Education standards.

Training for providers other than pediatricians varies widely. Physicians in other fields such as emergency medicine, family medicine, or gynecology, although they may practice in the field of child abuse, are not eligible to be certified through the ABP. To date, no medical specialty other than pediatrics has formal subspecialty certification in child abuse.

Practitioners other than physicians are active in the field of child abuse. PAs may specialize in pediatrics, but as of 2019 there is no formal certification process for PAs to specialize in child abuse. Training can be obtained under the guidance of an experienced mentor, and typically the PA will work closely with an experienced child abuse physician to further refine skills, develop expertise, and engage in peer review. Similarly, although nurse practitioners may specialize in pediatrics, no child abuse certification specifically for NPs is available. Most who specialize in child abuse work closely with a child abuse physician.

In 2015 Florida legally established a training requirement for medical directors for its child protection teams. Any established medical director had 4 years to pass the Department of Health's examination; new directors have 2 years. Chapter 39.303 states that "within 2 years after the date of employment as a child protection team medical director, obtains a subspecialty certification in child abuse from the American Board of Pediatrics or within 2 years meet the minimum requirements established by a third-party credentialing entity recognizing a demonstrated specialized competence in child abuse pediatrics."[23] This examination has also been taken by other physicians and NPs within the child protection team (CPT) system as an indication of competence. Each medical provider also must take 8 hours of continuing medical education in child abuse each year.

There is also a state program in Missouri called SAFE-CARE Providers. Missouri statute 334.950 in 2014 requires SAFE-CARE providers to receive Missouri-based initial intensive training regarding child maltreatment from the SAFE-CARE network, ongoing education, peer review, and access to resource centers. Providers include: physicians, advanced practice nurses, or physician's assistants licensed in Missouri who provide medical diagnosis and treatment to children suspected of being victims of abuse.[24] Reimbursement for examinations is contingent on being part of this system.

The National Children's Alliance (the organization responsible for Children's Advocacy Centers) also has minimum qualifications for various types of providers within their organization.[1] However, these are not legal requirements and in most instances more training and experience would be desirable.

SANEs may be advanced- or non–advanced-degree nurses. Because nursing school curricula do not cover sexual assault in great detail, nurses must seek additional training. Registered nurses may be trained and certified both in adult or adolescent assault and pediatric assault evaluations in courses that range from a few days to several weeks in length. The International Association of Forensic Nurses offers a 43-hour course for nurses to get certification in sexual assault nursing and outlines the clinical training and the hours of patient contact needed to receive the certificate. Successful completion of the certification process acknowledges objective validation of nurses' expertise. The process also enhances professional development and opportunities for professional growth. (For more information, see https://forensicnurses.org.) Although ongoing patient contact and continuing education are necessary to maintain skills, no national governing body monitors the quality of the training or continuing education of nurses. Because the training times for SANEs can be as little as a few days, SANEs should seek the most qualified medical director available to them.

Training and Education

As the field of child abuse pediatrics grows, and as research continues to show the inadequacy of resident training in abuse, efforts toward standardized curricula for pediatric residency training are beginning to emerge. Similarly, pediatric fellowships have developed standardized curricula, ensuring that fellowship-trained pediatricians enter the field with a well-defined knowledge base. However, these education efforts are directed at pediatricians, not at the family doctors, emergency physicians, and gynecologists who may be involved in the evaluation of these children. Given the diversity of professionals who provide child abuse examinations, these efforts to train pediatricians are not sufficient.

Most medical skills and knowledge require long-term commitment to develop and maintain. A health care provider who does not see sexual abuse cases on a regular basis may not be able to maintain a comfort level with the examination process. The inexperienced or low-volume examiner, in many instances, needs access to an expert second medical opinion. Because inexperienced examiners are more likely to make a diagnostic error suggesting that a finding is present when it is not, second opinions should be obtained in cases where a medical finding diagnostic of sexual abuse is being considered.[8,9]

Experts

For the courts, an expert is defined as someone who is qualified through expertise, training, and special knowledge regarding a subject. What qualifies an expert in a courtroom is not what qualifies an expert in the examination room. Although physicians are readily acknowledged as experts in the interpretation of human physical and physiological processes, there is tremendous variability in their knowledge in any specific area. An expert general pediatrician or family physician may have limited training or knowledge of child sexual abuse.

An expert medical consultant in child sexual abuse is generally a physician, PA, or NP with considerable experience in the medical evaluation and photodocumentation of children suspected of being abused. This person ideally should be involved in scholarly pursuits in the field of child sexual abuse, including conducting original research studies, publishing, and speaking at regional or national conferences on topics involving the medical evaluation of children with suspected abuse. Experts typically have a large clinical practice and often practice at academic medical centers. Their medical knowledge base is broad and encompasses all aspects of sexual abuse, including evaluation of chronic cases and knowledge of the differential diagnosis of mimics of abuse.

In many cases the qualifications of an NP or other provider may exceed the qualifications of local physicians, and the most qualified expert in the area may not be a physician. SANEs, although experts in sexual assault nursing, may have very little training in or knowledge of broader aspects of nonacute sexual abuse and evaluation of non–abuse-related medical concerns. Non-advanced practice nurses also may be limited in the scope of their practice by their state nurse practice acts. SANEs should practice with a qualified expert medical director.

Every medical provider, regardless of expertise, should have a method for oversight and review to increase the accuracy and validity of findings and ensure continued refinement of skills. Some professional settings will have expert examiners as full- or part-time staff. In these settings, internal review among all the medical providers can play an important role in the quality review process as well as the continuing education of the providers. Some programs must obtain this expertise through affiliation with local hospitals or other facilities. Programs in smaller or more rural communities may not have direct access to qualified examiners and may develop mentoring or consultative relationships with experts in other communities. The use of telemedicine technologies can play a valuable role in this form of consultation.

Programs with geographically isolated examiners, programs with inexperienced examiners, and non-advanced practice SANE programs should have a system in place for continuing review. At a minimum, these examiners should seek secondary review of all cases considered to be abnormal or diagnostic of abuse. The ongoing mentorship of an expert is beneficial and provides both support and ongoing education to the more inexperienced examiner.

Ongoing Education

The field of child sexual abuse medicine is evolving, and information can quickly become obsolete. The examiner should obtain continuing education on a routine basis to stay abreast of new developments. A health care provider who trained many years ago may have incomplete or inaccurate knowledge and need an update to remain current and consistent with standards of best practice. Dedication to remaining current in the field is mandatory to maintain a relevant knowledge base. It is mandatory for health care providers to interact with local and national experts to become apprised of updates in the field. In addition to this formal continuing education, providers should be able to demonstrate that they have kept up to date with published research studies on findings in abused and nonabused children as well as sexual transmission of infections in children. Current guidelines and recommendations for the evaluation of sexually abused children are available from national professional organizations such as the American Academy of Pediatrics (AAP) and the Centers for Disease Control and Prevention (CDC).

Conclusion

A variety of health care professionals are trained to examine children for sexual abuse, each with individual training and talents in the field. It is imperative to continue to strive for the best-educated, most qualified, and best-trained individuals to provide medical services to child victims of abuse. Examinations by unqualified professionals are a disservice to both the children and their families. Although communities differ in the types of professionals they have in place, the common goal is the health and well-being of the children. To that end, national standards are necessary to ensure that abused children receive the quality of care they deserve.

In many health care settings, communication and collaboration among health care professionals can bring excellent outcomes to the assessment and care of a child and family. Different professionals bring different, often complementary skill sets to a particular situation. Allowed to work in unison, the skill sets can be additive, resulting in optimal communication with child welfare workers, law enforcement personnel, prosecutors and defense lawyers, and others in a community system, as well as a best outcome for the patient and family.

References

1. National Children's Alliance. *Standards for Accredited Members*. Washington, DC: National Children's Alliance; 2017.

2. Ladson S, Johnson CF, Doty RE. Do physicians recognize sexual abuse? *Am J Dis Child*. 1987;141(4):411-415.

3. Lentsch KA, Johnson CF. Do physicians have adequate knowledge of child sexual abuse? The results of two surveys of practicing physicians, 1986 and 1996. *Child Maltreat*. 2000;5(1):72-78.

4. Hornor G, McCleery J. Do pediatric nurse practitioners recognize sexual abuse? *J Pediatr Health Care*. 2000;14(2):45-49.

5. Adams JA, Wells R. Normal versus abnormal genital findings in children: how well do examiners agree? *Child Abuse Negl*. 1993;17(5):663-675.

6. Paradise JE, Finkel MA, Beiser AS, Berenson AB, Greenberg DB, Winter MR. Assessments of girl's genital findings and the likelihood of sexual abuse: agreement among physicians self-rated as skilled. *Arch Pediatr Adolesc Med*. 1997;151(9):883-891.

7. Paradise JE, Winter MR, Finkel MA, Berenson AB, Beiser AS. Influence of the history on physicians' interpretations of girls' genital findings. *Pediatrics*. 1999;103(5 pt 1):980-986.

8. Makoroff KL, Brauley JL, Brandner AM, Myers PA, Shapiro RA. Genital examinations for alleged sexual abuse of prepubertal girls: findings by pediatric emergency medicine physicians compared with child abuse trained physicians. *Child Abuse Negl*. 2002;26(12):1235-1242.

9. Dubow SR, Giardino AP, Christian CW, Johnson CF. Do pediatric chief residents recognize details of prepubertal female genital anatomy: a national survey. *Child Abuse Negl*. 2005;29(2):195-205.

10. Heisler KW, Starling SP, Edwards H, Paulson JF. Child abuse training, comfort, and knowledge among emergency medicine, family medicine, and pediatric residents. *Med Educ Online*. 2006;11(1):4600. doi:10.3402/meo.v11i.4600.

11. Jenny C, Crawford-Jakubiak JE; Committee on Child Abuse and Neglect, American Academy of Pediatrics. The evaluation of children in the primary care setting when sexual abuse is suspected. *Pediatrics*. 2013;132(2):e558-567.

12. Limbos MA, Berkowitz CD. Documentation of child physical abuse: how far have we come? *Pediatrics*. 1998;102(1 pt 1):53-58

13. Finkel MA, Alexander RA. Conducting the medical history. *J Child Sex Abus*. 2011;20(5):486-504.

14. Bernard D, Peters M, Makaroff K. The evaluation of suspected pediatric sexual abuse. *Clin Pediatr Emerg Med*. 2006;7(3):161-169.

15. Cronch LE, Viljoen JL, Hansen DJ. Forensic interviewing in child sexual abuse cases: current techniques and future directions. *Aggress Violent Behav*. 2006;11(3):195-207.

16. Westcott HL, Kynan S. Interviewer practice in investigative interviews for suspected child sexual abuse. *Psychol Crime Law*. 2006;12(4):367-382.

17. Adams JA, Kellogg ND, Farst KJ, et al. Updated guidelines for the medical assessment and care of children who may have been sexually abused. *J Pediatr Adolesc Gynecol.* 2016;29(2):81-87.

18. Gavril AR, Kellogg ND, Nair P. Value of follow-up examinations of children and adolescents evaluated for sexual abuse and assault. *Pediatrics.* 2012;129(2):282-289.

19. Christian CW, Lavelle JM, De Jong AR, Loiselle J, Brenner L, Joffe M. Forensic evidence findings in prepubertal victims of sexual assault. *Pediatrics.* 2000;106(1 pt 1):100-104.

20. Young KL, Jones JG, Worthington T, Simpson P, Casey PH. Forensic laboratory evidence in sexually abused children and adolescents. *Arch Pediatr Adolesc Med.* 2006;160(6):585-588.

21. Kellogg N; American Academy of Pediatrics Committee on Child Abuse and Neglect. The evaluation of sexual abuse in children. *Pediatrics.* 2005;116(2):506-512.

22. Adams JA, Starling SP, Frasier LD, et al. Diagnostic accuracy in child sexual abuse medical evaluation: role of experience, training, and expert case review. *Child Abuse Negl.* 2012;36(5):383-392.

23. The 2018 Florida statutes: 39.303: child protection teams and sexual abuse treatment programs; services; eligible cases. Online Sunshine Web site. http://leg.state.fl.us/Statutes/index.cfm?App_mode=Display_Statute&Search_String=&URL=0000-0099/0039/Sections/0039.303.html. Accessed December 11, 2018.

24. Title XXII occupations and professions: chapter 334. Missouri Revisor of Statutes Web site. http://revisor.mo.gov/main/OneSection.aspx?section=334.950. Published August 28, 2014. Accessed December 11, 2018.

Chapter 13

The Multidisciplinary Team and Child Sexual Abuse

Mark Hudson, MD
Rich A. Kaplan, MSW, MD, FAAP†

Background and Rationale

The concept of an interdisciplinary approach to medical care is certainly not novel. It has traditionally meant the bringing together of several medical and ancillary specialties in response to medically complex diagnoses such as spina bifida or craniofacial malformations. With respect to child abuse in general and sexual abuse specifically, the concept of a multidisciplinary team (MDT) is significantly broader. In 1962, in their landmark article *The Battered-Child Syndrome*, Kempe and colleagues[1] noted that the physician should be acquainted with "facilities available in private and public agencies that provide protective services for children." They go on to recommend "an evaluation of the psychological and social factors in the case." There is also reference to law enforcement and the courts. In 1976, Fontana and Robison[2] described a system that used nonmedical community services to treat and prevent child abuse.

Formal research regarding the effectiveness of MDTs is somewhat limited and hampered by the complex nature of sexual abuse cases and the attribution of outcomes to particular elements of an MDT response. This is particularly true as it relates to child and family outcomes. Though limited, the existing evidence supports the efficacy of the MDT response.[3]

Members of the Multidisciplinary Team

The MDT concept in child maltreatment cases goes far beyond the traditional interdisciplinary treatment model. It is often considered a vehicle for performing investigations and arresting and incarcerating sexual perpetrators. The MDT concept goes beyond this as well. It has the potential to involve professionals from child protective services (CPS), law enforcement, the courts, and the mental health sector in a process that ideally minimizes trauma to the child victim and creates a synergy that meets the professional mandates of all constituents and, above all, the complex needs of young victims.

Child Protective Services

The notion that the protection of children is a government responsibility is relatively new. In the 18th century and much of the 19th century, maltreated children were placed in institutions known as almshouses. Mainly for orphaned, abandoned, or unwanted children of the poor, these facilities generally made for a crowded, chaotic, and unwholesome environment.[4] In the late 19th century there was a more evolved social apparatus for the protection of animals than for the protection of child victims. In 1874, the Society for the Prevention of Cruelty to Animals (SPCA) filed a writ of habeas corpus to secure the removal of 9-year-old Mary Ellen Wilson from her abusive home. At that time, there was no private or governmental agency to act on behalf of abused children.

Although the Wilson case is widely known, it was not an isolated event. There is an account of a previous attempt by the SPCA to protect an abused child 3 years earlier.[5] Following the case involving Mary Ellen Wilson, the New York Society for the Prevention of Cruelty to Children was formed. Ultimately, quite a number of these societies were formed as part of the American Humane Society. As the child welfare movement evolved into government-provided child protection programs, a healthy dialog developed between the at-times disparate approaches of investigation/placement and family service/support. This debate continues today as the pendulum swings between a "traditional" investigative response and an "alternative" or "assessment" response reported to be less adversarial and more likely to result in voluntary services.[6]

CPS plays a role in the evaluation and the response phases of child sexual abuse cases. In the early stages of a response, CPS will assess for risk to the child who may have been abused as well as the child's siblings and assess the need for ongoing services. This initial assessment is often performed in concert with a law enforcement investigation but may be undertaken separately. Rather than being directed toward criminal prosecution, the CPS evaluation often leads to voluntary services or a juvenile or civil legal proceeding involving protection, placement, and long-term disposition. Additionally, a service or program component of CPS is often involved in the provision of long-term services and support to a victim's family. This component of the CPS response may involve a different CPS worker, rather than the CPS worker who conducted the initial assessment. It should be noted that CPS involvement is often predicated on abuse being intrafamilial, perpetrated by a caregiver, or the result of inadequate parental supervision.

Law Enforcement

The role of law enforcement is central in the evaluation of cases of child sexual abuse. From the community perspective, law enforcement is charged with maintaining public safety. This is usually perceived as the apprehension of criminals. From the MDT perspective, the role of law enforcement is much broader and more complex. In nearly all jurisdictions, law enforcement personnel have the statutory authority to immediately protect children who are in imminent danger. From the standpoint of gathering a history, the police may have exclusive access to the scene of the abuse. In acute cases they can gather material that may contain biologic or physical evidence that may be diagnostically significant. In nonacute cases, they can identify details at the scene, such as computer data, photographs, or physical details, that may add to or reduce a possible victim's credibility. Law enforcement also has access to private data pertaining to past alleged or adjudicated criminal activity that may be pertinent.

It is simplistic to characterize law enforcement in a one-dimensional manner. As in the field of health care, there are varied roles and competencies. The uniformed officer is often the first contact and is responsible for stabilizing the scene and, at times, taking an initial statement from a possible child victim. This role is extremely sensitive and ideally requires specialized training. In a growing number of communities this initial interaction is protocol driven by various interagency agreements. There are also clear differences among child sexual abuse investigators, including the perception of their roles and the techniques they use.[7] An investigator's attitude and beliefs can affect case decisions, but attitude is malleable and can be influenced by intensive education.[8]

There are broad social variables as well. The degree of specialization varies depending on police department size as well as the police and municipal administration's commitment to the support of child abuse services. It is not uncommon for services to children to be cut when budgets are tight, which means that the investigator primarily responsible for a child sexual abuse case may lack the time or experience to perform optimally. Given the lack of physical or corroborative evidence in the vast majority of cases of child sexual abuse, the investigator's skill and ability to compile collaborative evidence or obtain an admission of responsibility from an offender may be one of the most important elements in the protection of a child and the community.

The Courts

With respect to child maltreatment, the court system has 2 different and often quite separate systems. One, the criminal court, is geared toward the charging and trying of individuals believed to be child abusers. The other, the civil or child protection court, is involved with the determination of abuse or neglect by caregivers or custodians of the child and with decisions regarding child safety and well-being, parental rights, and guardianship. Although the most visible element in child abuse cases is the criminal prosecution of offenders, with the exception of extra-familial sexual assaults, this aspect is unlikely to have the most impact on the child victim or the family. It is the child protection court that often has the most profound effect on the child.

The milieu of the child protection court is much more amenable to the assimilation of medical and scientific material into the decision-making process for several reasons. First, in most jurisdictions the proceeding is held only in front of a judge, which generally limits polemics and drama. In addition, there is usually more opportunity for a medical provider to provide complex medical answers to complex legal questions. Finally, the standard of proof is different. Civil decisions are more likely to be determined by a preponderance of evidence or clear and convincing evidence, both of which are less stringent than the "beyond a reasonable doubt" standard held in criminal court. Physicians should learn the specific legal parameters for the jurisdiction(s) in which they practice. They should also be aware of special situations that may impact procedural rules (eg, the Indian Child Welfare Act, which mandates additional procedures and different standards of proof).

This is not to imply that there is little or no value in criminal justice. The community has a stake in the status of potentially dangerous pedophiles in their midst. There is also strong evidence that recidivism is high among sexual offenders; therefore, separating them from the community protects children. What is not known is the impact that criminal proceedings have on the child victim. Despite the fact that more than 100 000 children appear in court each year, there has been relatively little study of the short- and long-term consequences associated with court proceedings. It is clear that children, like adults, experience great anxiety related to court proceedings. Postponements increase anxiety and repeated testimony can result in poor long-term mental health outcomes. As such, victims need psychosocial support for the potential trauma of legal proceedings in addition to the support needed for the sexual abuse. The provision of testimony can also result in positive outcomes with some victims experiencing decreased anxiety, a greater sense of control, and decreased feelings of victimization.[9] Regardless of the relative impact of legal proceedings on the patient, it is incumbent on the child abuse medical provider to have complete knowledge of the system.

Mental Health

Mental health professionals are involved in the evaluation and treatment of possible child sexual abuse victims. The possible behavioral consequences and emotional impact of abuse on the child are evaluated. This evaluation is useful in assessing the possible therapy needs for the victim and the victim's family. It is also helpful in developing an understanding of a child and caregiver's reaction relative to a disclosure or lack of disclosure. In 1983, Roland Summit[10] described common behavioral manifestations of sexual maltreatment in children. With the development of the Child Sexual Behavior Inventory (CSBI), the late Dr. William Friedrich and colleagues[11] provided a remarkable tool for the interpretation of sexualized behaviors and their relationship to a history of sexual abuse. Currently many members of the MDT understand that there is a correlate between increased sexual behaviors and sexual abuse. The interpretation of sexualized behaviors in any particular patient, however, is complex and requires consideration of individual, family, and cultural variables.[12] For a child who is demonstrating behavioral signs of abuse or for whom there are other reasons to be concerned about abuse, therapy may provide a safe environment in which to discuss abuse issues or may provide reassurance that there is no indication of abuse. Similarly, the mental health profession is often best suited to interpret and treat the highly variable reaction of nonoffending caregivers. Understanding a caregiver's response and formulating appropriate intervention is critical for the well-being of the child and requires consideration of a multitude of factors, including general caregiver attributions and abuse-specific cognition.[13]

Victims of child sexual abuse suffer a myriad of short- and long-term consequences and exhibit more internalizing and externalizing problems than non-sexually abused children.[14] If the collective goal of the response to child sexual abuse is to ensure the well-being of the abused child, it follows that referral to effective psychotherapy is a critical element in the response to sexual abuse. The notion of efficacy is critically important. To refer a child to counseling without having details or outcome data is somewhat akin to referring a child to an intensive laetrile therapy center for acute lymphoblastic leukemia (ALL). There is a growing collection of data supporting the fact that specialized trauma therapy is effective in treating child victims of sexual abuse (see Chapter 20, "Therapy for the Child Sexual Abuse Victim"). Cognitive behavioral therapy (CBT) has proven effective in the treatment of childhood PTSD, but the data remains mixed on which particular variant of CBT is most effective. Mental health professionals can earn certification in trauma-focused CBT (TF-CBT), an evidence-based treatment developed specifically for child sexual abuse victims.[11-13,15]

The greatest barrier to effective therapy may be the availability of a trained therapist. The limited number of skilled practitioners and the restrictive third-party payer environment make it difficult for some to secure appropriate mental health therapy.

The Health Care Provider

The health care provider's role in cases of child sexual abuse is multifaceted. First and foremost is the provision of skilled, compassionate health care. This is similar to the care provided to other patients, but special skills and competencies, along with a specialized knowledge base, need to be acquired, updated, and subjected to peer review. This care includes a careful diagnostic assessment utilizing history and physical examination data and, when needed, laboratory and imaging studies. In some settings the health care provider will rely on some of the historical data obtained by another team member during the forensic interview. In other settings the health care provider performs the entire history-taking. Either way, the history serves as a basis for guiding physical examination and determining need for laboratory or other testing. This includes the development of a differential diagnosis that includes possible mimics of abuse.

The medical professional is also responsible for providing other team members with an understandable assessment of the medical and scientific issues specific to each case (eg, an explanation to an inexperienced team member about the lack of diagnostic utility of a normal genital examination or the lack of probative clarity of a human papillomavirus infection). This means that the health care provider must be available to the MDT for consultation regarding medical issues. The health care provider is also responsible for providing necessary referrals for follow-up primary and specialty care as well as participating in the referral to appropriate mental health resources. Finally, the health care provider needs to act as a liaison between nonmedical team members and the medical/hospital community. The child sexual abuse medical provider must educate the rest of the health care team regarding the legal and social issues involved in these cases and must also work within the health care system to develop procedural guidelines that minimize trauma to possible child victims. Systems need to be developed that will prevent examinations by inexperienced practitioners, obviate the need for multiple evaluations, and provide a safe and child-friendly setting for the physical examination.

Multidisciplinary Team Function

In order for an MDT to function in a productive manner, several requisite conditions need to be in place. First, team members must clearly articulate their areas of professional competence, the mandate under which they function, and their perception of their role on the team. Second, these perceptions need to be addressed in light of other team member expectations. For example, medical team members need to explain why it is necessary to gather a medical history that may overlap with a previous interview or explain the reasons for performing a genital examination in addition to discovering physical evidence. This need for a clear understanding of disciplinary competencies and mutual expectations provides the basis for the trust that is the cornerstone of effective teamwork. Team functioning is, however, certainly not static. All constituent agencies are fluid, and change is inevitable (eg, an experienced investigator is promoted, a new DA is elected, budget cuts devastate CPS). As long as the fundamental articulation of expectations and roles is continued and trust is maintained, the team can function effectively.

That being said, there will be conflicts that occur for a variety of reasons. The following issues are sources of team conflict:

— Who is most suited to conduct an interview?[16]

— How will law enforcement and CPS work together?[17]

— Why are some cases not referred for charging?[18]

— Why wasn't a child informed of the need for an examination?[19]

Maintaining a productive and effective MDT is not easy. It takes patience, energy, and an unflagging commitment to the safety and well-being of child victims.

Conclusion

The MDT evaluating and intervening in cases of child abuse may include professionals from medicine, nursing, mental health, CPS, and law enforcement. Each member of the team contributes unique knowledge and expertise. Flexibility and an understanding of each others' role on the team are essential to functioning effectively to minimize trauma and meet the complex needs of young victims.

References

1. Kempe CH, Silverman FN, Steele BF, Droegemueller W, Silver HK. The battered-child syndrome. *JAMA*. 1962;181:17-24.

2. Fontana VJ, Robison E. A multidisciplinary approach to the treatment of child abuse. *Pediatrics*. 1976;57(5):760-764.

3. Herbert JL, Bromfield L. Better together? A review of evidence for multi-disciplinary teams responding to physical and sexual child abuse [published online ahead of print March 6, 2017]. *Trauma Violence Abuse*. doi: 10.1177/1524838017697268.

4. Schene PA. Past, present, and future roles of child protective services. *Future Child*. 1998;8(1):23-38.

5. Lazoritz S, Shelman EA. Before Mary Ellen. *Child Abuse Negl*. 1996;20(3):235-237.

6. Piper KA. Differential response in child protection: how much is too much? *Child Youth Serv Rev*. 2017;82:69-80.

7. Froum AG, Kendall-Tackett KA. Law enforcement officers' approaches to evaluations of child sexual abuse. *Child Abuse Negl*. 1998;22(9):939-942.

8. Darwinkel E, Powell M, Tidmarsh P. Improving police officers' perceptions of sexual offending through intensive training. *Crim Justice Behav*. 2013;40(8):895-908.

9. Pantell RH; Committee on Psychosocial Aspects of Child And Family Health. The child witness in the courtroom [published online ahead of print February 20, 2017]. *Pediatrics*. doi: 10.1542/peds.2016-4008.

10. Summit RC. The child sexual abuse accommodation syndrome. *Child Abuse Negl*. 1983;7(2):177-193.

11. Friedrich WN, Fisher JL, Dittner CA, et al. Child sexual behavior inventory: normative, psychiatric, and sexual abuse comparisons. *Child Maltreat*. 2001;6(1):37-49.

12. Miragoli S, Camisasca E, Di Blasio P. Child sexual behaviors in school context: age and gender differences. *J Child Sex Abus*. 2017;26(2):213-231.

13. Runyon MK, Spandorfer ED, Schroeder CM. Cognitions and distress in caregivers after their child's sexual abuse disclosure. *J Child Sex Abus*. 2014;23(2):146-159.

14. Lewis T, McElroy E, Harlaar N, Runyon D. Does the impact of child sexual abuse differ from maltreated but non-sexually abused children? A prospective examination of the impact of child sexual abuse on internalizing and externalizing behavior problems. *Child Abuse Negl*. 2016;51:31-40.

15. Sege RD, Amaya-Jackson L; American Academy of Pediatrics Committee on Child Abuse and Neglect; Council on Foster Care, Adoption, and Kinship Care; American Academy of Child and Adolescent Psychiatry Committee on Child Maltreatment and Violence; National Center for Child Traumatic Stress. Clinical considerations related to the behavioral manifestations of child maltreatment. *Pediatrics*. 2017;139(4):e20170100.

16. Drummond R, Gall JA. Evaluation of forensic medical history taking from the child in cases of child physical and sexual abuse and neglect. *J Forensic Leg Med*. 2017;46:37-45.

17. Cross TP, Chuang E, Helton JJ, Lux EA. Criminal investigations in child protective services cases: an empirical analysis. *Child Maltreat*. 2015;20(2):104-114.

18. Baiden P, Fallon B, den Dunnen W, Black TL. Police charging decisions in child maltreatment investigations: findings from the 2008 Ontario Incidence Study of Reported Child Abuse and Neglect. *J Public Child Welf*. 2017;11(2):211-230.

19. Muram D, Aiken MM, Strong C. Children's refusal of gynecologic examinations for suspected sexual abuse. *J Clin Ethics*. 1997;8(2):158-164.

Chapter 14

Child Sexual Abuse: An International Perspective

Marcellina Mian, MDCM, MHPE, FAAP, FRCPC

Introduction: Commercial Sexual Exploitation of Children

Commercial sexual exploitation of children (CSEC) is a crime and a severe betrayal of childhood that many find difficult to comprehend and confront. Yet it is critical that all of society have a better understanding of the kind of entrapment and misery that some children—too many children—endure on a daily basis, so that steps can be taken to prevent it. There are many actors on the global stage, including the United Nations (UN) and other international organizations, governmental and nongovernmental agencies, and those involved in grassroots projects, whose aim is to protect children from CSEC. Some of these will be identified in the sections that follow.

Definitions

In 2016, to facilitate communication among and between all stakeholders working to uphold child rights, an interagency working group published their conclusions on recommended terminology related to child rights.[1] The working group reviewed legally binding documents, including the Convention on the Rights of the Child (CRC)[2] and its Optional Protocols[3,4] and nonbinding instruments such as resolutions of the UN General Assembly and Human Rights Council (UNHRC).

Child

CRC Article 1 defines a ***child*** as "every human being below the age of eighteen years."[2] The CRC has been ratified by all states in the world except for the United States of America.[5]

Child Marriage

The United Nations International Children's Emergency Fund (UNICEF) defines ***child marriage*** as the "a formal marriage or informal union before age 18."[1] This definition applies even in countries where the age of majority is reached before age 18. ***Early marriage*** (sometimes used interchangeably) is a broader term that may include individuals older than 18 years who do not have the capacity to comprehend the meaning of marriage. In certain circumstances, such as the payment of a debt, child marriage may be considered a form of sexual exploitation.[6]

Child Labor

Child labor is a more restricted category than "economically active children" or "working children" because it excludes all children working legally in accordance with International Labour Organization (ILO) Conventions 138 and 182.[7,8] The worst forms of child labor are defined in Article 3 of Convention 182 (*Convention Concerning the Prohibition and Immediate Action for the Elimination of the Worst Forms of Child Labour*). These include[8]:

(a) all forms of slavery or practices similar to slavery, such as the sale and trafficking of children, debt bondage and serfdom and forced or compulsory labour, including forced or compulsory recruitment, of children for use in armed conflict;

(b) the use, procuring or offering of a child for prostitution, for the production of pornography or for pornographic performances;

(c) the use, procuring or offering of a child for illicit activities, in particular for the production and trafficking of drugs as defined in the relevant international treaties;

These practices are also termed "unconditional worst forms of child [labor]."[9]

Slavery: Forced Labor, Serfdom, and Debt Bondage

Child slavery has been defined as "children being in a hazardous situation and being exploited for someone else's gain, often under threats and/or use of violence, such as children who are used for profit through prostitution or pornography, forced begging, petty theft; children who are used for child labour; children who are used to take part in armed conflict; and child domestic workers/children in domestic servitude."[1]

Child Trafficking

Child trafficking is the "recruitment and/or transport, transfer, harbouring, and receipt of a child by others with the intent of exploiting the child through various means, like prostitution, begging, child labour, etc."[1] The intent to exploit differentiates "trafficking" from "sale of children," which is a broader term that always involves some form of commercial transaction in the transfer of a child from one person to another but does not necessarily involve exploitation (eg, illegal adoption where the adoptive parents plan to treat the child well), though there is considerable overlap.[1] Appropriate application must be done on a case-by-case basis. Child trafficking may include child marriage, illegal adoption, sale of child organs, and the recruitment of child soldiers. In some cases (eg, illegal adoptions into a loving family), the child may actually benefit from the transaction despite its illegality.

Commercial Sexual Exploitation

ECPAT International defines ***exploitation*** as "the unfair use of something/someone for one's own advantage or benefit" and ***commercial sexual exploitation (CSE)*** as "a form of sexual exploitation where the focus is specifically on monetary benefit, often relating to organised criminality where the primary driver is economic gain."[1] ***Commercial sexual exploitation of children (CSEC)*** includes child prostitution, child pornography, and sexual exploitation of children in the context of travel and tourism. Domestic minor sex trafficking refers to CSEC affecting children who are US citizens or legal residents victimized within US borders.[10] Child marriage and online child sexual exploitation may involve forms of CSEC. In cases of CSEC, the intended commercial gain need not be obvious, nor does it require the exchange of money. In some situations, such as child marriage, the exploitation involves contractual or commercial exchange, gain of prestige, land transfer, or other services. Conversely, child trafficking, child sales, and child slavery may all involve sexual abuse and exploitation, even if that was not the original or primary intent. The key element of CSEC, as opposed to other forms of child sexual abuse (CSA), is that it involves a commercial transaction or exchange in which one or more parties makes a gain. The beneficiaries of these transactions are the adults immediately involved in them, as well as the larger circle of facilitators. ***Facilitators*** are those who enable the sexual crimes, even if they do not themselves commit the abuse. They may be strangers, family members (including parents), and even children who are coerced to recruit their peers. Commercially exploited children may benefit from some transactions, but usually to a much lesser degree than the adults involved. Such benefits may be no more than what should be the child's by right (eg, protection, shelter, food). A child might agree to sexual favors in exchange for these benefits, but that agreement does not in any way imply true consent.

Sexual Exploitation of Children in Travel and Tourism

"Child sex tourism" is no longer considered an acceptable term. Per ECPAT International, "Terms such as ***sexual exploitation of children in travel and tourism*** [emphasis added] appear more appropriate; this explicitly says that the child is being exploited and adequately broadens the focus from the actions of offenders to a wider perspective on the settings in which the exploitation takes place."[1]

Sexual Exploitation of Children in/for Prostitution

Child prostitution is a form of exploitation that "consists of a child performing a sexual act in exchange for (a promise of) something of value," though the child is often not the recipient of that benefit.[1] The alternate term ***sexual exploitation of children in/for prostitution*** conveys the activity more accurately without stigmatizing the child. To avoid the risk of shifting the blame onto the child, "child prostitute" and similar terms should be avoided. This issue is relevant even for children who may "voluntarily" engage in prostitution, because under international law, children do not have the capacity to consent to their own exploitation and should always been seen as victims of exploitation.[1]

Use of Children for Sexual Performances

Child pornography is a term widely used in international legal documents; however, the term *use of children for sexual performances* is more accurate. With regard to the pornographic material itself, there is movement toward use of the term ***child sexual abuse material (CSAM)*** in order to emphasize that the material depicts the sexual abuse of a child. Again, the intent is to remove any suggestion of responsibility on the part of the child.[1]

Child Soldiers

A ***child soldier*** is "any person under 18 years of age who is part of any kind of regular or irregular armed force or armed group in any capacity, including but not limited to cooks, porters, messengers and anyone accompanying such groups, other than family members. The definition includes girls recruited for sexual purposes and for forced marriage. It does not, therefore, only refer to a child who is carrying or has carried arms."[11]

Scale of the Problem

Due to limitations in data collection, including variable definitions, problems with study design or feasibility, and the concealment of CSEC, the number of children who are involved in CSEC in its various manifestations is difficult to validate. With that in mind, the following estimates have been derived.

Child Marriage

Data from 2014 indicate that more than 700 million women worldwide were married as children and that about 250 million were married before reaching 15 years of age.[12] As reported by the United Nations International Children's Emergency Fund (UNICEF), the highest rates of child marriage worldwide have been found in sub-Saharan Africa, where 38% of girls were married before age 18 years and 12% before age 15 years, while in Eastern Europe and Central Asia, these rates were 11% and 1% respectively.[13] In 7 countries (Cuba, Marshall Islands, Comoros, Honduras, Nauru, Lao People's Democratic Republic, and Madagascar), the percentage of men aged 20 to 24 years who were first married or in union by age 18 years ranged between 11% and 13%. In the Central African Republic, the rate was 28%.

The median age for marriage is gradually increasing, but this increase is limited to higher income families.[12] Despite modestly encouraging data, UNICEF projects that unless significant efforts are made to magnify the decline, population growth in countries where early marriage is a common practice may offset the slight drop in prevalence, potentially keeping the number of child brides constant through 2050.

Child Labor, Trafficking, and Sexual Exploitation

Between 2000 and 2008, child labor in the 5- to 17-year age group declined globally from about 246 million to 215 million, representing a decline of 12.6% in incidence rate.[14] This downward trend continued through 2016, where the the number dropped to about 152 million children or a decline of 38% over the 16 years. **Figure 14-1** shows the estimate for children who are employed, those who are engaged in child labor, and those who are engaged in hazardous work.[14,15]

International Labour Organization (ILO) figures from 2016 indicate that worldwide, 218 million children aged 5 to 17 years were employed.[16] Of these children, 152 million children (58% boys) were involved in child labor, with the largest segment being 114 million children aged 5 to 14 years who were included as child laborers because of their young age. The majority (71% of the total) worked in agriculture. Roughly 73 million children performed hazardous work and other, worst forms of child labor, including forced recruitment for armed conflict, commercial sexual exploitation, and illicit activities (eg, drug trafficking, organized begging). According to this report, the highest prevalence of child labor is in Africa (19.6%), followed by Asia and the Pacific (7.4%), with the Arab states having the lowest (2.9%). UNICEF reports that sub-Saharan Africa had the highest prevalence of child labor and that in the least developed countries, about 25% of children aged 5 to 17 years are engaged in work that poses a risk to their health and development.[17] An estimated 5.5 million children constitute roughly 26% of all people who live under various forms of modern slavery, including debt bondage and trafficking for labor exploitation.[18,19]

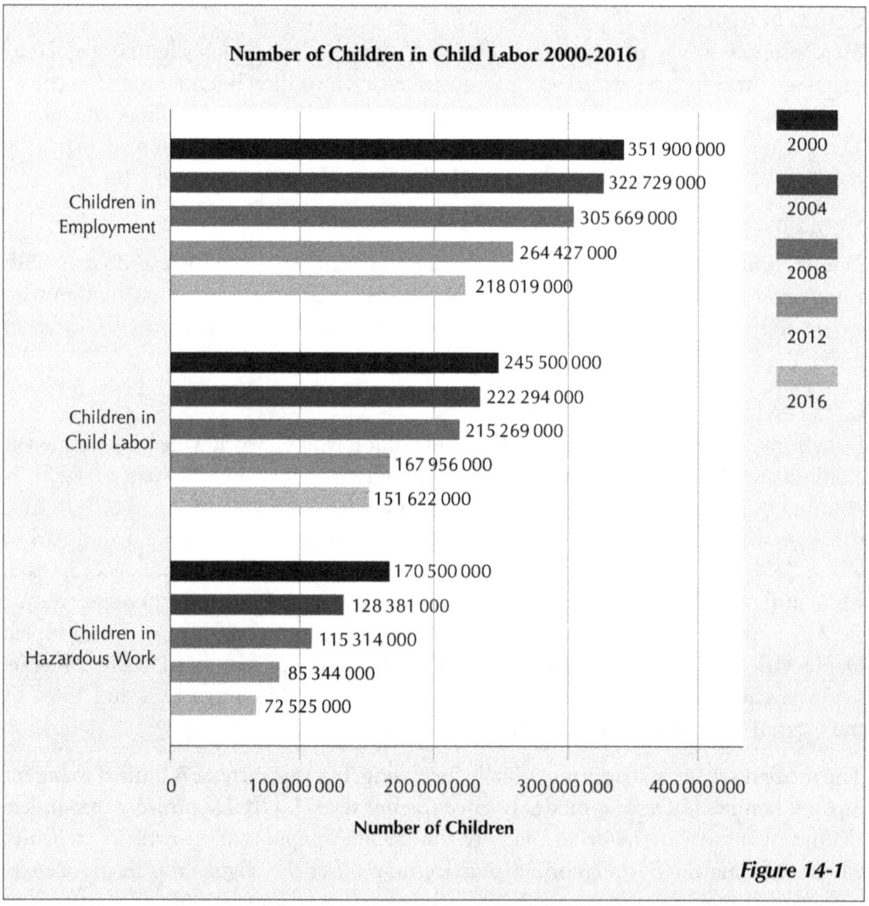

Figure 14-1. *Number of children in child labor from 2000 to 2016. Data from International Labour Organization.*[14,15]

Not all exploited children are trafficked across international borders to neighboring countries or other continents. Children can be taken from their parents and remain within their home country.[10,20,21] The International Organization for Migration (IOM) assisted 2040 child victims of human trafficking in 2011 (a 27% increase from 2008).[20] Children represented a little more than one-third of these cases. According to the IOM, "International trafficking cases fell 13% to 3531 in 2011, down from 4066 in 2008. But domestic cases shot up 140% from 713 in 2008 to 1708 last year." They attributed the decrease in international trafficking to tighter border security measures. Any country can be a country of origin, a destination, or both. Considering all victims, the top 3 destination countries were the Russian Federation, Haiti, and Yemen. The top 3 countries of origin were Ukraine, Haiti, and Yemen.

The greatest demand for children for exploitation in the context of travel comes from developed countries. Tourists, who may hold positions of trust in their own countries, seek the anonymity of foreign countries to engage in sex with children.[22] They represent all socio-economic backgrounds and travel to developing countries because of the availability of children in prostitution and because of weak law enforcement and corruption.[23]

People seeking sex with children no longer have to travel abroad. Previously thought to be confined to foreign soil, Americans are realizing that ***domestic sex trafficking of minors*** now conservatively involves 150 000 to 300 000 US citizens or legal immigrants.[10] This is thought to be an underestimate, particularly for boys, due to several factors, including the use of different definitions and the secrecy that surrounds this activity.

Contributing Factors

The World Report on Violence and Health applies an ecological model to explain susceptibility to violence.[24] **Figure 14-2** illustrates how risk factors pertaining to the individual nest within those related to the family and other personal relationships, which in turn nest within community risk factors, which lie within those that exist in society at large. Factors contributing to violence at each level influence those at all other levels and determine the degree of risk related to violence.

In child marriage, child labor, and CSEC, contributing factors are present in all levels of the ecological model. The root causes are multifactorial and include poverty, lack of education, gender inequality, dysfunctional families, conflicts and humanitarian crises, demand, criminality, cultural practices, and violations of the rights of the child.[12,13,16,25]

Birth Registration

Globally, the stage for the commercial sexual exploitation of a child may be set at birth. Article 7 of the CRC states, "The child shall be registered immediately after birth and shall have the right from birth to a name, the right to acquire a nationality and, as far as possible, the right to know and be cared for by his or her parents."[2] Notwithstanding this obligation, the births of only 71% of the world's children are registered before their fifth birthday, with African countries having the lowest rate of registration (41% to 45%).[26] However, even among registered children, a large number of children worldwide (around 290 million or 45% of all children younger than the age of 5) do not have a birth certificate. Boys and girls are equally likely to have birth certificates, but children living in affluent communities and in urban centers with ready access to registration facilities are more likely than others to have birth certificates.

A child who has a birth certificate has an identity registered in law. Without one, the child does not exist in law, has no proof of identity, age, or parentage, and cannot have valid identity documents (eg, a passport).[27] This means the child remains in the margins

Figure 14-2. *Ecological Model to Understand Violence. Reprinted with permission from* World Report on Violence and Health*; 1st ed; Krug EG, Dahlberg LL, Mercy JA, Zwi AB, Lozano R; Violence: a global public health problem; 1-22; 2002.*

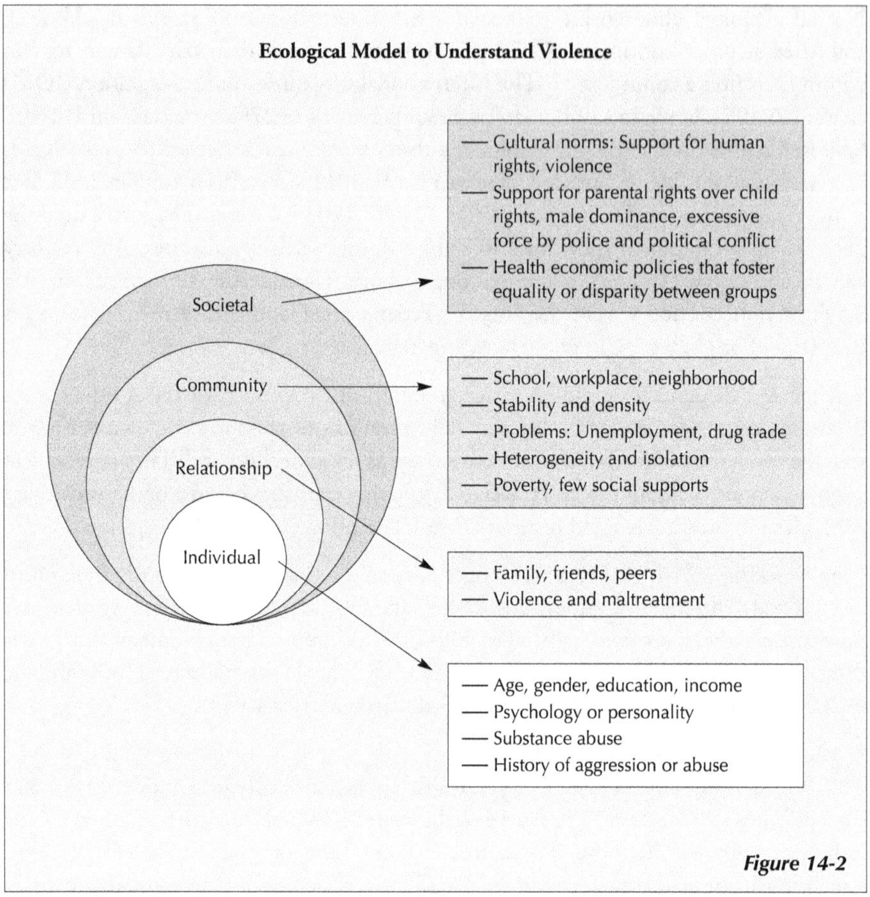

of society, unable to access its benefits, including education, health care, and many social programs. A child in this situation can be more easily neglected, abused, and exploited. For example, in places with laws pertaining to a minimum age for working children and marriage, absence of a birth certificate allows employers and families to marry young children and put them to work more easily. Lack of registration and nationality are considered significant risk factors for child trafficking and exploitation, because unregistered children are more easily hidden or passed off as young adults. A child can be hired ostensibly as a young adult domestic worker and then made to work in the sex trade. In places where the law recognizes the special status of young offenders, not having a birth certificate exposes youth to prosecution as an adult, incarceration with hardened criminals, and potentially to harsh penalties, including death.

Age, Gender, and Other Individual Factors

Gender and age are risk factors that determine the type of abuse to which children will be more vulnerable. Sexual violence affects girls more than boys, particularly adolescents.[28] Boys are more likely to be trafficked for forced labor on commercial farms, in the drug trade, or in petty crime.

Girls are more likely to be trafficked for commercial sexual exploitation and domestic service. Most child domestic workers are girls between 12 and 17 years of age, but girls as young as 8 may be hired as domestic workers.[29] Youth are recruited for domestic sex trafficking in the United States at 12 to 16 years of age.[10]

As a group, girls work longer hours than boys because in addition to their work outside the home, they are also expected to do domestic work at home. **Figure 14-3** demonstrates this difference, where boys appear to be working more if only economic activity is counted, but girls are shown to work far more when household chores are included.[30]

Children of parents with a history of CSA are at higher risk for sexual abuse, as are children who have witnessed sexual abuse of a peer.[31] Recruitment strategies may also take advantage of the normal developmental tendencies of adolescents (eg, desire for independence from parents, sexual experimentation, impulsivity).[10]

Poverty and Education

Poverty is the first among a number of factors cited as contributing to child labor in general, CSEC, and child marriages. According to the United Nations Population Fund, "Human trafficking is a global phenomenon that is driven by demand and fueled by poverty and unemployment."[32] Affluent countries contribute by the demand they create for children as sex objects, either by seeking CSAM or sex with children. Affluent individuals who might be too inhibited or frightened of legal consequences to engage in sex with children in their own community may travel to other communities, countries, or continents in order to indulge their pleasure. However, as noted above, domestic CSEC is increasingly common, making children in affluent countries vulnerable as well.

As reported by UNICEF, child marriage is most common among the poorest 40% of the general population compared to the richest 40%.[25] In that same report, women 20 to 24 years of age who had attended primary school or primary and secondary school were found to be less likely to be married by age 18 years than those who had not. Husbands are often much older than the child-bride. In Burkina Faso, 65% of the girls had a husband who was more than 15 years older. An older, better-educated man is or may be seen to be more likely to be able to look after his wife and family, or he may simply be in a better position to procure a young wife.

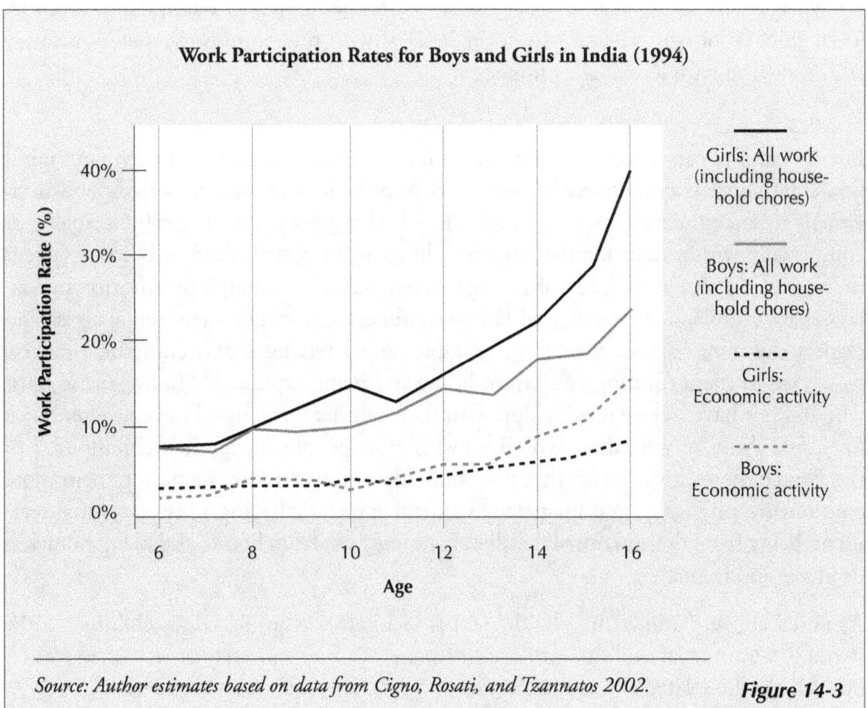

Figure 14-3. *Work participation rates for boys and girls in rural India (1994). World Bank. 2005. Gender Issues in Child Labor. PREM Notes; No. 100. World Bank, Washington, DC. © World Bank. https://openknowledge.worldbank.org/handle/10986/11210 License: CC BY 3.0 IGO.*

Poor children may choose to enter dangerous settings thinking those settings will offer opportunities and because they are not aware of the dangers they will face. As stated by Isabelle Guitard, Director of Programs at Child Soldiers International, "It is deeply shocking to see that, because their families cannot afford to pay school fees, some girls see joining an armed group as their only option, and decide to throw themselves in harm's way."[33]

Improving education contributes to improved economic well-being, later marriages, fewer children, and better protection of children in general.[34,35] Children who go to school are more likely to learn how to stay healthy and have fewer sexually transmitted infections (STIs), including human immunodeficiency virus (HIV). They are less likely to be trafficked, exploited, or suffer abuse or violence.[9,29] The education of girls is especially beneficial because it also benefits the next generation.[34] Educated girls are more likely to have healthier children who are better nourished and better educated.

When subsistence becomes a critical issue for families, the need for all members to contribute to the family's economic survival comes to weigh on even its youngest members. Options for gainful employment may be quite limited in economically disadvantaged countries. When families have to borrow, they may give a child in exchange or use the child to discharge an outstanding debt. Debt bondage is akin to slavery in that bonded individuals find the debt cannot ever be fully repaid, because of practices such as exorbitant interest rates or not applying the value of the work to the liquidation of the debt.[36] The choices made by families to have their children go to work as domestics, to be given as security for a debt, or to be married young may not be fueled by greed but rather by the desire to ensure the child's well-being. The family may view their choice as giving their children an opportunity they would not otherwise have if they remained with their families.[37]

Both at the individual and community level, education is a factor inversely related to degree of risk for victimization.[24] Children and parents with little schooling and knowledge of the world at large are at greater risk for being victimized. At the community level, child labor is more likely to occur in areas with no compulsory, quality primary education and with low rates of literacy.[38]

Family

Loving families can be protective of their children, but in dysfunctional, violent families, child abuse is more likely to occur.[24] A prior history of violence predisposes individuals to encounter violence again. Children who are abused physically, sexually, or emotionally within their families are more likely to be revictimized or become violent themselves.[24] In a recent study of young women exploited through prostitution in Malaysia, about 94% had experienced family dysfunction, including emotional abuse and neglect, substance abuse, gambling, unstable family relations, and domestic violence, which led to them running away from home and being exploited.[39] In Swaziland, girls who did not have a close relationship with their mother were found to be at higher risk for sexual abuse, as were those who lived with more people during their childhood.[31] In the United States, risk factors that put children at higher risk by rendering them more emotionally, physically, and financially vulnerable include having a history of maltreatment, being from dysfunctional families, running away from home, and being homeless or in a group home.[10]

As noted above, families may be the actual facilitators who introduce children to the world of commercial exploitation. This is frequently due to poverty or lack of education but can also be related to cultural factors and practices such as ritual slavery.[40]

Setting

The urban setting is a risk factor for sexual abuse for girls in Swaziland.[31] As reported by the World Health Organization, homelessness and living on the streets is a definite risk factor for youth exploited in prostitution.[41] In Iran, Pakistan, and South Africa 40% to 50% of street youth reported exchanging sex for money, goods, shelter, or protection.

The setting of the child's employment may also contribute to abuse, violence, and exploitation. In many countries, child domestic work is viewed in a positive light and is a preferred form of employment, especially for girls.[42] However, domestic work may also be designated a worst form of child labor, as children live and work in an environment completely controlled by the people who have power and authority over them.[37] They work hard and long days (up to 16 hours in some cases) and may have to handle heavy or dangerous material. They may be physically and sexually abused, deprived of food, and may experience emotional distress due to constantly being treated as inferior, insulted, belittled, or deprived of peer relations. If they displease their employer, they may be arbitrarily transferred to another home. They may also be denied their rights to education, health care, rest, recreation, being cared for, and to regular contact with their parents and peers.[42]

Natural disasters increase opportunities for the abuse and trafficking of children. In Nepal, for example, the amount of trafficking in children increased after the earthquakes of April 15, 2015.[21] Children were not only trafficked to India and other foreign destinations as domestic sex slaves and forced laborers, but also to orphanages within Nepal where they are at risk for illegal adoptions and exploitation.

Cultural Factors

Cultural practices and myths contribute to the sexual exploitation of children. In India and Ghana, girls are given to priests as a ritual form of slavery.[37,40,43] In India, these girls and women are known as "Devadasi." Nowadays, the practice is limited to the poor, illiterate, and to marginalized groups. The practice is based on a mixture of mythologies and is supported by the belief that a family's provision of a Devadasi will confer spiritual favor upon it, by the family's economic need, and by the lower status of girls, which renders them vulnerable to abuse.[40] Similarly, in Ghana, the underlying pretext for religious ritual slavery is the belief that a virgin daughter's dedication to a deity as a "Trokosi" will atone for any sins committed by a family member and provide protection for the family.[43] In both situations, girls are "married" to a deity and become available to the priest of the shrine to work as he directs and to submit to his sexual needs and potentially those of other men until about age 30, when they are no longer seen as desirable. Children born out of those relations may be considered children of the shrine or may not be recognized as children of the priest. Appropriate health care may not be provided either to the mother or the children.[40,43] Laws have been enacted in both countries against these practices, but they persist, especially in more remote areas. It is estimated there are 17000 to 23000 in each of 2 provinces in India and just under 5000 in the southern states of Ghana.

Legal and cultural factors affect what is considered appropriate or acceptable in terms of the treatment of children. Customs or religious doctrines that condone child marriage are juxtaposed against the adequacy of legislation against it and the ability to enforce that legislation to influence the persistence of the abusive practices.[25] Similarly, child trafficking is more likely to flourish if parents and other relatives, friends, peers, and teachers are complicit in allowing, encouraging, or benefiting from it. Negligent authorities and a systemic failure to respond also contribute to the problem.[44]

Community mores influence the treatment of domestic workers and the maltreatment of children, including child sexual exploitation.[42] Minimally, the community at large may not place sufficient moral sanctions on such behavior. They may view some behaviors as harmless (eg, CSA through pornography may be seen as "just looking at pictures"). The community may feel the child deserved the maltreatment or that it is none of their business. They may also become inured to the harshness of the children's circumstances, as may happen in refugee camps or among sex trade workers and their children. This is in part due to the stigmatization of exploited children, wherein the community does not consider them worthy of any attention, let alone positive intervention.

Armed Conflict

Armed conflicts, and the disruption, displacement, and disorientation they provoke affect many areas of the world. In 2016, millions of children in Syria, Nigeria, South Sudan, and Gaza fled the country or were internally displaced. These represented only a small fraction of the total number worldwide, many of whom are not accompanied by their families.[45] These situations lead to further violence, including what the UN has named the "6 grave violations" against children during armed conflict: (1) killing or maiming, (2) recruitment or use of child soldiers, (3) rape and other forms of sexual violence, (4) abduction, (5) attacks against schools or hospitals, and (6) denial of humanitarian access.[46]

Rape may be used as a means of terrorizing civilians in a factional conflict. Refugees are subjected to violence and rape, particularly if they go outside the camp perimeter to collect firewood, water, or other resources or if the latrines are positioned close to the camp's perimeter.[32] Gangs attack the camps to recruit or abduct children as combatants and girls as sexual slaves, cooks, and cleaners. Adult male refugees, unemployed and stressed by their circumstances, may become more aggressive, particularly toward adolescents and young women. Unfortunately, even some humanitarian workers use physical and sexual violence against refugees, in some cases demanding sex in exchange for supplies (including staples like food and water) and services. In 2002, relief workers (mostly local recruits but also international personnel) from a number of agencies working in refugee camps in Guinea, Liberia, and Sierra Leone were found to be using relief supplies to procure sex with underage girls.[47] In 2016, the Secretary-General on Children and Armed Conflict also reported disturbing cases of sexual abuse and exploitation by UN forces in 2015.[45]

Refugee children, especially unaccompanied children, face danger all along their journey. In the first 6 months of 2017, a total of 12 239 refugee children arrived in Italy, of whom about 93% were unaccompanied and separated children, mostly from Western Africa and Bangladesh.[48] According to UNICEF, besides drowning, they risk "dehydration, kidnapping, robbery, rape and extortion, as well as detention and beatings by the authorities or militias."[49] Both boys and girls were sexually abused and some girls had been impregnated as a result of that abuse. Criminal elements see the migration crisis as fertile ground for preying on vulnerable children for trafficking.

Virtually all nations with armies do not conscript children younger than 18 years of age, though some allow volunteers (sometimes requiring parental consent) at 16 or 17 years of age.[50] However, there are 63 nonstate parties listed by the Special Representative of the Secretary General for Children and Armed Conflict that recruit or use children in conflict, and 59 of them are considered persistent perpetrators.[45] Data on their recruitment efforts are difficult to confirm, but UNICEF estimates that tens of thousands of children are used in conflicts worldwide, including an estimated 17 000 children recruited in South Sudan and nearly 10 000 in the Central African Republic since 2013, while in Nigeria and neighboring countries, nearly 2000 children were recruited by Boko Haram in 2016 alone.[51]

Human Immunodeficiency Virus/Acquired Immunodeficiency Syndrome

Human immunodeficiency virus/acquired immunodeficiency syndrome (HIV/AIDS) is another source of devastation for children that leaves them orphaned, homeless, and without protection. The Joint United Nations Programme on HIV/AIDS (UNAIDS) reported that the number of orphans due to HIV/AIDS has been on a slow decline from 2010 to 2015, as seen in **Figure 14-4.**[52] However, according to UNICEF data, that trend did not hold for 2016. As of 2016, an estimated 16.5 million children have lost 1 or both parents due to AIDS, more than 80% of whom (13.8 million) live in sub-Saharan Africa.[53,54]

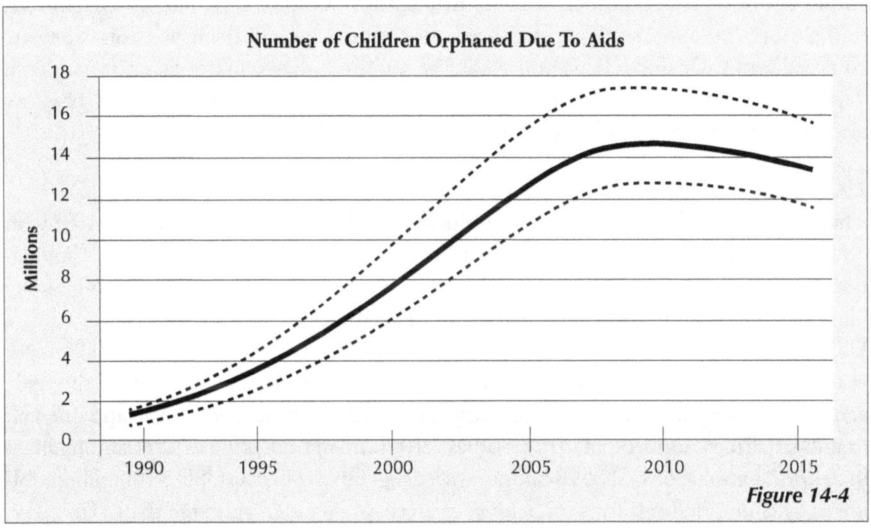

Figure 14-4. Number children orphaned due to AIDS (global). Reprinted with permission from Joint United Nations Programme on HIV and AIDS.[52]

Being orphans places these children at a disadvantage in terms of economic stress, inadequate nutrition, anxiety, depression, and missing out on their education, although trends in that last regard appear to be improving. Orphaned children in all low- and middle-income countries are now 83% as likely to attend school as their nonorphaned peers (96% in sub-Saharan Africa).[53] Significantly, orphaned children also start being sexually active earlier than their nonorphan peers. In an effort to address some of their needs, some of these vulnerable youths become involved in selling sex, thus exposing themselves to a greater risk of developing HIV/AIDS. Among homeless adolescent girls selling sex in Iran, only half knew the use of condoms could prevent HIV.[41] In Lahore, 40% of adolescent male street children exchanged sex for food or shelter, of whom two-thirds reported having sex with adult males and virtually none reported using condoms.[41]

Getting Involved in Commercial Sexual Exploitation of Children

For the reasons previously given, a family may be ready to send a child out to work, and adolescents may wish to seek employment or opportunities to improve their education. The family or youth may then respond to advertisements for babysitting, modeling, domestic work, or marriage as a mail-order bride and unintentionally become involved in the world of CSEC.[32] Conversely, recruiters, who are sometimes family members or other youth involved in CSEC, may actively search for and enlist children and adolescents who are ready and willing to go for the promise of a better life. At first, youth are recruited and kept in exploitative situations through seductive means and offers of love and security. Later, they are kept through fear, coercion, and in some case, forced drug use. Peers may be a powerful tool in recruitment, and the Internet plays a major role in luring children into a relationship or group that eventually leads to exploitation.[10] Finally, children may simply be abducted from their homes and communities.

Children's entry into CSEC may be swift if the initial encounter is with someone whose direct intention is to sell children's sexual services or traffic them for that reason. Personal accounts reveal that being conscripted as a child soldier can be brutal. Some are made to kill a family member(s), receive severe beatings, and some are made to feel unclean and isolated from the main group before eventually being made to feel part of the group.[55] For others, their descent into the CSEC world may be slower, passing through a phase of seduction followed by the use of fear and coercion or through other forms of child labor that expose them to maltreatment, unwanted pregnancy, eviction from their employer's home, homelessness, and stigmatization.[10] Once children are in the clutches of the people who intend to exploit them, they are in a very difficult position. They are confined and their documents and whatever resources they had are taken from them. They may be drugged and are frequently raped and beaten into subjugation.[32] They are often sold, resold, and trafficked again to other destinations.

Economics

The estimated profitability of human trafficking and its relative value as compared with other illicit industries varies from source to source. In 2006, the United Nations Population Fund (UNPF) reported that human trafficking ranked third after the 2 top-grossing illicit industries: arms and drug trafficking.[32] First-time transactions were reported as a USD $7 billion to USD $12 billion per year business. An additional USD $32 billion per year was generated in the destination countries through resale and the avails of the trade generated by sex trade workers. Reportedly, one third was generated in Asia and one half in industrialized countries. In 2010, Forbes listed human trafficking as sixth among illicit industries at a value of USD $28 billion, with drugs ranked first at USD $300 billion, followed by counterfeiting, arms trafficking, cigarette smuggling, and cargo theft.[56] In 2011, 24/7 Wall St. ranked human trafficking second among illicit industries at USD $31.6 billion, after illicit drugs (USD $300 billion).[57] Another, more recent estimate placed human trafficking at number 3 (or possibly number 2) among illicit trades, after drugs.[58] Regardless of its exact ranking, trafficking in human beings, including children, is big business.

Global profits related to using children for a pornographic purpose range from USD $3 billion to USD $20 billion.[59] In 2012, the Hill reported that "Molesting a child in front of a live webcam can earn a criminal $1000 a night."[59] America produces half of all CSAM, again indicating that CSEC is very much a lucrative domestic business in the United States, besides being an international money maker.

Consequences of CSEC

There are a multitude of potential acute and long-term physical and mental health consequences for people who suffer sexual violence as children. This is especially true for children who have been involved in CSEC, which carries a greater likelihood of violence and other hardships, as described in the sections above. Some assaultive physical injuries such as fractures or head trauma may be acute, while other injuries may have more long-term consequences, such as maiming, blindness, deafness, brain injury, or organ damage.[60] Additionally, children involved in child labor and CSEC are subject to malnutrition, dental problems, and substance abuse. Injury and infections of the reproductive organs may result from cases of sexual assault.

Victims of CSEC are at risk for HIV/AIDS related to multiple sexual partners and violent sexual encounters, which may result in tissue injury.[60] Additionally, a number of factors interfere with behaviors that could safeguard them from HIV/AIDS or allow them to receive care once infected, even if they are free to seek such help. Among these are ignorance of the preventive value of condoms or an inability to negotiate their use.[41]

Victims may also have a low perception of risk or a desire to avoid stigma, and they may experience denial associated with the fear that death is inevitable and/or lack trust in health care personnel and procedures.[61] Youth may keep away from health facilities out of fear of police harassment or of being sent to an institution.[62] There may also be practical considerations, such as difficulty in getting to a health facility or the scarcity of condoms.

Pregnancy is a serious consequence for adolescent girls involved in any form of CSEC.[12,60,63] Having not reached full maturity and potentially being malnourished, they have a 2- to 5-fold higher risk for complications and death than women in their 20s.[12,63,64] Furthermore, pregnancy under these conditions is unlikely to be followed appropriately by health care personnel, compounding the risk for the pregnant child and the child she carries. These babies may be stillborn or die within the first month of life.[12,63]

Mental health consequences may also be acute or long-term. Children under stress will feel anxiety and depression and may actually attempt suicide. They may develop posttraumatic stress disorder, dissociation, self-harm behaviors, and personality disorders among many other diagnoses.[60] Part of the mental anguish for victims of the worst forms of child labor is losing their innocence. Norman, a 12 year old in Uganda who was forced to kill at 12 years of age said, "'When you kill for the first time, automatically, you change ...Out of being innocent, you've now become guilty.'"[55] A 15-year-old boy abducted by Boko Haram recounted how the children who had been abducted were made to watch the rape of women and girls. They were instructed on how to hold them down, so they too could 'have fun' after capturing more victims.[65]

The Adverse Childhood Experiences (ACEs) Study has shown that the higher the score (ie, the more ACEs an individual suffers), the higher the chance that person will experience risky health behaviors, chronic health conditions, low life potential, and early death.[66] ACEs include physical, emotional, and sexual abuse, neglect, and household violence.[67] Chronic health conditions associated with ACES include chronic obstructive pulmonary disease, ischemic heart disease, and liver disease. **Figure 14-5** depicts the ACE Pyramid, which illustrates the connection between the ACE through disrupted neurodevelopment; social, emotional, and cognitive development; adoption of health risk behaviors; disease, disability, and social problems; and finally, to early death.

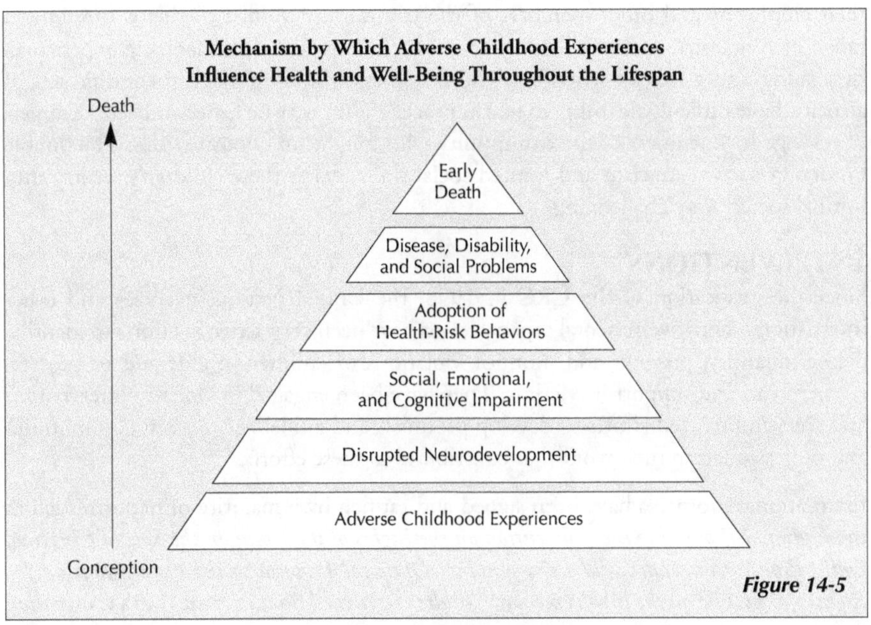

Figure 14-5. *The ACE Pyramid. Reprinted from Centers for Disease Control and Prevention.*[67]

Even if victims of CSEC can be freed from their exploiters, their suffering is not over.[60] Compounding their physical and mental health consequences, there is the problem of trying to lead a life free of abuse. They may or may not be able to return to their community of origin or their own home. Child brides are expected to stay in their new home and family. Children without valid documents, especially those taken from their families at a young age, may have lost any clear concept of their original identity or place of residence. Locating their families may be difficult, especially if they have no resources with which to accomplish the task. There may be difficulties with criminal and immigration laws.

In the case of children who were child soldiers or were otherwise exploited during times of conflict or disaster, reunification may be impossible because the families may no longer be alive, or they may have been displaced and relocated. Their families may also reject them because of what they have done, perceived alliances with enemies, pregnancy or HIV, or psychosocial difficulties.[68] In the case of sex workers, the families may not be prepared to take them back because of the shame they would bring to their families.[37]

With sexual exploitation, there is the stigma attached to being considered a prostitute. This stigma affects not only the child but also the family.[69] Even if it was the family that led a child to exploitation, as in the case of the Devadasi or Trokosi, the family may not be happy to take their daughter back.[40,43] While at the shrine, the girls are deprived in most cases of any education, any affection, and any chance at a true marriage and family. Outside the shrine, despite their supposed exalted religious status, they are often treated as prostitutes. Any children they have join their mother's fate, working and living at the priest's pleasure, unable to exercise any of their rights. Trokosi freed from their bondage worry that leaving the shrine removes any protection it provided to the family and fear for the well-being of their relatives. Having had children may make returning to a childhood home particularly difficult, because the new generation is evidence of a shameful experience. This stigma may affect them even if the community is well aware that the children were abducted and forced to do the things they did. A young girl who was abducted by Boko Haram found herself shunned after being liberated and returning home with a baby, who was the product of repeated rape by her abductor.[70]

Child workers have very low self-esteem, resulting from the treatment they receive from their employers and other members of the community. Added to this is the limited range of functional social skills they may have due to the dehumanizing experiences they suffer and a lack of schooling. Child soldiers who are forced to commit acts of atrocity, have difficulty learning to live in peace.[71] They may be feared or become targets of revenge for members of the community who fought on opposite sides. The double burden of social ostracism and limited social skills makes these children's reentry into normal society very challenging.

Interventions

Since the ratification of the CRC in 1990, the United Nations agencies and other international nongovernmental organizations have been very active in efforts to identify, define, quantify, prevent, and monitor violations of children's rights and to protect, rescue, treat, and support its victims. They have been engaged in violence intervention and have emphasized efforts to develop protocols and guidelines to assist communities and professionals in their work that contributes to these efforts.

International protocols have been signed and ratified by a majority of nations, such as the *Optional Protocol to the Convention on the Rights of the Child on the Sale of Children, Child Prostitution and Child Pornography*[3]; *Optional Protocol to the Convention on the Rights of the Child on the Involvement of Children in Armed Conflict*[4]; the ILO's *Convention*

Concerning the Prohibition and Immediate Action for the Elimination of the Worst Forms of Child Labour[8]; and a number of recommendations made by UN agencies (eg, UNICEF, UNPF, ILO, WHO) and other international and national nongovernmental agencies, a number of which are cited in this chapter. These agencies have also provided reports on the progress being made in the prevention of war, while cautioning that much work remains to be done.

A critical initiative of the United Nations was the development of the Millennium Development Goals (MDG 2015), which were followed by Sustainable Development Goals (SDG 2030). The 8 MDGs, with 18 associated targets, were to[72]:

1. Eradicate extreme poverty and hunger.
2. Achieve universal primary education.
3. Promote gender equality and empower women.
4. Reduce child mortality.
5. Improve maternal health.
6. Combat HIV/AIDS, malaria, and other diseases.
7. Ensure environmental sustainability.
8. Develop a global partnership for development.

Several of these contribute to the prevention of CSEC by eliminating its risk factors.

The MDG 2015 report on global achievements showed a reduction in extreme poverty from 1.9 billion to 836 million people from 1990, bringing the poverty rate down from 47% to 13% in 2015.[73] This was associated with a drop in the rate of malnutrition from about 23% to about 13%. The primary education enrollment rate increased from 83% in 2000 to 91% in 2015, with a similar increase in literacy rate in youth aged 15 to 24 years and narrowing the gap between men and women. There were fewer primary school-aged children out of school, the number having dropped from 100 million to 57 million. Sub-Saharan Africa showed great gains in increasing primary school enrollment from 52% in 1990 to 80% in 2015. Gender equality was achieved in primary, secondary, and tertiary school education in developing regions.[73] In South Asia, girls overtook boys, going from 74% to 103% enrollment in primary school compared to boys. Girls could also look to women having made gains in employment: a higher rate of employment outside the agricultural sector, fewer women in vulnerable employment, and gains in parliamentary representation in 90% of 174 countries over 20 years.

Globally, the number of under-5 child deaths dropped from 90 to 43 per 1000 live births between 1990 and 2015, reducing the number of deaths in this age group from 12.7 million in 1990 to almost 6 million in 2015. A 45% drop was also seen in maternal mortality from 1990 to 2015, associated with a doubling of the proportion of women having 4 or more antenatal visits to 89% between 1990 and 2014 in Northern Africa. There was a rise in the use of contraceptives by married women aged 15 to 49 from 55% to 64% worldwide. New HIV infections dropped by 40% between 2000 and 2013, with 13.6 million people receiving antiretroviral therapy for HIV in 2014, representing 12.8 million more than in 2003.

Building on the success of the MDG 2015, the 17 Sustainable Development Goals for the period 2015-2030 "are broader in scope and go further than the MDGs by addressing the root causes of poverty and the universal need for development that works for all people."[74] The 17 global goals have a number of targets that are to be achieved by

2030 with 230 indicators for tracking them. Of these, 8 goals and some of their targets are relevant to CSEC, either directly or by addressing its risk factors[75]:

— Goal 1: End poverty in all its forms everywhere.

— Goal 2: End hunger, achieve food security and improved nutrition, and promote sustainable agriculture.

— Goal 3: Ensure healthy lives and promote well-being for all at all ages.

— Goal 4: Ensure inclusive and equitable quality education and promote life-long learning opportunities for all.

— Goal 5: Achieve gender equality and empower all women and girls. This goal includes targets very specific to CSEC, including: "Eliminate all forms of violence against all women and girls in the public and private spheres, including trafficking and sexual and other types of exploitation."; "Eliminate all harmful practices, such as child, early and forced marriage and female genital mutilation."; "Recognize and value unpaid care and domestic work through the provision of public services, infrastructure and social protection policies."

— Goal 8: Promote sustained, inclusive, and sustainable economic growth; full and productive employment; and decent work for all. This goal also includes 1 target specific to CSEC: "Take immediate and effective measures to eradicate forced labour, end modern slavery and human trafficking and secure the prohibition and elimination of the worst forms of child labour, including recruitment and use of child soldiers, and by 2025 end child labour in all its forms."

— Goal 10: Reduce inequality within and among countries.

— Goal 16: Promote peaceful and inclusive societies for sustainable development; provide access to justice for all; and build effective, accountable, and inclusive institutions at all levels. This goal includes targets specific to CSEC: "Significantly reduce all forms of violence and related death rates everywhere."; "End abuse, exploitation, trafficking and all forms of violence against and torture of children."; and "Provide legal identity for all, including birth registration."

A progress report published in 2017 shows that progress has been made but must be accelerated to achieve its targets.[76]

Violence against children, especially the worst forms of child labor, requires integrated interventions, including practical programs, advocacy, and data collection.[37] Depending on the community, its resources, the size of the problem in that community, and the agency that is intervening, different responses may be set in motion. Emergency responses, such as the immediate rescue of children requiring shelter, may involve a small-scale project, while international agencies will need more complete and extensive programs that may include components aimed at preventing children from being abused in the first place.

Given the importance of poverty and low level of education as risk factors for CSEC and the link between them, it is worth considering how to correct these problems. An International Programme on the Elimination of Child Labour (IPEC) study estimated the cost and gains involved in replacing child labor with education.[77] It was based on the hypothetical application of an action plan and the study of the economic impact of each element of the program. The net benefit of replacing child labor with education as a percentage of gross national product would be 22% globally, with the greatest increase in Sub-Saharan Africa (more than 54%), and 5% in transitional countries changing from a centrally planned economy to a free market. From 2001 to 2020, the total global cost would be USD 760 billion (using currency values at the time of publication), while the accrued benefit would be more than USD 5 trillion. This represents an internal rate of return of about 44%, with benefits exceeding costs by a ratio of 6.7 to 1. The benefit-cost ratio would be highest in North Africa and the Middle East (8.4:1) and lowest in Sub–Saharan Africa (5.2:1). The cost of the program would exceed its return for approximately 15 years and then turns dramatically positive. After 2020, assuming the plan had started in 2000, there would be no more costs, only benefits. In currency value at the time of publication, the average annual cost of the program was estimated to be USD 55 billion in the first decade and USD 136 billion in the second. This represents 11% and 28%, respectively, of the annual global spending for the military (USD 493 billion) and 5.5% and 14% of debt service (USD 1 trillion).

These figures indicate that even without considering the considerable benefits in human and social terms, economically, the cost of CSEC is higher than the cost of eliminating it. The difficulty is that different people stand to benefit from the continuation or elimination of CSEC. Further, CSEC results in fairly immediate profits, while reaping the benefits of an investment in prevention takes a period of time that often exceeds the term of an elected official's or government's term in office.

Efforts have been directed at each of the forms of CSEC. Among the measures to reduce CSEC has been the attempt to reduce demand by focusing on prosecution of offenders beyond the national boundaries of their home states.[3] At least 40 countries have provisions for extraterritorial prosecution of individuals who engage in child sexual exploitation when away from their home country, so the offender who commits such a crime abroad is prosecuted at home, thereby losing the protection previously afforded by anonymity, weak law enforcement, and corruption.[78] In the United States, prosecution of these crimes have been deemed constitutionally sound.[22] The US Department of Immigration and Customs Enforcement's Child Exploitation Investigations Unit "uses cutting edge investigative techniques to bring justice to consumers, producers and distributors of child pornography, as well as to predators engaging in child sex tourism."[79] Potential penalties are: up to 30 years in prison for possessing, manufacturing, or distributing CSAM, or for being involved in any capacity in child sexual exploitation in the context of travel; and up to life in prison for sex trafficking children for the purpose of prostitution. Global trafficking reports collected from 2011 to 2017 by the State Department show with some fluctuation (due to a number of challenges in collecting data), an increase in the number of prosecutions from 7909 to 17 880, in convictions from 3969 to 7045, and in victim identifications from 42 291 to 100 409.[80]

Also helpful in this regard are the efforts of the tourist industry to eliminate sexual exploitation in its context. The global Code of Conduct for the Protection of Children from Sexual Exploitation in Travel and Tourism is an initiative developed through a collaborative effort involving several organizations and spread internationally through partnerships with the ECPAT network, the United Nations World Tourism Organization, and UNICEF.[81] There are currently more than 1500 travel companies with operations worldwide that have signed the Code.[82] The 6 essential steps to which a company agrees upon joining the Code are to (1) establish policies and procedures to protect children from CSEC; (2) train their employees on child rights, CSEC, and how to report suspected cases; (3) include a clause in contracts throughout their chain stating a zero tolerance for CSEC; (4) provide information to travelers on child rights, CSEC, and how to report suspected cases; (5) work with stakeholders to prevent CSEC; and (6) report annually on the implementation of the Code.[83]

UNICEF's *Cape Town Principles and Best Practices* provided a foundation for the 2007 Paris commitments aimed at ending the use of children in conflict.[11,84] In the intervening 10 years, the initial 58 countries who endorsed the Paris commitments grew to 105, and by 2017 at least 65 000 children had been released from armed forces and armed groups.[51]

As a means of disrupting the lucrative business of CSAM, the Financial Coalition Against Child Pornography (FCACP) was formed in 2006 by the International Centre for Missing & Exploited Children (ICMEC) and the National Center for Missing and Exploited Children (NCMEC), as a cooperative initiative between the financial and Internet industries to interfere with how financial transactions are conducted. It now includes 34 leading banks, credit card companies, third-party payment companies (these constitute 90% of the US payments industry), and Internet services companies.[85] It has resulted in the virtually total inability to conduct any credit card purchases online for CSAM, making Web sites selling such material to resort to more complicated payment methods.[85] Despite this success, and with new technologies appearing all the time, ongoing vigilance is necessary.

Knowing of the vulnerability of children during conflict and displacement, governments and nongovernmental organizations have taken steps to address the protection of children as part of disaster relief planning.[23,86] In the meantime, following the reports of abuse by aid workers in West Africa in 2002, UNICEF announced an education program for aid workers to prevent further occurrences.[47]

Once exploited children have been identified and located, contact needs to be made with them to remove them to safety. Possible means to this end are hotlines and peer-to-peer contact in public places, such as churches, parks, or shops, where the child workers go when they are off duty.[37] The removal of the children from exploitative situations requires skilled intervention so the child is not further traumatized. In an emergency, this may require rescue operations; in more stable situations, there may be time for more considered action. For child soldiers, any peace agreements must acknowledge their involvement in the war so that there can be effective plans for them on a national scale. To date few peace agreements have addressed child soldiers directly and none have addressed demobilization, disarmament, and reintegration and the elimination of impunity for those who conscripted them.[68]

The rehabilitation of children must include attention to their physical and mental health needs.[37] Programs must help children establish lives based on their individual capabilities and experiences. Because exploitation interferes with children's normal physical, emotional, and intellectual development, they need to be provided with an environment that fosters dignity and self-respect.[37] Good relations with a supportive family are beneficial, but some families may not be able to provide it. Settings that provide peer group living and are integrated into communities are viable alternatives to institutions.

Victims of CSEC may present for medical attention for a variety of reasons. Health care providers must be prepared to identify and treat them and take the appropriate steps to begin their integration into a life free from exploitation. This is no easy task, as these youths may be unable or unwilling to speak of their experiences, as well as the fact that good screening tools are not available.[60] Some possible indicators include having an unexplained injury, being accompanied by a domineering adult, and a psychosocial history of risky behaviors. If the youth cooperates, a careful medical history is helpful, especially covering sexual and reproductive history, abuse and injuries, substance misuse and abuse, and mental health history. Assessment and treatment of any abnormal condition (including testing for drugs and STIs as appropriate) is critical, as is documentation of any and all injuries and other findings. Anticipatory guidance, such as HIV protection, is crucial even if the youth appears unreceptive to hearing it. Mandatory child abuse reporting requirements must be followed. If the health care professional is unsure about the appropriate course of action, consultation with more experienced practitioners is recommended. In the United States, the National Human Trafficking Resource Center Hotline (1-888-373-7888) is a helpful resource.

Other professionals in the course of their professional activities, or lay people in the course of daily life, may encounter a situation suspicious for CSEC or a child who seems to be exploited. Without endangering their own safety, these individuals should try to address the situation. How to do this will depend on specific circumstances, and expert consultation may be required. Here, again, the National Human Trafficking Resource Center Hotline may be a helpful resource.

Monitoring intervention efforts in the child labor movement has shifted in focus from the industry to the child so as to ensure that children removed from work are provided with satisfactory alternatives with which to reenter mainstream society.[9,37] Coordinated efforts involve the identification, referral, verification, and tracking of children. This approach focuses on monitoring long-term changes in all types of child labor within specific geographical areas and includes all aid agencies and organizations working within a given geographical area. With these data, a better understanding of children's experiences with all types of violence can be garnered, which will improve future prevention strategies.

Conclusion

Globally, much has been learned and accomplished in efforts to eliminate any expression of CSA, especially CSEC. Much more still needs to be done through collaborative efforts, careful data gathering and analysis, and monitoring of any interventions taken to ensure the most effective means of protecting children, especially in areas where resources are scarce. Public awareness campaigns may be helpful in raising public knowledge of the problem and enlisting community support for vigilance and prevention. Residents of more affluent nations can no longer assume that CSEC is something that happens elsewhere; rather, they must be aware and vigilant in order to address this scourge in their own communities.

References

1. End Child Prostitution and Trafficking International. Terminology and guidelines for the protection of children from sexual exploitation and sexual abuse. https://www.ilo.org/wcmsp5/groups/public/---ed_norm/---ipec/documents/instructionalmaterial/wcms_490167.pdf. Accessed January 24, 2019.
2. Office of the United Nations High Commissioner for Human Rights. Convention on the rights of the child. https://www.ohchr.org/en/professionalinterest/pages/crc.aspx. Accessed January 24, 2019.
3. Office of the United Nations High Commissioner for Human Rights. Optional protocol to the convention on the rights of the child on the sale of children, child prostitution and child pornography. https://www.ohchr.org/EN/ProfessionalInterest/Pages/OPSCCRC.aspx. Accessed January 24, 2019.
4. Office of the United Nations High Commissioner for Human Rights. Option protocol to the convention on the rights of the child on the involvement of children in armed conflict. https://www.ohchr.org/EN/ProfessionalInterest/Pages/OPACCRC.aspx. Accessed January 24, 2019.
5. Office of the United Nations High Commissioner for Human Rights. Status of ratification interactive dashboard. http://indicators.ohchr.org/. Office of the United Nations High Commissioner for Human Rights Web site. Accessed January 24, 2019.
6. Office of the United Nations High Commissioner for Human Rights. Report of the office of the United Nations High Commissioner for Human Rights on preventing and eliminating child, early and forced marriage. https://www.ohchr.org/EN/HRBodies/HRC/RegularSessions/Session26/Pages/ListReports.aspx. Accessed January 24, 2019.

7. International Labour Organization. C138 - Minimum Age Convention, 1973 (No. 138): convention concerning minimum age for admission to employment. https://www.ilo.org/dyn/normlex/en/f?p=NORMLEXPUB:12100:0::NO::P12100_ILO_CODE:C138. Accessed January 24, 2019.

8. International Labour Organization. C182 - Worst Forms of Child Labour Convention, 1999 (No. 182): convention concerning the prohibition and immediate action for the elimination of the worst forms of child labour. https://www.ilo.org/dyn/normlex/en/f?p=NORMLEXPUB:12100:0::NO::P12100_ILO_CODE:C182. Accessed January 24, 2019.

9. International Labour Organization. The end of child labour: within reach: ILO global report on child labour 2006. https://www.ilo.org/ipecinfo/product/viewProduct.do?productId=2419. Published January 6, 2006. Accessed January 24, 2019.

10. Moore JL, Kaplan DM, Barron CE. Sex trafficking of minors. *Pediatr Clin North Am.* 2017;64(2):413-421.

11. United Nations International Children's Emergency Fund. Cape Town principles and best practices. https://www.unicef.org/emerg/files/Cape_Town_Principles(1).pdf. Accessed January 24, 2019.

12. United Nations International Children's Emergency Fund. Child protection from violence, exploitation and abuse: child marriage. United Nations International Children's Emergency Fund Web site. https://www.unicef.org/protection/57929_58008.html. Updated November 27, 2018. Accessed January 14, 2019.

13. United Nations International Children's Emergency Fund. Child marriage is a violation of human rights, but is all too common. United Nations International Children's Emergency Fund Web site. https://data.unicef.org/topic/child-protection/child-marriage/. Updated March 2018. Accessed January 24, 2019.

14. International Labour Office. Marking progress against child labour: global estimates and trends 2000-2012. https://www.ilo.org/wcmsp5/groups/public/---ed_norm/---ipec/documents/publication/wcms_221513.pdf. Accessed January 24, 2019.

15. International Labour Office. Global estimates of child labour: results and trends, 2012-2016. https://www.ilo.org/wcmsp5/groups/public/@dgreports/@dcomm/documents/publication/wcms_575499.pdf. Accessed January 24, 2019.

16. International Labour Office. *Global Estimates of Child Labour: Results and Trends 2012-2016.* Geneva, Switzerland: International Labour Office; 2017.

17. United Nations International Children's Emergency Fund. In the world's poorest countries, around 1 in 4 children are engaged in child labour. United Nations International Children's Emergency Fund Web site. https://data.unicef.org/topic/child-protection/child-labour/#. Accessed January 24, 2019.

18. International Labour Organization. Marking progress against child labour: global estimates and trends 2000-2012. https://www.ilo.org/wcmsp5/groups/public/---ed_norm/---ipec/documents/publication/wcms_221513.pdf. Accessed January 24, 2019.

19. International Labour Organization. ILO IPEC+ flagship strategy: international programme on the elimination of child labour and forced labour. https://www.ilo.org/global/about-the-ilo/how-the-ilo-works/WCMS_528938/lang--en/index.htm. Accessed Accessed January 24, 2019.

20. Child trafficking and labour trafficking cases rising: IOM [news release]. Geneva, Switzerland: International Organization for Migration; April 2, 2012. https://www.iom.int/news/child-trafficking-and-labour-trafficking-cases-rising-iom. Accessed January 24, 2019.

21. Nepal earthquakes: UNICEF speeds up response to prevent child trafficking [news release]. New York, NY: United Nations International Children's Emergency Fund; June 19, 2018. https://www.unicef.org/media/media_82328.html. Accessed January 24, 2019.

22. Caliendo A. What happens abroad does not stay abroad: *United States v. Pendleton* and Congress's constitutional authority to regulate child sex abuse abroad. *Seton Hall Circuit Review*. 2014;10:375-408. Seton Hall University eRepository Web site. https://scholarship.shu.edu/cgi/viewcontent.cgi?referer=&httpsredir=1&article=1132&context=circuit_review. Accessed January 24, 2019.

23. United States Department of State. Trafficking in persons report: June 2005. https://www.state.gov/documents/organization/47255.pdf. Revised June 2005. Accessed January 24, 2019.

24. Dahlberg LL, Krug EG. Violence – a global public health problem. In: Krug EG, Dahlberg LL, Mercy JA, Zwi AB, Lozano R, eds. *World Report on Violence and Health*. Geneva, Switzerland: World Health Organization; 2002:1-22. http://apps.who.int/iris/bitstream/handle/10665/42495/9241545615_eng.pdf;jsessionid=63248283252A4ED946D7EC1923C6D8C3?sequence=1. Accessed January 24, 2019.

25. United Nations International Children's Emergency Fund, Early marriage: a harmful traditional practice. https://www.unicef.org/publications/files/Early_Marriage_12.lo.pdf. Accessed January 24, 2019.

26. United Nations International Children's Emergency Fund. The births of around one fourth of the global population of children under five have never been registered. https://data.unicef.org/topic/child-protection/birth-registration/#. Updated January 2018. Accessed January 24, 2019.

27. United Nations International Children's Emergency Fund. Without birth registration, children are shut out of society altogether. https://www.unicef.org/protection/57929_67803.html. Updated February 11, 2013. Accessed January 24, 2019.

28. Runyan D, Wattam C, Ikeda R, Hassan F, Ramiro L. Child abuse and neglect by parents and other caregivers. In: Krug EG, Dahlberg LL, Mercy JA, Zwi AB, Lozano R. *World Report on Violence and Health*. Geneva, Switzerland: World Health Organization; 2002:57-86. World Health Organization Web site. http://apps.who.int/iris/bitstream/handle/10665/42495/9241545615_eng.pdf;jsessionid=63248283252A4ED946D7EC1923C6D8C3?sequence=1. Accessed January 24, 2019.

29. United Nations International Children's Emergency Fund. The state of the world's children 2007: women and children: the double dividend of gender equality. https://www.unicef.org/publications/files/The_State_of_the_Worlds__Children__2007_e.pdf. Accessed January 24, 2019.

30. The World Bank. Gender issues in child labor: developing effective policies against child labor requires attention to gender differences among working children. http://www1.worldbank.org/prem/PREMNotes/premnote100.pdf. Published August 2005. Accessed January 24, 2019.

31. Breiding MJ, Reza A, Gulaid J, et al. Risk factors associated with sexual violence towards girls in Swaziland. *Bull World Health Organ.* 2011;89(3):203-210.

32. United Nations Population Fund. State of world population 2006: a passage to hope: women and international migration. https://www.unfpa.org/sites/default/files/pub-pdf/sowp06-en.pdf. Accessed January 24, 2019.

33. Education crucial in preventing recruitment of girls [news release]. London, UK: Child Soldiers International; November 14, 2016. https://www.child-soldiers.org/news/press-release-drc. Accessed January 24, 2019.

34. International Labour Organization, International Programme on the Elimination of Child Labour. Give girls a chance: tackling child labour, a key to the future. https://www.ilo.org/ipecinfo/product/viewProduct.do?productId=10290. Published January 6, 2009. Accessed January 24, 2019.

35. Klugman J, Hanmer L, Twigg S, Hasan T, McCleary-Sills J, Santamaria J. Voice and agency: empowering women and girls for shared prosperity. World Bank Group Web site. https://openknowledge.worldbank.org/handle/10986/19036. Accessed January 24, 2019.

36. Jordan A. Slavery, forced labor, debt bondage, and human trafficking: from conceptional confusion to targeted solutions. Issuelab Web site. https://www.issuelab.org/resources/15356/15356.pdf. Published February 2011. Accessed January 24, 2019.

37. United Nations. Violence against children: United Nations Secretary-General's study. https://www.unicef.org/violencestudy/. Accessed January 24, 2019.

38. Allais FB, Hagemann F; International Labour Organization. Child labour and education: evidence from SIMPOC surveys. https://www.ilo.org/ipecinfo/product/viewProduct.do?productId=8390. Published January 6, 2008. Accessed January 24, 2019.

39. Lukman ZM, Nasir R, Fauziah I, et al. The relationship between dysfunctional family and the involvement of children in prostitution. *World Applied Sciences Journal.* 2011;12:7-12.

40. Black M. Women in ritual slavery: Devadasi, Jogini and Mathamma in Karnataka and Andhra Pradesh, Southern India. *Pakistan Journal of Women's Studies.* 2009;16(1/2):179-205.

41. World Heath Organization. Technical brief: HIV and young people who sell sex. http://apps.who.int/iris/bitstream/handle/10665/179868/WHO_HIV_2015.7_eng.pdf;jsessionid=0B7B5C2128FE89AEF3904AE25190A50F?sequence=1. Accessed January 24, 2019.

42. International Labour Organization. Child labour and domestic work. International Labour Organization Web site. https://www.ilo.org/ipec/areas/Childdomesticlabour/lang--en/index.htm. Accessed January 24, 2019.

43. Ohrt M. *Conflicting Discourses on the Trokosi Practice in Ghana: Exploring Tensions in the Global/Local Human Rights Translation* [master's thesis]. Hague, Netherlands: International Institute of Social Studies; 2011.

44. International Labour Organization. Every child counts: new global estimates on child labour. https://www.ilo.org/ipec/Informationresources/WCMS_IPEC_PUB_742/lang--en/index.htm. Issued December 1, 2002. Accessed January 24, 2019.

45. United Nations General Assembly Security Council. Children and armed conflict: report of the secretary-general. http://www.un.org/ga/search/view_doc.asp?symbol=s/2016/360&referer=/english/&Lang=E. Published April 20, 2016. Accessed January 24, 2019.

46. United Nations, Office of the Special Representative of the Secretary-General for Children and Armed Conflict.The six grave violations against children during armed conflict: the legal foundation. https://childrenandarmedconflict.un.org/publications/WorkingPaper-1_SixGraveViolationsLegalFoundation.pdf. Updated November 2013. Accessed January 24, 2019.

47. Moszynski P. Unicef sets up programme to prevent sex abuse by aid workers. *BMJ.* 2002; 325(7367):732.

48. International Organization for Migration. Migration flows to Europe—2017: quarterly overview: June. http://migration.iom.int/docs/Q2_2017_Overview_Arrivals_to_Europe.pdf. Accessed January 24, 2019.

49. United Nations International Children's Emergency Fund.Danger every step of the way: a harrowing journey to Europe of refugee and migrant children. https://www.unicef.org.uk/publications/danger-every-step-of-the-way-a-harrowing-journey-to-europe-for-refugee-and-migrant-children/. Accessed January 24, 2019.

50. Central Intelligence Agency. The world factbook. Central Intelligence Agency Web site. https://www.cia.gov/library/publications/the-world-factbook/fields/2024.html#139. Accessed January 24, 2019.

51. At least 65,000 children released from armed forces and groups over the last 10 years, UNICEF [news release]. New York, NY: United Nations International Children's Emergency Fund; February 21, 2017. https://www.unicef.org/media/media_94892.html. Accessed January 24, 2019.

52. Joint United Nations Programme on HIV/AIDS. AIDS by the numbers: AIDS is not over, but it can be. http://www.unaids.org/sites/default/files/media_asset/AIDS-by-the-numbers-2016_en.pdf. Accessed January 24, 2019.

53. United Nations International Children's Emergency Fund. Protection, care and support for children affected by HIV and AIDS. https://www.unicef.org/aids/index_armedconflict.html. Accessed January 24, 2019.

54. United Nations International Children's Emergency Fund. The AIDS epidemic continues to take a staggering toll, but progress is possible. United Nations International Children's Emergency Fund Web site. https://data.unicef.org/topic/hivaids/global-regional-trends/. Updated July 2018. Accessed January 24, 2019.

55. Storr W. Kony's child soldiers: 'When you kill for the first time, you change.' *The Telegraph*. February 12, 2014. https://www.telegraph.co.uk/news/worldnews/africaandindianocean/uganda/10621792/Konys-child-soldiers-When-you-kill-for-the-first-time-you-change.html. Accessed January 24, 2019.

56. Vardi N. The world's biggest illicit industries. *Forbes*. June 4, 2010. https://www.forbes.com/sites/oracle/2019/01/08/the-right-culture-the-invisible-pervasive-force-thats-key-to-cloud-success/#601dff561533. Accessed January 24, 2019.

57. 24/7 Wall St. The 12 most profitable international crimes. 24/7 Wall St. Web site. https://247wallst.com/investing/2011/02/10/the-12-most-profitable-international-crimes/. Published February 10, 2011. Accessed January 24, 2019.

58. Greenberg J. Yes, human trafficking ranks no. 3 in world crime.Politifact Web site. https://www.politifact.com/truth-o-meter/statements/2016/jul/26/amy-klobuchar/yes-human-trafficking-ranks-3-world-crime/. Published July 26, 2016. Accessed January 24, 2019.

59. Handrahan L. IRS should take a closer look at child porn industry finances.The Hill Web site. https://thehill.com/blogs/congress-blog/economy-a-budget/260731-irs-should-take-a-closer-look-at-child-porn-industry-finances. Published October 8, 2012. Accessed January 24, 2019.

60. Greebaum VJ. Commercial sexual exploitation and sex trafficking of children in the United States. *Curr Probl Pediatr Adolesc Health Care.* 2014;44(9):245-269.

61. Musheke M, Ntalasha H, Gari S, et al. A systematic review of qualitative findings on factors enabling and deterring uptake of HIV testing in Sub-Saharan Africa. *BMC Public Health.* 2013;13:220.

62. McClure C, Chandler C, Bissell S. Responses to HIV in sexually exploited children or adolescents who sell sex. *Lancet.* 2015;385(9963):97-99.

63. United Nations International Children's Emergency Fund. The state of the world's children 2009: maternal and newborn health. https://www.unicef.org/sowc09/report/report.php. Accessed January 24, 2019.

64. United Nations Population Fund. State of the world population 2005: the promise of equality: gender equity, reproductive health and the millennium development goals. https://www.unfpa.org/sites/default/files/pub-pdf/swp05_eng.pdf. Accessed January 24, 2019.

65. Obaji P Jr. Boko Haram teaching child soldiers to rape. *The Daily Beast.* December 27, 2016. https://www.thedailybeast.com/boko-haram-teaching-child-soldiers-to-rape. Accessed January 24, 2019.

66. Centers for Disease Control and Prevention. Adverse childhood experiences (ACEs). Centers for Disease Control and Prevention Web site. https://www.cdc.gov/violenceprevention/acestudy/index.html. Updated April 1, 2016. Accessed January 24, 2019.

67. Centers for Disease Control and Prevention. About the CDC-Kaiser ACE study. Centers for Disease Control and Prevention Web site. https://www.cdc.gov/violenceprevention/acestudy/about.html. Updated June 14, 2016. Accessed January 24, 2019.

68. Mukhar R. Child soldiers and peace agreements. *Annual Survey of International & Comparative Law.* 2014;20(1):73-100. https://digitalcommons.law.ggu.edu/annlsurvey/vol20/iss1/8/. Accessed January 24, 2019.

69. United Nations International Children's Emergency Fund. Sexual violence against children. United Nations International Children's Emergency Fund Web site. https://www.unicef.org/protection/57929_58006.html. September 28, 2018. Accessed January 24, 2019.

70. Patta D. Boko Haram victim shunned by community after having rapist's baby. CBS Evening News Web site. https://www.cbsnews.com/news/boko-haram-victim-shunned-by-community-after-having-rapists-baby/. Published December 21, 2015. Accessed January 24, 2019.

71. Steel M. Child soldiers. *Vision.* Fall 2008. http://www.vision.org/visionmedia/social-issues/child-soldiers/6684.aspx. Accessed January 24, 2019.

72. United Nations. Sustainable development goals: 17 goals to transform our world. https://www.un.org/sustainabledevelopment/blog/2015/12/sustainable-development-goals-kick-off-with-start-of-new-year/. Accessed January 24, 2019.

73. United Nations.The millennium development goals report: 2015. http://www.un.org/millenniumgoals/2015_MDG_Report/pdf/MDG%202015%20rev%20(July%201).pdf. Accessed January 24, 2019.

74. United Nations. The sustainable development agenda. United Nations Web site. https://www.un.org/sustainabledevelopment/development-agenda/. Accessed January 24, 2019.

75. United Nations. Final list of proposed sustainable development goal indicators. https://sustainabledevelopment.un.org/content/documents/11803Official-List-of-Proposed-SDG-Indicators.pdf. Accessed January 24, 2019.

76. United Nations.The sustainable development goals repost: 2017. https://unstats.un.org/sdgs/files/report/2017/TheSustainableDevelopmentGoalsReport2017.pdf. Accessed January 24, 2019.

77. International Labour Organization. Investing in every child: an economic study of the costs and benefits of eliminating child labour. https://www.ilo.org/global/publications/books/WCMS_071311/lang--it/index.htm. Issued December 1, 2003. Accessed January 24, 2019.

78. End Child Prostitution and Trafficking International. Creating a united front against the sexual exploitation of children in travel and tourism. http://www.ecpat.org/wp-content/uploads/legacy/ecpatjournaljune2009.pdf. Published June 2009. Accessed January 24, 2019.

79. US Department of Immigration and Customs Enforcement. Child Exploitation Investigations Unit. https://www.ice.gov/predator. Accessed January 24, 2019.

80. United States Department of State. Trafficking in persons report: June 2018. https://www.state.gov/documents/organization/282798.pdf. Accessed January 24, 2019.

81. Code of Conduct for the Protection of Children from Sexual Exploitation in Travel and Tourism. History. Code of Conduct for the Protection of Children from Sexual Exploitation in Travel and Tourism Web site. http://www.thecode.org/about/history/. Accessed January 24, 2019.

82. Code of Conduct for the Protection of Children from Sexual Exploitation in Travel and Tourism. Signatories. Code of Conduct for the Protection of Children from Sexual Exploitation in Travel and Tourism Web site. History Web site. http://www.thecode.org/who-have-signed/signatories/. Accessed January 24, 2019.

83. Code of Conduct for the Protection of Children from Sexual Exploitation in Travel and Tourism. About. Code of Conduct for the Protection of Children from Sexual Exploitation in Travel and Tourism Web site. http://www.thecode.org/about/. Accessed January 24, 2019.

84. United Nations International Children's Emergency Fund. Paris principles and Paris commitments. United Nations International Children's Emergency Fund Web site. https://www.unicef.org/protection/57929_58012.html. Updated December 6, 2013. Accessed January 24, 2019.

85. International Centre for Missing and Exploited Children. U.S. Financial Coalition Against Child Pornography. International Centre for Missing and Exploited Children Web site. https://www.icmec.org/fcacp/. Accessed January 24, 2019.

86. World Health Organization.Violence and disasters. https://www.who.int/violence_injury_prevention/publications/violence/violence_disasters.pdf. Accessed January 24, 2019.

Chapter 15

Adolescent Issues in Sexual Abuse and Assault

Nancy D. Kellogg, MD
Natalie N. Kissoon, MD, FAAP

Introduction

The medical care of adolescents who are suspected victims of sexual abuse or assault presents unique challenges for the health care provider. When sexual abuse is first suspected, there is often some confusion as to where the adolescent should go for a medical assessment. Pediatricians typically provide care for children and teens up to at least age 17 years. Menarcheal adolescents are often referred to adult sexual assault programs for forensic examinations. Although an adolescent may achieve adulthood in terms of physical and sexual maturity by age 13, and some may reach menarche as early as 10 years old, cognitive development, including comprehension of complex and abstract concepts, is still incomplete. In addition, the psychological responses and needs of sexually victimized adolescents are distinctly different from those of adult victims.

The clinical approach to the adolescent is further complicated by issues of confidentiality and consent. What if an adolescent does not want her parent to know she was a victim of date rape? What if the patient does not consider his sexual relationship with a 23-year-old abusive, but the parent does? Under what circumstances should a clinician report sexual experiences involving an adolescent as abuse? Establishing an approach to the examination also raises questions: Are speculum examinations always indicated or appropriate for female adolescents who are suspected victims of abuse? If the adolescent is sexually active, should testing for sexually transmitted infections (STIs) be done? If so, what kinds of tests should be used?

What is known is that adolescent victims of sexual abuse or assault face a greater likelihood of health-risky behaviors, which include running away, delinquency, drug and alcohol use, unprotected or early sexual activity, and teen pregnancy. Prevention of these deleterious sequelae and behaviors begins with the medical assessment. It is incumbent on medical providers to address not only the emergent issues of medical needs and forensic collection but also the long-term outcomes that may compromise the adolescent's development into a healthy adult.

Sexual abuse is a clinical diagnosis with legal, cultural, and health implications. The definition of sexual abuse is variable and encompasses a spectrum of circumstances including "date rape," incest, sexual activity that is consensual but illegal, sexual harassment, and online solicitation of a minor for sex. The diagnosis of sexual abuse in a clinical setting is often made based on the medical history because injuries, forensic evidence, and STIs are uncommonly present or helpful in determining whether sexual abuse or assault has occurred. Nonetheless, addressing the adolescent's medical and mental health concerns is critical in the management and prevention of short- and long-term deleterious effects of sexually abusive experiences.

Definitions and Victim Perceptions of Abusive Experiences

Although most clinicians understand their legal obligation to report suspected abuse, issues surrounding "the age of consent" and rights to confidential health care obfuscate the physicians' role in providing for the health and well-being of their adolescent patients. All states have laws that mandate reporting of suspected child abuse, and generally individuals are immune from liability as long as the report is made in good faith. However, the legal definition of which sexual acts are considered criminal and prosecutable varies somewhat from state to state. For example, if an adult fondles the buttocks of a child, this may be considered sexually abusive in some regions, but in other states such contact is not considered "indecency with a child" unless the anus is also touched. Most states use age parameters to define a "minor," and most states clearly indicate that any sexual activity between a minor and an adult is abusive and reportable. With regard to sexual activity between 2 consenting adolescents, some states require the clinician to make a report if it is their professional judgment that the contact is abusive (eg, lack of consent, drug-facilitated sexual assault), whereas other states require reporting based solely on age criteria. Still other states provide age criteria for reporting sexual assault but alter legal definitions for sexual assault among adolescents. For example, in one state, any sexual contact involving at least one minor younger than age 17 may be illegal and reportable, but if the adolescents are mutually consenting and both are between 14 and 17 years old, these conditions could be claimed as a defense during criminal proceedings.

Some consider such laws significant deterrents to adolescent health care. Reporting all sexual activity involving minors would breach adolescents' right to confidential health care and make them reluctant to seek or maintain health care. The care of adolescents who are sexually active and in need of health maintenance and prevention for pregnancy and STIs could be significantly compromised. There are no current data to support that age-based reporting laws would deter sexual activity among adolescents, but there is evidence that such laws would negatively affect an adolescent's willingness to share sexual health information with their health care provider.[1,2] The long-term effects of such laws could be detrimental to the health of adolescents if they do not seek health care and STIs and pregnancies are undetected and untreated. In Kansas, for example, physicians filed suit and successfully opposed the attorney general's attempt to reinterpret child abuse laws based solely on age criteria.[3] The clinician, however, is responsible for following reporting laws, not penal code laws that define the parameters of a crime. Clinicians should be aware of reporting laws in the state in which they practice. The Child Welfare Information Gateway is a good resource for further information.[4]

In a clinical setting, sexual abuse may encompass a variety of contact and noncontact sexual encounters that affect the health and well-being of the patient. For example, sexual harassment may result in significant anxiety and school refusal in some adolescents, yet it is not defined as a reportable act or crime. Teens may fabricate symptoms to avoid going to school. Such harassment now extends to the Internet because students may receive sexually explicit or insulting material from others. One study found that approximately one-third of adolescents have sent a nude image of themselves through electronic means, approximately one-half have been asked to send a nude image, and approximately one-third have asked for someone else to send a nude image to them.[5] This form of communication is known as "sexting." In the same study, most adolescents reported being bothered by being asked to send the nude image. Another study found that 20% of adolescents were solicited for sex by strangers through the Internet.[6]

Although medical and mental health consequences are commonly associated with sexual abuse or assault, symptoms and severity vary considerably. Adolescents are often embarrassed and ashamed, but some present clinically behind a veneer of apparent nonchalance in speaking about their abuse, consistent with feelings of invincibility common to mid-adolescence. The clinician should not allow a cavalier or obstinate demeanor in an adolescent who is a suspected victim of sexual abuse to dissuade her or him from this diagnosis.

The victim's perception is yet another facet of how abuse is defined and identified. For example, many adolescents feel that rape must include a beating or body injury and that the absence of such means the act was not abusive and therefore not reportable. Many do not realize that a verbal refusal is sufficient to establish the parameters of a rape. About one-third of all sexual abuse victims blame themselves to some degree for the assault or abuse.[7] Self-blame can, in turn, influence whether a victim labels a sexual assault as abuse. Self-blame can derive from illogical ideas such as "If I weren't there, it would not have happened." In a study of 5829 ninth graders in Denmark, 1.3% of boys and 4.5% of girls had sexual experiences with a person at least 5 years older but did not perceive the experiences as abusive.[8] Clinicians can play a key role in helping victims appropriately recognize sexually abusive experiences.

Clinical Presentations

About 90% of sexual assault or abuse is first detected when a victim discloses the abuse to a third party.[9] In most cases the disclosure occurs sometime after the actual abuse has occurred. Kellogg et al[10] found that children and adolescents abused by family members had a longer average disclosure time than those who were abused by non-family members. Cultural factors and use of threats by the abuser may also influence the average time to disclosure. The most common reason for not telling about the abuse in this patient population was a fear of consequences, not only for the victim but for the abuser and family members as well. It is important for the clinician to understand how these factors influence the disclosure process.

Sexual abuse is uncommonly diagnosed when a patient presents to a clinical setting with symptoms or signs of anogenital trauma or infection. A recent study of 1763 patients found that only 8.8% of patients had acute anogenital injuries, and gonorrhea or *Chlamydia* was found in 16% of adolescents and fewer than 3% of children younger than 12 years.[11] In addition, the presence of visible anogenital trauma does not necessarily differentiate consensual and abusive causes. The severity or number of anogenital injuries may not correlate with the likelihood that the assault was nonconsensual. The injuries should be interpreted within the context of a medical history. Body injury, such as ligature marks or bruises on the victim's forearms sustained during an attempt to protect his or her face from an attacker's blows, may provide more specific evidence of assault. Additionally, adolescents who present to clinical settings with signs of alcohol or drug toxicity should be questioned carefully about the possibility of sexual assault. Many state laws include provisions for drug-facilitated sexual assault when a person is unable to consent because of impairment from such substances. The clinician should be especially concerned by the possibility of sexual assault if the patient gives a history of drinking small amounts of alcohol or another drink followed by a rapid onset of altered mental status or brief alternating periods of impairment and lucidity. Such symptoms suggest drink spiking with intent to facilitate sexual assault. Some adolescents presenting for sexual assault examinations may be involved in sex trafficking. Clinical signs that a patient may be trafficked include the presence of an adult who speaks for the patient and is not the guardian; alternatively, the adolescent may be deferential to, or fearful of, the accompanying adult. Additional signs that are concerning for trafficking include false or changing demographic information, an accompanying adult paying for the patient's visit in cash, a history of running away from home or involvement with child protective services, a history of multiple sexual partners in a short period, or multiple prior STIs or pregnancies.[12]

Victims occasionally present with STIs. These infections are rare in adolescents who are not sexually active but common among sexually active adolescents and young adults. The presence of an STI in a patient who is sexually active and also sexually assaulted has no forensic significance as the origin of the STI cannot be reliably determined. However, sexual abuse in childhood is correlated with earlier and unprotected sexual activity in adolescence. The presence of an STI should prompt the clinician to ask the adolescent about the type and nature of all previous sexual contact, including nonconsensual and abusive encounters. It is important to remember that the presence of an STI does not always imply sexual contact as the only mode of transmission. Familiarity with different modes of transmission will assist the clinician in the appropriate interpretation of results of laboratory tests for STIs.

Adolescent victims of sexual assault are rarely detected based on an assessment of behavioral symptoms, although it is widely acknowledged that many adolescents do have behavioral symptoms caused by sexual abuse and may not disclose their abuse even when queried directly. Many victims are also asymptomatic, accommodating to the abuse and effectively hiding their symptoms of anxiety, depression, and posttraumatic dissociation. Mood swings typical of adolescence may mask or conceal symptoms attributable to victimization. As with detection of an STI, behavioral changes and problems should prompt the clinician to ask screening questions regarding abuse and violence, including sexual assault.

If a patient presents with a history of sexual abuse or assault, or the patient reveals sexual abuse during the course of a medical assessment, the clinician should be aware of the options and resources available in deciding the best course of action. When the assault has occurred within the previous 72 hours, the patient should be referred immediately for forensic evidence collection. These examinations are usually conducted at regional hospitals by sexual assault nurse examiners (SANEs) or physicians. Very rarely, a victim may present with genital injuries that require hemostasis and laceration repair. These patients should also be referred at once to a hospital setting, preferably one with an established sexual assault program.

Most adolescent victims of sexual assault, however, do not require immediate medical attention and many present for examinations more than 72 hours after sexual contact, obviating the need for forensic evidence collection. The urgency of the medical assessment for these patients depends primarily on emotional and physical symptoms, as well as the need for establishing a safety plan to protect the victim from further abuse. There are many well-established programs that provide medical evaluations, victim assistance, and crisis counseling for victims of sexual abuse. In the United States, medical evaluations of children and adolescents are usually conducted by experienced and trained pediatricians or nurses, as well as gynecologists, emergency medicine physicians, and family practitioners. In regions where such programs are available, the clinician should refer the patient for complete medical assessment and treatment. A report to child protective services or law enforcement should be made immediately. *Referral to a specialty program does not preclude the clinician's legal obligation to report.*

Programs that specialize in the assessment and treatment of pediatric sexual assault or abuse victims can provide valuable guidance to clinicians. Many parents present to clinicians with the concern that their teen has been sexually abused based on an observed physical or behavioral symptom. The TEAMHEALTH model provides some general approaches for the medical history that can also be used in situations when abuse is suspected but the adolescent has not disclosed.

Clinical Evaluation

The TEAMHEALTH approach (**Table 15-1**) outlines the scope of clinical care for adolescents who are suspected victims of sexual abuse or assault and encompasses the medical history, clinical assessment, treatment, and follow-up care. The components are not presented as an inclusive protocol or in a suggested sequence. Although some adolescents may benefit from a rapport-building introduction to the medical history that includes discussion of less embarrassing or intrusive topics, other adolescents may respond better to a direct approach, beginning with the reason for the office visit. In the latter situation, the clinician may gather a brief medical history before asking what the adolescent's understanding of the purpose of the visit is. After gathering information about the abuse, the remainder of the medical history, including behavioral and emotional responses to the abuse, can be gathered.

Table 15-1. The TEAMHEALTH Approach

Medical History	
T	**T**ell them your agenda
E	**E**arn trust
A	**A**ssure safety — Family history, support by non-abusive parent, protection of abuser or concern for integrity of family — Health-risky behaviors, including drug and alcohol use, runaway tendencies, self-harm behaviors, and unsafe sexual activity
M	**M**edical history — Medical and gynecological history — Physical and emotional symptoms — Sexual or physical victimization — Behavioral symptoms
Medical Examination	
H	**H**ead-to-toe examination
E	**E**vidence collection — Clothing and linens — Orifice swabs — Foreign debris — Serological testing
A	**A**ssess for body, oral, anal, and genital injury
L	**L**essen embarrassment and anxiety (keep parts of body not being examined draped)
T	**T**est — Sexually transmitted diseases — Pregnancy — Toxicological testing for drugs, alcohol
H	**H**ealing — Referral for counseling, mental health assessments, crisis support — Treatment of injuries, STIs, intoxication — Prophylaxis for STIs, pregnancy — Follow-up to ensure healing, complete assessment for STIs with prolonged incubation periods

Because most adolescents do not have injuries, forensic evidence, or an STI that provides specific evidence of sexual assault or abuse, medical diagnosis and treatment often relies on the patient's history. The extent to which a medical history is gathered depends on clinician expertise and comfort level, the local investigative procedures for interviewing victims, the victim's willingness to talk, and the context within which the victim first discloses. For example, if an adolescent discloses sexual abuse for the first time within a clinical setting, the clinician may encourage and support the patient by allowing him or her to share any information as wished but may defer the complete assessment to an experienced sexual abuse unit. The clinician still needs to gather the information necessary to assess the patient's immediate medical, psychological, and safety needs. Such information is best gathered from the patient directly, out of the presence of family members. Family members may be supportive, distraught, unsupportive, or disbelieving, all of which can affect the victim's willingness to disclose information to the clinician.

Medical History

Tell Them Your Agenda

The clinician should begin the interview by stating his or her role in the adolescent's health care and what is known about the reason for the adolescent's visit. ("As your doctor, it's my job to find ways to help you keep healthy and safe. I understand something sexual or physical may have happened to you. I'd like to ask some questions so we can come up with a plan that can help you.") If abuse has not been disclosed, the clinician might instead say, "I am going to ask you some questions about how your body is doing, how your feelings are doing, how your life is going, and about any hurtful or uncomfortable things that may have happened to you. The reason I am asking these questions is so I can figure out what I need to check you for, what tests I might need to do, and how I can best help you with your health." In addition, it is important for the clinician to explain the limits of confidentiality to the adolescent: "If we talk about something that places you or someone else in danger, I may have to share this with your parents or someone else who can make sure everyone is safe."

Earn Trust

Because a victim's trust is often violated during abuse, it is important for the clinician to establish rather than expect trust. Truthfully disclosing the clinical agenda (see earlier) is the first step, as is providing an explanation of the procedures and of the purpose of the various components of the medical assessment. The cooperative nature of the medical evaluation should be stressed because some adolescents may view the process as something they are undergoing for their parents, the police, the authorities, or the physician, rather than for themselves. A nonjudgmental, clinically focused approach reduces anxiety in the patient and facilitates information sharing.

When the adolescent confides their feelings and reactions to abuse, the clinician should acknowledge these feelings. Adolescents may describe shame, guilt, fear, or embarrassment about their victimization, family life, criminal behavior, and health-risky lifestyle. They will be sensitive to the responses of health professionals as they disclose and share feelings about these circumstances. Clinicians should maintain a nonjudgmental demeanor, restate their reasons for asking such questions, and acknowledge that such feelings are normal among children in similar circumstances: "I know this is hard for you to talk about. I have talked with other teens about this, and it is hard for them too. These questions will help me decide whether I should check you for sexually transmitted infections. If you feel more comfortable, you can write down or whisper your answers instead of saying them out loud. I really need your help before I can decide how to best help you."

Assure Safety

Family History, Support by Nonabusive Parent, Protection of Abuser, or Concern for Integrity of Family

In one study more than half the children and teens evaluated in a sexual abuse clinic reported past or present domestic violence in their home.[9] Risk of serious injury and death may arise if an adult victim of violence leaves his or her abuser when it is discovered that the abuser has also sexually assaulted one or more of the children in the home. In addition, up to 40% of mothers of sexual abuse victims either don't believe their child or are unsure that abuse occurred.[9] In these circumstances, teens may recant their abuse history to avoid jeopardizing the parent-child relationship and to preserve the integrity of the family. Similarly, one-third of victims feel ambivalent toward their abuser and may withdraw their statements of abuse to protect the abuser or the integrity of the family. Clinicians may uncover these concerns by asking adolescents how much they think their nonabusive parent believes or supports them and by asking what outcome or outcomes victims would prefer for their family and the abuser. If victims appear protective of their abuser and disclose only low-risk types of sexual contact, the clinician may wish to test for STIs anyway in the event that not all abuse details have been disclosed. In addition, clinicians should explicitly ask whether victims are afraid of their parents or of going home.

Another area that adolescents may have concerns about is the effect of their abuse on siblings. The clinician may ask how siblings are responding to recent family changes or how they are responding to the abuse (if they are aware it took place).

Health-Risky Behaviors

Adolescent victims of abuse may suffer suicidal thoughts and may engage in unhealthy activities, including cutting, overdosing on medications or recreational drugs, unprotected sex, sexual activity with multiple partners, runaway behavior, criminal activity, and drug or alcohol abuse. Substance use and sexual assault are strongly associated. In one large study sample, drug abuse and alcohol intoxication among adolescents was associated with a risk of sexual assault 1.5 to 4.7 times greater than that among adolescents who did not abuse drugs or alcohol.[13] Substance abuse tends to be a peer group activity, and it is not uncommon for such a peer group to engage in other health-risky behaviors, including unprotected sexual activity and sexual assault. **Appendix 15-1** provides a useful screening tool for adolescent substance abuse.

Medical Issues

The components of the medical history that are pertinent to sexual assault are not significantly different from any other medical care and include the following:

- ***Medical history*** includes chronic medical conditions that may affect the anogenital examination findings. Examples include neurological conditions that affect anorectal or pubic muscle laxity, labial adhesions, and Crohn's disease.
- ***Gynecological history*** begins with menarche (years of menstruation correlates with regularity of cycles) and addresses last menstrual period (need for pregnancy testing), regularity of cycles and menstrual volume (need for pregnancy testing), and prior gynecological examination and tampon use (ability to tolerate sexual abuse/assault examination. Painful tampon insertion has been associated with hymenal findings).[14]
- ***Sexual history*** details types of prior sexual contact with male or female partners, last consensual and last abusive contact (STI risk; interpretation of examination findings with regards to abuse or assault—acute findings may be specific to assault

only if consensual contact is remote), and use of barrier contraception (STI risk). When gathering a sexual history, it is important to acknowledge the possibility of alternative sexual identity or orientation in the adolescent. For example, the clinician may inquire whether the adolescent has ever had or thought about having sexual experiences with male or female partners, or both, and what questions or concerns the adolescent might have about those thoughts.

— ***Current and past sexual victimization*** includes the type or types of sexual contact (sites for STI and forensic evidence collection), the time since the last sexual contact (timing of STI testing), the frequency of intervals between sexual contact (STI risk), the number of abusers (STI risk, interpretation of examination results), the penetrative types of sexual contact (pain or bleeding may be associated with penetration but are not necessarily signs of physical injury), the use of lubricant (may decrease likelihood of injury), the use of condoms (may decrease STI risk), and any abuser risk factors if known (intravenous drug user, multiple sexual partners of same or different gender, gang member: more extensive STI testing recommended).

— ***Physical symptoms and concerns*** include conditions that may obscure examination findings (eg, encopresis and obesity may make it more difficult to visualize the hymen and vestibule), conditions that may be sequelae of abuse (eg, dysuria after genital contact, pain or bleeding after penetration, painful defecation, and vaginal or anal discharge as signifiers of a potential STI), and symptoms reported by patients that may reflect anxiety or concerns related to abuse rather than medical causes (eg, genital pain, discharge, enlarging stomach, and nausea as potential indicators of pregnancy). Although examination findings often do not reflect reported symptoms, the clinician needs to provide appropriate reassurance.

— ***Behavioral symptoms*** are also a cause for concern. More commonly reported symptoms include sleeping difficulties such as nightmares, trouble falling or staying asleep (symptoms of anxiety, intrusive memories), and school or work difficulties that may include trouble concentrating or staying on task because of intrusive thoughts of abuse. Adolescents should also be screened for anxiety, depression, self-injurious behaviors, eating disorders, and dissociative symptoms.

Medical Examination

Although it is preferable to conduct the interview out of the presence of family members and friends, the patient should be allowed to have a support person present during the examination portion. Many adolescents prefer not to include a parent but may opt for the presence of a sibling or friend.

Head-to-Toe Examination

It is important for the clinician to not focus solely on the genitals during the sexual assault examination. Many adolescents have some degree of anxiety regarding the examination because it is embarrassing or because they expect discomfort, and they may have been told that a speculum examination would be done. In many cases the adolescent has not had a health maintenance examination for years, and the clinician may use this opportunity to perform a needed health screening, including immunizations. Performing the general and more familiar pediatric examination may also facilitate cooperation and lower anxiety as the examination progresses to include the abdomen, genitals, and anus.

Evidence Collection

Most states provide standardized evidence collection kits with detailed instructions for collecting, processing, packaging, and maintaining the chain of forensic evidence. If the clinician determines that sexual assault likely occurred within the previous 72 hours, a prompt referral to a specialized program with trained sexual assault examiners is strongly urged. Evidence collection requires not only expert examiners and adherence to state protocols, but also specialized equipment and sufficient space to ensure appropriate processing and maintenance of a chain of custody for forensic materials. Clinicians who opt to collect evidence must familiarize themselves with all necessary procedures and protocols before conducting any part of the examination. Forensic material is time sensitive, so collection must occur as soon as feasible.

In general, evidence collection should be done before other examination procedures. Most protocols require the victim to unclothe over paper or a sheet, which is submitted for debris analysis. Then samples are taken from the oral cavity, head hair, pubic hair, fingernails, genitals, genital orifices, anus, and any areas potentially containing apparent dried secretions or bite marks are swabbed. The areas sampled depend on the specific protocol instructions, the history of assault, and prior examination findings.

Samples are air-dried, sealed, and signed in accordance with chain of custody procedures. Typically the sealed kit is retained in a locked, secured freezer until it is retrieved by law enforcement. State forensic laboratories process the contents for DNA and genetic markers. Some laboratories process the samples with less sensitive or specific tests such as acid phosphatase and P30 protein. Forensic analysis of samples continues to evolve and improve and will likely affect the procedures and time frame for forensic evidence collection in the future.

Assess for Body and Oral, Genital, and Anal Injuries

Victims of acute assault should be examined carefully for bruises, especially involving the face, neck, and head (more common sites for blows) as well as the forearms and lower extremities (more common sites for defensive injuries). Although areas of tenderness may be noted, the clinician should be cautious in attributing such findings to trauma without accompanying erythema, ecchymoses, or edema. Muscle strain and anxiety are other possible causes. **Table 15-2** provides examples of body injuries that have been associated with sexual assault. See **Figures 15-1** through **15-9** for examples of genital and anal injuries.

Forced oral-penile penetration may result in intraoral injuries, possibly accompanied by grasp marks or bruises to the cheeks or neck. Petechial hemorrhages associated with forced penetration generally occur at the junction of the soft and hard palate, near the uvula.

Genital injuries from sexual assault are uncommon. Although erythema and superficial excoriations of the vestibule and vulva are often noted, such findings are nonspecific for trauma. Acute injuries of sexual assault most often occur in the posterior vestibule, between the posterior attachment of the hymen and the posterior commissure. Other acute injuries include lacerations of the hymen, bruising of the hymen, and abrasions and bruising of the vestibule or inner labia minora folds. Findings that indicate healed penetrative trauma of the hymen include lateral and posterior clefts (defects in the hymen between the 3 o'clock and 9 o'clock positions that extend the entire width of the hymen at a discrete point) and scarring in the posterior vestibule (scarring that is palpable or causes contraction of surrounding tissue).[14] An evidence-based classification system indicates that a deep notch that extends nearly to the base of the posterior hymen is classified as a "no consensus" finding among an expert panel of reviewers.[15] The majority of acute injuries heal without sequelae or scarring in a matter of a few days. In one large patient series of children and adolescents who were examined for acute and nonacute sexual assault, 96% had normal or nonspecific findings of penetrative trauma.[16] Although "it's normal to be normal," "normal" does not mean "nothing happened."[17] In a study of 36 adolescents undergoing sexual abuse examinations while pregnant, 82% had normal "intact" hymens and no scarring.[18]

Table 15-2. Nongenital Injuries in Assault Victims

Type	Possible Mechanisim
Perioral or intraoral injuries, especially erythema or petechiae near junction of hard and soft palate	Hand restraint (voice muffling) Forced penile-oral penetration
Neck bruises, "hickies"	Choke by hand or ligature Suction/bite
Oval or semicircular bruises to neck, chest, breasts, extremities	Bite
Bruises to face, body, especially lips and eyes; intra-abdominal hematomas or organ rupture	Blunt force trauma such as blow with fist
Bruises to extensor surfaces of upper or lower arms, knuckles	Defense injuries (victim tries to protect head with arms)
Traumatic alopecia, subgaleal hematoma	Hair-pulling
Numerous small (2-3 cm) bruises on shoulders, arms, thighs, face	Hand restraint bruises or grab marks
Ligature marks to wrists or ankles	Restraint with rope or wire
Abrasions, friction injuries to bony prominences of back	Victim struggle while restrained in supine position on firm surface

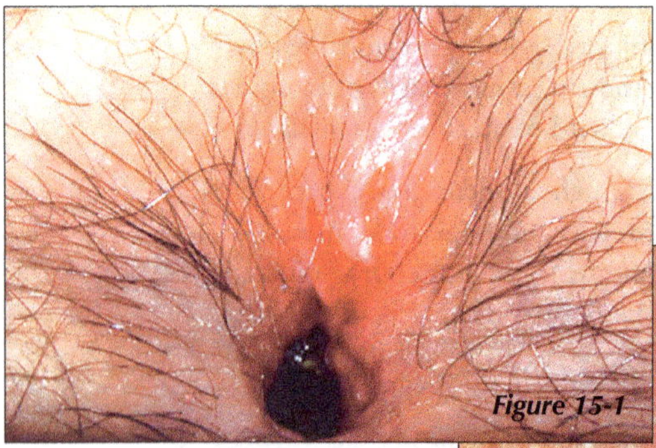

Figure 15-1

Figure 15-1. *Adolescent who denied anal penetration and denied any pain or bleeding in her anal area. In the prone knee-chest position, 2 tears are seen at 12 o'clock and 1 o'clock.*

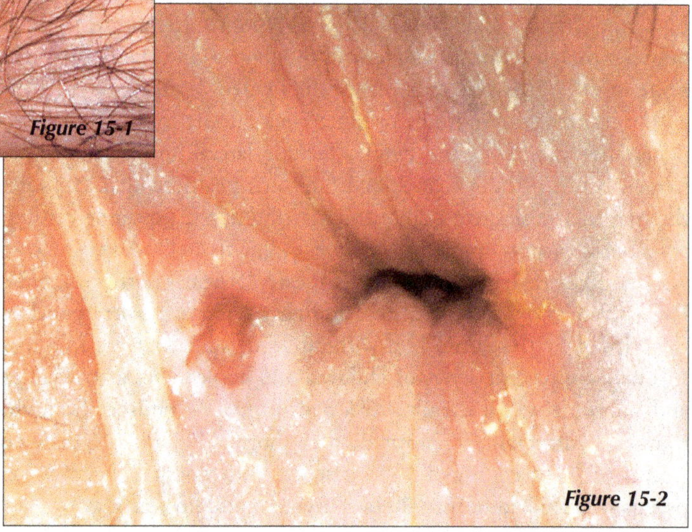

Figure 15-2

Figure 15-2. *A 14-year-old girl with a history of anal penetration occurring 3 days prior. Note tear at 9 o'clock. Patient is in left lateral decubitus position.*

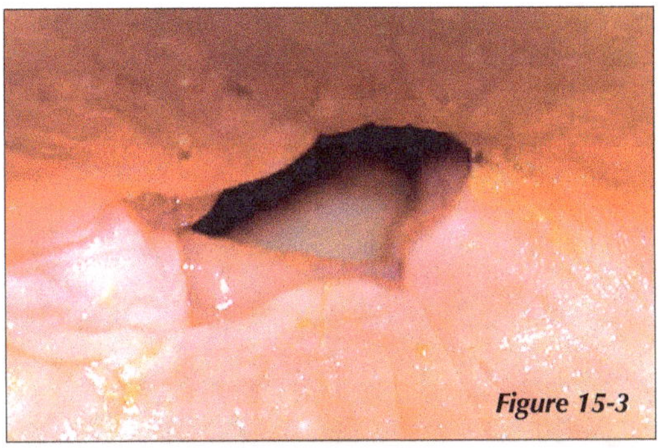
Figure 15-3

Figure 15-3. A 15-year-old adolescent boy with a long-term history of anal-penile penetration. Note laxity of anal opening and scar tissue at 9 o'clock. Patient is in the lateral decubitus position.

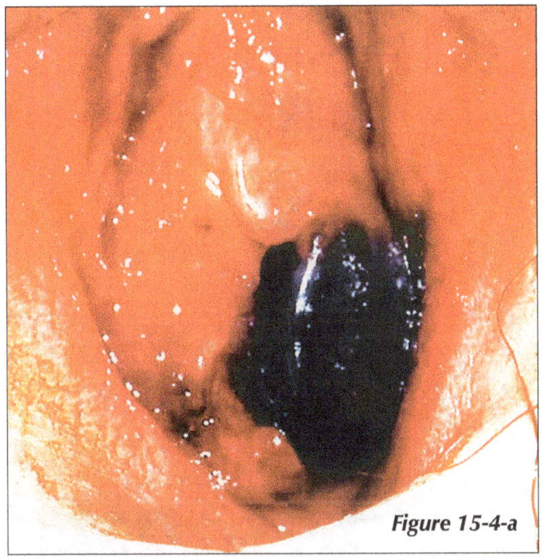
Figure 15-4-a

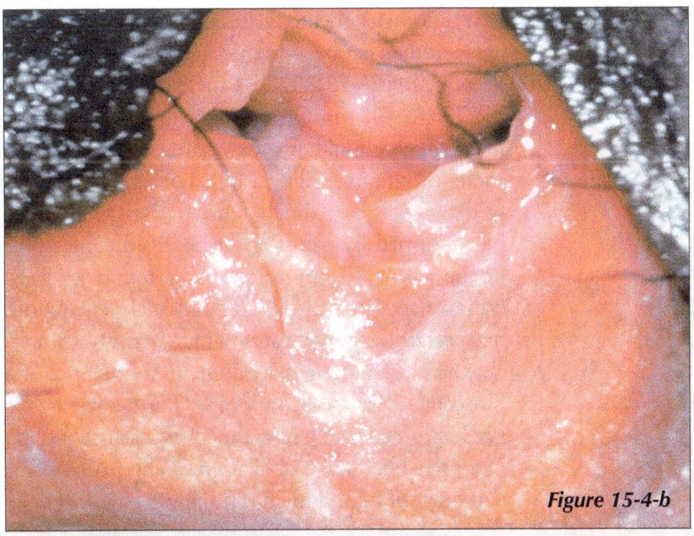
Figure 15-4-b

Figure 15-4-a. Hematoma. A 15-year-old victim of vaginal-penile penetration 36 hours previously.

Figure 15-4-b. Same patient, 5 days after initial examination.

Figure 15-5. A 5-year-old girl victim of vaginal-penile penetration occurring 36 hours earlier. Complete hymenal tear at 6 o'clock, and posterior vestibule tear with bruising.

Figure 15-6. Adolescent girl with several hymenal clefts, resulting in isolated "clumps" of hymen (caruncles). There is no visible hymenal tissue from 4 o'clock to 8 o'clock.

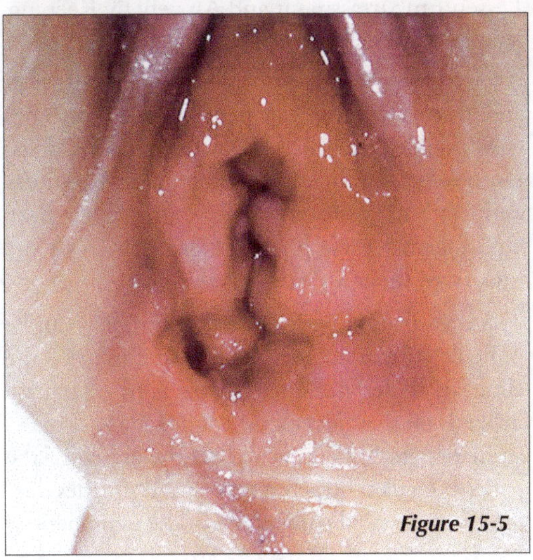
Figure 15-5

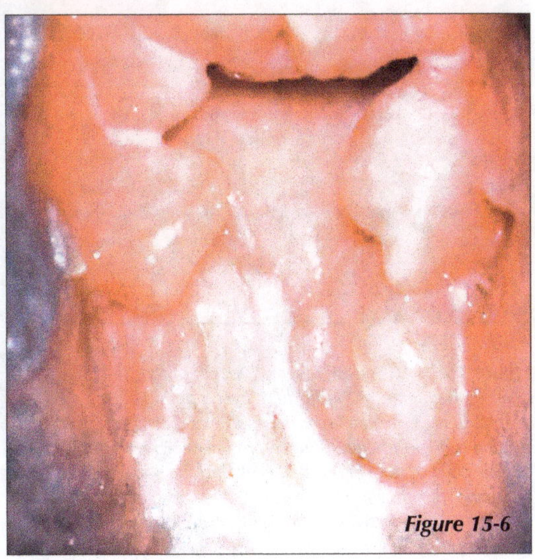
Figure 15-6

Figure 15-7. *Healed tear, or cleft, from 5 o'clock to 7 o'clock.*

Figure 15-8. *Posterior vestibule scar and large area from 4 o'clock to 8 o'clock with no visible hymenal tissue.*

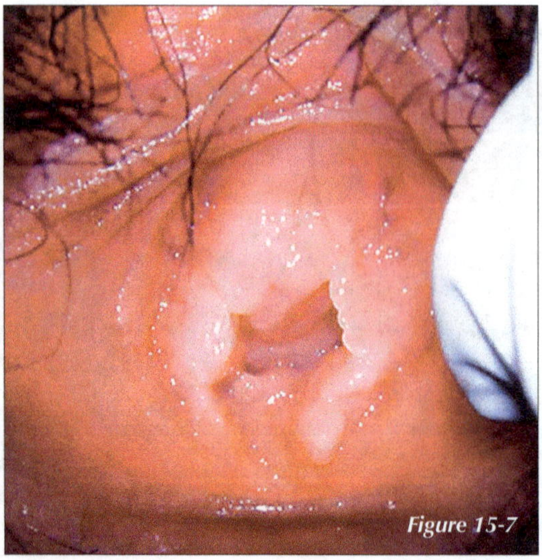

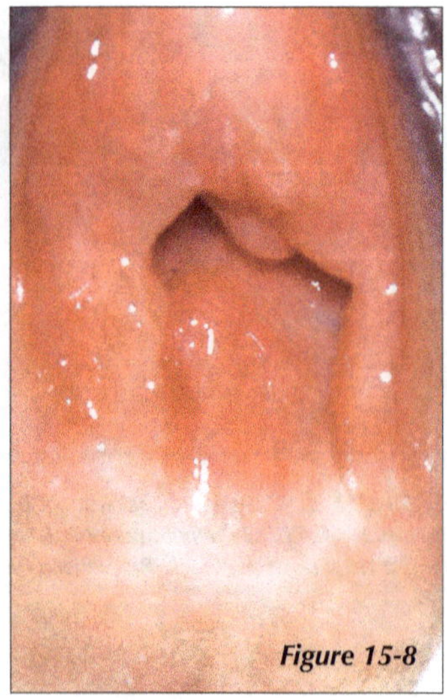

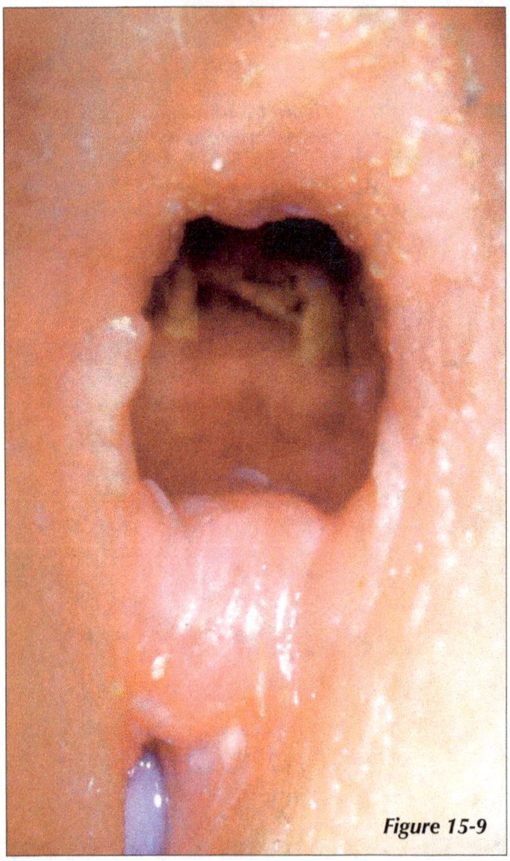

Figure 15-9. *A 13-year-old female victim of repeated anal-penile penetration by 2 individuals over a period of 3 to 4 years. Extensive perianal scarring and immediate anal sphincter dilation is noted (patient is in the prone knee-chest position). The absence of stool in the anal vault and the presence of other traumatic findings supports trauma as the cause of this dilation. The child also reported some difficulty with fecal incontinence over the past year.*

Anal findings of acute or healed penetrative trauma are rarer than genital findings. Acute findings include deep anal tears, usually in a stellate pattern close to the 12 o'clock and 6 o'clock midline, and hematomas, which should not be confused with hemorrhoids or venous pooling. Healed penetrative trauma of the anus is exceedingly rare. Any scarring should be confirmed by palpation or observed contraction of the tissue. Recent studies have found an association between anal dilation and anal penetration; however, these studies caution that care must be taken when interpreting this finding in the absence of a disclosure of anal penetration.[19,20] Further research is needed to determine how these new data should be interpreted because anal dilation can be attributed to a number of nontraumatic and physiological causes.

Lessen Embarrassment and Anxiety by Keeping Parts of Body Not Being Examined Draped

Adolescents are self-conscious and embarrassed about various features of their bodies. Most have considerable reluctance and, in some cases, resistance to having their genitals, anus, or breasts examined. Such concerns can be partly assuaged by ensuring that these private areas of the body are uncovered for as little time as possible.

The examination positions and techniques can be difficult to master effectively. The ability of the clinician to see the often subtle signs of trauma depends on their technical and judicious use of examination techniques as well as the ability of the patient to relax the pelvic and gluteal muscles during the anogenital component of the examination.

Testing for STIs, Pregnancy, Drugs, and Alcohol

STI Testing

When an adolescent presents within 72 hours of a sexual assault, forensic evidence, including swabs of orifices, should be collected before conducting tests for STIs. Appropriate testing for STIs requires consideration of the time since the assault, symptoms, risk factors, the purpose of the test, availability of the test, and the cooperation of the adolescent. A recent study supported the longstanding recommendation to test for gonorrhea and *Chlamydia* based on the type of sexual contact and regardless of symptoms. In addition, this study suggested that testing anal and oral sites should also be considered even if there is no history of sexual contact at those sites.[11] The optimal time to test for STIs depends on the incubation period of the STI in question. For example, most initial medical assessments for sexual assault involve testing for gonorrhea, *Chlamydia*, and sometimes *Trichomonas*, because these are the more common STIs and because infected individuals are often asymptomatic. Based on the incubation periods of these infections, an optimal time to test is at least 10 to 14 days after the sexual assault. If the sexual contact has occurred over several weeks or months, adolescents can be tested at the time of their evaluation even if the most recent sexual abuse occurred within 10 days. A positive test in an adolescent presenting for an acute sexual assault could represent a prior infection but could also be infective assailant secretions from the recent assault.[21] Variable testing schedules reflect variable incubation periods. Chapter 10 discusses STIs in more depth.

A sexually assaulted adolescent who presents with symptoms or signs such as dysuria, genital discharge, ulcers, or verrucous lesions may require more extensive testing for STIs. Adolescents with symptoms often presume the worst and a negative test may provide reassurance. Similarly, adolescents may worry that they have an infection even when they are asymptomatic, especially if the assailant is a stranger or if the teen has heard that the assailant has an STI. It is important for the clinician to address these concerns, and testing may be the most effective way to provide reassurance.

The primary role of the clinician is to provide for the health and well-being of the patient, although each procedure and test can be subjected to legal scrutiny in a court of law. These dual roles of clinical and forensic assessment present some controversy, particularly when selecting diagnostic tests for gonorrhea and *Chlamydia*. This choice is most difficult when testing for *Chlamydia*. Although the culture is considered the legal "gold standard," its sensitivity is low, averaging 60% to 70%. Nucleic acid amplification tests are more sensitive and more readily available than culture. The Centers for Disease Control and Prevention (CDC) previously required 2 nucleic acid amplification tests, targeting different genomes of the organism, to equate the result to a gold standard, but based on recent studies, routine retesting is no longer recommended unless indicated by the product insert.[22] In a significant majority of cases, the diagnosis of sexual abuse is based on the victim's history, not the examination findings. If clinicians feel confident in their diagnosis before conducting the examination, then they may wish to use the STI tests to optimize their *management* of the patient rather than to *diagnose* sexual abuse; in which case, clinicians should become familiar with the test they use so that the rationale for choosing the test can be adequately explained if court testimony is required. If the clinician wishes to legally confirm the diagnosis of sexual abuse, then the gold standard may be the appropriate test. In victims with prior sexual contact with another abuser or with a partner, testing for STIs no longer has forensic significance to the abuse, so the most sensitive and specific test is appropriate.

Before selecting the type of STI diagnostic test, the clinician should become familiar with the equipment and materials needed at the clinical site to conduct the test, the capability of local laboratories to process the test, and the expertise of laboratory personnel in processing and interpreting such tests. In some hospitals, for example, *Chlamydia* culture is no longer available, whereas other regions lack the capability to process nucleic acid amplification tests.

Finally, it is important to consider the adolescent's ability and willingness to cooperate with the examination. Adolescents may deny penetration that has, in fact, occurred, and refuse the examination because they think the doctor will be able to determine from the examination that they have had sex. Others refuse the examination because of extreme embarrassment and shame. Some may become distraught during the genital portion of the examination. If the patient cannot cooperate, the clinician may opt to defer the tests until later, not test, or send a urine nucleic acid amplification test for gonorrhea and *Chlamydia* (if available). Similarly, vaginal swabs can be obtained instead of cervical samples if the adolescent is anxious and has not had a speculum examination before the sexual assault examination.

Other Diagnostic Tests

The clinician should evaluate the need for pregnancy and drug testing, depending on the history and clinical presentation of the victim. If the adolescent is menarcheal, a pregnancy test should be conducted and confirmed as negative before giving emergency contraception. Because adolescents do not always report their menstrual history with accuracy, the clinician should test for pregnancy whenever there is a concern.

A drug test (urine or serum or both, depending on the time frame and symptoms) or an electrolyte panel should be submitted whenever the victim reports ingestion of a substance that altered their mental status or there are signs of intoxication on examination. Drug-facilitated sexual assault is a recognized entity, and although alcohol remains the single most commonly used substance in such cases, drugs such as alprazolam (Xanax), ketamine, flunitrazepam (Rohypnol), γ-hydroxybutyric acid, and even insulin have been employed by assailants. Clinicians should become familiar with which substances are detected in the urine toxicology screens provided by their facility, as some drugs, including flunitrazepam, are not routinely detected. The clinician should ensure that confirmatory testing is ordered for any positive drug screen.

Serological tests for syphilis, HIV, and hepatitis should be done when risk factors in the abuser are present or unknown, if the patient or family requests it, or if the patient is found to have at least one STI. Because most adolescents have been immunized for hepatitis B, serological testing is rarely needed, but if immunization status is unknown, adolescents can be given 1 dose of the vaccine as prophylaxis. Serologic testing for hepatitis C is recommended. HIV prophylaxis remains controversial but can be given when the assailant is known to be HIV positive and the victim presents within 72 hours of the assault. Baseline tests for renal and bone marrow function are also required at the time of the initial medical evaluation.

Healing

Healing for the adolescent victim of sexual abuse or assault is the most comprehensive phase of the TEAMHEALTH model. Although the focus tends to be on the components that take minutes to gather—injuries, STIs, and forensic materials—the health harms of sexual abuse can extend for years. For example, once the abuse has been reported and the initial medical assessment completed, it can take up to 3 years or longer for the criminal trial to occur. During this time, the adolescent and his or her family receive numerous subpoenas and trial reset notices, constant reminders of the abuse, and potential triggers for emotional distress. During this period, the clinician can provide reassurance and be a resource for the adolescent and his or her family.

Comprehensive, long-term management of the sexual abuse or assault survivor must encompass the medical, mental health, and safety needs of the victim. Immediate medical needs include surgical or medical management of acute injuries, STI prophylaxis (**Table 15-3**), and emergency contraception in cases where the sexual assault involves penile

Table 15-3. Management of Uncomplicated Sexually Transmitted Diseases in Adolescent* Victims of Sexual Abuse

Organism	Prophylactic Treatment	Treatment of Confirmed Disease
Gonorrhea	Ceftriaxone 250 mg IM x 1 or cefixime 400 mg PO† x 1 PLUS treatment for *Chlamydia*	Same as for prophylaxis
Chlamydia	Azithromycin 1 g PO x 1 PLUS treatment for gonorrhea	Azithromycin 1 g PO x 1 or doxycycline 200 mg/d (BID) x 7 days
Hepatitis	Begin or complete hepatitis B immunization	None
Trichomonas, bacterial vaginosis	Metronidazole 2 g PO x 1 or tinidazole 2g PO x1	Metronidazole 2 g PO x 1 or 500 mg BID x 7 days
Syphilis‡	(Gonorrhea prophylaxis has efficacy against incubating syphilis)	Benzathine penicillin G 2.4 million U IM x 1 or doxycycline 200 mg/d (BID) PO x 14 days
Herpes simplex virus	None	*Initial episode:* Acyclovir 1000-1200 mg/d (3-5 x/d) PO x 7-10 d or Valacyclovir 1gm bid PO x 10 d *Recurrent episodes:* Acyclovir 400 mg PO tid x 5 d or Valacyclovir 500 mg PO bid x 3 d
Human papillomavirus	None, although immunization with HPV vaccine for individuals who are unimmunized or partially immunized may be beneficial	*Patient administered*: Podofilox 0.5% solution or gel or imiquimod 5% cream *Clinician administered*: Bichloroacetic acid/trichloroacetic acid 80%-90% solution, cryotherapy, surgical excision, or intraluminal interferon
Human immunodeficiency virus	Consider if high-risk contact occurs: 3-drug regimen of emtricitabine/tenofovir and raltegravir for 28 days if patient presents within 72 hours of contact (with baseline HIV, CBC, and chemistry serologies)	Consult with infectious disease specialist

**Includes preadolescents weighing > 100 lbs.*
†Abbreviations: PO=orally, IM=intramuscularly, BID=2 times daily, TID=3 times daily.
‡CSF examination is recommended for those with central nervous system symptoms.
Data from American Academy of Pediatrics. 2018 Red Book: Report of the Committee on Infectious Diseases. *31st ed. Itasca, IL 60143: American Academy of Pediatrics; 2018.*

contact or penetration occurring within 5 days of the examination and the pregnancy test is negative. Plan B, Plan B One-Step, and its generic counterparts such as Next Choice One Dose or Take Action are available over the counter without age restrictions in the United States. It is the most common form of nonprescriptive emergency contraception. Ovral and Lo Ovral have also been approved for this purpose but are not readily available in packets specifically intended for emergency contraception. Patients must be directed on how to take multiple pills and approximate the necessary dose from a packet that is intended for cyclic use.

Victims of acute sexual assault may also be candidates for STI prophylaxis against *Chlamydia*, gonorrhea, and, in some cases, *Trichomonas* and HIV. Prophylaxis for HIV is determined by assessing the risk of the patient contracting HIV based on perpetrator risk factors and details of the sexual assault or abuse. Prophylaxis is costly and requires several weeks of antiviral medication with some side effects, although they are generally well tolerated in children. The efficacy of this prophylaxis has not been studied; however, it is based on occupational postexposure prophylaxis, which was associated with an 81% reduction in the risk of acquiring HIV.[23]

It is important to provide appropriate medical follow-up, especially for victims of acute sexual assault, given the prolonged incubation period of some STIs, such as human papillomavirus (HPV). **Table 15-4** provides guidelines for medical follow-up

Table 15-4. Follow-up Considerations for Victims of Sexual Trauma

2 Weeks
1. Healing of injuries
2. Type 2 herpes simplex virus: 3-10 days incubation
3. *Trichomoniasis*, bacterial vaginosis, *Chlamydia*, gonorrhea: 10-14 days incubation (if no initial prophylaxis given)
4. Pregnancy (if oral contraception is not provided at initial evaluation)
5. Psychological support and reassurance of patient and family
6. Drug and alcohol monitoring or treatment (if coordinated with specialist)
2-3 Months
1. HIV testing: repeat at 4 weeks, 3 months, 6 months, 1 year
2. Syphilis and hepatitis: 6-8 weeks incubation
3. Human papillomavirus: 2-3 months average incubation; up to 20 months incubation in rare cases
4. Psychological support of patient and family
5. Drug and alcohol monitoring (if coordinated with specialist)

Adapted from Kellogg ND, Sugarek NJ. Sexual trauma. Atlas of Office Procedures. *1998;1(1):181-197.*

evaluations. The CDC recommends 2 doses of the HPV vaccine in all female sexual abuse or assault victims until age 26 years.[23] Follow-up examinations also provide opportunities for the clinician to reassure the victim of injury resolution and to assess any need for further mental health services. The adolescent should be screened for depression and self-injurious thoughts and behaviors during follow-up appointments.

The clinician can play a key role in the emotional recovery of the victim and the family. Victims and family members may have a number of fears and anxieties, some of which can be alleviated by the clinician. For example, victims and family members may be wondering whether the victim is still a "virgin," or may believe the abuse did not occur when they are told the examination is "normal." Clinicians may clarify such terms and provide reassurance that "normal" does not mean "nothing happened." Some victims feel guilty because they delayed their disclosure; the clinician can reassure them that most victims delay their disclosure because of a variety of valid fears. The clinician can also provide encouragement that recovery from sexual assault and return to normalcy is possible.

It is critically important for the clinician to encourage and facilitate the use of community supports and services for victims and their families. Children's advocacy centers and regional rape crisis organizations often provide crisis services or referrals to victims of sexual abuse or assault, which can be of significant benefit to victims and family members immediately after the assault and in the difficult weeks and months that follow. Therapists trained and skilled in treating adolescent sexual assault victims are another valuable resource.

Documentation

Documentation during all phases of the TEAMHEALTH model is essential, especially because any of the information gathered may become significant in court proceedings. To the extent that it is possible, clinicians should document their questions and the patient's answers as direct quotations. This is particularly important if the victim is disclosing abuse for the first time, because the circumstances of the "first outcry" are critical to the investigation and legal proceedings that follow. Examination findings should be carefully documented, with extensive details of any visible injuries supported by high-quality photographs. Location, size, color, and characteristics such as bleeding and abrasions should be noted on body or anogenital findings. The clinician should provide a meaningful interpretation of the findings for nonmedical professionals involved in the investigation. If the medical diagnosis of sexual abuse is based primarily on the patient's history, the physician should document this, adding that most examinations of sexually abused adolescents are normal or nonspecific.

Conclusion

The medical assessment of an adolescent who is a suspected victim of sexual abuse or assault presents challenges that are distinctly different from evaluations of prepubertal children or adults. The TEAMHEALTH model provides a framework for gathering the medical history, conducting a thorough examination for injuries, using the appropriate diagnostic tests, and providing for the physical and emotional healing of the adolescent victim. In meeting these challenges of clinical care, the clinician is also presented with an opportunity to facilitate recovery and to promote a transition into healthy adulthood. TEAMHEALTH is a reminder that restoring health after sexual assault or abuse is achieved through a cooperative bond between the physician and his or her adolescent patient.

Appendix 15-1: The CRAFFT Interview

The CRAFFT Interview (version 2.1)

To be orally administered by the clinician

Begin: *"I'm going to ask you a few questions that I ask all my patients. Please be honest. I will keep your answers confidential."*

Part A

During the PAST 12 MONTHS, on how many days did you:

1.	Drink more than a few sips of beer, wine, or any drink containing **alcohol**? Put "0" if none.	☐ # of days
2.	Use any **marijuana** (weed, oil, or hash by smoking, vaping, or in food) or "**synthetic marijuana**" (like "K2," "Spice")? Put "0" if none.	☐ # of days
3.	Use **anything else to get high** (like other illegal drugs, prescription or over-the-counter medications, and things that you sniff, huff, or vape)? Put "0" if none.	☐ # of days

Did the patient answer "0" for all questions in Part A?

Yes ☐	No ☐
↓	↓
Ask CAR question only, then stop	**Ask all six CRAFFT* questions below**

Part B

		No	Yes
C	Have you ever ridden in a **CAR** driven by someone (including yourself) who was "high" or had been using alcohol or drugs?	☐	☐
R	Do you ever use alcohol or drugs to **RELAX**, feel better about yourself, or fit in?	☐	☐
A	Do you ever use alcohol or drugs while you are by yourself, or **ALONE**?	☐	☐
F	Do you ever **FORGET** things you did while using alcohol or drugs?	☐	☐
F	Do your **FAMILY** or **FRIENDS** ever tell you that you should cut down on your drinking or drug use?	☐	☐
T	Have you ever gotten into **TROUBLE** while you were using alcohol or drugs?	☐	☐

***Two or more YES answers suggest a serious problem and need for further assessment. See back for further instructions →**

NOTICE TO CLINIC STAFF AND MEDICAL RECORDS:
The information on this page is protected by special federal confidentiality rules (42 CFR Part 2), which prohibit disclosure of this information unless authorized by specific written consent. A general authorization for release of medical information is NOT sufficient.

Reprinted from CeASAR: The Center for Adolescent Substance Abuse Research. The CRAFFT. CeASAR Web site. https://ceasar.childrenshospital.org/crafft/. Accessed October 19, 2010.

For more information, contact ceasar@childrens.harvard.edu

References

1. Miller CA, Tebb KP, Williams JK, Neuhaus JM, Shafer M. Chlamydial screening in urgent care visits: adolescent-reported acceptability associated with adolescent perception of clinical communication. *Arch Pediatr Adol Med.* 2007;161(8):777-782.

2. Klein JD, Wilson KM. Delivering quality care: adolescents' discussion of health risks with their providers. *J Adolesc Health.* 2002;30(3):190-195.

3. *Aid for Women, et al v Nola Foulston, et al,* 427 F Supp 2d 1093 (D Kan 2006).

4. Crawford-Jakubiak JE, Alderman EM, Leventhal JM; Committee on Child Abuse and Neglect, Committee on Adolescence. Care of the adolescent after an acute sexual assault. *Pediatrics.* 2017;139(3):e20164243.

5. Temple JR, Paul JA, van den Berg P, Le VD, McElhany A, Temple BW. Teen sexting and its association with sexual behaviors. *Arch Ped Adolesc Med.* 2012;166(9):828-833.

6. Mitchell KJ, Finkelhor D, Wolak J. Risk factors for and impact of online sexual solicitation of youth. *JAMA.* 2001;285(23):3011-3014.

7. Kellogg ND, Hoffman TJ. Unwanted and illegal sexual experiences in childhood and adolescence. *Child Abuse Negl.* 1995;19(12):1457-1468.

8. Helweg-Larsen K, Bøving Larsen H. The prevalence of unwanted and unlawful sexual experiences reported by Danish adolescents: results from a national youth survey in 2002. *Acta Paediat.* 2006;95(10):1270-1276.

9. Kellogg ND, Menard SW. Violence among family members of children and adolescents evaluated for sexual abuse. *Child Abuse Negl.* 2003;27(12):1367-1376.

10. Kellogg ND. "Why didn't you tell?" Helping families and children weather the process following a sexual abuse disclosure. In: Teti DM, ed. *Parenting and Family Processes in Child Maltreatment and Intervention.* Basel, Switzerland: Springer Nature; 2017:35-43.

11. Kellogg ND, Melville JD, Lukefahr JL, Nienow SM, Russell EL.. Genital and extragenital gonorrhea and *Chlamydia* in children and adolescents evaluated for sexual abuse. *Pediatr Emerg Care.* 2018;34(11):761-766.

12. Greenbaum VJ. Commercial sexual exploitation and sex trafficking of children in the United States. *Curr Probl Pediatr Adolesc Health Care.* 2014;44(9):245-269.

13. Raghavan R, Bogart LM, Elliott MN, Vestal KD, Schuster MA. Sexual victimization among a national probability sample of adolescent women. *Perspect Sex Reprod Health.* 2004;36(6): 225-232.

14. Adams JA, Botash AS, Kellogg ND. Differences in hymenal morphology between adolescent girls with and without a history of consensual sexual intercourse. *Arch Pediatr Adolesc Med.* 2004;158(3):280-285.

15. Adams JA, Kellogg ND, Farst KJ, et al. Updated guidelines for the medical assessment and care of children who may have been sexually abused. *J Pediatr Adolesc Gynecol.* 2016;29(2):81-87.

16. Heger A, Ticson L, Velasquez O, Bernier R. Children referred for possible sexual abuse: medical findings in 2384 children. *Child Abuse Negl.* 2002;26(6-7):645-659.

17. Adams JA, Harper K, Knudson S, Revilla J. Examination findings in legally confirmed child sexual abuse: it's normal to be normal. *Pediatrics*. 1994;94(3):310-317.

18. Kellogg ND, Menard SW, Santos A. Genital anatomy in pregnant adolescents: "normal" does not mean "nothing happened." *Pediatrics*. 2004;113(1 pt 1):e67-69.

19. Hobbs CJ, Wright CM. Anal signs of child sexual abuse: a case-control study. *BMC Pediatr*. 2014;14:128.

20. Myhre AK, Adams JA, Kaufhold M, Davis JL, Suresh P, Kuelbs CL. Anal findings in children with and without probable anal penetration: a retrospective study of 1115 children referred for suspected sexual abuse. *Child Abuse Negl*. 2013;37(7):465-474.

21. Seña AC, Hsu KK, Kellogg ND, et al. Sexual assault and sexually transmitted infections in adults, adolescents, and children. *Clin Infect Dis*. 2015;61(Suppl 8):S856-S864.

22. Papp JR, Schachter J, Gaydos CA, Van Der Pol B; Centers for Disease Control and Prevention. Recommendations for the laboratory-based detection of *Chlamydia trachomatis* and *Nisseria gonorrhoeae*—2014. *MMWR Morb Mortal Wkly Rep*. 2014;63(RR-02):1-19.

23. Workowski KA, Bolan GA; Centers for Disease Control and Prevention. Sexually transmitted diseases treatment guidelines, 2015. *MMWR Morb Mortal Wkly Rep*. 2015;64(RR-03):1-137.

Chapter 16

CHILD SEXUAL EXPLOITATION

Jordan Greenbaum, MD
Sharon W. Cooper, MD, FAAP
Dan D. Broughton, MD

INTRODUCTION

Child sexual exploitation (CSE) is a broad term that includes many acts that violate the basic human rights of children around the world. With increasing public awareness of child trafficking and of Internet-based sexual exploitation, CSE has gained the public's interest, raising major concerns regarding child safety. *Child sexual exploitation* refers to any act in which a person younger than 18 years of age "takes part in a sexual activity in exchange for something (eg, gain or benefit, or even the promise of such) from a third party, the perpetrator or by the child her/himself."[1] This may involve the exchange of money, drugs, food, shelter, or luxury or other items. The critical element in this definition is the idea of an exchange. Because child sexual abuse (CSA) may involve promises of treats, attention, or gifts, there is significant overlap between CSA and CSE. CSE may take several forms, as outlined in **Table 16-1**. In addition, victims* may experience more than one form of exploitation,[2] such as, for example, a 15-year-old girl who is sexually solicited online by a male adult, shown nude photos of the perpetrator, and enticed to perform sexual acts in front of her Web cam at the direction of the perpetrator, who records the activities.

TYPES OF CHILD SEXUAL EXPLOITATION

CHILD SEX TRAFFICKING

As indicated in Table 16-1, US federal law defines child sex trafficking (CST) very broadly, such that it includes a variety of acts that lead to a commercial sex act with a minor.[3,4] Commercial sex acts may involve prostitution (including "survival sex"), production of child sexual exploitation materials, inducing a minor to perform sex acts in a sexually oriented venue, or any other sex act that accompanies the exchange of something of perceived value. There may or may not be a third party involved (ie, a trafficker), and movement of the victim is *not* required. Similarly, force, fraud, or coercion is not required to prove child sex trafficking because the person's young age prevents them from being able to give informed consent. Although much public attention has been focused on trafficking in the form of forced prostitution of adolescent girls by traffickers, it is important to realize that CST involves a much more diverse population including boys and girls, and transgender youth, and activities beyond prostitution.[5]

Those who are sex trafficked may be of any age, but most studies document a mean age between 12 and 16 years.[5-8] One may argue that all youth are at risk for CST because their stage of brain development favors risk taking and immediate gratification over careful analysis of pros and cons and consideration of the long-term effects of their actions.[9,10] However, some youth are at increased risk for 1 or more reasons that may be associated with individual, relationship, community, or societal factors.[11] A list of vulnerability factors is presented in **Table 16-2**.

**When the term "victim" is used in this chapter, it is used in its objective and legal sense, indicating a person who has been harmed as a result of some event or action or who has suffered because of someone else's actions. It does not refer to how the person may feel or perceive himself or herself as a result of the event(s) in question and is not intended to label that person. The words "child" or "children" refer to persons younger than 18 years of age.*

Table 16-1. Types of Sexual Exploitation

Type of Exploitation	Definition*	Example of Exploitation
Child sex trafficking	— Per US federal law, recruiting, harboring, transporting, providing, obtaining, patronizing, or soliciting a child (< 18 years) for a commercial sex act.[3,4]	— A 16-year-old girl is prostituted by 25-year-old man who pretends to be her boyfriend. — A 15-year-old girl dances in a strip club for the owner, who gives her food and a place to stay.
Exploitation in prostitution	— Child engaging in sex act in exchange for something of value (or promise of). A third party may or may not be involved with exchange.	— Homeless 15-year-old boy agrees to have sex with a stranger in exchange for a place to spend the night. — A 16-year-old girl has sex with men at the direction of her "boyfriend," who keeps some of the earnings from these activities.
Child sexual exploitation materials (formerly called "child pornography")	— Material depicting child sexual abuse and other sexualized content depicting children.	— Audio file of child being sexually assaulted. — Web cam recording of child exposing genitals.
Solicitation of child for sexual purposes ("grooming")	— Acts that aim to persuade a child to engage in sexual activities (may occur online or offline).	— A 35-year-old man meets a 14-year-old girl in an online chatroom, befriends her, and convinces her to meet him at a motel to have sexual intercourse.
Exploitation in the context of travel or tourism (formerly called "sex tourism")	— Sexual exploitation "that is embedded in a context of travel, tourism or both."[1] — Includes domestic and foreign perpetrators and includes travel for tourism, business, work, military, and other purposes.	— An American tourist travels to a resort town on the coast of West Africa to purchase sex with a 9-year-old boy. — An Italian man attends a business convention in Rome and purchases sex with 14-year-old girl.
Live sexual performances (online child sexual abuse or live performances in sexually oriented businesses)	— Child performs sexual acts at a sex-oriented venue (eg, exotic dance club) or child performs sex acts that are transmitted live through ICT.† — Observers are offsite and may be dictating child's acts.	— A 15 year old dances unclothed at a "gentlemen's club." — A mother advertises sexual acts with her 9-year-old daughter online. Buyers all over the world request performances and pay according to acts requested and time allotted. The child performs acts in the home in front of a Web cam.

**With the exception of sex trafficking, the definitions listed reflect the Luxembourg terminology guidelines[1] and do not necessarily reflect specific state/national/international laws and treaties. The international Interagency Work Group was convened to clarify terms related to child sexual exploitation and child sexual abuse that are inconsistently defined among various treaties and laws. These guidelines are the product of their extensive research and collaboration.*

†Information communications technology

Table 16-2. Vulnerability Factors for Child Sex Trafficking

Individual Level	Relationship Level	Community Level	Societal Level
Homeless/runaway/ told to leave home	Intrafamilial violence	Adult sex work in area	Cultural beliefs and stigmas
History of abuse, neglect, or sexual exploitation	Poverty, unemployment	Transient male populations	Gender-based violence and discrimination
LGBTQ* status[1]	Limited maternal education	High crime rate (especially organized crime)	Weak recognition of child rights
Mental health, behavioral problems, or intellectual disabilities	Family dysfunction (substance misuse, criminality, mental health issues)	Tolerance of sexual exploitation	Political and social upheaval
Substance misuse	Parent involved in commercial sex work	Lack of community resources or support	Law enforcement or political corruption
Involvement with juvenile justice or child protection system	Forced migration	Gang activity	
Unaccompanied status	Peers involved in CSE†	Low community awareness of CSE†	
Lack of documentation (eg, immigration, birth certificate)	Intimate partner violence		

**Lesbian, gay, bisexual, transgender, queer*
†Child sexual exploitation
Data from Cimino AN, Madden EE, Hohn K, et al[2]; Cole J, Sprang G[5]; Goldberg AP, Moore JL, Kaplan DM, Barron CE[7]; Greenbaum VJ, Dodd M, McCracken C[12]; Murphy LT[13]; Macias Konstantopoulos W, Ahn R, Alper EJ, et al[14]; Fedina L, Williamson C, Perdue T[15]; Reid J[16]; Reid J[17]; Reid JA, Baglivio MT, Piquero AR, Greenwald MA, Epps N.[18]

Traffickers who recruit or manage victims may be male or female; adolescents or adults; and of the same or different racial group, ethnicity, or nationality as the victim.[6,8,19,20] They may be family members, intimate partners, acquaintances, or strangers.[5,6,20-23] In one study of trafficked adolescent girls, 29% were recruited by a relative, 28% by a stranger, 28% by an established boyfriend, 10% by a girlfriend, 3% by a drug dealer, and 2% by an employer.[6] Traffickers may use any of a variety of methods to recruit victims, including but not limited to false romance; false promises of jobs; promises of a better life; promises of free assistance that later requires some form of sexual payback,;economic manipulation and deceit (debt bondage); and abduction, force, or threats.[6,24] Characteristically, traffickers identify and then proceed to fill the victim's needs,[25] be they tangible (eg, material goods, drugs, assistance in a specific situation) or intangible (eg, love, a father figure, acceptance, a sense of family).[25] Traffickers may work alone, with 1 or a few partners, or within a larger network.[20] There may be varied levels of organization and sophistication in these networks, with the most well developed having many members and separate roles for members (eg, recruiter, manager, transporter, investor).[19]

Living conditions may vary considerably in the lives of trafficked victims. Children may be allowed to live at home or may live with their trafficker, on the streets, or elsewhere.[13,26] They may have considerable freedom to come and go, or they may be forbidden to leave the premises on their own or be closely monitored (eg, alarms on doors and windows, locks, mobile phone confiscated or number changed).[6,20,23,24] There may be intermittent or constant violence incurred at the hands of traffickers, buyers, or community members or among the trafficked persons themselves.[6,20,23,24,27-30] Children may be required to earn quotas each night (eg, minimum amounts of money, often ranging from hundreds to a few thousand dollars), with violence or deprivation delivered by the trafficker if the quota is not met.[31] Drugs and alcohol may be used, sometimes provided by the trafficker.[5,24,32]

Although conditions vary, uncertainty, unpredictability, and loss of control are ubiquitous, creating substantial and chronic stress for the child. Not surprisingly, levels of posttraumatic stress disorder (PTSD) and suicidality are very high.[32,33] In one study of exploited girls and boys, 78% were identified as having PTSD and 50% reported having attempted suicide in the past year.[8] In addition, victimized youth may experience acute inflicted injury, sexually transmitted infections (STIs), HIV/AIDS, unwanted pregnancy, complications of abortions, chronic pain conditions, exhaustion, and malnutrition.[7,12,14,20,28,29,32-34] Commercially sexually exploited girls in one study reported a history of STI (33% of cases), prior pregnancy (32%), and multisubstance use (58%). Forty-seven percent were diagnosed with an STI at the time of medical evaluation.[12]

Child Exploitation in Prostitution

Child exploitation in prostitution may involve a child engaging in sex acts to obtain the means of existence (survival sex), a child exchanging sex for nonessential material goods, or a child exchanging sex for money or another valued item that is destined for a third party (commonly referred to as a pimp or trafficker). Survival sex is a relatively common experience among homeless, runaway, and ***throwaway children*** (ie, children who are told to leave the home or told they cannot return).[13] Estimates of the prevalence of survival sex among this population vary according to the characteristics of study samples but generally range from 9% to 32%.[35-40] Risk factors for engaging in survival sex include, among others, older age; lesbian, gay, bisexual, transgender, or queer (LGBTQ) status; young age at time of first runaway episode; antisocial behavior; substance misuse (especially injection drug use); and a history of sexual abuse.[35-41]

Children and youth may become involved in commercial sex through a variety of means. They may be introduced to the practice by peers on the streets, relatives, or would-be clients,[22,42] or they may learn by observation of others.[41] In one study of LGBT youth and young adults in New York City, 46% reported being introduced into commercial sex by a peer or friend, 26% were approached by someone offering the exchange, and 4% were introduced by a family member.[42] Most youth engaging in commercial sexual exploitation while living on the streets do not report being controlled by a trafficker. In a study of street youth in New York City, only 16% of girls, 9% of boys, and 0% of transgender youth reported ever having been controlled by a third person.[22] However, many youths report working with peers as facilitators who assist in identifying buyers and help protect the youth and who may or may not accept money for their services. The relationship is reportedly nonexploitative and friendly, with youths perceiving it as a business partnership.[42] The true proportion of prostituted youth who are or have been controlled by a trafficker is uncertain, and the issue is clouded by the subjectivity of interpretation of *facilitator* versus *trafficker*. In a study of women involved in prostitution, 48% of those who had been initiated into commercial sexual exploitation as minors reported ever having a pimp.[2] This number is considerably greater than that reported by street youths.[22,42]

Extricating oneself from exploitation through prostitution may be quite difficult, whether it involves escaping a life of survival sex when homeless or being controlled by a third-party trafficker.[2,25,43] Economic hardships and lack of education and job skills, feelings of hopelessness, an overwhelming sense of stigma and social rejection, job discrimination (eg, against transgender youth), substance dependence, threats or violence from traffickers, failure to perceive one's exploitation, and reluctance to return to a dysfunctional home may all drive youths back into exploitation when removed or keep them embroiled in the exploitation for years.[6,20,22,25,26,41,42] In a study of Canadian boys and young men engaging in commercial sex, 69% reported that when they began they felt the exploitation would be a transient activity only, leading to something better. However, the mean duration of sex exploitation through prostitution was 9 years.[41]

Child Sexual Exploitation Materials (Formerly "Child Pornography")

Child pornography is a term used widely in international laws and treaties, although the exact definition varies. Because of concerns that *pornography* may somehow imply consent or legitimacy, there are efforts to replace this term with others, such as *child sexual exploitation materials* or *child sexual abuse materials*. ***Child sexual exploitation materials (CSEM)*** encompasses materials that depict CSA but also includes other types of materials that reveal child sexual exploitation, even if the materials lack specifically criminal content.[1] Materials can include photographs or videos, audio recordings, drawings, and written material.

Offenders may use CSEM for a variety of purposes, including the following[44,45]:

— Sexual arousal and gratification

— Desensitizing a child to sex and sexual activities during the grooming process

— Normalizing sexual behavior, including sex between an adult and a child

— Teaching a child various sex acts

— Blackmailing a child into silence or compliance with additional sex acts

— Obtaining a profit or access to CSEM belonging to others

— Advertising children for prostitution or other sex acts

The total numbers of CSEM offenders and of victims are unknown, although tip lines operating throughout the world document very high numbers of reports of suspected CSEM each year.[46] The Internet Watch Foundation (IWF)[47] accepts tips from the public and professionals through its Web site and 16 portals around the world, as well as proactively searching for CSEM and removing it from the Internet. In 2016, the IWF identified 57335 URLs that contained CSEM, had links to it, or advertised it. These URLs were traced to 50 countries. The 5 most common countries identified were, in descending order, (1) the Netherlands; (2) the United States, (3) Canada, (4) France, and (5) Russia. These accounted for 92% of all the CSEM URLs identified. The year 2016 marked a significant shift in offender geographic distribution as the most often documented location changed from the United States to Europe.[47] CSEM was found most commonly on image hosting sites (41364) and much less often on Web sites (914) or social networking sites (634).

In contrast to studies of online grooming, in which the vast majority of victims are aged 13 to 17 years old,[48,49] evidence from tip lines suggests that CSEM may be more likely to include young children, as well as adolescents. The IWF documented that in 2016, 53% of sexual exploitation URLs depicted children aged 10 years or younger and 2% of URLs showed children aged 2 years or younger. The remaining 45% involved children estimated to be between 11 and 15 years of age (technique for estimating age not described). Similar results were found in an analysis by the Canadian CyberTipline of 46859 child victims: 49.6% were deemed to be younger than age 8 years (using Sexual Maturity Rating criteria[50]), 28.7% were age 8 to 11 years, and 21.7% were estimated to be age 12 to 18 years.[46]

Child victims of CSEM may be of any gender, but one Canadian study found they were much more likely to be girls than boys (30.4% versus 19.6% respectively; no transgender youth documented).[46] In this same study, 87% of children appeared to be Caucasian, with only 7.7% appearing East Asian or Southeast Asian and 5.2% appearing to be of other ethnicity. However, it must be remembered that this involves data from a Canadian tip line, so results may not be generalizable to global populations of CSEM victims.

Child sexual exploitation images vary in severity of depicted abuse. Analysis of more than 43000 images and videos identified 31.8% of severity level 1 (sexual posing), 18.2% severity level 2 (extreme sexual posing), 47.8% severity level 3 (explicit sexual activity or assaults), and 2.2% severity level 4 (extreme sexual assaults).[46] The highest proportion of materials that were rated level 3 or 4 within an age group were found among toddlers (59.7% of group), with the lowest occurring in older children (43.9% in children aged 12 to 17 years). Boys were more likely to have high levels of severity than girls (59.4% versus 50.9%), although the highest proportion of severe material depicted both genders (75.3%). Sexual acts recorded varied considerably, including adults committing a sexual assault on a child (53.6% of the 12600 individuals recorded engaging in sex acts), children engaging in sex acts alone (26.1%), multiple children engaged in sex acts (19.8%), and children engaged in sex acts with animals (0.4%).

There is no strict profile of CSEM offenders,[45] although studies do indicate a propensity for offenders to be Caucasian, young to middle aged (25 to 50 years), employed, and often with some level of higher education.[51-53] Many have access to children, either through living arrangements or work.[53] There is heterogeneity in the degree and type of psychopathology (eg, depression, obsessive-compulsive disorder [OCD]), presence and degree of low self-esteem or loneliness, levels of antisocial characteristics (eg, low moral choice internal values, psychopathic deviation), and interpersonal problems such as low assertiveness and decreased empathy.[45,54] Some CSEM offenders also engage in contact child sexual offenses,[44,45,55] and there is evidence suggesting that crossover behavior from CSEM to contact offenses may be associated with low victim empathy, increased cognitive distortions, and prior criminal convictions,[53,56] as well as living with a partner and children[53] and having a history of childhood difficulties.[56]

Houtepen[45] discusses particular types of CSEM offenders, including the "periodically prurient" and the "fantasy-driven" offenders. The former includes those who have a more general interest in pornography but who obtain child sexual exploitation material impulsively or out of curiosity. The fantasy-driven offenders are thought to be motivated by a sexual interest in children or youth. Within each group there is diversity in levels of psychopathology and interpersonal issues, although it is thought that risk factors for periodically prurient offenders tend to be associated with features of criminal behavior (impulsivity, lack of self-control, engaging in cognitive distortions), whereas those in the fantasy group have risk factors more associated with sexual deviance or fantasy (problems with intimacy and loneliness).

Solicitation of a Child for Sexual Purposes ("Grooming")

Those wishing to engage a child in sexual activity typically need to overcome external inhibitors in the environment as well as the child's inhibitions and resistance.[57] Such preparations of victims and their environments may occur online or offline. Increasing attention is being paid to online sexual solicitation, although research is still limited. This section focuses on Internet-related sexual solicitation of children; offline grooming is well described elsewhere.[58]

Online sex offenders may identify and make contact with victims using a number of strategies, including participating in chatroom conversations (creating their own profile to attract the type of child they prefer or lurking in the chatroom and then introducing themselves to a specific child of interest), reviewing online child profiles and bulletin board postings, searching social networking sites, and participating in online gaming activities.[59-61] In a study of convicted offenders who had used the Internet to meet and groom child victims in preparation for contact sex offenses, 81% reported using chatrooms as a venue for meeting minors, whereas 48% viewed online profiles posted by children.[59]

Youths who are subjected to online sexual solicitation may have a number of risk factors. In a study of sex offenders arrested for Internet-related crimes in which they engaged in online sexual communications with minors, 90% of the victims were between 13 and 17 years of age and 90% were female.[49] The vast majority of victims had no history of status offenses (85%) or problems with substance misuse (87%). Factors associated with increased risk of online solicitation may include trigger events that introduce vulnerability or compromise resilience, such as parental conflict, family illness, bullying, or some other event leading to "a low point in life."[62] Offline sexual or physical abuse increases the risk of online victimization,[63,64] as do certain online behaviors, such as sharing personal information with people met online, talking about sex online, making hostile comments to others online, and frequently embarrassing people online.[63] Additionally, there is evidence that multiple risky online behaviors have a cumulative effect on risk. In one study of Internet users aged 10 to 17 years, those who engaged in at least 4 high-risk online behaviors were 11 times more likely to report online interpersonal victimization than those reporting no risky behaviors.[63] In another study, online sex offenders reported being attracted to children and youth who mentioned sex online (eg, in their screen name), those who appeared "needy" in their online communication, and those whose age was readily identifiable.[59]

Contrary to popular stereotype, those attempting to sexually exploit youths online typically do not deceive their victims about their age or their motivation to have sex with youths. In one study, only 5% of offenders pretended to be younger than 18 years old, and although 21% misrepresented their motives, these deceptions typically involved false claims of love and romance, rather than deceptions about their desire to engage in a sexual relationship.[65] Additionally, among the 74% of cases involving face-to-face contact between victim and offender, a sexual offense was committed in 93% and these encounters only rarely involved violence or threats of such (5%) or coercion (ie, victim being pressured to perform sexual acts) (16%). Abduction was also rare (3%).

Online sex offenders may or may not be interested in engaging a youth in offline sexual activity. In some cases their motives for engagement may be related to sexual gratification through the online communication itself.[66] Briggs[66] identified 2 groups of Internet-initiated sexual offenders: contact-driven and fantasy-driven perpetrators. Although there were significant commonalities in behaviors between the 2 groups—100% in each group engaged in sexually explicit conversations with the victims, and most offenders in each group sent victims nude photographs of themselves—there were clear differences in others (**Table 16-3**). An analysis of offender characteristics found high rates of mental health disorders in both groups (73.3% contact-driven, 76.2% fantasy-driven with an Axis I diagnosis), especially depressive disorder (33.3% of each group). None were diagnosed with pedophilia or hebephilia. The vast majority of each group were employed, had at least a high school degree or general equivalency degree (GED), and were without prior sex offense convictions. Most were white, non-Hispanic (70% contact, 90.5% fantasy).

Table 16-3. Chat Room Behaviors of Contact-Driven Versus Fantasy-Driven Online Sex Offenders

Online Activity	Contact-Driven Offenders (%)	Fantasy-Driven Offenders (%)
Offender masturbated during conversation with victim	16.7	76.2
Engaged victim in cybersex	6.7	81.0
Tried to teach victim sexual behaviors	13.3	66.7
Scheduled face-to-face meeting	93.3	14.3
Engaged in exhibitionism on Web cam	6.7	66.7

Data from Briggs et al.[66]

Multiple models have been proposed to describe the grooming process.[60,67,68] O'Connell[60] describes 6 stages of "cybersexploitation" but emphasizes that offenders may skip stages, repeat stages, or change the order of stages. Variations depend to some extent on the motivation of the offender (offline contact or online sexual gratification). The stages are described in **Table 16-4**.

Table 16-4. Stages of Cybersexploitation

Stage of Cybersexploitation	Activities Involved
Friendship-forming stage	Makes initial contact; initiates nonsexual relationship; may ask for nonsexual photograph
Relationship-forming stage	Expansion of friendship-forming stage; asks questions about child's life; establishes self as friend or confidant of child
Risk assessment stage	Asks questions about environmental circumstances under which child is communicating (assess risk of detection)
Exclusivity stage	Establishes close relationship with victim; may bring up idea of trust
Sexual stage	Sexual topics or activities introduced using a variety of methods of psychological manipulation; this stage may be very emotionally intense for child; activities vary depending on motivation of offender and desire to have or not have lasting relationship
Conclusion stage	"Hit and run" (abrupt cessation of relationship) or more gradual withdrawal with efforts to ensure secrecy of relationship

Data from O'Connell R.[60]

There may be a great deal of variation in manipulation strategies used by the offender in the sexual stage, ranging from gentle suggestions for sexual activity, to explicit requests, to threats. The offender may couch the sexual activities in the guise of a mentor-pupil relationship or place them in the context of expressing love and trust.[60] Offenders may use strategies such as praise, reverse psychology, role reversal, and strategic withdrawal to manipulate the victims.[68]

Online solicitation (grooming) may overlap with other forms of exploitation, such as producing and exchanging CSEM (eg, offender sending nude photographs of himself and asking the victim to do the same), "sextortion" (sexual exploitation that "occurs primarily online and in which non-physical forms of coercion are utilized, such as blackmail, to acquire sexual content [photos/videos] of the child, obtain money from the child or engage in sex with the child"),[69] or engaging in live online sexual exploitation (eg, instructing the child to perform a sexual activity for the offender, using a Web cam).

Exploitation in Context of Travel or Tourism (Formerly "Sex Tourism")

Travel and tourism are major factors in the global economy. In 2016, they accounted for 10.2% of the global gross domestic product and involved 292 million jobs.[70] Although they bring economic prosperity and employment to some areas, they also bring adverse consequences, including child sexual exploitation in the context of travel and tourism (SECTT). This may encompass several types of exploitation, including prostitution, online grooming, live-streaming, and production of CSA materials.[71,72] Formerly referred to as sex tourism, the definition has been expanded to include the many other contexts in which travelers may sexually exploit children (**Table 16-5**). SECTT occurs all over the world, in large cities and remote regions, largely with the aid of information communications technology.[71,73] Although much public attention has been given to Western men traveling to Southeast Asia and other regions for the purpose of having sex with children, evidence indicates that offenders are more likely to originate from the same country as the child victim or from a country within the same region.[71,73] Most identified SECTT offenders are men, but women and child perpetrators have been described.[71] Evidence suggests most offenders are not pedophiles or other preferential offenders but may be more likely to be situational offenders[71]; that is, they do not travel with the goal of sexually exploiting a child and do not have specific sexual inclinations toward children but instead may react to the environment and the available opportunities to exploit children and youths. Such an opportunity may present itself in an environment in which children have few rights, poverty is widespread, commercial sexual exploitation is normalized (eg, business meetings that include alcohol and sexual entertainment), tourists are treated with special privileges (eg, in countries with a heavy dependence on the tourist industry), or the risk of adverse consequences is viewed as minimal (eg, in settings of widespread law enforcement corruption or where there are ambiguous or unenforced laws).[71,74] If the local culture is viewed as different or somehow inferior, traveling offenders may be able to use cognitive distortions to justify their behavior and overcome internal inhibitions ("It's normal for these people to sell their kids for sex."; "If it weren't for me, this child would go hungry.").[71,75] Additionally, cultural attitudes and beliefs that support gender bias and violence, the view that masculinity is associated with sexual prowess, the belief that boys cannot be victims of sexual violence, and the view that children must economically support the family set the stage for child sexual exploitation and may help SECTT offenders feel justified in their actions.

Table 16-5. Potential Settings for Child Sexual Exploitation in the Context of Travel and Tourism

Tourism
— Vacation travel by domestic or foreign tourists
— Organized sex tours
— Volun-tourism (eg, at orphanages, children's homes)
— Special zones (eg, casinos, resorts, and other businesses built to attract tourists and business travelers)
— Peer-to-peer accommodation services (eg, Airbnb, home stays)
Other Travel
— Business travel (eg, short-term or relocation for extended period)
— Industry in remote areas (eg, mining, oil industry)
— Military service
— Crisis relief work, peacekeeping missions

Data from Hawke A, Raphael A.[71]

Factors that render children vulnerable to SECTT include those that increase the risk of sex trafficking (see earlier), as well as a variety of environmental factors such as living in a tourist destination or near a special zone that has been created to attract business travelers and tourists.[71] Children living near areas where large groups of men are employed (eg, mines) are at risk, as are children living near military bases. Those children exposed to "volun-tourists" (tourists whose travel involves some sort of volunteer work) or living near places advertised as home-stays or other temporary housing situations potentially are at risk as well.

Information communication technology has increased access to victims by SECTT offenders because victims may be advertised online, groomed online, and made to give live sexual performances online.[73] Child sexual abuse materials may be created and distributed online, prompting a SECTT offender to seek face-to-face contact with the victim. An American man may use the Internet to locate and request online sexual performances of a 9-year-old boy in the Philippines, to maintain contact with the victim over time, and to arrange to have sex in a hotel in Manila when he arrives for his vacation. Additionally, online chatrooms for offenders provide the means of exchanging advice on SECTT activities, sharing information regarding ideal places to find certain types of children, and providing encouragement and support among offenders.[75] The rapid globalization of the economy, tremendous growth of tourism, and very rapid increase in Internet availability around the world all increase the risks for SECTT.[71,73]

Live Sexual Performances (Online Child Sexual Exploitation or Live Performances in Sexually Oriented Businesses)

Live online performance of sex acts involving Web cam streaming or other technology may be considered a form of sexual exploitation in the context of travel and tourism,[72,74] and on-site sexual performances fall under this category in some cases, depending on the clientele at the business (ie, tourist or traveler). The rapid rise in Internet use has laid a foundation for online sexual exploitation as many more vulnerable children and families are accessible to offenders using computers in faraway places.[76] Much of the existing information about live online sexual exploitation comes from the Philippines,[73] although it is highly doubtful that this practice is not also present in many other countries. The percentage of individuals using the Internet in the Philippines rose from slightly less than 6% in 2007 to nearly 40% in 2014.[77] The prevalence of online sexual exploitation via Web cam streaming is unknown, although numbers are likely quite high. A study by Terre des Hommes Netherlands involving Dutch researchers posing as prepubertal Filipino girls in 19 public chat rooms yielded more than 20 000 people from 71 countries who endeavored to purchase a Web cam sex show within a period of 10 weeks.[74]

Victims of online sexual abuse may be male or female, may be transgender, and tend to be aged 10 to 18 years.[76] They may live in isolated rural areas or urban centers, with families, or on the streets. Poverty is a common driving factor.[74,76] Children may be involved as individuals (often hoping to meet a foreign "boyfriend" who will marry them or give money and gifts[76]) and may use computers at home or in Internet cafes; they may be exploited by family members, typically at home; or they may be exploited by "den" owners who exploit or traffic multiple children.[74] These owners may belong to criminal organizations of varying sophistication; they may be Filipino or foreign nationals. Buyers of live-streaming child sexual exploitation may locate child victims in chat rooms, social networking sites, dating sites, or adult Web cam sites.[74] Sex acts performed range from nude posing to sexual intercourse, group sexual acts, and other activities, at the direction of the buyer. Shows commonly last 15 to 30 minutes and are customized to the buyer's desires. If the victim or operator (ie, the person accompanying child) does not understand the buyer's language, he or she may use Google Translate.

Sexual exploitation of children may also involve engaging a child in the performance of sexual acts in dance clubs, gentlemen's clubs, strip clubs, and other sexually oriented venues.[78] Sexual dancing in public may be used as part of the initiation process before a trafficker begins prostituting the child, as a way to normalize sexual acts with strangers and decrease inhibitions. Additionally, sex clubs and other venues may serve as recruitment sites for sex traffickers to identify new victims. To date, there is little formal scientific research on this specific form of sexual exploitation.

Adverse Effects of Child Sexual Exploitation

The myriad adverse effects associated with sex trafficking and exploitation through prostitution are enumerated earlier in this chapter. When there is an online component of child sexual exploitation, victims may face additional consequences. Sexual material that has been disseminated online can never be completely removed, and the victim is exploited indefinitely and repeatedly each time someone views the material. Exploiters may number in the millions and be located worldwide. Victims may worry that sexual material will surface far in the future, damaging chances for university admission or job applications, harming future relationships, and causing public humiliation. They may worry about being subjected to blackmail by someone who obtains the materials or being stalked by someone who decides to try to meet them. Few studies have examined the prevalence and degree of psychosocial adversity associated with the online component of sexual exploitation. Information from studies in the Philippines regarding the effects of live online sexual exploitation (Web cam streaming) suggests that it is associated with shame and dishonor, as well as depression, powerlessness, and stigma.[76] Children expressed fear of sexual images being spread on the Internet and fear of being arrested for illegal activity. They scored significantly higher than control participants on scales measuring symptoms of PTSD, low self-esteem, sexualized behavior, and self-destructive behavior.

Prevention of Child Sexual Exploitation

Following a social-ecological model, health care providers may address primary prevention of child sexual exploitation at the individual, relationship, community, and societal levels.[11]

Given the ubiquitous nature of the Internet and the numerous ways sex offenders can victimize children online, educating children and youth, as well as their parents, about Internet safety may be very helpful. As discussed earlier, increased risky online behaviors in which a youth engages are associated with increased risk of online sexual victimization[63]; therefore, education about safe and unsafe Internet behavior is indicated (especially *patterns* of high-risk online behavior). Speak with adolescents about the legal consequences of distributing and receiving sexual images, about the possibility of their sexual images being posted on the Internet, and about the nature of adult-child sexual relationships initiated online (eg, frequency of false romance as a method of luring victims, strategies of psychological manipulation practiced, frequent abrupt end to relationships, multiple youths often being targeted by a single offender).[48]

Health care professionals may also educate children and youth about the risks of child sex trafficking, including common recruitment methods used by traffickers and situations that pose an increased risk for exploitation. General anticipatory guidance on healthy relationships may help change attitudes about sexual objectification of girls and decrease gender bias while facilitating respect for others. Such guidance targets potential victims and potential offenders.

Counseling on self-protection is important for children and youth. However, health professionals may also educate them to be aware of risky behaviors in others and to take steps to report concerns they might have over the behavior of friends or acquaintances.[48] Although education of parents certainly has a role, many youth who are particularly vulnerable to online exploitation may not be in a position to listen to advice from parents and may benefit more from hearing the same information from others, including peers. Finally, although girls make up the majority of victims of online sexual exploitation, boys and transgender youth may be affected as well, so any prevention messages should be addressed to all groups.[64]

High-risk youths may be able to avoid CSE if provided with critical resources that address their vulnerabilities. The health professional may provide resources such as information about homeless shelters, LGBTQ support organizations, drug rehabilitation programs, food banks, and free or low-cost mental health services. Providers with a well-rounded knowledge of their community resources are in a good position to help.

Moving beyond education of patients and families, health care professionals may help reduce CSE by increasing awareness among the health community and the general public. They may assist in creating specific protocols for their health facility, so that all practitioners are aware of common risk factors and possible indicators of CSE; know how to work with potential victims in a trauma-informed, victim-centered way; and are able to make appropriate referrals for assistance. Finally, health care professionals can support community and national programs and policies that address vulnerability factors for CSE, as well as health and social needs of victims. They can advocate for child rights, gender equality, and violence prevention.

Conclusion

Child sexual exploitation encompasses a variety of behaviors that manipulate the vulnerability of youth for the gain of others. A victim may be exploited in multiple ways, including prostitution, production of sexual exploitation materials, online solicitation, and live or online sexual performances. They may be exploited by strangers or those very close to them. There is no stereotype of a CSE victim although certain risk factors are consistently identified. These factors occur at the individual, relationship, community, and societal levels. CSE may be associated with a spectrum of physical and mental health consequences ranging from physical injury to STIs and substance misuse, from PTSD to major depression and suicidality. Health professionals have a role in preventing CSE and identifying victims so that assistance may be offered and long-term adverse consequences minimized.

References

1. Interagency Working Group on Sexual Exploitation of Children. *Terminology Guidelines for the Protection of Children from Sexual Exploitation and Abuse.* Luxembourg City, Luxembourg: ECPAT International; 2016.
2. Cimino AN, Madden EE, Hohn K, et al. Childhood maltreatment and child protective services involvement among the commercially exploited: a comparison of women who enter as juveniles or as adults. *J Child Sex Abus.* 2017;26(3):352-371.
3. Trafficking Victims Protection Act of 2000, Pub L No. 106-386, 114 Stat 1464.
4. Justice for Victims of Trafficking Act of 2015, Pub L No. 114-22, 129 Stat 227.
5. Cole J, Sprang G. Sex trafficking of minors in metropolitan, micropolitan, and rural communities. *Child Abuse Negl.* 2015;40:113-123.
6. Reid JA. Entrapment and enmeshment schemes used by sex traffickers. *Sex Abuse.* 2016;28(6):491-511.
7. Goldberg AP, Moore JL, Houck C, Kaplan DM, Barron CE. Domestic minor sex trafficking patients: a retrospective analysis of medical presentation. *J Pediatr Adolesc Gynecol.* 2017;30(1):109-115.
8. Edinburgh L, Pape-Blabolil J, Harpin SB, Saewyc E. Assessing exploitation experiences of girls and boys seen at a child advocacy center. *Child Abuse Negl.* 2015;46:47-59.
9. Smith AR, Steinberg L, Chein J. The role of the anterior insula in adolescent decision making. *Dev Neurosci.* 2014;36(3-4):196-209.
10. Steinberg L. A dual systems model of adolescent risk-taking. *Dev Psychobiol.* 2010;52(3):216-224.
11. Centers for Disease Control and Prevention. The social-ecological model: a framework for prevention. Centers for Disease Control and Prevention Web site. https://www.cdc.gov/violenceprevention/overview/social-ecologicalmodel.html. Accessed June 28, 2018.
12. Greenbaum VJ, Dodd M, McCracken C. A short screening tool to identify victims of child sex trafficking in the health care setting. *Pediatr Emerg Care.* 2018;34(1):33-37.
13. Murphy LT. Labor and sex trafficking among homeless youth: a ten-city study executive summary. Covenant House Web site. https://www.covenanthouse.org/sites/default/files/inline-files/Loyola%20Multi-City%20Executive%20Summary%20FINAL.pdf. Accessed January 3, 2019.
14. Macias Konstantopoulos W, Ahn R, Alper EJ, et al. An international comparative public health analysis of sex trafficking of women and girls in eight cities: achieving a more effective health sector response. *J Urban Health.* 2013;90(6):1194-1204.

15. Fedina L, Williamson C, Perdue T. Risk factors for domestic child sex trafficking in the United States [published online ahead of print July 1, 2016]. *J Interpers Violence*. doi:10.1177088626051666230б.

16. Reid JA. An exploratory model of girls' vulnerability to commercial sexual exploitation in prostitution. *Child Maltreat*. 2011;16(2):146-157.

17. Reid JA. Exploratory review of route-specific, gendered, and age-graded dynamics of exploitation: applying life course theory to victimization in sex trafficking in North America. *Aggress Violent Behav*. 2012;17(3):257-271.

18. Reid JA, Baglivio MT, Piquero AR, Greenwald MA, Epps N. Human trafficking of minors and childhood adversity in Florida. *Am J Public Health*. 2017;107(2):306-311.

19. United Nations Office on Drugs and Crime. Global report on trafficking in persons: 2014. United Nations Office on Drugs and Crime Web site. http://www.unodc.org/res/cld/bibliography/global-report-on-trafficking-in-persons_html/GLOTIP_2014_full_report.pdf. Accessed January 3, 2019.

20. Raymond JG, Hughes DM. Sex trafficking of women in the United States: international and domestic trends. National Criminal Justice Reference Service Web site. https://www.ncjrs.gov/pdffiles1/nij/grants/187774.pdf. Published April 17, 2001. Accessed January 3, 2019.

21. Anderson PM, Coyle KK, Johnson A, Denner J. An exploratory study of adolescent pimping relationships. *J Prim Prev*. 2014;35(2):113-117.

22. Curtis R, Terry K, Dank M, Dombrowski K, Khan B. Commercial sexual exploitation of children in New York City: volume one: the CSEC population in New York City: size, characteristics, and needs. National Criminal Justice Reference Service Web site. https://www.ncjrs.gov/pdffiles1/nij/grants/225083.pdf. Published December 2008. Accessed January 3, 2019.

23. Raphael J, Reichert J, Powers M. Pimp control and violence: domestic sex trafficking of Chicago women and girls. *Women Crim Justice*. 2010;20(1):89-104.

24. Polaris. More than drinks for sale: exposing sex trafficking in cantinas and bars in the US. Polaris Project Web site. https://polarisproject.org/sites/default/files/Cantinas-SexTrafficking-EN.pdf. Accessed January 3, 2019.

25. Smith L, Vardaman S, Snow M. *The National Report on Domestic Minor Sex Trafficking: America's Prostituted Children*. Arlington, VA: Shared Hope International; 2009. Shared Hope International Web site. http://sharedhope.org/wp-content/uploads/2012/09/SHI_National_Report_on_DMST_2009.pdf. Accessed June 28, 2018.

26. Greenbaum VJ. Commercial sexual exploitation and sex trafficking of children in the United States. *Curr Probl Pediatr Adolesc Health Care*. 2014;44(9):245-269.

27. Shannon K, Kerr T, Strathdee SA, Shoveller J, Montaner JS, Tyndall MW. Prevalence and structural correlates of gender based violence among a prospective cohort of female sex workers. *BMJ*. 2009;339;b2939.

28. Ottisova L, Hemmings S, Howard LM, Zimmerman C, Oram S. Prevalence and risk of violence and the mental, physical and sexual health problems associated wtih human trafficking: an updated systematic review. *Epidemiol Psychiatr Sci*. 2016;25(4):317-341.

29. Oram S, Stöckl H, Busza J, Howard LM, Zimmerman C. Prevalence and risk of violence and the physical, mental, and sexual health problems associated with human trafficking: systematic review. *PLoS Med.* 2012;9(5):e1001224.

30. Nixon K, Tutty L, Downe P, Gorkoff K, Ursel J. The everyday occurrence: violence in the lives of girls exploited through prostitution. *Violence Against Women.* 2002;8(9):1016-1043.

31. Williamson C, Prior M. Domestic minor sex trafficking: a network of underground players in the midwest. *J Child Adolesc Trauma.* 2009;2(1):46-61.

32. Heilemann T, Santhiveeran J. How do female adolescents cope and survive the hardships of prostitution? A content analysis of existing literature. *J Ethn Cult Divers Soc Work.* 2011;20(1):57-76.

33. Willis BM, Levy BS. Child prostitution: global health burden, research needs, and interventions. *Lancet.* 2002;359(9315):1417-1422.

34. Lederer L, Wetzel C. The health consequences of sex trafficking and their implications for identifying victims in healthcare facilities. *Ann Health Law.* 2014;23:61-91.

35. Stoltz JA, Shannon K, Kerr T, Zhang R, Montaner JS, Wood E. Associations between childhood maltreatment and sex work in a cohort of drug-using youth. *Soc Sci Med.* 2007;65(6):1214-1221.

36. Walls N, Bell S. Correlates of engaging in survival sex among homeless youth and young adults. *J Sex Res.* 2011;48(5):423-436.

37. Whitbeck LB, Chen X, Hoyt DR, Tyler KA, Johnson KD. Mental disorder, subsistence strategies, and victimization among gay, lesbian, and bisexual homeless and runaway adolescents. *J Sex Res.* 2004;41(4):329-342.

38. Kerr T, Marshall BDL, Miller C, et al. Injection drug use among street-involved youth in a Canadian setting. *BMC Public Health.* 2009;9:171-177.

39. Greene JM, Ennett ST, Ringwalt CL. Prevalence and correlates of survival sex among runaway and homeless youth. *Am J Public Health.* 1999;89(9):1406-1409.

40. Chettiar J, Shannon K, Wood E, Zhang R, Kerr T. Survival sex work involvement among street-involved youth who use drugs in a Canadian setting. *J Public Health (Oxf).* 2010;32(3):322-327.

41. McIntyre S. Under the radar: the sexual exploitation of young men—Western Canadian edition. Alberta Human Services Web site. http://www.humanservices.alberta.ca/documents/child-sexual-exploitation-under-the-radar-western-canada.pdf. Accessed January 3, 2019.

42. Dank M, Yahner J, Madden K, et al. *Surviving the Streets of New York: Experiences of LGBTQ youth, YMSM, YWSW Engaged in Survival Sex.* New York, NY: Urban Institute; 2015.

43. Ashley J. Prostitution study finds Chicago girls trafficked through coercion, violence. *Illinois Criminal Justice Information Authority.* 2008;7(1):1-4.

44. Shelton J, Eakin J, Hoffer T, Muirhead Y, Owens J. Online child sexual exploitation: An investigative analysis of offender characteristics and offending behavior. *Aggress Violent Behav.* 2016;30:15-23.

45. Houtepen JABM, Sijtsema JJ, Bogaerts S. From child pornography offending to child sexual abuse: a review of child pornography offender characteristics and risks for cross-over. *Aggress Violent Behav.* 2014;19(5):466-473.

46. Canadian Centre for Child Protection. Child sexual abuse images on the Internet: a Cybertip.ca analysis. Cybertip.ca Web site. https://cybertip.ca/pdfs/CTIP_CSAResearchReport_Summary_2016_en.pdf. Accessed June 28, 2018.

47. Internet Watch Foundation. IWF annual report 2016. Internet Watch Foundation Web site. https://www.iwf.org.uk/sites/default/files/reports/2017-04/iwf_report_2016.pdf. Accessed June 28, 2018.

48. Wolak J, Finkelhor D, Mitchell KJ, Ybarra ML. Online "predators" and their victims: myths, realities, and implications for prevention and treatment. *Am Psychol.* 2008;63(2):111-128.

49. Wolak J, Finkelhor D. Are crimes by online predators different from crimes by sex offenders who know youth in-person? *J Adolesc Health.* 2013;53(6):736-741.

50. Tanner JM. *Growth at Adolescence.* 2nd ed. Oxford, UK: Blackwell Scientific Publications; 1962.

51. Burke A, Sowerbutts S, Blundell B, Sherry M. Child pornography and the internet: policing and treatment issues. *Psychiatry Psychol Law.* 2002;9(1):79-84.

52. Seto MC, Wood JM, Babchishin KM, Flynn S. Online solicitation offenders are different from child pornography offenders and lower risk contact sexual offenders. *Law Hum Behav.* 2012;36(4):320-330.

53. McManus MA, Long ML, Alison L, Almond L. Factors associated wtih contact child sexual abuse in a sample of indecent image offenders. *J Sex Aggress.* 2015;21(3):368-384.

54. Henry O, Mandeville-Norden R, Hayes E, Egan V. Do Internet-based sexual offenders reduce to normal, inadequate and deviant groups? *J Sex Aggress.* 2010;16(1):33-46.

55. Bourke ML, Hernandez AE. The "Butner Study" redux: a report of the incidence of hands-on child victimization by child pornography offenders. *J Fam Violence.* 2009;24:183-191.

56. Babchishin KM, Hanson RK, VanZuylen H. Online child pornography offenders are different: a meta-analysis of the characteristics of online and offline sex offenders against children. *Arch Sex Behav.* 2015;44(1):45-66.

57. Finkelhor D. *Child Sexual Abuse: New Theory and Research.* New York, NY: Free Press; 1984.

58. Galbreath NW. *Child Molesters.* Saint Louis, MO: Elsevier; 2011.

59. Malesky LA. Predatory online behavior: modus operandi of convicted sex offenders in identifying potential victims and contacting minors over the internet. *J Child Sex Abuse.* 2007;16(2):23-32.

60. O'Connell R. A typology of child cybersexploitation and online grooming practices. Guardian Web site. http://image.guardian.co.uk/sys-files/Society/documents/2003/07/24/Netpaedoreport.pdf. Accessed June 28, 2018.

61. Mitchell K, Finkelhor D, Jones LM, Wolak J. Use of social networking sites in online sex crimes against minors: an examination of national incidence and means of utiliization. *J Adolesc Health.* 2010;47(2):183-190.

62. Whittle HC, Hamilton-Giachritsis CE, Beech AR. In their own words: young peoples' vulnerabilities to being groomed and sexually abused online. *Psychology.* 2014;5(10):1185-1196.

63. Ybarra ML, Mitchell KJ, Finkelhor D, Wolak J. Internet prevention messages: targeting the right online behaviors. *Arch Pediatr Adolesc Med.* 2007;161(2):138-145.

64. Mitchell KJ, Finkelhor D, Wolak J. Youth Internet users at risk for the most serious online sexual solicitations. *Am J Prev Med.* 2007;32(6):532-537.

65. Wolak J, Finkelhor D, Mitchell K. Internet-initiated sex crimes against minors: impliications for prevention based on findings from a national study. *J Adolesc Health.* 2004;35(5):424.e11-20.

66. Briggs P, Simon WT, Simonsen S. An exploratory study of Internet-initiated sexual offenses and the chat room sex offender: has the internet enabled a new typology of sex offender? *Sex Abuse.* 2011;23(1):72-91.

67. Williams R, Elliott IA, Beech AR. Identifying sexual grooming themes used by internet sex offenders. *Deviant Behav.* 2013;34(2):135-152.

68. Lorenzo-Dus N, Izura C, Pérez-Tattam R. Understanding grooming discourse in computer-mediated environments. *Discourse Context Media.* 2016;12:40-50.

69. National Center for Missing and Exploited Children. Trends identified in cybertipline sextortion reports. National Center for Missing and Exploited Children Web site. http://www.missingkids.com/content/dam/pdfs/ncmec-analysis/sextortionfactsheet.pdf. Accessed January 3, 2019.

70. World Travel and Tourism Council. Travel & tourism economic impact 2016. World Travel and Tourism Council Web site. https://www.wttc.org/-/media/files/reports/economic%20impact%20research/regions%202016/world2016.pdf. Accessed January 3, 2019.

71. Hawke A, Raphael A. *Offenders on the Move: Global Study on Sexual Exploitation of Children in Travel and Tourism 2016.* Bangkok, Thailand: ECPAT International; 2016.

72. National Rapporteur on Trafficking in Human Beings and Sexual Violence Against Children. Barriers against child sex tourism: summary report. National Rapporteur on Trafficking in Human Beings and Sexual Violence Against Children Web site. https://www.nationaalrapporteur.nl/binaries/dutch-rapporteur-on-trafficking-in-human-beings-and-sexual-violence-against-children.barriers-against-child-sex-tourism.a-summary-tcm64-537281_tcm23-34744.pdf. Accessed January 3, 2019.

73. End Child Prostitution and Trafficking. The use of information and communication technologies in connection with cases of child-sex tourism in East and Southeast Asia. End Child Prostitution and Trafficking Web site. http://www.ecpat.org/wp-content/uploads/legacy/ecpat_journal_mar2010_final_0.pdf. Accessed January 3, 2019.

74. Terre des Hommes. Webcam child sex tourism: becoming sweetie: a novel approach to stopping the global rise of webcam child sex tourism. Save the Children's Resource Center Web site. https://resourcecentre.savethechildren.net/node/8164/pdf/webcam-child-sex-tourism-terre-des-hommes-nl-nov-2013.pdf. Accessed January 3, 2019.

75. Malarek V. *The Johns: Sex for Sale and the Men Who Buy It.* New York, NY: Arcade Publishing; 2009.

76. Terre des Hommes. Fullscreen on view: an exploratory study on the background and psychosocial consequences of webcam child sex tourism in the Philippines. Terre des Hommes Web site. https://www.terredeshommes.nl/sites/tdh/files/uploads/research_report_2.pdf. Published November 4, 2013. Accessed January 3, 2019.

77. UN Data. Percentage of individuals using the Internet. UN Data Web site. http://data.un.org/Data.aspx?q=philippines+internet&d=ITU&f=ind1Code%3aI99H%3bcountryCode%3aPHL#f_3. Accessed June 28, 2018.

78. Office for Victims of Crime. What is human trafficking? Office for Victims of Crime Web site. https://ovc.ncjrs.gov/humantrafficking/about.html. Accessed June 28, 2018.

Chapter 17

Child Sexual Abuse of Children With Disabilities*

Nora J. Baladerian, PhD
Angela M. Kaufman, MA, CI/CT
Roberta A. Hibbard, MD
Sharon Cooper, MD

Introduction

Sexual abuse can affect any child from any family, regardless of age, gender, ethnicity, disability, or socioeconomic status. Both typically developing children and children with disabilities may be victims of sexual abuse. Service providers should be familiar with their affirmative obligations under the Americans with Disabilities Act (ADA),[1] which prohibits discrimination against individuals with disabilities in publically provided programs, services, and activities; Section 504 of the Rehabilitation Act of 1973,[2] which prohibits discrimination against individuals with disabilities on the basis of their disability in programs, services, or activities that receive federal financial assistance; and Section 1557 of the Patient Protection and Affordable Care Act,[3] which extends nondiscrimination protections to individuals participating in (1) any health program that receives funding from the US Department of Health and Human Services (HHS), (2) any health program or activity administered by the HHS, and/or (3) the Health Insurance Marketplace and all plans offered by issuers participating in the Marketplace.

Providers and practitioners of medical care are required to provide full and equal access to their health care facilities, equipment, programs, services, and activities. Additionally, practitioners must understand the distinct needs and circumstances of child abuse victims who have disabilities or who are deaf. This chapter addresses specific considerations for the evaluation and treatment of sexual abuse in children and adolescents who have disabilities or who are deaf.

The definition of disability used for this chapter is the definition developed for the United Nations 2014 Convention on the Rights of Persons with Disabilities[4]:

> The Convention does not provide a closed definition of who persons with disabilities are, but states that they "include" those who have long-term physical, mental, intellectual or sensory impairments which in interaction with various barriers may hinder their full and effective participation in society on an equal basis with others.
>
> The Convention recognizes that "disability" is an evolving concept resulting from attitudinal and environmental barriers. Consequently, the notion of "disability" is not rigid and can be adapted to the prevailing environment in a particular society (the focus will be on the type of attitudinal and environmental barriers present in those societies and ways to overcome them).

**The language standards used in this chapter are consistent with the mandates of Rosa's Law (Pub L No. 111-256, 124 Stat 2643) and person-first language standards. This is an effort to comply with best practices when discussing or describing individuals with disabilities.*

In the United States, both Section 504 and the ADA provide a federal definition of disability: "...a person who has a physical or mental impairment that substantially limits one or more major life activities, a person who has a history or record of such an impairment or a person who is perceived by others as having such an impairment." Rather than focus on any particular diagnosis, these definitions focus on how impairments affect an individual when carrying out daily life activities. Definitions of developmental disabilities and intellectual disabilities can be found in federal legislation and include adaptive skills.[5] Additionally, each federal program may have its own definition of disability in order to qualify for benefits.

Federal disability laws that apply most directly to the hospital and medical care community include:

— ***Section 504 of the Rehabilitation Act of 1973***: Requires that facilities, programs, or activities that receive federal financial assistance from the HHS are accessible to persons with disabilities.[2]

— ***ADA and Section 508 of the Rehabilitation Act of 1973***: Covers access to electronic and information technology.[2]

— ***Title III of the ADA***: Covers all facilities, programs, services, and activities of public entities, including health care and social services programs.[1]

— ***Title II of the ADA***: Covers all facilities, programs, services, and activities provided by state or local government entities, including health care and social services programs.[1]

— ***Section 1557 of the Patient Protection and Affordable Care Act (ACA)***[6]: Ensures that an individual is not excluded from, denied benefits of, or subjected to discrimination by any health program or activity (any part of which receives federal financial assistance), any program or activity administered by an executive agency, or any entity established under Title I of the Affordable Care Act or its amendments.

Programs and professionals serving the public are encouraged to learn their states' disability laws, which may also affect their services and activities. For example, under California law, a disability only needs to "limit" a major life activity as opposed to needing to "substantially limit" as defined under the ADA and 504.

In October 1990, the Individuals with Disabilities Education Act (IDEA)[7] was signed into law, amending the Education for All Handicapped Children Act of 1975. The importance of this law, in the context of this chapter, is that children with disabilities will most likely attend school (private or public) under the regulations of IDEA. Children with known disabilities are evaluated for eligibility to receive educational services mandated by IDEA. Children may also be evaluated by request of a parent or teacher. It can be useful to know the classification that identifies a child's special education eligibility, to be aware of evaluations on file regarding the child's well-being, the impact of his or her disabilities, and how his or her educational program provides support and specialized services and effectively communicates with the child. For example, a forensic examiner could request copies of such evaluations in order to discuss with a speech therapist how to best communicate with a specific child. Each child has an annual individual education plan (IEP) that addresses the child's strengths and deficits and how to help that child meet goals identified in the IEP. The examiner can learn a great deal about a child by obtaining copies of his or her IEP and supporting evaluation reports by occupational, physical, and speech therapists and physical education teachers as well as psychological reports and any other documents in the child's IEP file.

Epidemiology

There is currently no universally accepted definition of what constitutes a disability. The lack of a single uniform definition results in variable findings on the incidence, attributes, and experiences of children with disabilities. The Centers for Disease Control and Prevention (CDC) describes developmental disabilities as "a diverse group of severe chronic conditions that are due to mental and/or physical impairments" that result in "problems with major life activities such as language, mobility, learning, self-help, and independent living."[8] The ADA[1] defines disability as a physical or mental impairment (ie, "any physiological disorder or condition, cosmetic disfigurement, or anatomical loss affecting one or more body systems"; "any mental or psychological disorder such as intellectual disability, organic brain syndrome, emotional or mental illness, and specific learning disability") that substantially limits one or more major life activity (ie, "caring for oneself, performing manual tasks, seeing, hearing, eating, sleeping, walking, standing, sitting, reaching, lifting, bending, speaking, breathing, learning, reading, concentrating, thinking, writing, communicating, interacting with others, working, and the operation of a major body function"). This definition includes all types of disabilities (ie, physical disabilities; cognitive or learning disabilities; motor and sensory disabilities; mental illness; any other kind of physical, mental, or emotional impairment).[9] The phrase "children with special health care needs" is less limiting than some other phrases.[10]

Child sexual abuse can be conceptualized as any sexual activity that is considered inappropriate for a child's age. Sexually abusive acts may include exposure to sexually explicit materials; demands made online for photographs of a child's body; not respecting personal privacy in bathing or toileting; exhibitionism; simulation of sexual acts; fondling; oral, anal, or vaginal intercourse; incest; and other more extreme forms of sexual acts. It is important to recognize that any disability may increase a minor's risk for abuse and impact his or her response to victimization. During evaluation and treatment, abusive experiences may affect a child's communication and emotional needs.

Incidence

In July 2017, the Bureau of Justice Statistics publication "Crime Against Persons with Disabilities, 2009-2015—Statistical Tables" reported that crimes against individuals with disabilities aged 12 years and older were significantly more frequent than crimes against those without disabilities.[11] There was an overall increase in crimes against those with disabilities during this reporting period, as contrasted with an overall decrease in crimes involving the neurotypical population.

In 2015, the HHS reported that an estimated 683 000 children were determined to be victims of abuse or neglect.[12] More than 75% of child victims experienced neglect, slightly more than 17% were physically abused, and 8.4% were sexually abused. Of the 43 states that reported on disabilities, child victims who were reported to have one or more disabilities accounted for 10.6% of all victims. Victims with the following conditions were reported as having a disability:

— Intellectual disability (0.5%)

— Emotional disturbance (2.7%)

— Visual or hearing impairment (0.7%)

— Learning disability (1.2%)

— Physical disability (0.7%)

— Behavioral problems (3.7%)

— Other medical conditions (4.6%)

Other medical conditions include those not listed that significantly affect the functioning or development of the child or that require special medical care, such as chronic illnesses.[12] It is believed these conditions are underrecognized and underreported because not every child receives a clinical diagnostic assessment when child maltreatment is reported.

In March 2012, The Children's Bureau published their report *The Risk and Prevention of Maltreatment of Children with Disabilities*, updating incidence and prevalence as well as addressing identification, assessment, and response.[13] It indicates that "a special analysis of data from *Child Maltreatment 2004* revealed that children with a disability were 1.68 times more likely to experience abuse or neglect than children without a disability."

In 2000, Sullivan and Knutson[14] reported maltreatment in 9% of typically developing children and 31% of disabled children in a school setting. In this study of more than 4500 maltreated children, children with disabilities were 3.4 times more likely to be abused and neglected when compared to neurotypical children. The most common form of maltreatment for children with disabilities was neglect. Sexual abuse was found to occur 3.1 times more often among children with disabilities. Children with behavioral disorders were found to be at the highest risk for all types of maltreatment, which should be recognized as a cyclical problem. A 2005 study reported 18.5% of children with autism had been physically abused and 16.6% sexually abused.[15] In 1994, Sobsey[16] reported that 48.1% of perpetrators of sexual abuse against people with disabilities gained access to their victims through disability services. In 1993, Cross and colleagues[17] reported that disability itself directly contributed to child abuse in 47% of maltreated children with disabilities. The most common disabilities noted were emotional disabilities, learning disabilities, physical disabilities, and speech or language delay. However, it should not be concluded that children with disabilities are responsible for the abuse they suffer nor that they invite abuse in any way. It would be wrong to blame the abuse victim for the perpetrator's conduct, particularly in cases of sexual abuse, as it is well recognized that perpetrators seek victims who cannot or likely will not report them.

The Child Abuse and Prevention, Adoption, and Family Services Act of 1988 included a mandate to study the incidence of child maltreatment among children with disabilities. The National Center on Child Abuse and Neglect (NCCAN) reported that 14.1% of children whose maltreatment was substantiated by child protective services (CPS) workers in 35 states had one or more disabilities. Of the children who were abused, 17.2% had disabilities; of those sexually abused, 15.2% had disabilities. Children with disabilities were found to be at greater risk for abuse and neglect victimization than children without disabilities. Another study found the overall incidence of child maltreatment to be 39% in 150 children with multiple disabilities admitted to a psychiatric hospital. Of those children, 69% had been physically abused, 45% had been neglected, and 36% had been sexually abused; 52% of those children experienced multiple forms of maltreatment.[18] Deaf children seem to experience a particularly high level of sexual abuse. Kyam[19] found that deaf women in Norway reported childhood sexual abuse more than twice as often as the hearing population (39.6% as compared to 19.2%) and that deaf Norwegian men were more than 3 times as likely to have been abused (32.8% as compared to 9.6% in the general population). It is of note that there are relatively few studies of the incidence of abuse among children with disabilities, as compared to the number of studies of abuse of children who do not have disabilities. For this reason, extant studies are included in this chapter although they may seem outdated.

Risk Factors

There is no single risk factor that places a child at specific risk for abuse or neglect. A child with a disability may be more vulnerable to abuse because of society's beliefs or responses to their condition, rather than the condition itself. The interaction of factors seems to be most important. An integrated ecological model based on child development takes into account cultural and environmental factors as well as characteristics of the parent and child and their interactions.[16] Substance abuse on the caregivers' part is a well-known risk factor for maltreatment of all children. Other identified risk factors include parents' poor coping skills, psychiatric conditions, financial stressors, poor impulse control, and a history of violence. Parents who lack positive parenting role models and suffer from low self-esteem and depression are more likely to maltreat children.

Additional factors that influence risk of maltreatment of children with disabilities relate to communication, negative societal attitudes, stress, families, children, nonfamilial caregivers, and service providers. Some individuals believe that children with disabilities are unlikely to be abused, which results in a lack of awareness and less effort in providing protection. Although parents may worry about their children becoming victims of abuse, they may not have access to resources that would allow them to learn protective strategies on their children's behalf. Because they may be perceived as asexual or unable to understand sexual matters, children with disabilities may be offered less sex education or no sex education at all. Children who are deaf or hard of hearing often do not receive enough information to understand or report abuse. Lack of information about abuse contributes to higher risk for maltreatment. Children with disabilities could benefit from risk reduction programs intended to provide information about violations of sexual and legal conduct, sexual abuse, and sexual abuse response skills, including how to report sexual abuse and other assaults.

Isolating the child from general society increases risks by decreasing the child's knowledge and awareness of appropriate behaviors, which lessens the chance that other individuals will be aware of maltreatment, while maintaining privacy of contact with the child. Uninformed responders may consciously or subconsciously consider the child unreliable or an untrustworthy source of information, and they may be unable to establish effective communication with the child. The perception that all caregivers and service providers are inherently good results in lack of attention to signs or symptoms of child maltreatment and efforts to provide risk reduction guidance and support. Caregivers and service providers are trusted to provide good care and good service, and children are taught to obey authority figures without question, placing them at higher risk. Many caregivers and service providers for children with disabilities provide extensive physical care. Children who require assistance from caregivers or service providers for their physical needs may be accustomed to having their bodies, including their genitals, touched by adults on a regular basis and in private locations. Children with some disabilities require assistance for toileting and intimate care. A child may not be able to report abusive behavior, especially if taught to trust the provider to always know what is best. It may be very difficult for the child to comprehend the distinction between appropriate assistance in activities of daily living and behaviors that become abusive. The child is often dependent on the caregiver to put the nature of the behavior in context. If taught that the behavior or activity is normal or necessary, the child may be less likely to question it or to report it.

With respect to sexual abuse, infrequent contact between a child with disabilities and other children and adults may enable molestation because there is decreased opportunity for the child to develop a trusting relationship with an individual to whom he or she may disclose the abuse and decreased opportunity to learn to resist molestation.[9] On the other hand, children with disabilities who require multiple caregivers may have contact with numerous individuals in private, which increases the opportunity for abuse, including sexual abuse. However, an advantage of having a large number of caregivers is both the increased chance of someone detecting injuries or signs of abuse and additional assistance that lessens the amount of stress placed on the primary caregiver. The presence of multiple providers may heighten or reduce the risk. Risk may be minimized by adequate screening and selection of providers, sporadic and unscheduled monitoring of care, and keeping an open mind to recognizing that any child may become a victim of abuse. Furthermore, changes in the child's mood and willingness to be near particular caregivers are more likely to be noticed with multiple caregivers. On the other hand, too many individuals providing intimate care can be invasive and uncomfortable for the vulnerable child or teen.

Children with disabilities often have limited access to critical information pertaining to personal safety and sexual abuse prevention. Some parents have objected to their child being provided with education on human sexuality thus these children may not know how to explain what was done to them during a sexual assault. In regards to volitional sexual interaction, parents may believe that their children will never need this information because of their disabilities, without recognizing that children with disabilities experience sexual feelings and need to know what behavior is acceptable and what is not. Of course, sex education is not an antidote to assault, but it can be useful in that the child might have an understanding of what has been done to them and be better able to describe sexual acts done to them. Another essential factor is that children with disabilities are often conditioned to comply with authority at rates far beyond that expected of typically developing children, which could result in their failing to recognize abusive behaviors as maltreatment.[20] Children with disabilities are often perceived as easy targets or "good victims" because their intellectual limitations are expected to prevent them from being able to discern the experience as abuse; because they may not be able to communicate the experience; or because perpetrators believe that no one would believe the child if he or she tried to tell. The perpetrator may attempt to explain away the disclosed abuse as the child's misunderstanding of routine care.

Parents and other care providers often cannot imagine that their child might become a victim of abuse, thus missing opportunities to identify or prevent future abuse. The parent may hesitate to voice concern for fear it may result in dismissal from a program or services, and they might lose all assistance in providing care for a child with special needs. There are also fears of not wanting to accuse someone without proof that inappropriate activity actually took place. Yet, it is important to acknowledge that persons in any role who have access to children with disabilities might be abusers, including physicians, psychiatrists, psychologists, occupational therapists, speech therapists, interpreters, teachers and other education professionals, sports coaches, camp counselors, members of faith communities, and transportation providers.

In 1990, Sobsey and Mansell[21] outlined five "cultural myths" that contribute to the erroneous thinking about persons with disabilities. The acceptance of these myths may perpetuate psychological justification that a perpetrator may employ.

— ***Dehumanization myth:*** Labels such as "vegetative state" suggest that a person with the disability is something less than a full member of society and serves to dehumanize the individual. Perpetrators may rationalize their abusive behavior as not really injuring another person.

— ***Damaged merchandise myth:*** Similar to dehumanization, this myth asserts that the life of the individual with the disability is "worthless" and that he or she has nothing to lose. Such philosophy can lead to the justification of cessation of minimal support (ie, providing food, water, or medication) to a person who is otherwise relatively functional, especially after a catastrophic event such as a traumatic brain injury. This thinking is aligned with advocates for euthanasia of children with severe disabilities, who rationalize that such killing is in the best interests of the child.

— ***Feeling no pain myth:*** People with disabilities are thought of as having no feelings or as being immune to pain and suffering. There is no basis for this myth; individuals with disabilities experience the same range of emotions found in any person.

— ***Disabled menace myth:*** Perceived as different, individuals with disabilities are often considered unpredictable and dangerous, whether or not there is any foundation for the fear. Adherence to this myth may motivate people to prevent community facilities, such as group homes for adults with intellectual disabilities, from being developed in their neighborhoods.

— ***Helpless myth:*** Beliefs or perceptions that individuals with disabilities are helpless and unable to take care of themselves. These beliefs undermine self-esteem and the ability to make decisions related to daily life. Such thinking makes the individual with a disability more vulnerable to abuse and manipulation.

The prevalence of these myths with respect to the views of children with disabilities is unknown; however, in-depth case analysis of crimes against children with disabilities might direct prevention strategies to target these widely held misconceptions.

Clinical Presentation of Child Sexual Abuse

There is no typical clinical presentation of sexual abuse for a child with or without disabilities. Physical abuse and sexual abuse often occur together. Physical, psychological, and behavioral indicators of child maltreatment are similar, although they differ in manner of expression, form, intensity, and duration of the symptoms. Indicators of child sexual abuse may consist of behaviors, physical symptoms or signs, changes in moods, or a statement by the child. Such indicators suggest but do not prove the possibility of abuse. Child sexual abuse is most easily recognized when the child makes a clear, consistent statement about the activity; when the activity has been witnessed by others; or when there is clear forensic evidence. Unfortunately, these conditions are rare. As discussed above, the child with a disability may have difficulty or may be incapable of making a clear statement that describes the abuse. Compounding these difficulties, acts of abuse are rarely witnessed, and forensic evidence is unlikely to be present by the time sexual abuse is considered. Added diligence and recognition of the possibilities are necessary to identify the suspected child sexual abuse victim who has a disability. Any report of concern about sexual abuse must be carefully explored.

Behavioral Indicators

Behavioral indicators encompass a variety of patterns, all of which may be the abused child's response to the stress or distress of what they are experiencing. These are changes that occur subsequent to the first act of abuse, including grooming. Patterns may encompass but are not limited to new or unusual fear of specific individuals or places, aggression, withdrawal, regression in adaptive skills, change from usual behaviors, wariness of physical contact, and destructive behaviors. Defensive startle behaviors such as covering of the eyes or ears, extreme reluctance to accept assistance, onset of sleeping in the fetal position or needing to sleep with parents, withdrawal, and self-imposed isolation might signal abuse. Additional signs of abuse include onset of emotional lability, easy agitation, and fearfulness during bathing or toileting. The difficulty is that these behaviors are nonspecific and simply reflect the child's stress. They do not identify what the underlying stressor is (eg, maltreatment, death in the family, financial problems in the home, marital discord). Changes in mood and conduct, rather than any specific behavior or change, are usually of greater concern. However, if the child has been sexually abused for a long period of time, the behavior may have been evident for a prolonged period of time and is not recognized as a "new" behavior and, thus, not recognized as a sign of abuse. Reenacting sexually abusive or explicit conduct on others or oneself is a common sign that abuse has occurred. If the child is characterized as unreliable or not trustworthy, exhibited changes may go unrecognized. Careful and thoughtful attention to all possibilities is warranted.

Physical Signs and Symptoms

The physical signs and symptoms may be multivariate or completely absent. Multiple somatic complaints, including headaches, chest pain, abdominal pain, fatigue, and a general malaise, are not unusual in victims of child sexual assault. More specific symptoms referable to the genitourinary tract or an area of the physical assault may be present. Children may complain of discomfort in the genital area, dysuria, or painful defecation. They may have specific signs such as genital bleeding, vaginitis, or blood in the stool. The child may have bruises, "hickies," or bite marks that may indicate physical trauma coexistent with the sexual assault. It may be the physical findings of bruising, bleeding, anal tearing, or vaginitis that raise initial concerns of sexual abuse. Changes in the child's physical health and underlying medical problems must be explored. Vigilance is required to refrain from automatically assigning etiologies to the underlying disability without considering sexual abuse. Just as behavioral indicators may have multiple etiologies, so may the physical indicators. One must also recognize the importance of psychological changes. These may appear rather abruptly or emerge over time, and they are an essential part of the picture of how the child has been affected. In response to unrecognized abuse, the child may, among other responses, display frequent moodiness, sullenness, anger, terror, anxiety, and depression. Some children may have nightmares or daymares and traverse into reexperiencing. A psychiatric evaluation by practitioners experienced in PTSD and children with disabilities would be indicated. Children with disabilities require an appropriate and complete medical evaluation considering all possibilities in order to determine their association with possible child sexual abuse, abuse of other types, or other unrelated medical conditions. (Refer to the Rule Out Abuse Campaign at http://disability-abuse.com/rule-out-materials.pdf for more information.) Overall, the most important factor is recognition of changes in the child's normal health, habits, and moods.

Disclosure By The Child

A child's verbal disclosure about sexual contact, including disclosure using sign language, is typically the most helpful information in ascertaining what has happened to the child and who was involved. The child who has a disability that significantly influences communication skills or a cognitive disability is likely to have more difficulty communicating the activities that occurred and who was involved. Disclosures must be interpreted in the context of the child's cognitive and behavioral ability. Any physical disability (eg, motor, sensory, auditory, visual) may influence the timing and content of the disclosure as well as the child's reluctance or inability to disclose.

In documenting a history of sexual assault or child sexual abuse, an understanding of the method and content of disclosure is critical. If a child has a developmental level within the very early childhood range, the disclosure might be blurted out within the context of toileting or bathing. Some children who are cognitively less than 5 years old will not have learned the concept of a "secret" and may feel comfortable in revealing private information without hesitation, while others at the same developmental level may report that a perpetrator told them not to tell anyone about an abusive incident. Some examiners may discount such a disclosure if it constitutes a simple environmental contamination and seems to have no validity. However, if the child has not demonstrated sexually reactive or related behaviors in the past and has not had a habit of verbalizing in a sexually explicit manner, there is no reason to dismiss the factual nature of the information any more than one would disbelieve any other statement a child might make.[22]

A child's disclosure may be incomplete because of the level of understanding or interpretation of the specific events that took place. This is a developmental and cognitive function. Although a child with a developmental delay may not understand the concept of inappropriate touch, he or she might still be able to describe the incident within the context of its sensation. Identification of sensations and feelings are important to note as they describe and support that the event was experienced. Sensations of wetness, gagging or choking, or "gooiness" are among a variety of vivid descriptors. If a child with a developmental disability has been told a story about sexual contact, it is not likely that he or she would be able to describe the sensation that would accompany that activity. A detailed description of the feelings of touch, taste, sounds, and smell are unlikely to come from only hearing about these activities and most likely represent an accurate history about the event. Such detail in a disclosure significantly enhances its credibility. For example, one child's disclosure was not believed until the alleged perpetrator's wife learned of the child's description of the sounds and ritual behavior that she had observed in her husband for many years. When she heard the child's description, she knew the child had experienced the contact. This detailed information can be helpful to investigators in the field and at the scene, where they may find items that corroborate the child's disclosure.

Children with disabilities have disclosed extremely sexually explicit information, such as forced fellatio or anal penetration. Indication of such forms of abuse may be frankly stated, described, or demonstrated by gestures and reenactment. Such descriptions are beyond the normal range of psychosexual development and knowledge. It is unlikely these disclosures have been suggested by others. They should be documented verbatim and as descriptively as possible, along with a description of the demeanor in which it was made. Some children may have been exploited through exposure to a significant amount of pornography as a method of grooming for future abuse. This may have definite impact on the child's sexual knowledge and influence the interpretation of the disclosure. This form of desensitization by a perpetrator does not negate the reality of a true sexual assault and is exploitation by itself. It may also explain a delay in the disclosure or a feeling in the assault victim that their sexual behavior constitutes what grown-ups do. This may be offered to the child as justification for the activity by a perpetrator.

There is sometimes a concern that a child has fabricated a story of sexual abuse. Fabrication may occur in children with disabilities just as it may occur in children without disabilities. It is important to consider the basis of concern for sexual assault. For example, one must determine whether it is the actual content of the child's statement or the adult's interpretation of a statement or behavior. A well-intentioned adult may misinterpret a child's cues and behaviors. There often exists a good-faith concern on the part of a parent to ensure that nothing has happened to the child. Without investigation, however, no one will have a good understanding of the child's intent or experience. Clinicians who have experience in evaluating children for sexual abuse readily recognize the risk of false disclosure when there has been a threat or coaching of a statement by a parent. At the same time, such clinicians recognize that a description of sexual abuse cannot be "made up" by a child whose knowledge base does not include this information.

Children with disabilities, particularly developmental disabilities, are trained to behave in a more compliant manner than those who do not have disabilities. This results not only from parental behavior, but also from service providers who demand compliance with all instructions and orders without a balance of allowing the child to learn through personal experience. The fact that children learn best through experience, rather than blind obedience, has not yet taken hold. The concept of "the dignity of risk" has not yet been fully embraced by those providing educational services and other services to children with disabilities. Mandatory compliance is often practiced by parents and teachers to facilitate their children's social acceptability and ease of conformity. Children may agree to details that may not be accurate in order to please the adult asking questions. This should not be assumed, as the details may be accurate. It is important to remember that some inconsistencies and inaccuracies are to be expected from any child's statement. Inconsistencies must be interpreted in the context of all the available information and the degree of variance. Is the variation minor, major, or is the child talking about multiple different incidents? A coached statement may be too consistent at a level not expected of the child. The consistency of the disclosure, language used, and details can help sort out the veracity of the disclosure. However, recounting a coached statement would be extremely difficult for a traumatized child with a disability and should be considered unlikely.

The same set of guidelines and standards regarding obtaining a history from a child who does not have a disability should be used within the limitations of the availability and need for special services that may be required to interview the child. As with any child, the parent or caregiver of a child with a disability may provide background information and the reason for concern prior to an interview or interaction with the child. A family member or another individual who is accustomed to the abuse victim's communication style (and is neither a suspected perpetrator nor someone likely to interfere with the child's disclosure) can be invaluable in helping the examiner to understand what the child is communicating. These individuals may include special education teachers, speech therapists, occupational therapists, sign language interpreters, and other individuals who regularly interact with and understand the child's form of communication. That being said, it should be known that under ADA Title II[23] and Title III,[24] a public entity or public accommodation shall not rely on an adult accompanying an individual with a disability to interpret or facilitate communication. Therefore, although a parent or caregiver may be allowed to be present for the interview, they should not be within view of the child and should refrain from signaling or signing to the child after a question has been asked. A qualified interpreter [ie, "an interpreter who, via a video remote interpreting (VRI) service or an on-site appearance, is able to interpret effectively, accurately, and impartially, both receptively and expressively, using any necessary specialized vocabulary"][25] should be obtained. In cases involving child abuse victims, on-site interpretation is preferable to VRI, because VRI may hinder communication. In some areas, particularly rural areas, the interpreter and deaf community may be very small. All efforts should be made to ensure that an interviewed child is comfortable with the available interpreter. Furthermore, the interpreter should disclose any conflicts of interest (perceived or otherwise) with regard to the child or the child's family. An interpreter may not recognize a conflict until he or she is on site.

Specific Disabilities

Hearing Disability

There are various degrees of hearing loss. They range from mild to moderate to severe. In the United States, 2 to 3 out of every 1000 children are born with a detectable level of hearing loss in one or both ears.[26,27] Based on estimates reported to the US

Food and Drug Administration (FDA) by cochlear implant manufacturers, 38 000 cochlear implant devices had been implanted in American children as of December 2012.[28] More than 90% of deaf children are born to hearing parents.[29] Hearing parents of deaf children are more likely to physically abuse these children than are parents of hearing children.[30] Hearing parents often struggle to decide whether they should subject a deaf child to an operation for a cochlear implant or, rather, learn and use American Sign Language (ASL). Deaf children tend to miss out on learning experiences hearing children have through casual aural stimuli. In that sense, deaf children have access to less information and incidental learning than hearing children, but they are just as curious. Deaf children may be isolated or feel lonely, which makes them easy targets for abusers. Limited communication makes it harder for deaf children to disclose abuse, and abusers may target them in light of that fact. Deaf children may only be able to communicate with certain family members and caregivers. If a family member, caregiver, or teacher abuses a deaf child, the child may not feel safe disclosing to anyone. Data from an 8-year survey of college students at Rochester Institute of Technology indicate that the incidence of maltreatment, including neglect and physical and sexual abuse, is more than 25% higher among deaf and hard-of-hearing children than among hearing children.[31] The study also noted that having a deaf parent or a family member who signs or is part of the deaf community did not reduce the risk of childhood maltreatment.

Some deaf children will use sign language to communicate while others may lip read (although only 30% of English is visible on lips),[32-35] use a hearing aid, have a cochlear implant, or use a text device to communicate. If an abused child uses sign language, a parent or care provider should never be used as an interpreter, except in cases of emergency involving imminent threat to the safety or welfare of an individual or the public.[23,24] Instead, a qualified sign language interpreter should always be used, preferably on site rather than via VRI. Depending on the child's age and language fluency, practitioners should discuss with the interpreter agency the potential need for a Certified Deaf Interpreter (CDI). CDIs have specialized training and experience in the use of gesture, mime, props, drawings, and other tools to enhance communication. They possess native or near-native fluency in ASL and have an extensive knowledge and understanding of deafness, the deaf community, and deaf culture, which combined with excellent communication skills can lend added expertise to difficult interpreting situations.

When interviewing an abuse victim who is deaf or hard of hearing, especially a child, the practitioner should be seated at the patient's level and maintain eye contact. While asking questions and listening to answers, the practitioner should look at the child and not the interpreter(s). Before taking the sexual assault history, the clinician may need to take additional time for rapport-building and free-associative conversation, which helps to ensure effective communication. Neither the interpreter nor the child should sit with a window behind them. The practitioner should consider using coloring props, communication boards, or dolls and toys to assist communication. It is helpful to understand the patient's family dynamic and communication approaches used in the home and at school. It is important to ensure that the sign language interpreter is qualified to interpret in sexual assault cases. The interpreter should have training in medical settings, understand the protocols of a sexual assault examination, and be familiar with protocols for a law enforcement interview in a sexual assault nurse examiner (SANE) examination. The interpreter should also have experience working with deaf children or deaf teenagers. Best practices indicate that a team of sign language interpreters, including a hearing and a deaf interpreter, be provided for child SANE examinations in order to help ensure effective communication and reduce frustration and misunderstanding with the child. Interpreting for children and adults in everyday situations can be challenging. Being able to interpret effectively for a child who has experienced sexual abuse and trauma is crucial to accurately documenting the child's disclosure, which may influence whether a child will be deemed a credible witness.

Practitioners who have never treated a deaf child or worked with a sign language interpreter are encouraged to reach out to their state or local deaf services agency, local child abuse agency that serves the deaf community, or sign language interpreters in their area before ever needing to employ their services. You can find local interpreters and interpreter service agencies through the Registry of Interpreters for the Deaf (RID) Web site (https://www.rid.org/about-rid/about-interpreting/hiring-an-interpreter/). Interpreter service contracts requiring validation of medical interpreter training, law enforcement interpreter training, and precredentialing for qualified interpreters should be established prior to the need of the services. Some states require sign language interpreters to be licensed or certified. State-by-state regulations for interpreters and transliterators can be found at https://www.rid.org/advocacy-overview/state-information-and-advocacy/.

Regardless of language, culture, or ethnicity, all groups use names in a way to identify a specific individual. In deaf culture, name signs (ie, a sign used to identify a person in place of spelling out his or her given name) are provided to individuals.[36] Name signs are used for introductions and references to specific people, but in conversation, references to present individuals are made by gesturing.[37] Deaf parents will usually give their children name signs at birth, regardless of their children being deaf or hearing. Deaf children born to hearing parents may not receive their name sign until they start school. Depending on the child's age and education, the deaf sexual abuse victim may not know the perpetrator's name or how to spell it but may know the perpetrator's name sign, be able to provide a name sign he or she created for the perpetrator, or describe a dominant feature(s) of the perpetrator (ie, hair color, length, style; tattoos or piercings; status). An interpreter can describe such means of identification (eg, "The child is using a name sign for the perpetrator and is signing 'R' at the temple."; "The child is describing the perpetrator as having long, wavy, dark hair.").

Practitioners should discuss with the sign language interpreter the use of first- and third-person language. When interpreting for persons who are deaf or hard of hearing, the interpreter will usually speak in first person. At times, however, there may be dysfluency, use of home signs or signs the interpreter does not recognize, and it may become necessary to use the third person or to describe the child's language.

The sexual vocabulary of many deaf people may be colloquial or idiosyncratic. It is recommended in cases of child physical and sexual abuse that a team of interpreters [a hearing and a deaf (CDI) interpreter] be used to minimize frustration to the child and medical staff.

Visual Impairment

The information in a disclosure by a child who is blind or has a visual disability will include mostly nonvisual sensory information. Details such as the time of day or place of the assault should be explored in more depth based on the assault victim's usual means for making these determinations. The child who has a visual disability is at a disadvantage and may require direct and explicit instruction in gender differences. In our society, gender clues and descriptions such as hair color, length, and style; color and type of clothing; tattoos; scars; and names are vague. The obvious difference would lie in the genitalia and their function in the reproductive process. Children with visual disabilities are educated on those differences at different times and in different ways. Store mannequins and anatomically detailed models of all ages and both genders can be used to assist a child's descriptions. Examiners should also consider using variously textured clothing to determine what the child can remember feeling and also learning from parents or teachers what terms the child uses for sexual anatomy and what the child has been taught regarding touching and saying "no." As explained by Judith Davies,[38] in their efforts to "show" children with visual disabilities the world around them, caregivers often employ more touching than would be necessary for sighted children. As an unintended consequence, this additional touching, which is usually intended to be helpful, may render children with visual disabilities more vulnerable to abusive touching. For that reason, Davies advises that children with visual disabilities should, from an early age, be encouraged to say no to uncomfortable touching and that parents should discuss with such children the difference between inappropriate and appropriate touching (eg, unwarranted or uninvited touching of a child's body as opposed to touching during the normal course of a medical examination).

When interviewing a child who is blind or visually impaired, careful, step-by-step questioning may yield important historical details, such as unusual smells on the perpetrator or in the room, the sensation of facial hair, or the recognition of an unusual accent or inflection in the perpetrator's voice. If the perpetrator used a weapon during the abusive incident, the abuse victim may recall exactly where on the body the instrument was placed when it was used to touch or injure him or her. Such information may assist the examiner in locating and documenting marks or injuries associated with the weapon in question.

Children and adolescents who have lost their sight either from birth or very early in life may have early language delay. Expressive language in children with severe visual disability develops later than in sighted children.[39] Victims of sexual assault who have a visual disability are often able to describe auditory and olfactory details or recognize the perpetrator's voice, which may help to identify the perpetrator. If the perpetrator is known to the assault victim, the interviewer might ask how the victim knows the person in question and what role that person plays in the victim's life.

Children who lose their vision after 5 years of age have a higher level of independence and better language development. The lack of visual stimuli is a natural incentive for enhanced vocabulary acquisition in these children. One language parameter noted to be problematic is the incorrect use of personal and possessive pronouns (eg, confusing "his" and "their"). This may impact the ability of such an assault victim to clearly convey the history of the sexual assault; therefore, it is wise to screen language concepts in a child with a visual disability and ensure that the child responds reliably, consistently, and with expressive understanding. Identification of body parts might need to be done with tactile cues, so that the examiner will assuredly understand what the assault victim is saying. A review of behaviors and feelings should be conducted in a manner similar to that of the deaf or hard-of-hearing assault victim, with intentional verbal redundancy to ensure that the examiner has a clear understanding of the information being communicated about the assault of the individual.

When a visual disability accompanies other disabilities (eg, cognitive disability, physical disability, hearing loss), the victim may demonstrate tactile defensiveness after a sexual assault. This manifests as aversion to being touched and is another indicator that might lead investigators to believe the sexual assault could have occurred.

Motor Disabilities

Children with motor disabilities may present unique challenges. Motor disabilities may range from the central nervous system to the distant muscle fiber. Depending on the etiology of the motor disability, cognition may or may not be affected. Cerebral palsy (CP) is a category of static motor dysfunction that is most often present at or shortly after birth. Many children with CP have normal cognitive function, but may have speech disabilities and/or physical disabilities. The traumatic brain injury victim often has significant gaps in motor, cognitive, and behavioral functioning. Of individuals with hemiplegia, 85% have both normal intelligence and the capability of complete independent living. Children with athetosis also have a higher incidence of near-normal intelligence, although dysarthria may lead to difficulty with speech intelligibility and the observer may err in assuming that the child has an intellectual disability. Receptive language in such individuals is often consistent with their chronological age. It is important to keep this in mind when determining a victim's ability to respond to questions regarding his or her sexually assaultive experience(s).

Epilepsy

Children may have any of the various types of epilepsy. It is essential to know what type of epilepsy a child has, what medications have been prescribed, and if the child experiences "breakthrough" seizures. Stress is known to exacerbate the condition, and the sexual assault examination certainly could induce stress. The evaluator should be trained in how to respond when a seizure begins. Because signs of seizure vary from person to person as well as by type of seizure, the examiner should be familiar with a given child's typical signs prior to the examination or interview.

Intellectual Disability

The fifth edition of the *Diagnostic and Statistical Manual of Mental Disorders* (DSM-5) defines intellectual disability as "a disorder with onset during the developmental period that includes both intellectual and adaptive functioning deficits in conceptual, social and practical domains."[40] Areas include deficits in abstract thinking and needs for support in any adaptive functioning and social participation. Level or category of the impact of the disability are defined and described as "mild," "moderate," "severe," and "profound." In many cases, students have speech therapists at school who, prior to the interview, can help the practitioner by providing guidance to communicate with the child. Most children with intellectual disabilities can engage with normal verbal interaction, while others may require accommodations. Approaching the child in the usual manner (ie, using language that is clear and simple but not "baby talk") is usually effective. Matching one's vocabulary and pacing to that of the child is recommended. Detailed information on interviewing children with intellectual and communication disabilities is available from the Office for Victims of Crime.[41]

Autism Spectrum Disorders

The DSM-5 describes autism as including "persistent deficits in social communication and social interaction across multiple contexts."[40] Because there is such variety among individuals with autism, practitioners must inquire as to how the condition is expressed in each individual person. The practitioner should ask how the child best communicates, as some individuals with autism are nonverbal and communicate only through the use of a device (eg, a tablet) or the physical assistance of a trained communication specialist. When preparing the interview site, it is important to consider that children with autism may have a hypersensitivity to sensory stimuli. Some may engage in well-recognized actions that seem to help manage anxiety (eg, hand flapping). Usually, parents are excellent informants and may be able to offer information on how to best respond when unusual conduct occurs. It is of particular note that self-injurious behaviors are common among those with autism, as well as among those with other diagnoses.[42] These may increase following abuse.

Communication Disabilities and Augmentative and Alternative Communication

The ADA requires that services provided "to the public" be accessible to individuals with disabilities.[1] In addition to the ADA, practitioners providing services to children with disabilities should be familiar with augmentative and alternative communications (AAC) (ie, methods other than verbal communication used by individuals with disabilities as their primary form of communication). AACs include "unaided systems" (ie, methods of communication performed with one's own body, including gestures, body language, facial expressions, sign language) and "aided systems" (ie, methods of communication performed with the aid of a tool or device, including writing with pen and paper, pointing to letters or images on a board, interacting with speech-generating computers).[43] Familiarity with these methodologies is important for all practitioners serving the public.

Interview Techniques

Taking into consideration the above general information about the major categories of disabilities, standard interview techniques should be adapted to reflect an appropriate level of interaction for the child's cognitive or developmental level and needs. Adapt the interview space for a child's visual or hearing disability, physical disability, or developmental disability.[41]

Prior to the interview, it is important to create an inviting and accessible environment free of sensory "toxins." This would include, for example, replacing fluorescent light bulbs with full-spectrum lighting for those who are sensitive to the flickering of and sounds emitted by fluorescent lights, which can be quite distracting to those with heightened sensory sensitivity. Those present for the interview should not wear any scents (eg, perfume, shaving lotion, scented lotion, deodorant, laundry soap). Such toxins may stimulate sensitivities in the child abuse victim, such that the interview must be rescheduled or practitioners rotated out. External noises (eg, those from devices that beep or create loud distracting noises) should be eliminated or reduced. Seating accommodations and arrangements should enhance the child's comfort and ensure appropriate seating for the interpreter(s), if needed. If the child uses a wheelchair, adequate space should be made in advance of the child entering the room.

The first step in the forensic interview is to engage in rapport-building discussions. The practitioner should begin by introducing himself or herself and his or her role in the conversation. It is important to inform the child of the purpose of the interview before continuing the interview process. Appropriate communication supports must be in place prior to the interview. For example, when interviewing a child with a hearing disability who uses sign language, efforts should be made to employ an interviewer (deaf or hearing) who is fluent in ASL. If an interviewer who is fluent in sign language is not available, a qualified, certified sign language interpreter should be hired. Contracts for services should be in place, and interpreters under contract should be screened for prior education and training in medical, legal, law enforcement, and SANE settings, including interpreting during sexual abuse examinations and interviews.

During rapport building, it is preferable to ask the child questions to which he or she knows the answers. These may include questions regarding the child's home (eg, questions about family members, pets) or school (eg, questions about teachers, the classroom, the playground, favorite activities). Asking the child to write his or her name is recommended. Children with disabilities may have more difficulty shifting from topic to topic; therefore, the interviewer should create smooth transitions between areas of inquiry. If the abusive event occurred outside, asking about weather conditions may help corroborate the event. One can easily confirm whether the conditions described by the abuse victim reflect that day's weather report. Rephrasing questions allows one to ask the individual in several ways about the same information. One must be careful not to suggest answers to the questions asked and should avoid leading questions. When a victim provides the same answer to repeated questions, the examiner can feel secure that there is no confusion regarding the facts. However, the examiner should avoid excessive repetition of the same question, which can cause the child to wonder if the examiner does not believe or does not understand his or her answers. Simple questions are best. Complex sentences and sentences that run together in content and meaning are confusing and should be avoided. The child's receptive language age equivalent may be far less than his or her chronological age; therefore, the examiner should ask questions that approximate the child's measured age of language comprehension. A limited time for the interview based on the child's attention span must also be respected. It is critical to understand how the deaf or hard-of-hearing child communicates with their family members and school staff.

It is critical to use language that the child understands. It is best to use the child's terminology, once identified. The interviewer must be skilled at helping children describe all aspects of their experience. If the child does not know terminology or who a specific individual is, the examiner must be creative in helping the child convey as much detail as possible. The child may be able to describe the duties of an individual, what they look like, their name sign, or special occasions when they encounter that individual.

Conducting the Interview

It is important for the medical examiner to introduce himself or herself as a health care provider and be sure that the child is aware that he or she is at a medical facility. If the encounter is for medical diagnosis and treatment, establishing that fact is essential. In some states and jurisdictions, the hearsay exception associated with a medical history requires that the crime victim understands that he or she is taking part in a medical encounter.

When taking a history from a child abuse victim, it is important to consider a gradual approach to seeking information. Questions about daily routines, such as, "What do you do when you get up in the morning?" encourage open conversation in the rapport-building phase. They also establish the abuse victim's ability to recall activities of daily living. Prompts such as, "What happens after that?" afford the opportunity to evaluate spontaneous language content and the ability of the abuse victim to speak in terms of concrete actions versus abstract feelings. Questions such as, "Do you stay home all day?" can assist the abuse victim express place and person concepts. They may also allow him or her to speak of an alleged perpetrator in an indirect fashion, so the examiner might learn the terminology used in reference to this person. The examiner should use the same terms or signs the child uses. When utilizing an interpreter, the interviewer must note that the spoken words may be that particular interpreter's chosen English-language interpretation and not an actual word the child signed. Have a discussion with the interpreter prior to the interview to clarify terms and concepts, clarify use of first or third person, and to understand the interpreting process. The child's concept of time may not be fully developed; therefore, demonstrating concepts of yesterday, today, and tomorrow help establish whether the child has an understanding of time. Relating incidents to specific times of day (eg, before or after school, taking their morning or afternoon medicine, watching a favorite TV show) can help. Relating incidents to special events, holidays, or locations can assist in establishing a time frame.

Perpetrators of sexual assault and abuse are most commonly known to their victims (eg, a family member, family friend, other community member, authority figure). That being the case, sexual abuse victims, including victims with intellectual or developmental disabilities, may experience difficulty in reporting an abusive experience. Most children with a developmental disability are taught to be compliant with authority figures and to seek assistance from them. Although rare, some may not perceive that someone has hurt them or touched them in a bad way. However, most abuse victims will indicate that the event caused them to feel upset and that they know it should not have happened. Asking a child "What happened?" or to "Tell me more about that." encourages spontaneous and increased detail and avoids the introduction of interviewer assumptions. Questions should not be asked in a "yes-no" format if they can be avoided. However, if this is the only option, asking such questions must be done in a way that the opposite but equal question is also asked in the yes/no format. For example, "Did this happen only one time?" and "Did this happen more than one time?" can be asked.

Closing the Interview

It is essential to end the interview in a way that helps the child feel more comfortable. Reassuring the child that he or she is not at fault for what happened to him or her and that he or she did a good job during the interview (no matter what happened) is recommended. If a follow-up interview is likely, inform the child that you will meet again or that another interview will happen soon. If the next interview will be conducted by a new practitioner, the child should be made aware. Tell the child what will happen with the information he or she provided.

Post Interview

Corroborative information from family members or others who are frequently with the abuse victim should be obtained to support the victim's report. Such corroborative information could include the weather on the day of the assault; who was present in the residence, school, or facility; what time the assault may have taken place; and to whom the victim made a statement or comment about what happened.

Standard Procedure and Documentation

The medical evaluation of the suspected child sexual abuse victim who has a disability should progress along the same lines as any medical evaluation (ie, history taking, physical examination, impression, planning). The evaluation and physical examination must be tailored to the individual needs of the patient. Depending on the child's ability to make a disclosure and provide essential details of an abusive act, additional investigation by child protection services and law enforcement will follow. Implementing standard practices as described in generic SANE/SART protocols is recommended.

History

The purpose of the medical history is to understand what happened and to ascertain any medical consequences from a possible sexual contact. In some settings, the medical team obtains the history. In other settings, forensic interviewers not in the medical environment interview the child regarding the allegation or experiences. The details of the assault may then be shared with the medical providers, to assist in determining the appropriate medical steps. The interview techniques described in the previous section should be used when taking the medical history.

The child usually presents to health care either because of verbal disclosure, behavioral concerns of assault, or because there were suspicious circumstances leading to an evaluation. An assault victim with a disability may present with evidence of physical body harm, genital trauma, or pregnancy. The health care provider must obtain a concise yet detailed account of the history as given by the child or other observer. It is important to speak with someone knowledgeable of the child to understand the child's capabilities and typical behaviors and to identify physical complaints. A careful behavioral history is important because family members or care providers who know the child well can describe changes in the child's usual routines and identify disconcerting new behaviors. A child may not be able to name the person who committed the abuse, but may be able to describe the activity in which they engaged or a specific physical feature. A child who uses ASL may be able to provide the perpetrators name sign and describe the individual. Behavior and mood changes as well as a complete review of systems should be documented. Behavioral, psychological, and physical consequences of sexual contact should be detailed and distinguished from other medical conditions that may be confused with sexual assault.

Behavioral and psychological or mood changes may be the primary evidence warranting an initial evaluation for child sexual abuse in a victim with cognitive or communication disabilities. A care provider familiar with the usual functioning of the child should be included in the evaluation meetings. Although instruments have been devised to assess sexualized behaviors in typically developing children, no such studies have been devised for children with disabilities. Nonabused, typically developing children have more sexualized behaviors at younger ages. As they mature, fewer sexualized behaviors are seen. It is the developmental age equivalence of the child that is important in assessing the appropriateness of any behavior. This understanding of cognitive age equivalence is important in determining the approach to the interview. The approach must match the child's abilities for the examiner to obtain the cooperation of the child and revelation of meaningful information.

Physical Examination

The physical examination of the child sexual assault victim should be a complete, head-to-toe examination, including a detailed genital examination. Special attention should be paid to those parts of the body with signs or symptoms. It is important to evaluate the skin, mouth, and anogenital area of every sexual assault victim in order to look for evidence of new or old trauma, infection, or clues to underlying medical conditions. Sexual maturity will also influence medical considerations independent of cognition, specifically the possibility of pregnancy and sexually transmitted infections (STIs). (Refer to Chapter 10, "Sexually Transmitted Infections," for information about STI screening and treatment.)

The approach to the physical examination, like all other aspects of the evaluation for sexual assault, should be geared to the child's developmental, psychological, and physical or sensory disabilities. Adaptations for motor or physical disabilities will likely be necessary in considering examining equipment and positioning. As with all children, the child with a vision disability should be told what is happening at every step, and extra care should be taken in letting them feel and touch any instruments that might be used (eg, moistened cotton swab). The child who is deaf or hard of hearing should also see and touch any materials and equipment that will be used. Additionally, the examiner should explain the entire process, including every step of the examination, and demonstrate how examination equipment will be used in each step. The child should be allowed to ask questions about the explanation. When examining a child with an interpreter, the examiner should be aware that the child will need to look at the interpreter to understand what the examiner is saying during the examination. In order to gain their trust and cooperation, it is important to keep children informed of what is happening during the examination, whether or not they have a disability. Just as a typically developing child should not be coerced into an examination and held down against her will, neither should a child with a disability. Coercion depends on level of cognition. For example, an 18-month-old child may have to be coerced to have his or her ears examined. Most examinations can be easily performed by examiners experienced in cajoling and adapting the approach to fit the needs of the child. The benefit of an examination (often with no physical findings) must be weighed against the risks of further emotional trauma related to coercion. In rare situations, physical signs or symptoms that require immediate medical attention may warrant sedation or an examination under anesthesia. When examining a child who uses a wheelchair or other pieces of assistive equipment, the examiner should be aware of proper procedures to help the child safely transfer to the examination table and back.

Violence associated with sexual assault requires close surveillance for head and neck injuries, facial trauma, strangulation-related trauma, old trauma, and other body injuries. Although violence is not typical as part of the sexual assault of children, children who are physically abused are more likely than their peers to be sexually abused. If the abuse victim has communication disabilities, the clinicians must be very thorough in order to ensure discovery of all injuries. Defensive wounds, which usually occur to the upper extremities when the victim assumes a defensive posture, should be carefully noted. Injuries that result from defending against the perpetrator's hand or weapon can be seen in the upper outer arms, shoulders, or palms of the hand. Ligature marks about the wrists or ankles may be seen in the child who has been restrained. There may be marks about the neck from strangulation or choking. Injuries may result to the mouth as a result of oral-genital contact, and bruising may occur anywhere, especially the breasts and inner thighs. In sum, there may evidence anywhere.

In a sexual assault case, there are two "crime scenes": the victim and the site where the crime occurred. Both scenes deserve meticulous attention to ensure the integrity of results. Evidence collection is extremely important at the crime scene and from the child. Forensic collection from the child is recommended when the child presents to the health care system up to 72 or 96 hours of a sexual assault. Studies have shown the greatest yield for positive forensic evidence of the prepubertal child sexual assault victim is from the clothing gathered and submitted with the rape kit.[44] In a study by Christian et al,[45] the DNA evidence present in this material was found to be more reliable than those fluids found on the assault victim's body. Realization of this fact requires a careful retrieval of any and all articles of clothing the child was known to have been wearing at the probable time of the crime. From a crime scene perspective, this includes discarded diapers or clothes that might be present at the scene. Bed sheets and towels should also be examined.

Multidisciplinary Team Evaluation

The evaluation of children for possible child sexual abuse requires a team approach under all circumstances. There is no single profession or provider that has access to all the information necessary to make a determination of what happened, address medical consequences, interview witnesses and suspects, collect and process forensic evidence, and provide the abuse victim and his or her family with treatment as needed. Each team member has a distinct role in the case. CPS is responsible for ensuring safety and protection of the child; law enforcement is responsible for determining whether a crime has been committed; and the medical provider is responsible for assessing and treating the patient and collecting evidence from the patient's body.

The CPS social worker in the medical setting can be an invaluable source early in gathering background psychosocial information on the child and family. This may include information on domestic violence, previous child protection involvement, criminal histories, and possible confounding factors or additional risk factors (ie, living with a convicted sex offender) in the child's life. The social worker can also assess the level of anxiety and genuine concern for the child in balance with external issues of a parent who has not dealt with his or her own sexual assault or domestic violence in the past or may be using the allegation to seek custody of a child. A history of the child's functional, behavioral, and cognitive abilities can aid medical providers and social and legal investigators in determining the best approach to questions and examination of the child. The social worker can assist with abuse victim advocacy options if domestic violence, substance abuse, or homelessness are contributing factors. The social worker can facilitate referrals for mental health treatment for the child and family and assist in enrolling the abuse victim and his or her family members in the Victims of Crime program to pay for services required because of the crime. It is essential to note that there is a scarcity of specialized mental health treatment for child abuse victims with disabilities or who are deaf or hard of hearing.

Team decision-making processes are indicated, particularly when a victim of abuse has a disability. Many communities have established sexual abuse response teams or child advocacy centers to address the special issues of child victimization. However, most do not yet include a disability specialist on the team. The expertise of specially trained sexual assault investigators (child protection services, law enforcement, and prosecutors) in conjunction with medical providers with advanced training in sexual assault cases is invaluable. In the circumstances of the victim who has a disability, physical evidence of an acute sexual assault is self-explanatory. In the circumstance of a nonverbal child abuse victim from whom no forensic evidence has been collected and who may have no physical evidence of a sexual encounter, team reviews of all the information can be very helpful. Consultation with specialists who have expertise in working with children with disabilities is indicated. When a team documents that there has been attention to all of the possibilities explaining the presentation and discerns that enough evidence exists to discount other hypotheses, the credibility of the final decision is increased.

Investigation by law enforcement and CPS is important in determining what is hearsay and what observers directly report. When team members receive and share information, it is imperative to document the source of the original information so that investigators can identify and confirm the information from the original source. The sexual assault may have been witnessed or the victim may have been discovered very shortly after the event occurred. For example, if a child with a cognitive or communication disability is brought from a residential care facility, the provider accompanying the child may not have any direct information. Providers at the facility who have information should be personally interviewed. In some cases, a provider may initially deny any knowledge of the assault or concern. In such cases, CPS must seek out and interview other sources of information. Some may err in only interviewing the adult who accompanies the child, failing to directly interview the assault victim.

The investigator should go to the scene of the reported incident to look for evidence of what was described, such as possible forensic evidence on bed sheets and towels. The observations of many providers may be helpful in determining what actually happened.

Investigators can learn whether there are new fears the child has developed, of a specific room or area in the home or residence, similar to what is noted in children and adolescents who have no developmental disabilities. This may be useful insight into the possible location of an assault. It is not uncommon that the acute sexual assault victim comes for medical care after the most recent event in a series of recurrent episodes. Changes in the child's moods, cognition, behaviors, physical complaints, or other observations may be reported by other providers. This information should be added to the report of the findings of the examinations, interviews, and investigations.

Team members can also assist in establishing whether the child abuse victim is capable of giving a reasonable history. Care providers familiar with the child can provide information on the child's short- and long-term memory, reliability to recover normal facts, and their language abilities in comprehension and expression. Although a child with a disability may not be able to read, he or she may be able to consistently recall incidents that had a major impact on his or her memory.

Treatment

Children with disabilities who have been sexually assaulted have the same types of medical and mental health treatment needs as typically developing children who have been sexually assaulted. Considerations for medical care, pregnancy, and STI prophylaxis should be the same for all child abuse victims. All medical conditions identified should receive appropriate care and treatment. Each case of child sexual abuse that is confirmed or strongly suspected should include a multidisciplinary treatment plan, which includes a mental health assessment and treatment plan appropriate for the child's cognitive and developmental level. Counseling for the family members is a necessary component for their needs as presumed vicarious trauma victims, and to assist in helping their child. This child and family treatment plan should be integrated with other intervention plans that may have already been developed for the child. Children with disabilities require mental health services that are appropriately designed to match their individual needs—be it a developmental adaptation or sign language interpreter for psychotherapy treatment sessions. If a child uses ASL, it is recommended that a therapist who is fluent in ASL be assigned for direct communication, rather than using an interpreter.

Institutional policies should include prompt reporting of allegations of sexual abuse and screening and monitoring for employees and volunteers, sign language interpreters and other support providers, and chaperones and field trip supervisors. All children, including children with disabilities, should receive accurate information regarding sex education and personal safety.[46]

Psychological Post-Trauma Treatment

Children with disabilities experience the full range of feelings and emotions that are experienced by children without disabilities. It is an error to assume that a child with a disability does not comprehend an abusive experience and will not experience adverse effects as a result. It must be recognized that many children are identified as victims because of the behavioral manifestations of the assault. The mental health treatment provider should assess how the child has changed since the abuse and how the child understands or interprets the emotional impact of the experience. The therapist must individualize the treatment plan to meet the specific needs of the child. Multiple modalities of treatment, including play, art or music therapy, cognitive and educational methods, and psychoanalytic approaches, may be considered.[47]

Prevention

Prevention of child maltreatment and child sexual abuse specifically must be addressed in order to protect children with disabilities. The steps to prevention that any parent or professional can follow include the following[48]:

— Learning the risks and understanding facts

— Minimizing opportunities for the child to be molested by talking about prevention and sex education with their children

  — NOTE: Although sex education is not a protection or deterrent from sexual abuse, it can help the child learn terminology of sexual body parts and sexual acts, that could assist in reporting a sexual assault.

— Getting involved in community prevention efforts

— Becoming an "abuse-aware parent" and designing a risk-reduction plan for their family

Parents of children with disabilities should be informed of how to reduce risk for abuse, prepare their child in the event of an abusive incident occurring, and learn effective response methods. Parents can develop an individual response plan as described in *A Risk Reduction Workbook for Parents and Service Providers: Policies and Practices to Reduce the Risk of Abuse, Including Sexual Violence, Against People with Intellectual and Developmental Disabilities* (available from the Spectrum Institute's Disability and Abuse Project at http://disabilityandabuse.org/books/).[49] Use of the individual response plan has been effective in reducing the risk and impact of sexual abuse.

Societal Response to the Abuse of Children and Adults With Disabilities

At a national level, *A Call to Action: Ending Crimes of Violence Against Children and Adults with Disabilities* recommends establishing prevention as priority, determining the magnitude and scope of the problem, creating a plan of action and implementation, and instituting an evaluation plan.[50] Society should recognize children with disabilities as equal citizens with equal rights to services and protections.[51] Attitudes about children and youth with disabilities must change in order to empower their positions and decrease their vulnerability to abuse. The keys to success in reducing the risk and impact of abuse include informing parents about the reality of the problem and making children aware of the possibilities and empowering them all to have a viable plan to reduce the risk and impact of abuse. Knowledgeable providers with supportive programs should continue to provide ongoing education and services in these areas.

Future Efforts

Research has demonstrated that there are significant training needs for collaborative responses in the evaluation of children with disabilities who have been maltreated. Orelove et al[52] studied parents, educators, and investigators about their understanding of the needs in working with children with disabilities and child maltreatment. Respondents had a cursory awareness of some of the issues. A majority of the respondents were interested in training, and they ranked recognition of maltreatment of children with disabilities as a priority.

There should be future efforts to expand the recognition that children with disabilities are abused at rates exceeding those of typically developing children. There should be concentrated efforts to expand awareness of risk reduction and the impact of abuse. Research and training initiatives should incorporate a focus on children with disabilities in order to improve understanding of their unique responses to abuse and of effective treatments matching their cognitive and communication skills.

Conclusion

Sexual abuse occurs at a higher rate among children with disabilities than among children who do not have disabilities. Disabilities include intellectual and developmental disabilities, mental health conditions, vision disabilities and blindness, hearing disabilities and deafness, learning disabilities, physical disabilities, motor disabilities, behavioral problems, and other medical problems. Children with disabilities are more vulnerable to abuse as an outcome of numerous societal and cultural factors, lack of communication, and increased stress on parents and other caregivers. Sexual abuse may occur along with physical abuse or separately. When evaluating a child with a disability, modifications in communication and examination techniques are required. Physical and mental health care should be equal in quality and availability for children with and without disabilities. Increased awareness of the issues surrounding abuse of children with disabilities is needed. Society must recognize children with disabilities as equal citizens with equal rights to quality services and protections.

Appendix 17-1: Recommended Language Use When Discussing or Writing About People With Disabilities or Those Who Are Deaf or Hard of Hearing*

My lawn mower is disabled, my car is disabled. I am a person of short stature. I am not broken and do not need to be fixed.

—Billy Barty [actor and founder of Little People of America (LPA)]

...the difference between the almost right *word and the* right *word is really a large matter—'tis the difference between lightning bug and the lightning.*

—Mark Twain[53]

Introduction

The following guide provides essential up-to-date information on how to respectfully refer to or address people with a variety of disabilities or other conditions. The information is current as of 2017. It must be noted that most of the following preferred references come from those with disabilities or conditions and that preferences change over time. Thus is it essential for the professional serving the general public to stay aware of the changes.

As defined by the Americans with Disabilities Act (ADA), the term "disability" is defined as: "(a) a physical or mental impairment that substantially limits one or more major life activities of [an] individual; (b) a record of such an impairment; or (c) being regarded as having such an impairment." Language is powerful. Our words can teach, inspire, motivate, and uplift people; at the same time, they can oppress, demean, and hurt. People who are born with or acquire their disability early in life typically do not view the disability as a negative or something to be pitied. Disability or deafness is part of their identity, no less than their race, gender, ethnicity, citizenship or immigration status, religion, sexual orientation, or other identifying characteristics.

Person-first language focuses on the individual rather than his or her disability. Oftentimes, it is not even necessary to state an individual's disability. Additionally, through the years, some terminology has become outdated, inaccurate, derogatory, and offensive when addressing children and adults with disabilities. The term "person with a disability" replaced the outdated term "handicapped" with the 1990 passage of the ADA. Additionally, under Rosa's Law (Pub L No. 111-256, 124 Stat 2643), the terms "mental retardation" and "mentally retarded" were removed from federal health, education, and labor policy and replaced with "intellectual disability" and "individual with an intellectual disability."[54] Many state legislatures have also adopted the replacement of these terms in state laws and regulations. In California, Senate Bill No. 1381 ("Mental retardation: change of term to intellectual disability"), was signed into law on September 22, 2012 by Governor Jerry Brown.

When you are speaking to or writing about persons with disabilities in general, disability advocacy agencies and organizations recommend the use of person-first language. However, some persons with disabilities may refer to themselves using the term "disabled" or another outdated term. When interacting directly with a person with a disability, it is best to use his or her preferred terminology.

Table 17-1 identifies terms considered offensive by the disability and deaf communities and recommendations for alternate preferred language.

Table 17-1. Preferred and Outdated Terminology Referring to Persons With Disabilities

Disability	Preferred Term	Outdated Term(s)
Disability	— Person with (who has) a disability	— Handicapped — Disabled
Mental health disability	— Person with schizophrenia	— Schizophrenic
Developmental disability/cognitive disability	— Person with an intellectual disability — Person who has a cognitive disability — Person with a learning disability	— Retarded/mentally retarded — "Special Ed" — Slow — Brain-damaged
Physical/mobility disability	— Person with a physical disability — Person who uses a wheelchair — Wheelchair user — Person with a mobility disability	— Cripple — "Special" — Wheelchair-bound — Confined to a wheelchair — Lame — Gimp — Challenged
Health/medical condition	— Person with epilepsy or seizure disorder — Person with a medical condition	— Epileptic
Health/medical condition	— Person living with AIDS — Person who is HIV positive or living with HIV	— Suffering from stricken with AIDS or HIV
Health/medical condition	— Person with multiple sclerosis	— Afflicted by MS
Little person/short stature	— Little person — Person of short stature	— Dwarf — Midget
Deaf and hard of hearing	— Person who is deaf or hard of hearing	— Deaf-mute — Deaf and dumb
Cognitive disability	— Person who has a traumatic brain injury — Person who has an acquired brain injury	— Brain-damaged
Physical disability	— Accessible parking	— Disabled parking — Handicapped parking
Congenital disability	— Person who has a congenital disability	— Birth defect
Speech disability	— Person with a communication disability — Person who uses a device to communicate — Person with a speech disability — Person unable to speak — Person who uses synthetic speech	— Mute — Dumb — Speech-disabled

(continued)

Table 17-1. Preferred and Outdated Terminology Referring to Persons With Disabilities *(continued)*

Disability	Preferred Term	Outdated Term(s)
Mental health/ emotional/psychiatric disability	— Person with an emotional or behavioral disability — Person with a mental health or psychiatric disability	— Insane — Crazy — Psychotic — Mentally ill — Mental — Disturbed
Blind or visual disability	— Person who is blind or has a visual disability	— The blind

Meeting and Interacting With Persons With Disabilities

When initially meeting someone with a disability for the first time, one might feel nervous. The usual rules of etiquette still apply:

— Establish eye contact.

— When speaking with a child or a person in a wheelchair, try to sit at his or her eye level.

— Say hello, introduce yourself, shake hands, and then begin a conversation.

Keep in mind that a person who has a disability is a person like any other—entitled to dignity, consideration, respect, and basic human rights. When meeting a person with a disability in a practice setting, the practitioner should be familiar with the facility, including the locations of accessible restrooms, drinking fountains, and dog relief areas. If such facilities are not available or inaccessible, be ready to offer alternatives (eg, private or employee restrooms, a glass of water, a desk phone) or move the meeting to a location with accessible facilities. Consider adopting an indoor environmental quality policy. According to the Centers for Disease Control and Prevention's (CDC) *Indoor Environmental Quality Policy*, "Fragrance is not appropriate for a professional work environment, and the use of some products with fragrance may be detrimental to the health of workers with chemical sensitivities, allergies, asthma, and chronic headaches/ migraines."[55] To that end, the CDC encourages their employees to be as fragrance-free as possible when they arrive in the workplace.

When introduced to a person with a disability, it is appropriate to offer to shake hands. People with limited hand use or who use a prosthesis can usually shake hands. Note the following recommendations:

— Shaking with the left hand is acceptable.

— For those who cannot shake hands, find another way to welcome and acknowledge their presence.

— Treat adults in a manner befitting adults.

— Call a person by his or her first name only when extending that familiarity to all others present.

— When talking with a person with a disability, look at and speak directly to that person rather than through a companion, assistant, or interpreter who may also be present.

— Offer assistance in a dignified manner with sensitivity and respect. Be prepared to have your offer declined. Do not proceed to assist if your offer to assist is declined. Some people may be well able to help themselves. If the offer is accepted, listen to and accept any instructions.

— When offering to hand a coat or umbrella, do not offer to hand a cane or crutches unless the individual requests otherwise. Persons with disabilities should not be separated from their assistive devices.

— Use appropriate language.

— Do not treat the person like a hero.

— Do not sensationalize the disability.

— When writing or speaking about people with disabilities, emphasize abilities rather than limitations.

— Remember to keep in mind other cultural and gender issues with regard to hand shaking, touching, and eye contact.

The following sections offer case-specific recommendations for interacting with individuals who have different types of disabilities.

Persons With Physical and/or Mobility Disabilities

— A person in a wheelchair is a "wheelchair user" or "person who uses a wheelchair."

— Wheelchairs are part of a person's personal space; therefore, it is not appropriate to lean on, touch, or otherwise maneuver an individual's chair without permission.

— Always ask a person and wait for his or her response before pushing his or her wheelchair.

— Always ask a person if he or she needs assistance with opening a door or navigating a space before doing so.

— Never patronize people using wheelchairs by patting them on the head or shoulder.

— Keep mobility devices (eg, walkers, canes, crutches) within the reach of the person.

— It is ok to shake hands with someone who is a wheelchair user.

— Offer to hold or carry packages.

— Sit down or kneel when conversing for an extended period of time with an individual who uses a wheelchair.

— Ask before touching or petting a service animal, as petting may distract the animal from working.

Persons Who Are Blind or Have Visual Disabilities

— Identify yourself so a blind person knows you are in the room.

— If asked for assistance, let the blind person hold your arm as a guide, this will allow you to guide the individual instead of lead or propel the individual.

— Orient the individual to the environment, mentioning specific rooms, restrooms, water fountains, and other points of interest.

— When assisting a blind person, be descriptive: describe upcoming obstacles, let them know if the door is on the right or left, and warn them of possible hazards.

— Offer to assist with reading printed information or filling out forms.

— A person with a visual disability may ask for materials in alternative format (eg, large print, Braille, recorded tapes, files on a disk). Know the process for requesting and obtaining alternative formats.

— Ask before touching, petting, or verbally/visually interacting with a service animal, as such interaction may distract the animal from working.

— Announce when you or other individuals enter or leave a room.

— Inform the individual of what is transpiring if there are silences in conversation.

— Speak directly to the individual in a normal tone and speed.

— Describe people, objects, and places in detail.

Persons With Speech and/or Communication Disabilities

— Listen with respect and patience.

— Speak normally.

— Do not complete the individual's sentences.

— Do not pretend to understand or assume information. Ask the person to repeat what they have said if you do not understand or consider rephrasing what you did understand.

Persons Who Are Deaf or Hard of Hearing

— Speak in a normal tone and provide a clear view of your mouth.

— Do not exaggerate your mouth movements.

— Speak directly to the individual rather than addressing an interpreter. Always maintain eye contact with the person not the interpreter.

— You can touch a deaf or hard-of-hearing person on the shoulder, turn lights on and off, or tap a table or the floor to get their attention. Do not throw objects to gain their attention.

— Ask the individual if they need an interpreter. Respect the individual's choice of communication and requests for accommodation.

— A deaf or hard-of-hearing person may ask to write messages back and forth. Be prepared to provide a paper and pen or pencil, smart phone, tablet, or laptop.

— Speech reading or lip reading is not always effective. Even the most adept lip readers only receive about 33% of the information. Be aware of lighting, beards or moustaches, window glare, situation, accents, or speech disabilities of the interviewer.

— Have an assistive listening device system in place and available for the meeting.

— Keep in mind that English is often not a deaf individual's first language and that he or she may prefer a qualified sign language interpreter to communicate in ASL. Know the process and time frame necessary for obtaining qualified sign language interpreters.

— Ask the person to repeat himself or herself if you do not understand. Do not pretend to understand or assume information.

— Use facial expressions, body language, and pantomime.

— Never use a child to communicate with an adult.

— During conversation, describe or inform the individual of any other interrupting conversations or distractions.

Persons With Learning Disabilities

— During interviews, understand that occasional inattentiveness, distraction, or lack of eye contact is not unusual for individuals with learning disabilities. A quiet room with minimal distractions may help.

— Be aware that there may be some information-processing problems that might affect the individual's social skills, leading to inappropriate behavior and responses.

— Be aware that an individual may need extra time to process information or questions pertaining to the situation.

Persons Who Have Developmental or Intellectual Disabilities

— The term "intellectual disability" has replaced the term "mental retardation" at the federal and several state levels of government.

— "Developmental disability" is a legal term referring to a variety of disabilities that begin during childhood or adolescence. Among these are intellectual disability, cerebral palsy, autism, epilepsy, and other similar or related conditions.

— Adults with developmental disabilities are not children. They are adults and deserve to be treated as such.

— Take your time, do not rush the individual. Do not complete sentences or thoughts of the individual, allow them to finish on their time.

— Do not touch individuals except in response to their touch with the exception of normal hand shaking.

— Be aware of lighting. Fluorescent lighting is sometimes distressing or distracting; therefore, a room with a window and natural or full-spectrum lighting may be required.

— Avoid any distractions in the room (eg, phones, clocks, other conversations in the same space, public address (PA) systems, radios, flickering lights).

— Individuals may need to use a communication board or another type of equipment or technology to assist with communication.

Persons Who Have Acquired/Traumatic Brain Injury

— Help keep a conversation on track. People with brain injuries may digress or change course during a conversation. Redirect them using appropriate cues and reminders.

— Repeat important information or questions. Summarize and review where necessary.

— Offer to make notes for the person to take with them after the meeting.

— Keep the environment free of distractions.

— Certain individuals may exhibit impulsive, irritable, or egocentric behavior.

— If you did not understand the individual, ask for clarification. Do not pretend to understand or make assumptions.

Persons With Mental Health or Psychiatric Disabilities

— People with mental health disabilities do not necessarily have an intellectual or cognitive disability.

— Some people with mental health disabilities may experience difficulties with their attention span or discussing topics that produce anxiety.

— Some people with mental health disabilities may overreact to emotionally charged topics or conversations, which can lead to miscommunication or misunderstandings.

— Some people with severe mental health or psychiatric disabilities may have difficulty processing or expressing emotions.

— Some people may not be able to understand and process what is being said to them, due to interference of the mental health disability.

Persons With Hidden Disabilities

— Many people have a disability that is not obvious (eg, back injuries, medical conditions, mental health, traumatic brain injury or acquired brain injury).

— A person may have trouble following complex vocal or written instructions.

— A person may have a delay in their response to questions.

— Someone may seem angry, but they may only be frustrated, feeling vulnerable, or they may be experiencing pain.

References

1. Americans With Disabilities Act, 42 USC §12101 (1990).
2. Rehabilitation Act, 29 USC §701 (1973).
3. Patient Protection and Affordable Care Act, Pub L No. 111-148, 124 Stat 119.
4. United Nations. *The Convention on the Rights of Persons With Disabilities: Training Guide*. Geneva, Switzerland: United Nations; 2014. *Professional Training Series*; no 19.
5. Developmental Disabilities Assistance and Bill of Rights Act of 2000, Pub L No. 106-402, 114 Stat 1677.
6. Patient Protection and Affordable Care Act, Pub L No. 111-148, 124 Stat 119.
7. Individuals With Disabilities Education Act, Pub L No. 101-476, 104 Stat 1142.
8. Centers for Disease Control and Prevention. Key findings: trends in the prevalence of developmental disabilities in U.S. children, 1997-2008. Centers for Disease Control and Prevention Web site. https://www.cdc.gov/ncbddd/developmentaldisabilities/features/birthdefects-dd-keyfindings.html. Accessed January 18, 2018.
9. Ammerman RT, Baladerian NJ. *Maltreatment of Children With Disabilities*. Chicago, IL: National Committee to Prevent Child Abuse; 1993.
10. van Dyck PC, Kogan MD, McPherson MG, Weissman GR, Newacheck PW. Prevalence and characteristics of children with special health care needs. *Arch Pediatr Adolesc Med*. 2004;158(9):884-890.
11. Harrell E; US Department of Justice, Office of Justice Programs, Bureau of Justice Statistics. Crime against persons with disabilities, 2009-2015 - statistical tables. https://www.bjs.gov/content/pub/pdf/capd0915st.pdf. Published July 2017. Accessed January 7, 2019.
12. US Department of Health and Human Services; Administration for Children and Families; Administration on Children, Youth and Families; Children's Bureau. Child maltreatment 2015. https://www.acf.hhs.gov/sites/default/files/cb/cm2015.pdf. Accessed January 7, 2019.
13. Children's Bureau; US Department of Health and Human Services; Administration for Children and Families; Administration on Children, Youth and Families. The risk and prevention of maltreatment of children with disabilities. https://www.childwelfare.gov/pubPDFs/focus.pdf. Accessed January 7, 2019.
14. Sullivan PM, Knutson JF. Maltreatment and disabilities: a population-based epidemiological study. *Child Abuse Negl*. 2000;24(10):1257-1273.

15. Mandell DS, Walrath CM, Manteuffel B, Sgro G, Pinto-Martin JA. The prevalence and correlates of abuse among children with autism served in comprehensive community-based mental health settings. *Child Abuse Negl.* 2005;29(12):1359-1372.

16. Sobsey D. *Violence and Abuse in the Lives of People with Disabilities: The End of Silent Acceptance?* Baltimore, MD: Paul H. Brookes; 1994.

17. Cross S, Kaye E, Ratnofsky A, et al. *Report on the Maltreatment of Children with Disabilities.* Washington, DC: U.S. Department of Health; Administration for Children and Families; Administration of Child Youth and Family; National Center on Child Abuse and Neglect; 1993.

18. Ammerman RT, Van Hasselt VB, Hersen M, McGonigle JJ, Lubetsky MJ. Abuse and neglect in psychiatrically hospitalized multi-handicapped children. *Child Abuse Negl.* 1989;13(3):335-343.

19. Kyam MH. Sexual abuse of deaf children: a retrospective analysis of the prevalence and characteristics of childhood sexual abuse among deaf adults in Norway. *Child Abuse Negl.* 2004;28(3):241-251.

20. Sullivan P, Cork PM. *Developmental Disabilities Training Project.* Omaha, NE: Center for Abused Children with Disabilities, Boys Town National Research Hospital, Nebraska Department of Health and Human Services; 1996.

21. Sobsey D, Mansell S. The prevention of sexual abuse of people with developmental disabilities. *Dev Disabil Bull.* 1990;18(2):51-66.

22. Gil E, Johnson TC. *Sexualized Children Assessment and Treatment of Sexualized Children Who Molest.* Rockville, MD: Launch Press; 1993.

23. 28 CFR §35.160(c)(2).

24. 28 CFR §36.303(c)(3).

25. 28 CFR §35.104.

26. Centers for Disease Control and Prevention. Identifying infants with hearing loss—United States, 1999–2007. *MMWR Morb Mortal Wkly Rep.* 2010;59(8):220-223.

27. Vohr B. Overview: infants and children with hearing loss—part I. *Ment Retard Dev Disabil Res Rev.* 2003;9(2):62-64.

28. US Department of Health and Human Services, National Institute on Deafness and Other Communication Disorders. Cochlear implants. National Institute on Deafness and Other Communication Disorders Web site. https://www.nidcd.nih.gov/health/cochlear-implants. Updated March 6, 2017. Accessed January 7, 2019.

29. Mitchell RE, Karchmer MA. Chasing the mythical ten percent: parental hearing status of deaf and hard of hearing students in the United States. *Sign Language Studies.* 2004;4(2):138-163.

30. Knutson JF, Johnson CR, Sullivan PM. Disciplinary choices of mothers of deaf children and mothers of normally hearing children. *Child Abuse Negl.* 2004;28(9):925-937.

31. Dube W. Study: abuse rates higher among deaf and hard-of-hearing children compared with hearing youth. Rochester Institute of Technology University News Web site. https://www.rit.edu/news/story.php?id=48054. Published January 18, 2011. Accessed January 7, 2019.

32. Humphrey JA, Alcorn BJ. *So You Want to be an Interpreter? An Introduction to Sign Language Interpreting.* Amarillo, TX; H&H Publishers; 1994.
33. Lane H. *The Mask of Benevolence: Disabling the Deaf Community.* 2nd ed. San Diego, CA: Dawn Sign Press; 1999.
34. Padden C, Humphries T. *Deaf in American: Voices from a Culture.* Cambridge, MA: Harvard University Press; 1988.
35. Sacks OW. *Seeing Voices: A Journey Into the World of the Deaf.* Berkeley, CA: University of California Press; 1989.
36. Wilbur RB. *American Sign Language and Sign Systems: Research and Applications.* Baltimore, MD: University Park Press; 1979.
37. Isenhath JO. *The Linguistics of American Sign Language.* Jefferson, NC: McFarland & Company; 1990.
38. Davies J. Sexuality education for children with visual impairments. Texas School for the Blind and Visually Impaired Web site. https://www.tsbvi.edu/component/content/article/129-materials/3254. Accessed May 16, 2018.
39. McConachie HR, Moore V. Early expressive language of severely visually impaired children. *Dev Med Child Neurol.* 1994;36(3):230-240.
40. American Psychiatric Association. *Diagnostic and Statistical Manual of Mental Disorders.* 5th ed. Washington, DC: American Psychiatric Association; 2013.
41. US Department of Justice, Office of Justice Programs, Office for Victims of Crime. *Victims With Disabilities: The Forensic Interview.* Rev ed. Washington, DC: US Department of Justice, Office of Justice Programs, Office for Victims of Crime; 2011.
42. Brodie N, McColgan MD, Spector ND, Turchi RM. Child abuse in children and youth with special health care needs. *Pediatr Rev.* 2017;38(10):463-470.
43. American Speech-Language-Hearing Association. Augmentative and alternative communication (AAC). American Speech-Language-Hearing Association Web site. https://www.asha.org/public/speech/disorders/AAC/. Accessed January 7, 2019.
44. Christian CW, Lavelle JM, De Jong AR, Loiselle J, Brenner L, Joeffe M. Forensic evidence findings in prepubertal victims of sexual assault. *Pediatrics.* 2000;106(1 pt 1):100-104.
45. Parker T, Abramson PR. The law hath not been dead: protecting adults with mental retardation from sexual abuse and violation of their sexual freedom. *Ment Retard.* 33(4):257-263.
46. Adolescent Medicine Committee, Canadian Pediatric Society. Sexual abuse of adolescents with chronic conditions. *Pediatr Child Health.* 1997;2(3):212-213.
47. Allington-Smith P, Ball R, Haytor R. Management of sexually abused children with learning disabilities. *Adv Psychiatr Treat.* 2002;8(1):66-72.
48. Seven simple steps to keep your kids safe. From Darkness to Light Web site. https://www.d2l.org/seven-simple-steps-to-keep-your-kids-safe/. Accessed January 7, 2019.
49. Baladerian NJ. *A Risk Reduction Workbook for Parents and Service Providers: Policies and Practices to Reduce the Risk of Abuse, Including Sexual Violence, Against People with Intellectual and Developmental Disabilities.* 2nd ed. Los Angeles, CA: Spectrum Institute; 2014.

50. Marge, DK. *A Call to Action: Ending Crimes of Violence Against Children and Adults with Disabilities: A Report to the Nation 2003*. Syracuse, NY: SUNY Upstate Medical University; 2003.

51. Svevo K. Children with disabilities and child maltreatment. *Off Newsl Int Soc Prev Child Abuse & Negl.* 2005;14(2):8.

52. Orelove FP, Hollahan DJ, Myles KT. Maltreatment of children with disabilities: training needs for a collaborative response. *Child Abuse Negl.* 2000;24(2):185-194.

53. Bainton G. Methods: conscious and unconscious. In: Bainton G, ed. *The Art of Authorship: Literary Reminiscences, Methods of Work, and Advice to Young Beginners, Personally Contributed by Leading Authors of the Day*. New York, NY: D Appleton and Company; 1890:55-118.

54. Rosa's Law, Pub L No. 111-256, 124 Stat 2643.

55. Centers for Disease Control and Prevention. *Indoor Environmental Quality Policy*. Atlanta, GA: Centers for Disease Control and Prevention; 2009.

Additional Reading and Resources

Baladerian NJ. A guide on responding to suspected abuse of people with developmental disabilities: ten tips for parents or family members whose loved one receives school, residential, transportation, day program, vocational, or other direct or support services. Disability and Abuse Project Web site. http://www.disabilityandabuse.org/survey/10-tips.pdf. Accessed January 7, 2019.

Baladerian NJ. Recognition of a pattern, call for a response: a "rule out abuse campaign" for physicians (part 1). Disability and Abuse Project Web site. http://disabilityandabuse.org/rule-out-abuse-physicians.pdf. Accessed January 7, 2019.

Baladerian NJ. Rule out abuse campaign part 2. Disability and Abuse Project Web site. http://disabilityandabuse.org/rule-out-abuse-physicians-2.pdf. Accessed January 7, 2019.

Disability and Abuse Project. Home page. Disability and Abuse Project Web site. http://disabilityandabuse.org/. Accessed January 7, 2019.

Marshall S, Joffee E. ADA checklist: health care facilities and service providers: ensuring access to services and facilities by patients who are blind, deaf-blind, or visually impaired. American Foundation for the Blind Web site. http://www.afb.org/info/programs-and-services/public-policy-center/civil-rights/advocacy-resources/ada-checklist-health-care-facilities-and-service-providers/12345. Accessed January 7, 2019.

Myers L. *Communication Book for Individuals Who Are Victims of Violence and Abuse.* Milwaukee, WI: Independence First; 2005.

National Children's Advocacy Center. Extended forensic interview training. National Children's Advocacy Center Web site. https://www.nationalcac.org/extended-forensic-interview-training/. Accessed January 7, 2019.

Simpson KM, ed. Table manners and beyond: the gynecological exam for women with developmental disabilities and other functional limitations. The Lurie Institute for Disability Policy Web site. http://lurie.brandeis.edu/pdfs/TableMannersandBeyond.pdf. Accessed January 7, 2019.

US Department of Justice, Civil Rights Division, Disability Rights Section. *Americans with Disabilities Act Business Brief: Communicating with People Who Are Deaf or Hard of Hearing in Hospital Settings*. Washington, DC: US Department of Justice; 2003.

US Department of Justice, Civil Rights Division, Disability Rights Section; US Department of Health and Human Services, Office for Civil Rights. Americans with Disabilities Act: access to medical care for individuals with mobility disabilities. Americans with Disabilities Act Web site. https://www.ada.gov/medcare_mobility_ta/medcare_ta.htm. Published July 2010. Accessed January 7, 2019.

US Department of Justice, Office of Justice Programs, Office for Victims of Crime. Victims with disabilities: collaborative, multidisciplinary first response: techniques for first responders called to help crime victims who have disabilities. Office for Victims of Crime Web site. https://www.ovc.gov/publications/infores/pdftxt/VwD_FirstResponse.pdf. Revised January 2011. February 8, 2018.

US Department of Justice, Office of Justice Programs, Office for Victims of Crime. *Victims with Disabilities: Collaborative, Multidisciplinary First Response* [DVD]. Rev ed. Washington, DC: US Department of Justice, Office of Justice Programs, Office for Victims of Crime; 2011.

US Department of Justice, Office of Justice Programs, Office for Victims of Crime. Victims with disabilities: the forensic interview: techniques for interviewing victims with communication and/or cognitive disabilities. Office for Victims of Crime Web site. https://www.ovc.gov/publications/infores/pdftxt/VictimsGuideBook.pdf. Revised July 2011. Accessed January 7, 2019.

US Department of Justice, Office of Justice Programs, Office for Victims of Crime. *Victims with Disabilities: The Forensic Interview* [DVD]. Rev ed. Washington, DC: US Department of Justice, Office of Justice Programs, Office for Victims of Crime; 2011.

Chapter 18

The Medical Professional's Guide to Court Process and Procedures

Craig L. Barlow, JD

Introduction

Medical professionals who treat children who have been sexually abused face many challenges. Care of children and diagnosis of their injuries and conditions are activities for which medical professionals are prepared and well trained. In these situations, they function in a familiar setting. However, when allegations of child sexual abuse become part of the legal system, the nature of the challenges faced changes. At some point in their careers, most medical professionals engaged in cases of suspected child sexual abuse will be involved in some aspect of the legal system, whether as an expert witness or otherwise. Therefore, it is vital that these professionals prepare for the experience by having at least a rudimentary understanding of how the legal system works. It is even more important that medical professionals learn to function comfortably and competently in the courtroom setting.

The Legal System

Law is a complex body of knowledge, process, and application. Most of the concepts presented in this chapter are simplified in the interest of the reader's time. It is important that medical professionals who appear in court focus on the essentials. As such, the information contained here is abridged and streamlined, with little mention of areas of the law that have slight bearing on the issue of child sexual abuse. Additionally, this chapter focuses on so-called common law court systems, such as those in the United States, Canada, and the United Kingdom, as opposed to civil law systems, such as those found in continental Europe and other regions. Cases in which medical professionals evaluate child victims of sexual abuse can be either civil or criminal. Cases in juvenile court involving abuse, neglect, or dependency are considered part of the civil law system. In almost every American jurisdiction, a judge is the sole fact-finder in juvenile court. The parties in juvenile court are the petitioner and respondent, and the case is generally referred to as "in the matter of [juvenile's initials]," or "In re [juvenile's initials]." The party bringing a petition in juvenile court, which is almost always the state or local government's family services agency, must prove its case by a standard of "clear and convincing evidence." This level of proof is greater than a "preponderance of the evidence," which is the usual standard in other cases, but it is less than the standard of "beyond a reasonable doubt," which must be met in criminal cases. Cases involving Native American children usually apply the "beyond a reasonable doubt" standard. In criminal cases, the state, acting through a district attorney, county attorney, state's attorney, or attorney general, is the plaintiff and the person charged with the crime is the defendant. The cases are usually styled as *The State of [state's name] versus* (often written as "*v.*") *[defendant's last name]*.

In almost all criminal cases, juries act as fact-finders while the judge rules on questions of law (ie, motions and objections) and gives instructions to the jury on legal principles that apply to the case. In juvenile court, the decision is called an ***order*** or ***ruling***. In criminal court, the ultimate decision is called a ***verdict***. Because cases in juvenile court are considered civil, not criminal, either party may appeal the decision of the court. In criminal cases, with very few and rare exceptions, only the defendant can appeal an adverse verdict. The Double Jeopardy Clause of the United States Constitution prohibits the government from appealing if the defendant is acquitted.

A Practical Guide to Testifying in Court

Medical professionals usually become involved in child sexual abuse cases because they treated or diagnosed a child's injuries, illness, or medical condition(s). Such situations often result in medical professionals being asked to appear in court as expert witnesses.

The testimony of expert witnesses is governed by special rules in a jurisdiction's rules of evidence. These rules are generally uniform from one state to another. They provide that a witness qualified by knowledge, skill, experience, training, or education may testify about scientific and medical concepts in the form of an opinion or otherwise. Unlike fact witnesses who receive a standard witness fee, expert witnesses may receive payment for time spent preparing for and giving testimony. An expert witness is never paid "for her testimony." That would be improper. However, payment for an expert's time is entirely appropriate.

There are a number of rules, both formal and informal, that govern what an expert witness can say when testifying. These rules additionally dictate how an expert witness, or any witness, should testify.

Formal Rules

A jurisdiction's rules of evidence allow experts to testify about what they perceive, what they conclude, and about other opinions and information on which they reasonably and regularly rely in forming opinions, which includes consultations with other experts. Experts can testify about what other experts have told them or what other experts have written if that information helps develop the testifying witness's opinions. Statements made by those outside of the courtroom that are presented by witnesses in court for the truth of the matter asserted are generally considered hearsay and thus inadmissible. The Federal Rules of Evidence, specifically Rule 801(c), define hearsay as "a statement, other than one made by the declarant while testifying at the trial or hearing, offered in evidence to prove the truth of the matter asserted." States' definitions are similar in this regard.[1]

There are, however, many exceptions to the hearsay rule. For example, if a witness testifies in court that she was told that it rained in Philadelphia last week in order to prove that it did, in fact, rain in Philadelphia last week, the statement is deemed hearsay because the witness is trying to prove it rained. However, if the witness provides that testimony only to offer evidence that a conversation about the weather in Philadelphia last week took place and not to establish the truth of the statement, it would not be considered hearsay. In other words, in the second situation, the testimony does not serve to prove the truth or validity of the content of the conversation—it merely attests to the fact that a conversation did occur, regardless of the accuracy or veracity of the conversation's content.

The exception to the hearsay rule most applicable to medical professionals is related to statements for purposes of medical diagnosis or treatment. This exception to the hearsay rule, a version of which is found in every jurisdiction, states[2]:

803(4). Statements for the purpose of medical diagnosis or treatment. Statements made for the purpose of medical diagnosis or treatment and describing medical history, or past or present symptoms, pain, or sensations, or the inception or general character of the cause or external source thereof insofar as reasonably pertinent to diagnosis or treatment.

Thus, statements made to a medical professional by a child seen for purposes of diagnosis or treatment may be testified to in court by the medical professional as proof of the veracity of what the child said. Statements by children could include information about the abusers' identities. Identification of a child's abuser is essential to the treatment of that child because it is imperative that there is no further contact between the abuser and the child.

Another exception to the hearsay rule that is important in some cases are statements made outside of court conveying present sense impressions; containing excited utterances; or about then-existing mental, emotional, or physical conditions. These statements are not excluded by the hearsay rule and are often witnessed by others who are not medical professionals (eg, police officers, 911 operators). When a rule of evidence is involved in a case, the medical professional should consult with the lawyer who is calling the professional as a witness, prior to providing any testimony, about the application of the rule. There are other elements relating to the formal rules of evidence that might affect the testimony of medical professionals: namely, the testimony's relevance, the weight of the evidence (ie, its prejudicial versus probative value), and whether the testimony involves business records or learned treatises. It is not the responsibility of medical professionals to seek training in the law so that they can be effective witnesses. The lawyer calling medical professionals as witnesses should be thoroughly versed in the formal rules and other conditions of testifying. The lawyer should be the one to advise witnesses about the rules that will apply to their testimony.

It is important for medical professionals being called as witnesses to communicate quickly and directly with the lawyer calling them as witnesses. Medical professionals should anticipate that the lawyer will explain the nature of the case, the times and places where the professional will testify, and any special circumstances or legal issues affecting the testimony. If this information is not provided in a timely manner, it is appropriate for the medical professional to diplomatically insist on it from the lawyer. The better the communication between the medical professional and the lawyer, the more effective and useful the testimony will be.

Medical professionals who treat children should be sensitive to the social dynamics of cultural and ethnic diversity. In some cultures, for example, making eye contact with a stranger or an elder is considered rude and disrespectful. In other cultures, failure to make eye contact is indicative of deception or fear. Medical professionals who treat children from different cultural, religious, and ethnic backgrounds should actively learn about cultural differences so they can more meaningfully care for their patients. Of particular importance to medical professionals who treat children from sovereign tribes is the Indian Child Welfare Act of 1978 (ICWA).[3] This federal law governs all children who are enrolled or eligible to be enrolled in a recognized Native American nation and has particular relevance in child neglect, dependency, and abuse cases. The ICWA also raises the standard of proof in certain child welfare cases from "clear and convincing" to "beyond a reasonable doubt." The medical professional and the lawyer have a heightened need to communicate thoroughly when handling cases involving children of diverse cultural, religious, or ethnic backgrounds.

Informal Rules

Besides the formal rules of testifying, there are many important informal rules about how to be an effective witness. **Table 18-1** provides specific suggestions for witnesses, which help them prepare and understand what is expected of them.

Table 18-1. Informal Rules of Testifying

BEFORE THE TRIAL

— Be prepared, and know the case before the trial.

— Review and be familiar with notes and reports and any medical articles relied on to inform opinions.

— Meet with the lawyer before the hearing and trial (you should call the lawyer to arrange the meeting).

— Review the reports of other experts who are involved in the case and ensure that the attorney is aware of your own research in scholarly journals that pertains to the subject matter of your testimony.

— Assist the attorney with difficult words, phrasing, and concepts so that he or she can be sure to substitute them with simpler terminology at the trial.

DURING QUESTIONING

— First, listen to a question in its entirety then take a moment to think about the answer. Second, answer the question.

— Do not begin thinking about your answer until the question has been fully stated.

— Easy questions require no thinking (eg, "What is your name?", "What is your job?").

— Answer only the question asked, which is corollary to listening to the full question.

— Do not volunteer unrequested information.

— Always be truthful, regardless of the anticipated outcome of the testimony.

— Do not anticipate where the questioning is leading. If you are anticipating where the questioning is leading, you are not concentrating on listening to the questions.

— Bear in mind that it does not matter what you think about the direction of the questions.

— Be a vessel of truth and information.

— Realize that it is extremely rare that the answer to any one question changes the outcome of the proceeding or trial.

— If you either misunderstand or did not hear a question, you can ask for it to be repeated. However, do not ask for a question to be repeated because you do not understand its purpose.

— Remember that it is acceptable to say "I do not know" if you do not know the answer to a question.

— You are also permitted to say "I do not remember" if you are uncertain of the facts relevant to a question; however, this answer should be used sparingly to preserve your credibility.

— Use common sense when you answer. For instance, if the question is, "Did this incident occur on Thursday or Friday?" and your memory is that it occurred on Wednesday, Thursday, or Friday, but you are unsure which day, you should answer "I am not sure which day, but it was Wednesday, Thursday, or Friday." The answer should not be simply "No."

— When in court, address your answers to the fact-finder (ie, either the jury or the judge).

(continued)

Table 18-1. Informal Rules of Testifying *(continued)*

DURING QUESTIONING *(CONTINUED)*

— Give answers naturally, not theatrically or flamboyantly.

— Avoid using highly technical words and phrases, as it is critical that the fact-finder understands your testimony.

— Do not read from notes unless absolutely necessary.

— During cross-examination, if you are asked about an article, book, or study, you should ask to see it and read it before answering questions about it.

— Avoid overreaching in your offered opinions: that is, do not profess to have knowledge of topics outside your area of expertise. If you are asked a question that pertains to matters outside your area of expertise you should briefly state so, then remain quiet.

— When an objection is made, stop talking until the judge rules.

— Be reserved. Do not attempt to argue with, fence, debate, outguess, trick, engage in wordplay with, deceive, charm, or flirt with opposing counsel during cross-examination.

— Do not let the questioning become a contest between you and the lawyer.

— In formulating your answers, focus on the words in the question, not the tone of the lawyer.

— Do not think of an answer as either helping or hurting the opposing lawyer; instead, think of them as assisting the fact-finder.

— You should shun jokes and wisecracks. The general rule is that only the judge, not the lawyers or witnesses, is allowed to make jokes.

There are also rules about what medical professionals can and cannot say substantively when testifying. They are permitted to testify about what information a child provided to them at the time of diagnosis or treatment of the child. This does not mean that they should conduct a forensic interview of the child for the planned purpose of acting as a conduit for the child's testimony. In the US Supreme Court case *Crawford v. Washington*,[4] the court considered the question of whether an out-of-court statement sought to be introduced at trial was "testimonial" or "nontestimonial." The Supreme Court held that if the out-of-court statement is testimonial (ie, elicited with a purpose to develop testimony for trial), it is inadmissible because it violates the Confrontation Clause of the Sixth Amendment, which guarantees a defendant the right to be confronted with those providing testimony against him, unless the witness is available to be cross-examined at trial. Since *Crawford*, many courts have applied the *Crawford* ruling to various types of out-of-court statements. Of particular interest to medical professionals is whether statements made by a patient for purposes of medical diagnosis or treatment are now inadmissible under *Crawford*. Almost all courts considering the issue have concluded that statements made for purposes of diagnosis and treatment are nontestimonial and, therefore, still admissible. Medical professionals are well advised, however, to be certain that the interviews with children they see are solely for purposes of diagnosis and treatment. Medical professionals should not conduct investigation-like forensic interviews with children as a way of seeking to elicit more information than is necessary for diagnosis and treatment.

Medical professionals are allowed to testify that an evaluation of a child is consistent with sexual abuse. Medical professionals may say they cannot rule out sexual abuse and can even say that it is their professional opinion that a child has been sexually abused. However, medical professionals can neither testify that a particular person sexually abused a child, nor can they testify that a child or another witness is telling the truth or is believable. Experts generally cannot testify about the profile of a sexual abuser of children and its similarity to the defendant's profile.

Ultimately, when medical professionals testify in court as expert witnesses, their purpose is to tell the truth and inform the fact-finder about information relative to their area of expertise. An expert's role in this setting is not as an advocate for the child or any particular person. Rather, advocacy in this situation is the responsibility of the lawyer. When called as an expert witness, it is especially incumbent upon the medical professional to speak truthfully and objectively. If the medical professional is prepared and informed, the experience of testifying in court can be effective and rewarding.

References

1. Myers JEB. *Myers on Evidence in Child, Domestic and Elder Abuse Cases.* New York, NY: Aspen Publishers; 2005
2. Utah R. Evid. 803(4) (2008).
3. Indian Child Welfare Act of 1978, 25 USC § 1901.
4. *Crawford v. Washington*, 541 US 36 (2004).

Chapter 19

THE ADVERSE EFFECTS OF SEXUAL ABUSE

Randell Alexander, MD, PhD

HARMS OF SEXUAL ABUSE

Sexual abuse is widely considered harmful, and many countries and jurisdictions have laws regarding the sexual exploitation of minors. In the United States, age of consent varies from 16 to 18 years; elsewhere in the world, it varies even more widely (eg, the age of consent in the Philippines is 12 years). Age of consent may vary based on gender, may be lower if a minor is getting married, or vary if one of the persons involved is in a position of authority, such as a teacher (eg, in England, Wales, and Sweden). Historically, the effective "age of consent" in humans and other mammals has been puberty. More recent laws have tended to increase age of consent, with respect for the concern that children are not developmentally ready for sex and its emotional and psychological implications until at least mid-puberty.

In 1999, the World Health Organization (WHO) defined child sexual abuse as follows.[1]

> Child sexual abuse is the involvement of a child in sexual activity that he or she does not fully comprehend, is unable to give informed consent to, or for which the child is not developmentally prepared and cannot give consent, or that violates the laws or social taboos of society. Child sexual abuse is evidenced by this activity between a child and an adult or another child who by age or development is in a relationship of responsibility, trust or power, the activity being intended to gratify or satisfy the needs of the other person. This may include but is not limited to:
>
> — The inducement or coercion of a child to engage in any unlawful sexual activity
>
> — The exploitative use of a child in prostitution or other unlawful sexual practices
>
> — The exploitative use of children in pornographic performance and materials

In refining legal concepts about sexual activity and ages of consent, science can contribute to the understanding of what the specific harms of sexual abuse and assault might be and how those harms impact victims.

As a pediatric concern, sexual abuse is relatively common.[2] Prevalence rates are susceptible to a number of reporting biases, but overall, prevalence of sexual abuse appears, in some samples, to be more than 10% and may be as high as 40% globally, with differences between genders.[3] The prevalence rate of sexual abuse is higher than the rates of asthma or ADHD, which might be around 5% and no more than 10%. Few pediatric diseases are as common as sexual abuse or child abuse in general, and few pose a similarly significant population health burden. The following overview illustrates key areas of interest related to the adverse effects of sexual abuse, summarizes some of the hundreds of studies regarding those effects, and explains how those studies methodologically explore the problem.

Mechanisms of Harm

The brain is the primary target organ of sexual abuse. Decades after abusive events occur, it is the behavioral and psychological scars of abuse, reflected in physiologic and anatomic underpinnings, that are likely to be problematic, not the residuals of physical injury. Other underappreciated targets include the neurohormonal systems, the immune system, and genetics.

Genetics

Telomeres are the ends of DNA strands that assist DNA duplication and cell division. They can be conceptualized as aglets—the ends of shoelaces. Each time DNA divides to create 2 cells, the telomeres are shortened. This shortening, a natural effect of growth and aging, continues until the telomeres reach the Hayflick limit (ie, the point at which a cell will no longer divide). At that point, the cell becomes senescent. On a cellular level, this is akin to "old age." Thus, telomere shortening and cell division are of particular interest with regard to development of diseases related to aging and life span of organisms overall. Acceleration of telomere shortening beyond normal growth is one of the negative outcomes of abuse.

In 2010, Tyrka et al[4] examined 31 adults (22 women, 9 men) aged 18 to 64 years. From each subject, they obtained a medical history, physical and neurological examination, blood chemistries, electrocardiogram, and urine analysis and toxicology. They excluded anyone with a psychiatric disorder and anyone using medicines that might influence brain or neurohormonal function. After administering the Childhood Trauma Questionnaire to assess for childhood maltreatment, including sexual abuse, only 10 subjects were found to have been maltreated, of whom 2 experienced sexual abuse. Nevertheless, overall child maltreatment, particularly physical and emotional neglect, was found to result in significantly shorter telomeres. While preliminary, the authors speculated that a mechanism such as glucocorticoid oxidative stress might damage the telomeres. Subsequently, Glass and colleagues[5(ppe21-ppe22)] used data from a twin study of 123 cases and 1751 controls. Using a short questionnaire about physical, sexual, and emotional abuse, they found no difference in telomere length. They argued that Tyrka et al's findings might result from confounding factors such as smoking, obesity, lack of exercise, or social class. In response, Tyrka et al[5(ppe23-ppe24)] noted that the sample size reported by Glass et al was smaller than it appeared, although it did include 34 victims of sexual abuse. They argued that the Childhood Trauma Questionnaire, as opposed to the several questions used by Glass et al, was validated and noted that they did, in fact, control for confounding factors. As such, the authors concluded that the study by Glass et al did not disprove their results.

Shalev and colleagues[6] considered telomere erosion as a potential mechanism linking stress to cellular aging, disease, and mortality. Using a prospective longitudinal design, they examined 239 children who were part of a larger ongoing study using buccal DNA samples. The children (49% females) were assessed for telomere length at 5 years of age and then again at 10 years of age, using quantitative PCR. Three types of violence were assessed: (1) exposure to domestic violence (Conflict Tactics Scale), (2) frequent bullying victimization, and (3) physical abuse (standardized clinical interview protocol). Mothers were interviewed when the children were 5, 7, and 10 years of age in order to determine these occurrences. There were 236 children in the study. Of those children, 108 had been exposed to some form of violence, including 63 who were victims of physical abuse. Thirty-nine had experienced 2 or 3 forms of violence. The authors made adjustments for sex, socioeconomic status, and body mass index (BMI). Children who were exposed to 2 or more types of violence were found to have more telomere erosion than children who experienced no exposure or exposure to only 1 type of violence. Physical abuse was the only single type of violence that demonstrated a statistically significant association with telomere erosion, but the most significant results were for all forms of violence combined. The consequences of this advanced telomere erosion are likely to impact life-long health. Although sexual abuse was not examined, the same stress mechanisms would presumably exist, and the results would be similar.

Looking at long-term effects of negative experiences on telomeres, Savolainen et al[7] used 2 distinct measures: (1) separation from parents and (2) self-reported traumatic experiences. The Helsinki Birth Cohort Study was used to identify participants. During World War II, approximately 70 000 children were evacuated from Finland to other countries, primarily Sweden and Denmark. Thus, they were temporarily separated from their parents. Self-reported traumatic experiences were assessed by the Traumatic Experiences Checklist, which includes questions about emotional neglect and emotional abuse; physical abuse; and about bizarre punishments, pain, and threat to life. There were 1486 participants averaging 61.5 years of age at the time of telomere assessment via PCR. Of these, 215 had been separated from their parents in childhood. Emotional traumas were more common in those who had been separated, though physical traumas were not. Telomere length was not found to be related either to experience of separation or lack of such experience nor was it found to be related to self-reported traumatic experiences. However, those with a combination of traumatic separation from parents and self-reported traumas had shorter telomeres. Thus, a more complex association of experiences or an accumulation of different types of traumas may be key to shortened telomeres.

Also looking at an older population, Mason et al[8] used the Nurses' Health Study II, which ascertained child physical and sexual abuse histories in 2001. Using the Revised Conflict Tactic Scale, they assessed for physical abuse in 1135 participants who had PCR telomere assessments. Of that group, 470 had experienced no physical abuse, 184 had experienced mild physical abuse, 283 had experienced moderate physical abuse, and 193 had experienced severe physical abuse. Regarding a history of sexual abuse, 660 reported no history, 248 reported a history of abusive touching only, and 219 reported a history of forced sex. There was no dose-response relationship for the severity of physical abuse and telomere length, but there was when comparing moderate physical abuse versus no history of abuse. No association with sexual abuse was found. The authors speculated that studies finding telomere associations to child abuse usually involved younger individuals.

Blaze, Asok, and Roth[9] in a review of telomeres and epigenetics, concluded that early life stresses result in alterations in telomere length and that such changes may be long term. Whether telomere reductions develop later, improve later, and the exact mechanisms by which they develop are subjects of further research. Interestingly, telomeres themselves are subject to epigenetic regulation, but this too is not well studied.

In 2016, Tyrka and colleagues[10] examined 290 healthy adults aged 18 to 61 years for telomere length, mitochondrial DNA copy number, and childhood adversity. They measured childhood adversity by loss of a parent before age 18 years and by the Childhood Trauma Questionnaire, concerning physical, sexual, and emotional abuse and physical and emotional neglect. Childhood adversity and lifetime psychopathology were each associated with shorter telomeres and a higher mitochondrial DNA copy number. This implies that childhood adversity alters mitochondrial biogenesis as well as telomere length.

In a large review of chronic social stress and telomere length, Oliveira et al[11] found that chronic social stress accompanied telomere shortening for both child and adult exposures, with most studies showing a significant relationship.

Humphreys et al[12] examined telomere length in adult women who experienced intimate partner violence (IPV). In their study, 61 formerly abused women were found to have significantly shorter telomeres than 41 nonabused women, even when controlling for multiple potential confounders. Length of time in an abusive relationship and having children while in an abusive relationship were associated with shorter length. This may help to explain the continued health problems of IPV victims, even after the abuse has ended. The findings also suggest the impact of duration of abuse.

Other genetic markers besides telomeres might reflect abuse. York et al[13] considered that telomere shortening might be hastened by stress inflammation leading to perturbations in the regulation or expression of several genes (eg, interleukins, tumor necrosis factor). Hypothesizing that other chromosome abnormalities might occur, they looked at cytokinesis-block micronucleus assay as a biomarker for estimating chromosomal damage associated with environmental insults or exposures. Micronuclei can occur during cell division, accumulate with age, and increase in patients with cancer, cardiovascular disease, Alzheimer's disease, and Parkinson's disease. Micronuclei (MN) are small cellular structures outside the nucleus of a cell that contain damaged chromosome fragments or whole chromosomes that were not incorporated into the nucleus after cell division. MN may occur by defects in the cell repair machinery and accumulation of DNA damages and chromosomal aberrations.[14] Adult female identical twins were asked about sexual abuse prior to age 16 years. Seventeen pairs of twins who were discordant for childhood sexual abuse (ie, one twin reported a history of abuse while the other did not) were sampled. Age of first abuse ranged from 5 to 16 years of age. Compared to the non-sexually abused twins, the twins who were exposed to childhood sexual abuse had an average increase in their frequency of micronuclei by 1.63. The authors noted a significant interaction between child sexual abuse history and age and suggested that the biological effects of sexual abuse on micronuclei formation might be cumulative. Because the subjects were identical twins with the same genetics and a similar environment, the effects seemed to be specific to the abuse. Extrapolating from previous data from healthy people, the "biological age" of the sexually abused twins was estimated to be 9.9 years older than that of the non-sexually abused twins. Therefore, because of a history of sexual abuse, life expectancy would be less and the onset of "old age" diseases would occur earlier.

In summary, these studies most often show:

1. Childhood maltreatment (and some adult maltreatment) may have an impact on telomere length and other markers of cellular stress
2. Sexual abuse also negatively impacts telomere length.
3. Telomere length is a proxy for cellular aging and also appears to be related to early morbidity and mortality.
4. Childhood maltreatment leaves its footprints in genetic and cellular makeup.

Epigenetics

The prefix "epi-" derives from Greek and can be understood as meaning "above" or "beyond." Epigenetics includes any process that alters gene activity without changing the DNA sequence.[15] This occurs by means of chemical changes interacting with the DNA molecules that regulate gene expression. The consequence is a change in phenotype without a change in genotype. Epigenetic changes occur naturally, but are also influenced by age, disease, and environment. These epigenetic changes can be transmitted to "daughter cells" (ie, either of the 2 cells resulting from cell division), although reversal of epigenetic changes is possible. Some of the primary mechanisms of epigenetics include: DNA methylation, acetylation, phosphorylation, ubiquitylation, sumoylation, chromatin (histone) modification, and gene slicing associated with noncoding RNA.

DNA methylation is the addition or removal of a methyl group (CH_3) to DNA, which modifies function or gene expression (eg, turning the gene off or on). This occurs predominantly where cytosine bases occur consecutively. The methyl group may be added to the 5-carbon cytosine ring resulting in 5-methylcytosine—the "fifth base" of DNA. Projecting into the major grove of DNA, this inhibits transcription. A variety of enzymes are involved in such processes. This can lead to demethylation as well.

Ubiquitylation is the process of attaching a small molecule (ubiquitin) to a target protein that may mark it for degradation, alter the cellular location, affect activity, or enhance or prevent protein interactions. Ubiquitin is found in almost all tissues, hence it is "ubiquitous." Sumoylation is a posttranslational modification process that is like ubiquitylation but involves small ubiquitin-like modifiers (SUMOs) instead.

There are a variety of ways in which the expression of DNA can be modified by many molecules, which is not as simple as DNA leading to life functions alone. The opportunity for the environment to modify what DNA does provides a complex and wonderful opportunity for the organism to adapt at cellular and macro levels that DNA coding alone would not. However, it also provides the opportunity for cellular dysfunctions and short-term adaptations that are hurtful in the long term.

In 2011, Beach et al[16] studied epigenetic processes linking child sexual abuse to symptoms of antisocial personality disorder. Previously, they found that overall hypermethylation of the *5HTT* promoter region (a portion of the chromosome) was associated with sexual abuse, harsh parenting, and physical abuse.[17] The 2011 study used 155 randomly selected female participants from the Iowa Adoptee Study. They were surveyed about sexual contact before 16 years of age, using a scale ranging from 0 (no sexual contact with a relative), 1 (sexual contact with a relative other than parent or grandparent), and 2 (involvement with a parent or grandparent). Lymphoblast cell line DNA was examined for methylation at each of the 71 CpG residues in the *5HTT* promotor island. An average residue value was used for analysis. Multiple factors were assessed to determine a final effects model. The adults were assessed for antisocial personality disorder. Childhood sexual abuse history was significantly related to increased methylation of the *5HTT* promotor region, which was related to increased antisocial personality disorder. The authors concluded that child sexual abuse may create long-lasting changes in methylation that lead to increases in the risk for adult antisocial behavior. Psychologically, being a victim of sexual abuse and having antisocial personality may not come as a surprise, but this study helps to elucidate the biological mechanism.

Also drawing from the Iowa Adoptee Study, Vijayendran et al[18] examined methylation in lymphoblast DNA from 158 female participants. They looked at 16 CpG residues spread across the SLC6A4 locus and analyzed their relationship to gene expression for two SLC6A4 splice variants. Examination of the CpG residues showed that methylation of one splice variant was influenced by both genotype and sex abuse history, while the methylation of another splice variant was influenced only by sexual abuse history. At other CpG pairs, methylation was not influenced by these factors. Thus the effects of methylation on transcription appears to vary by splice variant. This is a genetic area of interest for future studies of the effects of environment on epigenetics, perhaps especially for sexual abuse.

Comparing 96 maltreated children removed from their parents due to some type of child maltreatment to 96 matched control children, Yang et al[19] studied the epigenetic effects of abuse. For the maltreated children, some abuse types overlapped. Twenty-four percent were sexually abused, of whom 83% experienced genital fondling, oral-genital contact, or vaginal or anal penetration. After controlling for multiple possible confounders (eg, race, gender, age), there were significantly different methylation values at 2868 CpG sites. The pattern across all 23 pairs of chromosomes was that maltreated children had higher methylation values at sites associated with typically low- to mid-range methylation values and reduced methylation at sites with typically high methylation values. The genes involved contained numerous markers of known diseases and biological processes related to health problems associated with early childhood adversity. This suggests that epigenetic mechanisms may be partially responsible for health problems later in life.

Weder et al[20] explored epigenetics as a possible mechanism that links child abuse to a wide range of health problems later in life. They looked at 94 children (aged 5 to 14 years) within 6 months of removal from their parents' care due to reports of child abuse or neglect, with an average of 3 substantiated child abuse reports prior to removal. This group was compared to 96 nontraumatized children. Of the abused children, 92% experienced more than 1 type of maltreatment, 65% experienced physical abuse, 24% experienced sexual abuse, 83% experienced neglect, 65% experienced emotional abuse, and 70% witnessed domestic violence. Using the Schedule for Affective Disorders and Schizophrenia, the researchers measured depression in each child and in 1 biological parent or relative caregiver per child. When no biological parent or relative caregiver was available to complete the Schedule for Affective Disorders and Schizophrenia ($n = 32$), a foster parent or a residential staff member completed the Child Behavior Checklist. The maltreated children also completed the Posttraumatic Stress Disorder Checklist. Teacher reports, the Mood and Feelings Questionnaire, and other measures were used to derive an overall assessment of the maltreated children's well-being. Posttraumatic stress disorder (PTSD) was seen in 50% of the maltreated children, depression in 35%, and behavioral disorders in 25%. Notably, 88% of the children with depressive disorder also met criteria for PTSD. DNA was collected from saliva. The researchers found that 3 genes emerged as significant predictors of depression: (1) *ID3* (DNA-binding protein inhibitor), *TPPP* (tubulin polymerization-promoting protein), and *GRIN1* (glutamate NMDA receptor, NR1 subunit). *ID3* is involved in stress response, *GRIN1* is involved in neural plasticity, and *TPPP* is involved in neural circuitry development. Hence methylation at these sites was considered biologically relevant. The combination of these genes coupled with child maltreatment was thought to pose a risk for depression. However, the authors note that such changes are not necessarily permanent and interventions might prove useful.

In a comprehensive review, Nemeroff[21] noted that it is well established that child abuse is associated with psychiatric and medical disorders and that biological substrates are transformed and mediate the vulnerabilities and risks. Epigenetic mechanisms transduce environment stressors into disease vulnerability.

In summary, these studies most often show:

1. Genetic vulnerabilities enabled or modulated by maltreatment and other environmental experiences may exist.
2. Epigenetics explains an important mechanism by which the effect of the environment (eg, maltreatment) alters the genes. This may be beneficial in the short run, but it can lead to genetic expressions that cause disease or dysfunction later.
3. A number of candidate genes have been identified across a large number of studies (more than can be reviewed here). Further clarification will occur in the future.
4. Child abuse, including sexual abuse, leads to biological changes at the cellular level and is reflected psychologically and behaviorally during childhood and adult life. This is not inevitable, but it poses a substantial risk.

Effects on the Brain

A logical concern when dealing with stressful events is to consider the hypothalamic-pituitary-adrenal axis (HPA). In 1994, De Bellis et al[22] looked at 13 sexually abused girls ranging from 7 to 15 years of age (referred from child protective services [CPS]) and compared them to 13 matched non-sexually abused girls. Three consecutive 24-hour urine collections for urinary free cortisol were performed, as well as blood testing. Psychiatric profiles were obtained. Findings include:

— The sexually abused girls had more suicidal ideation, suicide attempts, and dysthymia than the nonabused girls.

— The sexually abused girls had significantly lower basal plasma ACTH levels.

— The sexually abused girls had normal urinary free cortisol and plasma ACTH responsiveness to ovine CRH stimulation.

The authors interpreted these findings as showing dysregulatory disorder of the HPA axis, showing that sexual abuse affects more than psychiatric morbidity alone.

Sexual abuse induces a cascade of neurohormonal and physiological effects regarding the brain and neurohormonal axes. Anderson et al[23] reviewed research showing that child abuse was associated with clinically significant increased EEG changes in the left hemisphere, left hemisphere EEG incoherence, a smaller left (but not right) hippocampus, thinning of the middle portion of the corpus callosum (in males more than in females), and that excessive glucocorticoids (or stress) damages areas of the brain such as the hippocampus. They postulated that the cerebellar vermis similarly would be vulnerable since it has the highest density of glucocorticoid receptors during development and may be sensitive to stress. Sixteen adult control subjects were matched to 8 subjects with a history of at least 3 episodes of forced sexual contact prior to 16 years of age that were accompanied by threats of harm and feelings of terror. Functional magnetic resonance imaging (fMRI) was used to determine blood flow in the vermis. As compared to the controls, the sexually abused subjects had higher T2 relaxation times in the vermis but not in the cerebral or cerebellar hemispheres. The relaxation times correlated with the Limbic System Checklist ratings for temporal lobe epilepsy-like symptomatology. These symptoms have been shown to correlate with drug use. Overall, the findings indicate an area of the brain that can be altered by sexual abuse stress leading to psychiatric problems and involving an area of the brain that is associated with a risk for substance abuse.

Parts of the brain may be made smaller as a result of childhood sexual abuse. Anderson and colleagues[24] examined the effects of sexual abuse based on when the abuse occurred. They recruited adults between 18 and 22 years of age who experienced 3 or more episodes of forced sexual contact at least 2 years prior to enrollment. For the purposes of the study, the episodes had to include threats of harm or feelings of terror or fear. The Traumatic Antecedents Questionnaire was used to support this determination. A variety of exclusion criteria were used so that other brain injuries or conditions were not confounding. The study included 26 abused women and 17 healthy comparison subjects. Unlike some prior studies, PTSD was not a selection criterion. MRI was used to measure volumes in different areas of the brain. Findings include:

— Hippocampus size was reduced if sexual abuse occurred at ages 3 to 5 years or at 11 to 13 years.

— The corpus callosum was smaller if abuse occurred between 9 and 10 years.

— The frontal cortex was reduced if the sexual abuse occurred between 14 and 16 years.

Data from several of the subjects could not be used for each brain region. The immature hippocampus may be especially sensitive to corticotropin-releasing hormone (CRH) in early childhood. The hippocampus matures early, but the prefrontal cortex matures later, hence the period of sensitivity to environmental stress. Similarly changes in the corpus callosum reflect the age of sensitivity to sexual abuse. These windows of sensitivity may contribute to a better understanding of brain changes related to sexual abuse and how therapy or medications might be targeted.

Another study looked at the gray matter volume in the visual cortex of young women who were exposed only to sexual abuse, not accompanied by physical abuse, neglect, or witnessing domestic violence.[25] The study included 23 abused women and 14 control women between 18 and 22 years of age. Inclusion criteria required 3 or more episodes of forced sexual contact with fear or terror occurring before 18 years of age and at least 2 years before enrollment. Four of the abused women had major depression, 4 had PTSD, and 1 had depersonalization disorder. MRI imaging found 2 significant clusters of gray matter volume loss: (1) the left primary and secondary visual cortex (18.1%) and (2) a smaller cluster on the right side (12.6%). More specifically, gray matter volume was reduced in the left and right lingual and inferior occipital gyri. This reduction was significantly associated with the duration of sexual abuse before age 12 years but not after. This suggests a sensitive period of brain development in this area in which sexual abuse is adverse, as was found by Anderson et al in 2008.[24] The affected areas might be involved in sleep (eg, nightmares) and facial perception.

A German study examined structural and functional limbic changes related to child abuse.[26] Subjects were recruited by local newspaper ads and public notices. The researchers enlisted 148 subjects. Experienced psychologists screened the subjects and determined they had no history of psychiatric disorders, including acceptable scores on psychometric testing. Two subjects were excluded for anatomic abnormalities of the brain. Imaging was done with fMRI. A face matching paradigm was used to investigate amygdala responsiveness. The Childhood Trauma Questionnaire was used to assess maltreatment during childhood. Physical neglect, followed by emotional abuse, sexual abuse, physical abuse, and emotional neglect, were all highly associated with reduced hippocampal volume. Findings include:

— Strong associations between amygdala responsiveness to negative facial expressions (threat stimulating) and reduced hippocampal volumes.

— Strong association between child abuse scores and amygdala responsiveness as well as reduced gray matter volume in the hippocampus, insula, orbitofrontal cortex, anterior cingulate gyrus, and caudate.

The authors concluded that limbic hyper responsiveness and reduced hippocampal volume could be mediators between childhood adverse experiences and development of emotional disorders. They also noted that by selecting subjects without psychiatric problems, the results would more directly reflect the effect of abuses themselves, rather than coexisting conditions.

In a 2011 review of neurodevelopmental biology associated with sexual abuse, De Bellis et al[27] noted that sexual abuse may lead to biological stress system dysregulation or PTSD anxiety symptoms in childhood. In turn, brain development may be physically altered (likely adversely) with consequent compromised neurocognitive and psychosocial outcomes. Using the term "developmental traumatology," they described how multiple disciplines contribute to the understanding of genes and life experiences. Abuse is seen as an extreme form of dysfunctional family and interpersonal functioning.

Multiple environmental and experiential factors can cause the brain to develop in ways that are adverse. It is likely that adverse experiences in childhood are worse than trauma experiences in adulthood due to the cellular microenvironments of the young brain. Rates of PTSD in abused children are similar to children traumatized by war and homicide. If the child does not develop PTSD, there is still an increased risk it will manifest in adulthood. The sympathetic nervous system, limbic-hypothalamic-pituitary-adrenal axis (LHPA), and the serotonin system are the 3 major neurobiological stress response systems that may be altered. The locus ceruleus nucleus (the major center for norepinephrine neurotransmitters) and the sympathetic nervous system lead to fight, flight, or fright reactions. This is altered with sexual abuse. The amygdala responds to the locus ceruleus to initiate the LHPA axis. PTSD is thought to be a consequence, as well as physical health and other mental health problems. Hyper-responsiveness creates an overly aggressive or timid person. Myelinated areas of the brain are especially susceptible to early exposure to stress chemicals. This can lead to size decreases in the corpus callosum, prefrontal areas, and overall size of the brain. The results predict behavioral problems, cognitive problems, and other social effects of abuse.

Hart and Rubia[28] point out that the areas of decreased brain volume are accompanied by deficits in structural interregional connectivity suggesting neural network abnormalities. Research with child abuse and neuroimaging is complicated by the frequent occurrence of comorbidities. However, behavior and affect control seem to be the major effects, for which there is a physiologic correlate. Academic achievement, IQ, memory, emotion processing, working memory, attention, and response inhibition are consistently seen as impairments from abuse. Along with functional MRI, the authors hoped that diffusion tensor imaging (DTI) might elucidate affected pathways.

Looking at neurocognitive outcomes from maltreatment, De Bellis et al[29] compared 3 groups: (1) maltreated youth with PTSD (n=60), (2) maltreated youth without PTSD (n=38), and (3) 104 controls. Ages ranged from approximately 6 to 18 years of age. Maltreatment was defined as positive forensic investigations by CPS for physical, sexual, or emotional abuse or neglect. They excluded participants with an IQ of less than 70, disabilities that made an interview difficult, significant medical and mental health conditions, significant prenatal problems, or exposure to alcohol or substance use disorder. The research assessment took 6 to 8 hours to complete and consisted of a variety of clinical measures of behavior and functioning. Neuropsychological measures included IQ testing, fine motor, attention, language, visual-spatial, memory-learning, executive, and academic achievement domains. Archival records (birth records, pediatric records, school attendance, forensic and CPS records) were used to ascertain mental health symptoms, trauma, and medical history information to see if inclusion criteria were met. Children with maltreatment and PTSD had a higher level of dissociative symptoms, internalizing, and total behavior problems on the Child Behavior Checklist and lower levels of global functioning than the maltreated children without PTSD and the comparison group. Maltreated children with PTSD had significantly more lifetime types of maltreatment experiences and more physical abuse. The comparison group performed better in general than the maltreatment groups. Sexual abuse was negatively correlated with language and memory, suggesting poorer cognitive outcomes than other forms of maltreatment. Receptive language and general memory were the main negative effects. Small effects were seen on visuospatial abilities and PTSD. Cumulative lifetime maltreatment resulted in poorer academic achievement. The results indicate that maltreatment negatively affects neuropsychological functioning. The results are not surprising in light of prior research, but help to further define how bad child abuse is for the brain.

A study by Heim et al[30] found that sexual abuse results in brain changes and, therefore, changes in sexual dysfunction later in life. The authors recruited 51 healthy adult women without substance or alcohol abuse and free of medication or mental health concerns. They used the Childhood Trauma Questionnaire to determine what type of abuse (if any) the subjects had experienced. The study found that 55% of subjects had moderate to severe maltreatment and 45% had none to low maltreatment. Magnetic resonance imaging was performed to assess cortical thickness. Widespread cortical thinning was determined to have occurred as a result of childhood maltreatment, especially in the left hemispheric lateral somatosensory area in anatomical locations associated with sensory representations of the female clitoris and surrounding genital area and in the mouth area. When sexual abuse was specifically examined, it was highly specific and significant to these areas, whereas emotional abuse was associated with thinning in regions related to self-awareness and self-evaluation. It was hypothesized that childhood adversity was associated with pronounced neuroplastic changes, resulting in cortical thinning in areas associated with the sexual abuse experience. This may be a protective response, allowing children to adapt to adverse experiences, but in adulthood, it can lead to sexual dysfunction by which sensory representations for pleasure are diminished.

In a study of female twin pairs, reduced hippocampal volume was found associated with maltreatment.[31] Furthermore, if maltreatment was experienced later in childhood, the reduction was more severe. This might be related to neurodevelopment and a developmentally sensitive period of life. Alternatively, it could be that older children are better able to conceptualize what abuse, especially sexual abuse, entails; therefore, the stress may be more salient. The authors also conducted a meta-analysis of 49 studies of hippocampal volume and child maltreatment. They found that reduction of hippocampal volume was most pronounced if the maltreatment occurred in middle childhood versus early childhood or adolescence. This suggests the significance of a physiologically sensitive period for these neuroanatomical deficits.

In a study of 35 females sexually abused as children and 24 controls, Ben-Amitay et al[32] examined various psychophysiologic measures to determine if sexual abuse results in over-reactivity to stimuli.[32] Electroencephalography, frontalis electromyography, electrodermal activity and heart rate parameters were monitored while participants looked at a set of pictures representing various stimuli. The pictures were selected from the International Affective Picture System and consisted of neutral, positive, negative, and sexually allusive (ie, suggestive) themes. Each image was presented on a computer screen for 45 seconds followed by a rest period of 30 seconds. When viewing neutral pictures, abused females experienced higher heart rates than controls. Abused females also experienced higher heart rates, EMG, and theta waves when viewing sexually allusive pictures. The more time that had elapsed between abusive experiences and time of testing, the weaker the physiological reaction in the abused females. The authors note that the dysfunctional regulation of physiologic stress systems associated with child sexual abuse may endanger children with various stress and anxiety disorders.

In contrast, Nemeroff[21] found that amygdala volume is increased in individuals exposed to child maltreatment. This has been associated with elevated CRF concentrations. Amygdala reactivity is associated with anxiety states.

In summary, these studies most often show:

1. Child abuse and sexual abuse are associated with the development of smaller parts of the brain, including the hippocampus (which includes short term memory as one of its functions), corpus callosum, grey matter of the visual cortex, insula, orbitofrontal cortex, anterior cingulate gyrus, and caudate nucleus.

2. Child abuse and sexual abuse are associated with development of a bigger amygdala, which is a functional response to an environment in which stress or threats occur.
3. When compared to nonabused controls, the limbic system and neurophysiological systems in abused individuals are hyperreactive. This reflects a functional response to an environment in which stress or threats occur.
4. Although possibly adaptive in the short term, these changes lead to or reflect an increased risk for behavioral, emotional, and life-functional problems in the long term. They are a risk to health and even to life expectancy.

As noted by De Bellis and colleagues,[29] "all [CPS-identified] youth should be comprehensively examined for the integrity of their neuropsychological functioning and academic skills, regardless of the presence or absence of mental health symptoms." An even wider range of brain, physiologic, and life-impairing functions should also be assessed and treated. These results may not be completely reversible. Hence, prevention should be a priority.

Long-term Effects

Child sexual abuse encompasses life experiences ranging from anogenital penetration, genital contact, and other contact to exhibitionism and exposure to pornography. Given the range of experiences, the ages and relationships of those involved, and the duration and complexities of abuse, the outcomes of sexual abuse are diverse.[33] Depression in adults and sexualized behavior in children are among the best-documented outcomes. Prevention efforts often aim at teaching children to avoid or report abuse, but primary prevention directed at potential perpetrators is uncommon. Treatment, including trauma-focused cognitive behavioral therapy, has been better researched.

In a large study of 2759 sexually abused children assessed between 1964 and 1995, a public psychiatric database was linked to other health databases to determine outcomes.[34] Follow-up varied from 12 to 43 years after the assessment. This group was compared to a control group matched on gender and age groupings drawn from the national electoral database. Life-time contact with public mental health services was 23.3% in the sexually abused sample and 7.7% in the controls (ie, 3.65 times higher in the abused sample). Child sexual abuse accounted for 7.8% of all mental health contacts. These included psychosis, affective and anxiety disorders, substance abuse, and personality disorders. Risks were greater for individuals abused at older ages and for those exposed to penetration or multiple perpetrators.

Another long-term study from New Zealand[35] reviewed data from 987 members of a birth cohort from the Christchurch Health and Development Study. Participants were assessed for child sexual abuse at 18 and 21 years of age. They were assessed in terms of what occurred, how often it occurred, characteristics of the perpetrator(s), and other factors. A 4-point scale was derived:

1. No child sexual abuse (85.9% of the sample)
2. Noncontact abuse (2.7%)
3. Contact not involving attempted or completed sexual penetration (5.1%)
4. Attempted or completed sexual penetration involving oral, vaginal, and anal (6.3%)

Participants were questioned at ages 21, 25, and 30 years on a range of outcomes. Mental health problems at 30 years of age were worse the higher the participant scored on the scale. These problems included major depression, anxiety disorder, suicidal ideation, suicide attempt, alcohol dependence, illicit substance dependence, or any mental health problems. The severe sexual abuse group had about 2.5 times the number of problems compared to those who were not abused. Measures of well-being included the assessment of PTSD symptoms, self-esteem, life satisfaction, and partner relationship quality. All worsened with an increased sexual abuse score. Likewise, sexual risk-taking behaviors (eg, age of onset of sexual activity, number of sexual partners between 18 and 30 years of age, and number of unplanned pregnancies), physical health (eg, number of doctor or hospital contacts), and socioeconomic issues (eg, leaving school without qualifications, welfare dependence between 25 and 30 years, and gross income at 30 years) all worsened with an increased sexual abuse score. They found no difference between males and females. Although the individual effect sizes were small to moderate, the accumulative adverse effects on adult developmental outcomes were substantial. They emphasized that child sexual abuse has broad-ranging and complex sequelae that persist over time, which should be considered when providing long-term support and therapy. The authors also called for programs, policies, and interventions to prevent sexual abuse primarily.

In a review of the neurobiological effects of child abuse, Teicher and Samson[36] note that maltreatment is the most important preventable cause of psychopathology and accounts for up to 45% of the population attributable risk for childhood-onset psychiatric disorders. Sexual abuse, parental verbal abuse, and witnessing domestic violence affect brain regions such as auditory, visual, and somatosensory cortex and pathways associated with them. In contrast to volume reductions in the anterior cingulate, dorsal lateral prefrontal and orbitofrontal cortex, corpus callosum, and adult hippocampus, the amygdala has an enhanced response to emotional faces (over-reactivity) and a diminished striatal response to anticipated rewards (less happy). Various locations and pathways have time periods in which they are most vulnerable. Such changes should be seen as adaptive to adversity, facilitating survival and reproduction for the organism. However, they may be dysfunctional in nonabusive settings and for future adult functioning.

An Australian study examined a sample of 68 459 children from New South Wales.[37] Linking administrative data for children and their parents, any form of maltreatment was linked to developmental problems (physical, social, emotional, cognitive, and communication) by age 5. Children who were exposed to 2 or more types, with first maltreatment occurring after 3 years of age, were even more vulnerable on multiple domains. The idea of critical periods was considered.

In an extensive review of the neurobiological and clinical consequences of child abuse and neglect, Nemeroff[21] noted the multiple psychiatric and organ systems affected by abuse and related them to changes in the neuroendocrine and neurotransmitter systems. Proinflammatory cytokines, alterations in the brain, and gene and epigenetic consequences from abuse lead to disease vulnerability.

In response to the neurodevelopmental science and its effects on life-long health, the American Academy of Pediatrics (AAP) endorses an enhanced pediatric role in focusing on early childhood development, strategies to reduce toxic stress, and ways in which to mitigate the negative effects of abuse on development and health across the life span.[38,39] The AAP concludes that early experiences are built into bodies; significant adversity can produce physiologic disruptions or biological memories that undermine the development of the body's stress response systems and affect the developing brain, cardiovascular system, immune system, and metabolic regulatory controls; and these disruptions can persist into adulthood leading to lifelong impairments.[38] Training of physicians, medical homes, and advocacy are encouraged.

In summary, these studies most often show:

1. Sexual abuse and child abuse in general lead to long-term changes in adult functioning that appear to be dysfunctional even if they may have been adaptive at the time of the adversities.
2. There are underlying physical changes that help explain why certain health problems and behaviors are seen.
3. The effects are often persistent and may be permanent.
4. Prevention is, therefore, vital.

Adverse Childhood Experiences (ACEs)

One of the most visible conceptualizations about the impact of child abuse and other adversities arose from the Adverse Childhood Experiences study conducted by Vincent Felitti and Robert Anda.[40,41] Funded by the Centers for Disease Control and Prevention and conducted at Kaiser Permanente in San Diego, 17 337 adults were extensively queried about a variety of possible adverse childhood experiences which was then related to their health records. Ten categories of childhood adversity were identified: sexual abuse, physical abuse, psychological abuse, emotional neglect, physical neglect, alcoholism or drug use in the home, divorce or loss of biological parent, depression or mental illness in home, mother treated violently, or imprisoned household member. Not only were the individual adversities associated with worse health outcomes later in life, but the accumulation of categories of adversities dramatically and repeatedly increased risks for a wide variety of conditions. A major innovation in thinking about the impact of maltreatment was the creation of the Adverse Childhood Experience (ACE) score. The participants averaged 57 years of age. Instead of trying to ascertain how many times a child was sexually or physically abused (the neglect determination would be nearly impossible since most neglect is not a discrete event), instead they assigned a score of 0 (did not occur in childhood) or 1 (it did). The ACE score is the summation of each category. Thus, being sexually abused once or a hundred times equals a score of 1. As seen above, although multiple experiences within a category no doubt worsen outcome, the ACE score allows a summation across categories. This binary approach yielded impressive results.

There have been numerous studies in the United States and internationally that used the ACE approach or variations thereof. Findings typically include a dose-response relationship whereby as the ACE score increases, the dependent variable of interest increases as well. Examples include early-onset smoking, current adult smoking, and chronic obstructive pulmonary disease (ie, emphysema) increase as the ACE score increases. Alcoholism, intravenous drug use, chronic depression in women, suicide attempts, current depression, and rates of antidepressant prescriptions show the dose-response relationship. Impaired memory of childhood, hallucinations, serious job problems of a variety of sorts, and the likelihood of 3 or more marriages are related to ACEs. Heart disease, cancer, fractures, dying young, and numerous other health outcomes are strongly related to ACEs. The number of unexplained symptoms has a dose-response specifically to sexual abuse. ACEs is related to the likelihood of 50 or more sexual partners, and not surprisingly, the likelihood of sexually transmitted infection (STI).

In one study, Dong et al[42] looked at sexual abuse more specifically. They found that about 25% of women and 16 % of men had some sexual abuse experience and observed a strong relationship between sexual abuse and the other 9 categories of adversity, the strongest being with emotional abuse and other significant associations with physical abuse, physical neglect, and a mother treated violently. With such overlaps, the authors point out the need to assess for other forms of mistreatment besides child sexual abuse in isolation.

Dube et al[43] extended these findings using the same participants. They noted that men reported females as perpetrators of sexual abuse nearly 40% of the time, whereas women reported female perpetration only 6% of the time. The long-term impact on sexual abuse cut across multiple social and health problems, for both men and women. Suicide attempts were twice as likely for those sexually abused as children, who were also found to have a 40% increased risk of marrying an alcoholic and a 40% to 50% risk of current problems in a marriage. Thus, the impact of sexual abuse had no strong gender bias.

The impact of sexual abuse on a wide variety of conditions could be considered as a nonspecific risk factor for pathology of small to medium magnitude.[44] However, when considered in the context of the likelihood of multiple forms of maltreatment being present, the overall impact is large and persistent.[41]

By merely questioning about ACEs in clinical practice with over 100 000 adults, Felitti[41] found a 35% reduction in doctor visits and an 11% reduction in ER visits, without any substantial interventions such as therapy. Simply put, the opportunity to acknowledge one's childhood adversities in a clinical setting proved helpful to the Kaiser system, as a 35% reduction in doctor visits could translate into a savings of $2 billion in annual costs.

In summary, these studies most often show:

1. ACEs are one of the most powerful determinants of adult health.
2. Sexual abuse leads to numerous health and behavioral outcomes, some of which are not obvious.
3. Asking about ACEs alone in clinical practice may improve the health of patients. This does not reduce the need for therapy in serious cases. Given the numbers of people with adverse childhoods or who have experienced sexual abuse, attempting involvement in all such cases would simply overwhelm the treatment community.

Prevention of ACEs, including sexual abuse, could result in huge health care cost savings. More importantly, it could reduce human misery.

Intergenerational

For decades, researchers have known to test the effects of drugs on, not only the offspring of animals, but also the subsequent generations (F1 and F2 generations). With genetic and epigenetic changes in association with sexual abuse, and with brain and behavioral alterations, intergenerational effects seem possible.

Looking at the effects of maternal adverse childhood experiences on infant development, Racine et al[45] surveyed 1994 women averaging 31 years of age, who completed questionnaires at < 25 weeks and at 35 weeks gestation as well as at 4, 12, and 36 weeks of infant age. In addition to their ACE score at 36 months of infant age, pregnancy psychosocial risk, pregnancy health risk, postpartum psychosocial risk, infant health risk, maternal hostile behavior at 4 months of infant age, maternal socioeconomic, and child developmental outcome (Ages and Stages questionnaire at 12 months) were assessed. Path analysis determined that there was an association between maternal ACEs and infant development at 12 months via 2 pathways: biological health risk and psychosocial risk. The relationship to infant developmental outcomes begins prenatally suggesting supporting women with exposure to early adversity may improve outcomes for children.

Another study looked at both maternal and paternal ACEs and the association to infant development at 24 months of age.[46] Using a retrospective cohort design, 311 mother-child and 122 father-child pairs were enrolled. ACE scores were obtained from the parents at the 4 month visit. Resilience and postnatal depression scores were also obtained. The Ages and Stages Questionnaire was used at 24 months of age to determine suspected developmental delays of the infants. As the maternal ACE score increased, so did the estimated probability of infant delay. Increased paternal ACEs were also related to worse infant developmental outcomes. This suggests that assessing parent's ACE scores may be clinically relevant in pediatric primary care.

References

1. World Health Organization. *Report of the Consultation on Child Abuse Prevention.* Geneva, Switzerland; World Health Organization: 1999.

2. Pereda N, Guilera G, Forns M, Gómez-Benito J. The international epidemiology of child sexual abuse: a continuation of Finkelhor (1994). *Child Abuse Negl.* 2009;33(6):331-342.

3. Murray LK, Nguyen A, Cohen JA. Child sexual abuse. *Child Adolesc Psychiatr Clin N Am.* 2014;23(2):321-337.

4. Tyrka AR, Price LH, Kao HT, Porton B, Marsella SA, Carpenter LL. Childhood maltreatment and telomere shortening: preliminary support for an effect of early stress on cellular aging. *Biol Psychiatry.* 2010;67(6):531-534.

5. Glass D, Parts L, Knowles D, Aviv A, Spector TD. No correlation between childhood maltreatment and telomere length. *Biol Psychiatry.* 2010;68(6):e21-e22; author reply e23-e24.

6. Shalev I, Moffitt TE, Sugden K, et al. Exposure to violence during childhood is associated with telomere erosion from 5 to 10 years of age: a longitudinal study. *Mol Psychiatry.* 2013;18(5):576-581.

7. Savolainen K, Eriksson JG, Kananen L, et al. Associations between early life stress, self-reported traumatic experiences across the lifespan and leukocyte telomere length in elderly adults. *Biol Psychol.* 2014;97:35-42.

8. Mason SM, Prescott J, Tworoger SS, De Vivo I, Rich-Edwards J. Childhood physical and sexual abuse history and leukocyte telomere length among women in middle adulthood. *PLoS One.* 2015;10(6):e0124493.

9. Blaze J, Asok A, Roth TL. The long-term impact of adverse caregiving environments on epigenetic modifications and telomeres. *Front Behav Neurosci.* 2015;9:79.

10. Tyrka AR, Parade SH, Price LH, et al. Alterations of mitochondrial DNA copy number and telomere length with early adversity and psychopathology. *Biol Psychiatry.* 2016;79(2):78-86.

11. Oliveira BS, Zunzunegui MV, Quinlan J, Fahmi H, Tu MT, Guerra RO. Systematic review of the association between chronic social stress and telomere length: a life course perspective. *Ageing Res Rev.* 2016;26:37-52.

12. Humphreys J, Epel ES, Cooper BA, Lin J, Blackburn EH, Lee KA. Telomere shortening in formerly abused and never abused women. *Biol Res Nurs.* 2012;14(2):115-123.

13. York TP, Brumelle J, Juusola J, et al. Increased frequency of micronuclei in adults with a history of childhood sexual abuse: a discordant monozygotic twin study. *PLoS One.* 2013;8(1):e55337.

14. Luzhna L, Kathiria P, Kovalchuk O. Micronuclei in genotoxicity assessment: from genetics to epigenetics and beyond. *Front Genet.* 2013;4:131.

15. Weinhold B. Epigenetics: the science of change. *Environ Health Perspect.* 2006;114(3):A160-A167.

16. Beach SR, Brody GH, Todorov AA, Gunter TD, Philibert RA. Methylation at 5HTT mediates the impact of child sexual abuse on women's antisocial behavior: an examination of the Iowa adoptee sample. *Psychosom Med.* 2011;73(1):83-87.

17. Beach SRH, Brody GH, Todorov AA, Gunter TD, Philibert RA. Methylation at SLC6A4 is linked to family history of child abuse: an examination of the Iowa Adoptee sample. *Am J Med Genet B Neuropsychiatr Genet.* 2010;153B(2):710-713.

18. Vijayendran M, Beach SR, Plume JM, Brody GH, Philibert RA. Effects of genotype and child abuse on DNA methylation and gene expression at the serotonin transporter. *Front Psychiatry.* 2012;3:55.

19. Yang BZ, Zhang H, Ge W, et al. Child abuse and epigenetic mechanisms of disease risk. *Am J Prev Med.* 2013;44(2):101-107.

20. Weder N, Zhang H, Jensen K, et al. Child abuse, depression, and methylation in genes involved with stress, neural plasticity, and brain circuitry. *J Am Acad Child Adolesc Psychiatry.* 2014;53(4):417-424.

21. Nemeroff CB. Paradise lost: the neurobiological and clinical consequences of child abuse and neglect. *Neuron.* 2016;89(5):892-909.

22. De Bellis MD, Chrousos GP, Dorn LD, et al. Hypothalamic-pitutary-adrenal axis dysregulation in sexually abused girls. *J Clin Endocrinol Metab.* 1994;78(2):249-255.

23. Anderson CM, Teicher MH, Polcari A, Renshaw PF. Abnormal T2 relaxation time in the cerebellar vermis of adults sexually abused in childhood: potential role of the vermis in stress-enhanced risk for drug abuse. *Psychoneuroendocrinology.* 2002;27(1-2):231-244.

24. Andersen SL, Tomada A, Vincow ES, Valente E, Polcari A, Teicher MH. Preliminary evidence for sensitive periods in the effect of childhood sexual abuse on regional brain development. *J Neuropsychiatry Clin Neurosci.* 2008:20(3):292-301.

25. Tomoda A, Navalta CP, Polcari A, Sadato N, Teicher MH. Childhood sexual abuse is associated with reduced gray matter volume in visual cortex of young women. *Biol Psychiatry.* 2009;66(7):642-648.

26. Dannlowski U, Stuhrmann A, Beutelmann V, et al. Limbic scars: long-term consequences of childhood maltreatment revealed by functional and structural magnetic resonance imaging. *Biol Psychiatry.* 2012;71(4):286-293.

27. De Bellis MD, Spratt EG, Hooper SR. Neurodevelopmental biology associated with childhood sexual abuse. *J Child Sex Abus.* 2011;20(5):548-587.

28. Hart H, Rubia K. Neuroimaging of child abuse: a critical review. *Front Hum Neurosci.* 2012;6:52.

29. De Bellis MD, Woolley DP, Hooper SR. Neuropsychological findings in pediatric maltreatment: relationship of PTSD, dissociative symptoms, and abuse/neglect indices to neurocognitive outcomes. *Child Maltreat.* 2013;18(3):171-183.

30. Heim CM, Mayberg HS, Mletzko T, Nemeroff CB, Pruessner JC. Decreased cortical representation of genital somatosensory field after childhood sexual abuse. *Am J Psychiatry.* 2013;170(6):616-623.

31. Riem MM, Alink LR, Out D, Van Ijzendoorn MH, Bakermans-Kranenbrug MJ. Beating the brain about abuse: empirical and meta-analytic studies of the association between maltreatment and hippocampal volume across childhood and adolescence. *Dev Psychopathol.* 2015;27(2):507-520.

32. Ben-Amitay G, Kimchi N, Wolmer L, Toren P. Psychophysiological reactivity in child sexual abuse. *J Child Sex Abus.* 2016;25(2):185-200.

33. Putnam FW. Ten-year research update review: child sexual abuse. *J Am Acad Child Adolesc Psychiatry.* 2003;42(3):269-278.

34. Cutajar MC, Mullen PE, Ogloff JR, Thomas SD, Wells DL, Spataro J. Psychopathology in a large cohort of sexually abused children followed up to 43 years. *Child Abuse Negl.* 2010;34(11):813-822.

35. Fergusson DM, McLeod GF, Horwood LJ. Childhood sexual abuse and adult developmental outcomes: findings from a 30-year longitudinal study in New Zealand. *Child Abuse Negl.* 2013;37(9):664-674.

36. Teicher MH, Samson JA. Annual research review: enduring neurobiological effects of childhood abuse and neglect. *J Child Psychol Psychiatry.* 2016;57(3):241-266.

37. Green MJ, Tzoumakis S, McIntyre B, et al. Childhood maltreatment and early developmental vulnerabilities at age 5 years. *Child Dev.* 2018;89(5):1599-1612.

38. Shonkoff J, Garner AS; Committee on Psychosocial Aspects of Child and Family Health; Committee on Early Childhood, Adoption, and Dependent Care; Section on Developmental and Behavioral Pediatrics. The lifelong effects of early childhood adversity and toxic stress. *Pediatrics.* 2012;129(1):e232-e246.

39. Garner AS, Shonkoff JP; Committee on Psychosocial Aspects of Child and Family Health; Committee on Early Childhood, Adoption, and Dependent Care; Section on Developmental and Behavioral Pediatrics. Early childhood adversity, toxic stress, and the role of the pediatrician: translating developmental science into lifelong health. *Pediatrics.* 2012;129(1):e224-e231.

40. Fellitti VJ, Anda RF, Nordenberg D, et al. Relationship of childhood abuse and household dysfunction to many of the leading causes of death in adults: the adverse childhood experience (ACE) study. *Am J Prev Med.* 1998;14(4):245-258.

41. Felitti VJ, Anda RF. The lifelong effects of adverse childhood experiences. In: Chadwick DL, Giardino AP, Alexander R, Thackeray JD, Esernio-Jenssen D, eds. *Chadwick's Child Maltreatment: Sexual Abuse and Psychological Maltreatment.* Vol 2. 4th ed. Saint Louis, MO: STM Learning, Inc; 2014:203-215.

42. Dong M, Anda RF, Dube SR, Giles WH, Felitti VJ. The relationship of exposure to childhood sexual abuse to other forms of abuse, neglect, and household dysfunction during childhood. *Child Abuse Negl.* 2003;27(6):625-639.

43. Dube SR, Anda RF, Whitfield CL, et al. Long-term consequences of childhood sexual abuse by gender of victim. *Am J Prev Med.* 2005;28(5):430-438.

44. Maniglio R. The impact of child sexual abuse on health: a systematic review of reviews. *Clin Psychol Rev.* 2009;29(7):647-657.

45. Racine N, Plamondon A, Madigan S, McDonald S, Tough S. Maternal adverse childhood experiences and infant development. *Pediatrics.* 2018;141(4):e20172495.

46. Folger AT, Eismann EA, Stephenson NB, et al. Parental adverse childhood experiences and offspring development at 2 years of age. *Pediatrics.* 2018;141(4):e20172826.

Chapter 20

Therapy for the Child Sexual Abuse Victim

Jessica L. Griffin, PsyD*
Laura K. Murray, PhD
Judith A. Cohen, MD
Anthony P. Mannarino, PhD

Introduction

Child sexual abuse (CSA) is an all-too-common occurrence that transcends ethnicity, socioeconomic status, and gender.[1-3] The 2006 World Report on Violence against Children has estimated that, in a given year, approximately 150 million girls and 73 million boys are subject to CSA worldwide, including 1.2 million trafficked children and 1.8 million exploited through prostitution or pornography.[4]

There are multiple variables within a child sexual abuse case that complicate psychological treatment. First, the definition of CSA encompasses a wide range of activities such as intercourse, oral-genital contact, fondling, exposing children to sexual behavior, and the exploitation of a child via prostitution. Second, outcomes of abuse are affected by multiple characteristics such as the age and gender of the child; when the abuse occurred or began to occur; the age and gender of the perpetrator; the relationship between the perpetrator and the victim; the frequency, duration, and severity of the abuse; and the amount of threat or coercion. Third, the effects of CSA vary depending on a youth's vulnerability and resilience, preabuse functioning, risk and protective factors, and emotional support. Lastly, victims' often grave reluctance to disclose CSA or to bring CSA to the attention of authorities because of shame, fear and self-blame, or other cultural or sociological factors, makes treatment more difficult to navigate and the impact of CSA harder to ascertain.[5,6] Treatment should consider all these variables, addressing each client's needs while capitalizing on his or her strengths and resources.

This chapter begins by giving a brief overview of psychological symptoms commonly seen in children who have been sexually abused, within a framework that is useful in maximizing treatment approaches. Next, this chapter will outline the importance of early treatment and treatment engagement and the need for evidence-based, trauma-focused treatments that have demonstrated efficacy and effectiveness in well-designed studies. Finally, trauma-focused cognitive behavioral therapy (TF-CBT), the most rigorously scientifically tested trauma-focused child treatment to date, is briefly described.

Sequelae of Child Sexual Abuse

CSA can be a devastating experience causing negative short- and long-term consequences in the psychological and physical well-being of the victim; however, it is important to note that not all sexually abused children have serious ongoing psychological sequelae.[7,8] Research

**The author would like to thank Zlatina Kostova, PhD, Postdoctoral Associate at UMASS Medical School, for her assistance in the development of this chapter.*

shows that approximately 70% of initially asymptomatic children remain symptom-free over time, and approximately 30% go on to develop symptoms later.[9-11] Mannarino et al[11] have documented evidence of "sleeper effects," with serious symptoms not manifesting until a year after disclosure. By contrast, some studies have reported initial high levels of symptomology followed by a decline or fluctuation of symptoms over time.[12] For asymptomatic children, treatment focuses on prevention of further abuse incidences, safety planning, normalizing feelings, and psychoeducation for both the child and caregivers.

Unfortunately, the majority of sexually abused children do show psychological symptoms at some point. Research from both clinical and community samples continually demonstrates that sexually abused children exhibit more mental health symptoms than nonabused comparison children.[10,13-17] Furthermore, most often, CSA victims experience maltreatment of other types in addition to their sexual abuse. According to one estimate, up to 89% of sexual abuse cases occur in the presence of another type of child maltreatment,[18] making it difficult to isolate or identify the unique effects of CSA because symptoms are confounded with the impact of those other types of maltreatment or trauma.[19,20] Another implication, highlighted by Vaughn et al[21] is that the negative effect of childhood sexual abuse is exacerbated by its frequent co-occurrence with other types of maltreatment. A victim's psychopathological symptoms often have more to do with the extent—and the severity and chronicity—of abuse than with its specific type. Chronically, multiply maltreated children who experience an early age of onset of maltreatment within the caregiving environment are conceptualized as ***complexly traumatized.*** With increasing traumatic exposure comes increasing symptom and outcome complexity.[22] The cumulative impact of multiple traumatic experiences over an extended period is reflected in the range of interrelated social, emotional, and behavioral difficulties observed among complexly traumatized children, evidenced by disruptions across a variety of domains of development spanning attachment, biological processes, self-regulatory capacity, cognition, and self-concept.[23] Therefore, treatment must account for CSA co-occurring with other traumatic experiences, being part of cumulative trauma, or being one of multiple traumas occurring within complex trauma experiences and leading to complex trauma outcomes.

Because of this potential range of experiences, no one symptom denotes CSA. In fact, the effects of CSA commonly span both externalizing and internalizing symptoms and can vary significantly across developmental stages.[6,15,21] Symptoms may include anxiety; inappropriate sexual behavior and preoccupation[10,24-26]; anger, guilt, shame, and depression; and other emotional and behavioral difficulties.[27-34] Current research demonstrates that a high proportion of sexually abused children also suffer from posttraumatic stress disorder (PTSD),[25,35-38] with between 37% and 53% eventually meeting full diagnostic criteria for PTSD, and many more displaying partial criteria.[38-41] A diagnosis of PTSD is also associated with high suicide risk.[42-44] A history of childhood abuse or trauma more than doubles the likelihood of developing a major depressive episode[45,46] and conveys a markedly increased risk for suicide and suicidal behavior later in life.[47-52] For example, exposure to CSA was a significant predictor of suicidal ideation (holding constant the effects of combat exposure) among current and former US military service members.[53] Longitudinal studies have shown the persistence of this increased risk of suicidal behavior as a result of CSA.[54] In fact, even after controlling for other family problems such as caregiver mental illness, sexual abuse is found to account for almost 20% of the population-attributable risk for suicide attempts in young people.[48,49]

There is also now a substantial body of research literature that affirms the increased risk CSA victims have for various other mental health disorders and problems in their future, as well as the factors that tend to mediate these risks.[10,30,51,55-62] For example, one common consequence seen in individuals with CSA histories is adolescent or adult substance use.[44,63-65] Results from a cross-sectional psychiatric survey indicated that women experiencing nonconsensual intercourse before the age of 16 were—other things held constant—between 4 and 9 times more likely to have developed common psychiatric disorders such as depression, substance dependence, PTSD, and eating disorders.[44] Moreover, recently CSA has been associated with a greater vulnerability to cyberbullying. Rates are twice as high in sexually abused teens compared with nonvictims, and one of the forms of abuse most often reported by CSA victims is sexual harassment or exploitation via the Internet.[62,66]

CSA not only has deleterious effects on mental health but also alters victims' physical and neurobiological functioning. Research has demonstrated that CSA is related to a variety of physical conditions such as chronic pain, gastrointestinal diseases, irritable bowel syndrome, cardiovascular diseases, diabetes, metabolic syndrome, and sleep disorders.[67,68] Many studies have investigated the pathways between sexual abuse and adverse health outcomes, revealing multiple mechanisms.[69] The toxic stress caused by CSA may lead to lasting physiological changes in the body and brain. It aggravates allostatic load, which in turn increases the risk of illness.[70,71] The toxic stress of trauma may increase the body's immune response, leading to inflammation and contributing to an array of health problems.[72,73]

More recently, highly innovative research has also investigated neurological and neurocognitive effects of CSA, demonstrating that victims of CSA have more irregularities in the cortical and subcortical regions of their brains, which in turn affects their cognitive, behavioral, and psychological health.[74,75] Neuroimaging findings have opened up a new frontier in the investigation of the effects of child trauma, including CSA, showing that CSA can alter both structure and function of certain stress-susceptible regions in the brain. This has vastly improved our understanding of the neurobiological mechanisms in which psychiatric disorders result from child trauma.[76]

With regard to the treatment of sexually abused children who have this complex array of symptoms, it is often helpful to think in terms of 4 categories of symptoms—cognitive, emotional, behavioral, and relational—rather than only in terms of diagnoses. This allows a clinician or referring practitioner to better tailor treatment to the specific needs and strengths of each youth.

Cognitive Symptoms

Many sexually abused youth present with cognitive distortions or "unhelpful thoughts" that may lead to extreme distrust of others, feelings of self-blame, a negative view of the world, and so on.[77-79] A perceived lack of self-confidence and effective communication skills are also commonly found in maltreated youth.[80-82] Sexually abused youth also demonstrate unhelpful or inaccurate thoughts of low self-esteem and self-blame.[83-85] For example, youth may display dysfunctional ideas about relationships and difficulty with accurate judgment, which can interfere with their ability to assess risk and lead to poor decision making, impaired problem solving, and a distorted sense of reality.[80,86] In addition, many children who have been sexually abused report difficulty with attention and concentration in school or decreased academic performance.[87]

Emotional Symptoms

Emotional difficulties concomitant with CSA can include anxiety, sadness, anger, or guilt.[27,28,46] Deficits in affect regulation are consistently noted in sexually abused children.[88,89] In addition, shame and fear of rejection have been shown to be prominent in sexually abused children.[80,90-92] Depression symptoms are also highly correlated with child sexual abuse.[43,49,93-96]

Behavioral Symptoms

A wide variety of behavioral problems have been associated with CSA in general.[97] Numerous studies have found that sexually abused children exhibit sexualized behaviors more often than children in comparison groups.[24,98-100] Other behavioral problems may include aggression, violence, or impulsivity.[15,18,101-105] Donenberg et al[106] demonstrated that the sexual behavior among adolescent psychiatric patients who were sexually abused was impulsive and spontaneous, rather than a result of sound decision making. Impulsivity experienced by many CSA victims leads to increased suicide attempts, as well as other self-harming or life-threatening behaviors.[43] Youths who have experienced CSA are also more likely to show other maladaptive behavior patterns such as substance abuse[107] and higher numbers of sexual partners.[108] These two outcomes are intertwined in a way that complicates the sequelae of sexual abuse—victims are more likely to use drugs and alcohol to mitigate the intrusive thoughts, hyperarousal, or other symptoms related to CSA, which then increases their likelihood of sexually risky behaviors (eg, sex with high number of uncommitted partners, impulsive sex, other high-risk sexual behaviors).[108] In turn, this may increase the risk of further abuse, assault, or exposure to other traumatic situations. Evidence demonstrates that victims of CSA are at greater risk of sexual revictimization.[110]

Relational Symptoms

CSA occurs within a relational context and as such often results in feelings of betrayal and mistrust, difficulty establishing personal boundaries, and fear of establishing close relationships in the future. Current and future relationships are often affected for youth with CSA.[54,111] The impact on the relationship domain must be considered in treatment with CSA victims because treatment itself is conducted in a relational framework. Thus clinicians need to be cognizant of times in which the therapy relationship may serve as a trauma reminder for youth. Yet it is through the therapeutic relationship that healing from traumatic experiences can occur.[112]

Even with examining these clusters of symptoms to help guide appropriate intervention, the typical clinical picture varies widely within and across cases and is often very complex and severe. This can leave clinicians and referring professionals confused regarding where to start with treatment. The first step is for the therapist and families to understand the need for and importance of early treatment and then to engage families in therapy from the first contact with any professional.

Engagement of Families in Therapy

It is well documented in the United States that mental health services rarely reach those most in need.[113-119] Among families who do receive and attend treatment, 20% to 60% terminate treatment prematurely.[120-122] Traumatized populations are some of the most difficult to engage and maintain in treatment because of the common existence of avoidance symptoms, as well as parental stress and depression and severity of child dysfunction.[123,124] Moreover, many CSA survivors and their families will go to significant lengths to try to "simply forget," "move on," "leave the past behind," or "just deal with it." In the treatment of CSA, engagement needs to be at the forefront of delivery of services, whether that care is rendered by a clinician or any other professional who has contact with the family.

Research in the area of engagement has advanced since the late 1990s and has identified numerous barriers that prevent children and families from receiving the care they need.[125] For example, Fong et al[126] highlighted reasons that parents may not refer their child to mental health services after CSA, including a perceived absence of behavioral problems in their child as well as concerns that treatment would stigmatize or retraumatize the child. More generally, demographic and sociopsychological factors may play a role, alongside those perceptions of the benefits of and barriers to mental health services, in deterring caregivers from accessing treatment for their child. Another study of caregivers who did not link their abused children to mental health services suggested that not knowing where to access treatment (33% of respondents) and concerns about the cost (29%) were primary barriers.[127] Nock and Kazdin[128] found that parent expectancies were predictive of subsequent barriers to treatment participation and of premature termination from therapy. Family perceptions of the therapeutic relationship and the degree to which they are involved in service planning have also emerged as important issues in the continuation of treatment and in better outcomes.[129-131] McKay et al[132] have also shown that parental attitudes about mental health services; parental discipline effectiveness; family stress; and the presence of, or encouragement from, a social support network are significantly related to keeping a first appointment within an outpatient mental health program and to longer lengths of stay in services for urban youth and their families. Moreover, among adoptive parents there might be an under-recognition of mental health problems and a perception or fear that treatment will focus on parenting issues rather than understanding or acknowledging the child's specific problems.[133]

More recently there have been impressive strides in engagement strategies that address these barriers and significantly improve service usage for youth and their families, including reminders of appointments, and discussions during the initial telephone contact of overcoming potential barriers.[115,116,134,135] These strategies have resulted in an approximately 30% increase in attendance at an initial clinic appointment, a significant increase in the number of child mental health sessions, and fewer dropouts.[115] Thus treatment should include engagement during any and all contact with the child and adult caregiver. Interventions to streamline access to mental health services benefit from better informing caregivers about the specific benefits of treatment as well as proactively addressing their concerns.[126] In particular, caregivers should be informed about the potential gains from trauma-focused therapies, notably TF-CBT, as treatment directly addresses abuse experiences and associated negative cognitions.[102] Particularly with families that have experienced trauma and carry distrust, guilt, and shame, it is critical to begin addressing barriers and encouraging treatment immediately.

Responsibilities of Referring Practitioners and Families

The engagement of families, encouragement of treatment, and proper referral are intimately connected to knowledge about the treatment options for CSA victims. There is a need of interagency collaboration between the various mental health and child protection services in order to identify, assess, and refer children and their families to appropriate treatment.[136,137] Often when people are faced with a health-related problem or procedure, someone involved is asking a number of important questions such as what the procedure is, what the risks and benefits are, how long recovery is, how much pain is involved, if the doctor is qualified and experienced, and the number of successful outcomes. Referring professionals and even family members should begin to ask these same questions to mental health care providers. Professionals involved in the care of sexually abused children can effectively advocate for these children by referring them to programs or practitioners with the highest demonstrable treatment effectiveness.

Responsibilities of Mental Health Practitioners

Likewise, mental health care practitioners have a responsibility to choose and deliver the treatments that are most appropriate for their patients. Ours is a generation of "evidence-based" treatments, which have proven to be more appropriate and tailored for the specific symptoms presented by victims of childhood trauma.[102,138-141] Furthermore, these treatment strategies are not simply encouraged, they are quickly becoming mandated by many third party payers and federal and state funders and agencies. Nevertheless, many of the challenges of connecting science with real-world practice and policy have yet to be ironed out.[142,143] The successful implementation of evidence-based treatments is conditional on a number of factors, including characteristics of the providers and programs but also various features of the institutional context.[144-146] As such, it becomes even more important for practitioners themselves to be intimately familiar with the treatments available for particular populations and to be able to turn a critical eye toward the research behind them.

Clinical and Empirical Literature on the Treatment of CSA

Since the mid-1980s, the mental health treatment of child victims of sexual abuse has been examined by both the clinical and research communities. Theories have been developed that give direction to specific approaches for clinical intervention.[147,148] A large and rich body of clinical treatment literature has resulted, with descriptions of interventions that appear to be theoretically sound and have good clinical utility.[149-152] Most importantly, there now is a growing corpus of research literature detailing efficacy tests of mental health interventions in populations of sexually abused children.[8,102,153-162] Efficacy research within mental health treatment research is understood as laboratory-based studies that control for most variables, such as child and family diagnoses and characteristics, use of highly trained therapists, standardized assessments, strict adherence to a manual, and intensive supervision of therapists.[138,163]

Recent reviews describe certain treatment protocols for the treatment of sexually abused children that have yielded empirical data.[139,154] A Cochrane review assessed the effectiveness of psychological interventions in treating adolescents and children with PTSD, including PTSD resulting from sexual abuse.[164] Fourteen studies were reviewed, using 6 different therapies: (1) cognitive behavioral therapy (CBT); (2) exposure based; (3) psychodynamic; (4) narrative; (5) supportive counseling; and (6) eye-movement desensitization and reprocessing (EMDR). Of these, CBT was found to have the highest efficacy, with no adverse effects identified and significant reduction in PTSD and depression symptoms recorded for up to a year after treatment. A similar review[165] also evaluated randomized controlled trials (RCTs) of treatments for childhood trauma and found that trauma-focused cognitive behavioral therapy was the only one meeting criteria for a well-established treatment, based on Chambless and colleagues' categorization of evidence.[138,166]

Cognitive behavioral therapy is considered to be one of the most efficacious and well-supported interventions for sexual abuse.[141] This is not to say that other treatments are not effective; rather that CBT has the greatest empirical support, whereas other techniques have not been well evaluated or researched. For example, interventions based on attachment difficulties and emotional regulation (eg, attachment, self-regulation, competency—the ARC model) have also been found to be promising for complex trauma, although relatively few have been systematically evaluated and most are not yet considered evidence based.[167] Child-parent psychotherapy, a treatment targeted at young children ages 0 to 6 focusing on the parent-child dyad, has demonstrated positive outcomes across different types of child trauma (eg, exposure to domestic violence) and has a growing evidence base.[168] Allen et al[169] demonstrated significant improvement in sexual concerns and externalizing behavior among children with CSA history using another evidence-based intervention for childhood trauma, parent-child interaction therapy. That said, although the intervention showed positive results, it was focused on a young group of youths, children younger than 8 years old, and this study did not include a control group.

A meta-analysis[170] of children who were sexually or physically abused found that, when compared with other therapy (eg, play therapy[171]), TF-CBT consistently resulted in larger gains in fewer sessions. The median age ranged from 4 to 11 years with a maximum age of 18 years and a minimum age of 3 years. CBT for trauma consists of many well-established components initially developed for the treatment of fear and anxiety in adults[172,183] and commonly used with adult rape victims.[174,175] CBT has been adapted and applied to many problems in children and adolescents, such as depression and anxiety.[176-179] The shared components across disorders make sense given the range of symptoms that a sexually abused child might exhibit. Many cognitive behavioral treatment manuals for a particular disorder or symptom cluster are similar, and thus clinicians are often familiar with many of the components. However, in each evidence-based treatment, there is a particular theoretical basis, system, and flow to the order and application of the components. Most often, one component is designed to build on the next. In this way it is important to understand that the efficacy of each treatment modality is based on a certain amount of fidelity to the model.

In addition to efficacy trials—which test performance under ideal, controlled circumstances—some of these empirically supported treatments have benefited from effectiveness research, which involves shared, direct practice experience and feedback from thousands of clinicians providing these services, all of which created intervention models that were more flexible and applicable to the "real world" (see Schoenwald and Hoagwood[180] for a review of effectiveness and dissemination research). Effectiveness research is important in that it tests the performance of treatments under highly naturalistic conditions.[181,182] Still, researchers are finding that treatments validated by efficacy trials are not commonly offered in routine mental health practice settings.[183]

Empirical Reviews of Efficacious Treatments for Sexual Abuse

In recent reviews of treatments for abused children, only one model—trauma-focused cognitive behavioral therapy—was found to have enough empirical evidence to be deemed "well-supported and efficacious" by 2 independent groups.[184,185] The developers, Drs. Cohen, Mannarino, and Deblinger, began testing TF-CBT in the 1990s, and to date there have been more than 20 RCTs testing TF-CBT. In 1996, Deblinger et al[157] compared TF-CBT across 4 conditions: child only, parents only, both child and parent, and standard community care. The 2 conditions where children received treatment resulted in the greatest improvement of symptoms, with all TF-CBT conditions performing better than the standard community care. In the same year, Cohen and Mannarino[186] demonstrated that TF-CBT was superior to nondirective supportive therapy (NST) in reducing PTSD, internalizing, externalizing, and sexualized behavior symptoms in preschool children and their caregivers. An additional study by Cohen and Mannarino[156] found that TF-CBT was effective in improving depression and social competence in sexually abused children aged 8 to 14 years. A reduction in PTSD and dissociation symptoms was found in this population at a 1-year follow-up.[187] In a multisite RCT with 229 sexually abused children, TF-CBT was superior to child-centered supportive therapy in improving PTSD, depressive, anxiety, shame, and behavioral symptoms in children.[102] This study also demonstrated decreased depressive symptoms and an increase in parental support and positive parenting practices in the parents of sexually abused children. Since these initial treatment studies, there have been numerous RCTs by other independent researchers who have demonstrated that TF-CBT is superior to treatment as usual or to control groups at improving a variety of symptoms in sexually abused children.[188]

Over the last 10 years, the research base on TF-CBT has been growing exponentially across geographic, ethnic, religious, and socioeconomic groups and across treatment settings, demonstrating TF-CBT's proven effectiveness in reducing trauma symptoms and improving positive outcomes for young people who have been sexually abused as well as those who have had other traumatic experiences.[189] A recent randomized controlled study in Zambia comparing TF-CBT and treatment as usual among 257 orphan and vulnerable children found that children with a history of sexual abuse had disproportionate improvements after TF-CBT treatment, suggesting that it is a particularly effective treatment for the symptoms of CSA.[190] Another such study in Congo with girls who were victims of rape and sexual abuse in war found that group-based, culturally modified TF-CBT, even though delivered by facilitators without a mental health or medical background, significantly reduced PTSD, depression, and anxiety symptoms.[191] Underscoring the sustainability of the gains made through TF-CBT, these improvements were maintained at follow-up. Cohen et al[192] assessed the potential benefits and risks of adding a selective serotonin reuptake inhibitor (SSRI), sertraline, versus placebo to TF-CBT among 22 children who had experienced sexual abuse. Results demonstrated that both groups receiving TF-CBT improved significantly in PTSD and other clinical outcomes but to more or less the same extent, indicating that there was only minimal benefit in adding an SSRI to TF-CBT.

Clinically it is important to note that many of these studies included multiply traumatized children and children with complex trauma experiences and outcomes. In summary, several randomized controlled treatment trials and review studies have supported the efficacy of TF-CBT in treating the myriad symptoms common in sexually abused children as well as the multiple types of trauma comorbidly seen in sexual abuse victims.

TF-CBT has also been used in transportability, dissemination, and effectiveness studies that demonstrate its applicability and sustained effectiveness when used in a "real-world" setting. Through the efforts of The National Child Traumatic Stress Network[193] and the Medical University of South Carolina,[194] TF-CBT has been and continues to be extensively disseminated and implemented across the United States, resulting in ongoing effectiveness studies with culturally diverse children who have experienced varied types of traumatic life events. TF-CBT was also used in the Child and Adolescent Trauma Treatments and Services (CATS) Consortium, which is the largest youth trauma evaluation and treatment project associated with the September 11 attacks.[195]

TF-CBT has been adapted and used with several populations, including Latino/Hispanic populations,[196] Australians,[188] Africans,[159,190,191,197] Canadians,[198,199] and Europeans.[200-202] Alongside the evidence on sexual abuse reviewed earlier, other RCTs have found TF-CBT to be effective with other types of trauma, such as intimate partner violence,[203] adolescent pregnancy,[199] and single-incident trauma.[204,205] TF-CBT is also applicable and efficacious with children as young as 3[200,206] and has been adapted for the foster care system.[207]

A recent trial demonstrated the utility of an innovative delivery approach named Stepped Care TF-CBT. This is designed to provide first-line intervention and to ease some of the difficulties with standard treatment, conserve resources (notably therapists' time), and be easily accessible (through Web-based psychosocial information). Stepped Care TF-CBT proved not to be inferior to TF-CBT: it improved trauma-related symptoms (apart from externalizing symptoms) and maintained parent satisfaction.[208] The RCT conducted by Konanur et al,[209] with 113 children and their caregivers in different Canadian cities, demonstrated that TF-CBT can be successfully applied with demographically diverse populations in a community-based setting. This study also disproved the adage that time heals all wounds; children and families who were in the wait-list control group showed no clinical improvement, whereas those enrolled in TF-CBT reported significant reductions in posttraumatic stress symptoms.

TF-CBT has also been compared with another promising intervention for trauma, eye-movement desensitization and reprocessing.[210] EMDR is based on the desensitization of a traumatic memory while simultaneously concentrating on a distracting stimulus,[211] and has in recent years begun to be tested on youth with PTSD. Although the guidelines for PTSD by the National Institute for Health and Care Excellence[212] judged this treatment to show promising results, EMDR cannot yet be categorized as evidence-based in the same way as TF-CBT because it is not as well researched in children with PTSD. In the study reported by Diehle et al[210] 48 children were randomly assigned to EMDR or TF-CBT. Both treatments alleviated posttraumatic stress symptoms (PTSS), suggesting that both treatments are effective in this context. However, it is notable that parents in the TF-CBT group reported more positive treatment effects than parents in the EMDR group.

Recent evidence suggests that TF-CBT maintains its effectiveness with adaptations for different groups, or service and treatment settings.[213] It has demonstrated broad applicability and acceptability among ethnically diverse therapists with varied backgrounds and among children and parents.[214]

Treatment Description of TF-CBT and Its Components

TF-CBT is a components-based hybrid treatment model that integrates trauma-sensitive interventions; cognitive behavioral principles; and elements of humanistic, attachment, family, developmental neurobiology, and empowerment theoretical models and techniques into a treatment designed to address the unique needs of children with problems related to traumatic life experiences such as sexual abuse.[141] TF-CBT includes primary treatment components for children ages 3 to 18 years and for their nonoffending parents or primary caregivers. The mnemonic term ***CRAFTS*** spells out both the core values and the difficulties addressed by TF-CBT (**Table 20-1**). These are helpful in understanding the underlying foundation of TF-CBT and in balancing fidelity and flexibility when using this treatment.

There are 8 primary components of TF-CBT: **p**sychoeducation and parenting skills, **r**elaxation skills, **a**ffective expression and modulation skills, **c**ognitive coping skills, **t**rauma narration and processing, **i**n vivo mastery of trauma reminders, **c**onjoint child-parent sessions, and **e**nhancing future safety and development. These 8 elements spell out *PRACTICE* (**Table 20-2**). Many of these are common components found in many cognitive behavioral treatments for children and adolescents. Of note, gradual exposure to trauma is provided across treatment sessions.

Table 20-1. Difficulties Addressed by and Core Values of TF-CBT

Difficulties Addressed	Core Values
Cognitive problems	**C**omponents based
Relationship problems	**R**espectful of cultural values
Affective problems	**A**daptable and flexible
Family Problems	**F**amily focused
Traumatic behavior problems	**T**herapeutic relationship is central
Somatic problems	**S**elf-efficacy is emphasized

Table 20-2. Primary Components of TF-CBT
EIGHT COMPONENTS:
Psychoeducation and parenting skills
Relaxation skills
Affective expression and modulation skills
Cognitive coping and processing skills
Trauma narration and cognitive processing of trauma narration
In vivo mastery of trauma reminders
Conjoint parent-child sessions
Enhancing future safety and development

Each of these components has specific goals that should be achieved in order to maintain fidelity to the model. The flexibility comes in how a therapist actually achieves some of these goals. Additionally, although TF-CBT emphasizes its components-based approach, it is important to note that TF-CBT is also a phase-based intervention with 3 phases (safety and stabilization, trauma narration and processing, and integration and consolidation). For sexually abused youth who have complex trauma experiences and outcomes, TF-CBT treatment length may increase and additional modifications of treatment may be necessary (eg, moving safety to the beginning of treatment with a greater emphasis on safety and stability in the initial phases of treatment; focusing on "themes" in trauma narration rather than discrete incidents or traumatic experiences; other modifications as appropriate).[189]

The remainder of this chapter contains brief summaries of both goals and possible applications for each of the treatment components to give readers a basic understanding of an evidence-based cognitive behavioral treatment plan for sexually abused children. For a more complete understanding of TF-CBT, readers are strongly encouraged to visit the free online training in TF-CBT at the Medical University of South Carolina's Web site.[194]

Psychoeducation and Parenting Skills

Goals of Psychoeducation

— To normalize the child's and parent's (or parents') reactions to stress and trauma

— To provide information about sexual abuses and psychological and physiological reactions to stress and traumatic experiences

— To provide hope for child and family for healing and recovery after sexual abuse

— To educate the family about the benefits of and need for early treatment, as well as to present a clear plan (eg, how long treatment will last, treatment expectations)

— To discuss safety planning currently and for the future (if needed)

Application of Psychoeducation

Psychoeducation is a component that can be performed by anyone and should ideally begin with the patient's or caregiver's *first* encounter with any professional. The information provided to children and their families can take many forms and should vary with respect to the family and the child's developmental level. Some methods commonly used by practitioners include simply talking to the child and caregiver to give them information; asking them to read a book about how trauma (including sexual abuse) affects people; using the Internet to research the topic with the child or caregiver, including accessing handouts, videos, or apps for smartphones or tablets that have been developed on various topics (eg, natural disasters); or handing out written materials to parents. A clinician or referring practitioner talking about the many children he or she has seen with similar experiences and problems can provide information as well as normalize reactions to trauma. Every clinician and referring practitioner should provide families with information on the research behind the treatment choice, because doing so also achieves the goals of providing information, instilling hope, and educating the family about the need for early treatment. Psychoeducation may also include some information about what treatment will look like—for example, what the treatment schedule is and how long it will last. TF-CBT is a time-limited treatment with a beginning, middle, and end. Describing a plan and a timeline for treatment, with an emphasis that it is time limited (eg, will not take years), can help to assure families, take away any fear of the unknown, and promote attendance and treatment compliance.

Goals of Parenting Skills

— To explain the rationale for parent/caregiver inclusion in treatment

— To begin to establish the parent/caregiver as the person the child turns to for help in times of trouble

— To emphasize positive parenting skills and maximize effective parenting

Application of Parenting Skills

TF-CBT and CBT treatments in general view parents or caregivers as central therapeutic agents of change and include them in treatment because they can be the child's strongest source of healing.[141,147,155,157,186] Clinicians should convey that "a parent is the expert on their child." Emphasizing positive parenting practices, this component also includes working as needed on some parenting skills such as praise, selective attention, time outs, reward programs, use of functional behavioral analysis, and other behavior management techniques. Application of these behavioral techniques are done as needed in the family and are incorporated into the treatment by working on small goals throughout treatment rather than spending multiple full sessions on parenting skills alone.

Relaxation and Stress Management Skills

Goals

— To explain the body's responses to stress

— To reduce the physiological manifestations of stress and other trauma-related physiological symptoms

— To empower youth by increasing coping skills to better manage stress

Application

The key to application of relaxation is to make sure that the method taught is personally effective for each individual. Some of the most common relaxation techniques taught include progressive muscle relaxation, deep breathing, and positive self-talk; however, people relax using all types of methods. Other skills include exercise, yoga, meditation, guided imagery, gardening, spending time with pets or those close to the individual, dancing, and so on. Culturally relevant activities should be actively integrated into this component. Creative strategies and technology may be used within this component (eg, relaxation apps, music).

Affective Expression and Modulation Skills

Goals

— To accurately identify and describe a variety of emotions

— To understand the patient's (or caregiver's) feelings vocabulary

— To gain another way to talk about feelings (eg, as colors, objects)

— To understand the physical, concrete manifestation of emotions (eg, body, facial expressions)

— To comprehend different situations that correspond to the emotions

— To gain a sense of the strength and intensity of different feelings

— To express feelings more effectively rather than using maladaptive coping strategies

These goals might also be necessary:

— To teach control over thoughts that are negatively affecting emotions or functioning (eg, traumatic reminders, flashbacks)

— To increase positive emotions through positive self-talk

Application

This component can be achieved through a number of different techniques and can be altered depending on characteristics such as developmental age and culture. These may include board games (eg, feelings Jenga, memory games, feelings charades) or activities such as the "color your life" technique, which entails drawing a person and listing each emotion the child can come up with, asking which color "looks like" that feeling to them, drawing where in the body they feel it, and asking about a situation when they may have felt that way. Clinicians can use a child's interests in the Affective Expression and Modulation component (eg, books, music, movies, apps), encouraging the child to identify feelings in different characters. Thought-stopping techniques may be used when a child is having difficulty functioning because of traumatic reminders; such strategies might include visualizing a stop sign as a reminder to stop the intrusive thought and replace it with a more positive one. Thought stopping is done only on an as-needed basis (eg, when intrusive thoughts or images are so overwhelming they are unable to concentrate on daily tasks) and is not conducted with young children.

A clinician may also teach positive self-talk. Youth can learn to repeat a particular phrase such as "I am good at many things" or "Many people like me" to help regulate some of the negative emotions. This is also a very useful tool for parents. Parents of sexually abused children often feel great amounts of shame or guilt and may say things such as "I am a terrible parent" or "How could I not have protected my child?" Incorporating positive self-talk with caregivers—such as "I am helping my child in many ways"—can help them become more emotionally available to their children.

Cognitive Coping and Processing Skills: the Cognitive Triangle

Goals

— To help children and parents understand the cognitive triad: connections among thoughts, feelings, and behaviors, as they relate to everyday events

— To help children distinguish among thoughts, feelings, and behaviors

— To help youth and caregivers differentiate between accurate and inaccurate and helpful and unhelpful thoughts

— To help children and parents identify alternative thoughts and view events in more accurate and helpful ways

— To encourage parents to assist children in cognitive processing of upsetting situations and to use this in their own everyday lives to improve affective modulation

Application

To teach the connections among thoughts, feelings, and behaviors, the cognitive triangle is often used (**Figure 20-1**).

First, a clinician guides the child or parent to imagine a familiar situation that is not inherently emotional. For example, a social situation where a child walks into the lunch room and a group of friends are laughing could be used. On the other hand, a heated argument between a mother and a teenager who have a stressed relationship could still be very "raw" and may be more difficult to use in the initial teachings of the triangle.

The clinician walks the child or the caregiver through the triangle, asking what they were thinking during the situation, what they were feeling, and what their behaviors were, then points out the connections among them. A number of different scenarios are used so that the child or adolescent becomes aware of the interrelatedness of thoughts, feelings, and behaviors. For some youth, it may be helpful to also ask about experiences they had in their body (eg, heart racing, restlessness, other hyperarousal symptoms).

Trauma Narration and Processing

Goals

— To gain mastery over trauma reminders by unlinking thoughts, reminders, or discussions of the trauma from overwhelming emotions

— To resolve avoidance symptoms

— To correct distorted cognitions

— To model adaptive coping

— To identify and prepare for trauma or loss reminders

— To make meaning out of traumatic experiences

NOTE: The exposure component of processing a trauma is the component most often avoided in the treatment of CSA for a variety of reasons, including child discomfort, parent discomfort, and, most commonly, therapist discomfort. There is extensive literature indicating that gradual exposure treatment has demonstrated effectiveness in the treatment of a variety of anxiety-related illnesses.[174,175,215]

Application

This component is most often implemented in the form of a book that the child or adolescent creates; however, this so-called narrative can also be in the form of a poem, song, puppet show, computer presentation, interview, or other creative strategy. Regardless of the media chosen, the trauma narration often begins with designing a title page (or naming the puppet show, the song, etc.); in addition, for those children who are multiply traumatized (eg, polyvictimization, complex trauma), the creation of a table of contents or time line in which to lay out the periods of abuse or number of incidences or different types of traumatic experiences may be used. The first chapter (or first verse, act) includes innocuous information about the child such as his or

Figure 20-1. *A number of different scenarios are used so that the child or adolescent becomes aware of the interrelatedness of thoughts, feelings, and behaviors.*

The Cognitive Triangle

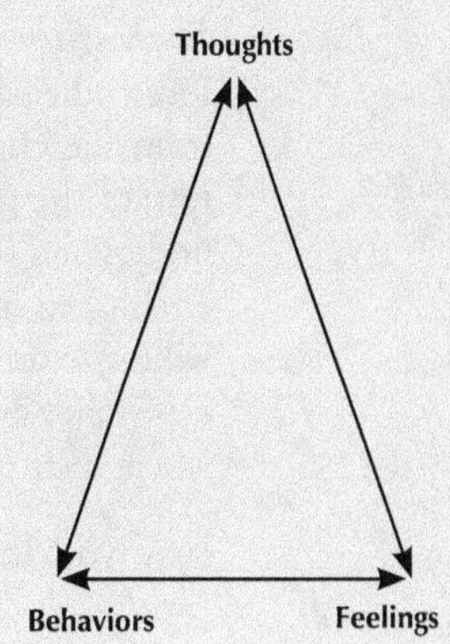

Figure 20-1

her name, age, school, or hobbies, through an "About Me" section. The child is then encouraged to talk about or write about his or her traumatic experience(s), starting with the easiest aspect to talk about, what happened first, or the event the child remembers the most, allowing for the youth to have control over where he or she would like to start. Over the course of several sessions, the child is encouraged to give more and more details of the traumatic experience(s). The therapist encourages the child, incrementally over time, to talk or write about increasingly more upsetting details, aspects, or events related to the trauma experience(s) so that each step is only slightly more difficult than the previous one. The exposure process inherent in the trauma narration should be *gradual.* Although at the end of treatment there will likely be a tangible "product" (eg, a book, song, poem), the heart of the trauma narration is the narration *process* (the back-and-forth gradual exposure conducted within the therapy relationship), not the actual narrative *product.*

The narrative is reread or reviewed during every session to gradually desensitize the child to the event over time. Once the youth has written a description of what happened during the sexual abuse or traumatic experience(s), the therapist will ask what the child was thinking, feeling, and doing at the time, walking the child around the cognitive triangle. Before moving on to cognitive processing of the trauma, the clinician will ask about the worst aspect of the trauma or the "yuckiest part." This is sometimes referred to as the "hot spot." Throughout the trauma narration process, youth are encouraged to use their coping skills (eg, psychoeducation, relaxation, affective regulation, cognitive coping [PRAC] skills) and the clinician monitors their level of distress using a Subjective Units of Distress Scale (SUDS) or some other means. Before ending each trauma narration session, the therapist will praise the child for all of his or her hard work and the child and therapist will engage in some neutral or positive activity (eg, play a game together, blow bubbles, practice grounding/reorienting strategies, take a walk). After the youth has developed a full draft of his or her narrative, the clinician will engage in cognitive processing of the trauma, returning to some of the thoughts that may be inaccurate or unhelpful (eg, "I should have known that would happen;" "It is all my fault") and trying to restructure them to a more accurate or helpful cognition. A variety of cognitive processing techniques may be used, including the cognitive triangle, Socratic questioning, best friend scenarios (eg, "What would you tell your best friend if they said their sexual abuse was all their fault?"), a responsibility pie chart, and other techniques. The last chapter or phase of the trauma narration is to assist the child in making meaning out of the traumatic experience(s) and may include information about what the child has learned in treatment and what the child wants other children to know about sexual abuse and trauma.

Sharing the Trauma Narration with the Parent

Ideally the narrative is shared with the parent after each session, after gaining permission from the child or adolescent to do so. Sharing the narrative with the parent moves toward the goals of desensitizing the parent to the trauma and helping the parent to understand the child's thoughts and feelings. In this way the parent or caregiver is being established as the one the child turns to when in need. The parents are most often willing to do this and are appreciative that they are able to hear the details of their child's experience gradually over time and with the therapist first, before the conjoint sessions where their child reviews the trauma narration with the parent and therapist together.

In Vivo Mastery of Trauma Reminders

Goals

— To desensitize a child to innocuous trauma reminders

— To resolve remaining avoidance symptoms

NOTE: The component of in vivo mastery as a whole may not be needed in all trauma cases and is the only TF-CBT component that is optional. Most children do not demonstrate overgeneralized fears of innocuous situations. This component should only be used for youth who are experiencing avoidance of situations, places, or cues that are innocuous or safe and in which the avoidance is markedly interfering with their functioning or daily life.

Application

Once the specific feared situation or place (eg, fear of sleeping in their own bed, fear of returning to places where trauma occurred such as school) is identified, there is a plan to have the child gradually remain in the situation or place for longer and longer periods. Behavioral reinforcement techniques are often added to help encourage and maintain the plan. For example, there should be praise for success, statements that the child can do this, and rewards once the child has succeeded. Each plan is highly individualized depending on the avoided situation or trauma reminder and the child's or adolescent's presentation, strengths, and severity of symptoms.

Conjoint Parent-Child Sessions

Goals

— To share the child's trauma narration

— To correct cognitive distortions (held by the child, the parent, or both)

— To encourage optimal parent-child communication and a question-and-answer situation between child and parent about trauma and other topics

— To prepare for future traumatic reminders and to suggest how the child and parent can optimally cope with these

— To model appropriate child support and redirection

— To praise for progress made

Application

This component includes the clinician preparing the parent or caregiver and child to share the trauma narration together. A list of questions is developed with both the child and caregiver, and the questions are reviewed in the joint session to help encourage open communication between the child and the caregiver. The clinician then meets with the parent and child and has the child review his or her trauma narration with the parent. The child reads the words and describes the pictures or color scribbles that represent the thoughts, feelings, and behaviors discussed throughout. Questions are also exchanged between the parent and child. Conjoint sessions provide opportunities to practice skills together, increase the comfort between child and caregiver or parent in talking about difficult things, and enhance the parent-child relationship. Conjoint sessions should not be conducted until the caregiver has demonstrated sufficient emotional control so that he or she is able to model healthy coping for the child and so that the sessions feel safe, healthy, positive, and supportive for youth.

Enhancing Future Safety and Development

Goals

— To review physical and psychological safety and identify sources of support

— To prepare plans for dealing with future trauma reminders or safety situations

— To prepare for termination of treatment and celebrate the completion of TF-CBT

Application

This component focuses on any remaining safety issues that may exist. Throughout treatment, as in any good practice, clinicians should be checking in with youth regarding their safety. Addressing safety issues at the beginning of treatment is critically important when there may be potential for ongoing trauma or for youth with complex trauma. The Enhancing Future Safety and Development component addresses physical and psychological safety concerns, healthy sexuality (when appropriate and with parental support), and assertiveness training. Safety skills are reviewed in the presence of caregivers and may include a variety of materials or strategies (eg, handouts, body safety books, discussion of Internet safety, role playing, more formal individualized trauma-informed safety plans). The final session(s) of treatment include moving toward termination and review of treatment; planning for the future, including future trauma reminders and identifying sources of support; a graduation ceremony or ritual that celebrates the child's successful completion of treatment; and bringing treatment to a close.

Conclusion

CSA is a highly variable experience that can have myriad widely devastating and long-term consequences. The resulting symptoms and impact on victims and families are equally diverse, making the treatment of CSA challenging at best. Throughout the 1990s and 2000s, extensive research has resulted in a number of identified treatments that have been found via RCTs to have efficacy. More recent efforts have been focused on extending these empirically sound treatments into the mainstream and testing their ability to perform under more naturalistic conditions. Available research suggests that, to date, TF-CBT is the most rigorously researched treatment and is most efficacious in treating sexually abused children and their varied, complex symptoms. It is important for both clinicians and other involved professionals to familiarize themselves with the most efficacious treatments now available for addressing the complex needs of sexual abuse victims.

However, although TF-CBT is currently considered one of the most efficacious and well-supported treatments for sexually abused children, it is also clear that effective psychotherapeutic treatment consists of more than a clinician executing the components of a manual for a particular disorder. In fact, rather than a cookie cutter approach, treatment must be an interdisciplinary effort to weave together treatment engagement, therapeutic alliance, the retention of families, an understanding of child development and attachment, trauma-informed and trauma-sensitive practices, and the theory and practice of a treatment, while capitalizing on the strengths of a child and family. As such, it is becoming increasingly important for all professionals involved in sexual abuse cases to become familiar with the treatments available, the research behind them, and what elements are included in trauma-informed, trauma-focused, evidence-based treatments. Collaboration across practitioners and researchers is necessary to deliver optimal services to sexually abused youth and their families.

References

1. Finkelhor D. *Sexually Victimized Children*. NY, New York: Free Press; 1981.
2. Finkelhor D. Epidemiological factors in the clinical identification of child sexual abuse. *Child Abuse Negl.* 1993;17(1):67-70.
3. Singh MM, Parsekar SS, Nair SN. An epidemiological overview of child sexual abuse. *J Fam Med Prim Care.* 2014;3(4):430-435.
4. United Nations General Assembly. World report on violence against children: United Nations Secretary General's study. https://www.unicef.org/violencestudy/reports/SG_violencestudy_en.pdf. Published August 29, 2006. Accessed January 28, 2019.

5. Vaillancourt-Morel MP, Godbout N, Bédard MG, Charest É, Briere J, Sabourin S. Emotional and sexual correlates of child sexual abuse as a function of self-definition status. *Child Maltreat.* 2016;21(3):228-238.

6. Murray LK, Nguyen A, Cohen JA. Child sexual abuse. *Child Adolesc Psychiatr Clin N Am.* 2014;23(2):321-337.

7. Finkelhor D. Early and long-term effects of child sexual abuse: an update. *Prof Psychol Res Pr.* 1990;21(5):325-330.

8. Finkelhor D, Berliner L. Research on the treatment of sexually abused children: a review and recommendations. *J Am Acad Child Adolesc Psychiatry.* 1995;34(11):1408-1423.

9. Kendall-Tackett K. The effects of childhood maltreatment and of exposure to early toxic stress. In: Contre JR, ed. *Child Abuse and Neglect Worldwide*. Santa Barbara, CA: Praeger; 2014:155-179.

10. Kendall-Tackett KA, Williams LM, Finkelhor D. Impact of sexual abuse on children: a review and synthesis of recent empirical studies. *Psychol Bull.* 1993;113(1):164-180.

11. Mannarino AP, Cohen JA, Smith J, Moore-Motily, S. Six and twelve month follow-up of sexually abused girls. *J Interpers Violence.* 1991;6(4):494-511.

12. Berliner L, Elliott DM. Sexual abuse of children. In: Myers JEB, Berliner L, Briere J, Hendrix CT, Jenny C, Reid TA, eds. *The APSAC Handbook on Child Maltreatment.* 2nd ed. Thousand Oaks, CA: Sage Publications; 2002:55-78.

13. Browne A, Finkelhor D. Impact of child sexual abuse: a review of the research. *Psychol Bull.* 1986;99(1):66-77.

14. Mannarino AP, Cohen JA, Gregor M. Emotional and behavioral difficulties in sexually abused girls. *J Interpers Violence.* 1989;4(4):437-451.

15. Lewis T, McElroy E, Harlaar N, Runyan D. Does the impact of child sexual abuse differ from maltreated but non-sexually abused children? A prospective examination of the impact of child sexual abuse on internalizing and externalizing behavior problems. *Child Abuse Negl.* 2016;51:31-40.

16. Clarke K, Patalay P, Allen E, Knight L, Naker D, Devries K. Patterns and predictors of violence against children in Uganda: a latent class analysis. *BMJ Open.* 2016;6(5):e010443.

17. Witt A, Münzer A, Ganser HG, Fegert JM, Goldbeck L, Plener PL. Experience by children and adolescents of more than one type of maltreatment: association of different classes of maltreatment profiles with clinical outcome variables. *Child Abuse Negl.* 2016;57:1-11.

18. Vachon DD, Krueger RF, Rogosch FA, Cicchetti D. Assessment of the harmful psychiatric and behavioral effects of different forms of child maltreatment. *JAMA Psychiatry.* 2015;72(11):1135-1142.

19. Scott-Storey K. Cumulative abuse: do things add up? An evaluation of the conceptualization, operationalization, and methodological approaches in the study of the phenomenon of cumulative abuse. *Trauma Violence Abuse.* 2011;12(3):135-150.

20. Finkelhor D, Ormrod R, Turner H, Hamby SL. The victimization of children and youth: a comprehensive, national survey. *Child Maltreat.* 2005;10(1):5-25.

21. Vaughn MG, Salas-Wright CP, Underwood S, Gochez-Kerr T. Subtypes of non-suicidal self-injury based on childhood adversity. *Psychiatric Q.* 2015;86(1):137-151.

22. Cloitre M, Stolbach BC, Herman JL, et al. A developmental approach to complex PTSD: childhood and adult cumulative trauma as predictors of system complexity. *J Trauma Stress.* 2009;22(5):399-408.

23. Cook A, Spinazzola J, Ford J, et al. Complex trauma in children and adolescents. *Psychiatr Ann.* 2005;35(5):390-398.

24. Cosentino CE, Meyer-Bahlburg HF, Alpert JL, Weinberg SL, Gaines R. Sexual behavior problems and psychopathology symptoms in sexually abused girls. *J Am Acad Child Adolesc Psychiatry.* 1995;34(8):1033-1042.

25. Deblinger E, McLeer SV, Atkins MS, Ralphe D, Foa E. Post-traumatic stress in sexually abused, physically abused, and nonabused children. *Child Abuse Negl.* 1989;13(3):403-408.

26. Friedrich WN, Grambasch P, Damon L, et al. Child Sexual Behavior Inventory: normative and clinical comparisons. *Psychol Assess.* 1992;4(3):303-311.

27. Cohen JA, Mannarino AP. Psychological symptoms in sexually abused girls. *Child Abuse Negl.* 1988;12(4):571-577.

28. Koverola C, Pound J, Heger A, Lytle C. Relationship of child sexual abuse to depression. *Child Abuse Negl.* 1993;17(3):393-400.

29. Wozencraft T, Wagner W, Pellegrin A. Depression and suicidal ideation in sexually abused children. *Child Abuse Negl.* 1991;15(4):505-511.

30. Briere JN, Elliott DM. Immediate and long-term impacts of child sexual abuse. *Future Child.* 1994;4(2):54-69.

31. Conte JR, Schuerman JR. Factors associated with an increased impact of child sexual abuse. *Child Abuse Negl.* 1987;11(2):201-211.

32. Einbender AJ, Friedrich WN. Psychological functioning and behavior of sexually abused girls. *J Consult Clin Psychol.* 1989;57(1):155-157.

33. Nalavany BA, Ryan SD, Hinterlong J. Externalizing behavior among adopted boys with preadoptive histories of child sexual abuse. *J Child Sex Abuse.* 2009;18(5):553-573.

34. Tyler KA. Social and emotional outcomes of childhood sexual abuse: a review of recent research. *Aggress Violent Behav.* 2002;7(6):567-589.

35. Cohen JA, Mannarino AP. Factors that mediate treatment outcome of sexually abused preschool children: six- and 12-month follow-up. *J Am Acad Child Adolesc Psychiatry.* 1998;37(1):44-51.

36. McLeer SV, Deblinger E, Henry D, Orvaschel H. Sexually abused children at high risk for post-traumatic stress disorder. *J Am Acad Child Adolesc Psychiatry.* 1992;31(5):875-879.

37. McLeer SV, Callaghan M, Henry D, Wallen J. Psychiatric disorders in sexually abused children. *J Am Acad Child Adolesc Psychiatry.* 1994;33(3):313-319.

38. McLeer SV, Deblinger E, Atkins MS, Foa EB, Ralphe DL. Post-traumatic stress disorder in sexually abused children. *J Am Acad Child Adolesc Psychiatry.* 1988;27(5):650-654.

39. Copeland WE, Keeler G, Angold A, Costello EJ. Traumatic events and posttraumatic stress in childhood. *Arch Gen Psychiatr.* 2007;64(5):577-584.

40. Trask EV, Walsh K, Dilillo D. Treatment effects for common outcomes of child sexual abuse: a current meta-analysis. *Aggress Violent Behav.* 2011;16(1):6-19.

41. Walsh K, Galea S, Koenen KC. Mechanisms underlying sexual violence exposure and psychosocial sequelae: a theoretical and empirical review. *Clin Psychol (New York).* 2012;19(3):260-275.

42. Oquendo M, Brent DA, Birmaher B, et al. Posttraumatic stress disorder comorbid with major depression: factors mediating the association with suicidal behavior. *Am J Psychiatry.* 2005;162(3):560-566.

43. Daray FM, Rojas SM, Bridges AJ, et al. The independent effects of child sexual abuse and impulsivity on lifetime suicide attempts among female patients. *Child Abuse Negl.* 2016;58:91-98.

44. Jonas S, Bebbington P, McManus S, et al. Sexual abuse and psychiatric disorder in England: results from the 2007 Adult Psychiatric Morbidity Survey. *Psychol Med.* 2011;41(4): 709-719.

45. MacMillan HL, Fleming JE, Streiner DL, et al. Childhood abuse and lifetime psychopathology in a community sample. *Am J Psychiatry.* 2001;158(11):1878-1883.

46. Lindert J, von Ehrenstein OS, Grashow R, Gal G, Braehler E, Weisskopf MG. Sexual and physical abuse in childhood is associated with depression and anxiety over the life course: systematic review and meta-analysis. *Int J Public Health.* 2014;59(2):359-372.

47. Brent DA, Baugher M, Bridge J, Chen T, Chiappetta L. Age- and sex-related risk factors for adolescent suicide. *J Am Acad Child Adolesc Psychiatry.* 1999;38(12):1497-1505.

48. Brown J, Cohen P, Johnson JG, Smailes EM. Childhood abuse and neglect: specificity of effects on adolescent and young adult depression and suicidality. *J Am Acad Child Adolesc Psychiatry.* 1999;38(12):1490-1496.

49. Fergusson DM, Horwood LJ, Lynskey MT. Childhood sexual abuse and psychiatric disorder in young adulthood: II. psychiatric outcomes of childhood sexual abuse. *J Am Acad Child Adolesc Psychiatry.* 1996;35(10):1365-1374.

50. Kaplan SJ, Pelcovitz D, Salzinger S, Mandel F, Weiner M. Adolescent physical abuse and suicide attempts. *J Am Acad Child Adolesc Psychiatry.* 1997;36(6):799-808.

51. Mullen PE, Martin JL, Anderson JC, Romans SE, Herbison GP. The long-term impact of the physical, emotional, and sexual abuse of children: a community study. *Child Abuse Negl.* 1996;20(1):7-21.

52. Maniglio R. The role of child sexual abuse in the etiology of suicide and non-suicidal self-injury. *Acta Psychiatr Scand.* 2011;124(1):30-41.

53. Youssef NA, Green KT, Dedert EA, et al. Exploration of the influence of childhood trauma, combat exposure, and the resilience construct on depression and suicidal ideation among US Iraq/Afghanistan era military personnel and veterans. *Arch Suicide Res.* 2013;17(2):106-122.

54. Trickett PK, Noll JG, Putnam FW. The impact of sexual abuse on female development: lessons from a multigenerational, longitudinal research study. *Dev Psychopathol.* 2011;23(2):453-476.

55. Beitchman JH, Zucker KJ, Hood JE, daCosta GA, Akman D, Cassavia E. A review of the long-term effects of child sexual abuse. *Child Abuse Negl.* 1992;16(1):101-118.

56. Duncan RD, Saunders BE, Kilpatrick DG, Hanson RF, Resnick HS. Childhood physical assault as a risk factor for PTSD, depression, and substance abuse: findings from a national survey [published correction appears in *Am J Orthopsychiatry.* 1997;67(1):161]. *Am J Orthopsychiatry.* 1996;66(3):437-448.

57. Felitti VJ, Anda RF, Nordenberg D, et al. Relationship of childhood abuse and household dysfunction to many of the leading causes of death in adults: the Adverse Childhood Experiences (ACE) Study. *Am J Prev Med.* 1998;14(4):245-258.

58. Polusny MA, Follette VM. Long term correlates of child sexual abuse: theory and review of the empirical literature. *Appl Prev Psychol.* 1995;4(3):143-166.

59. Saunders BE, Kilpatrick DG, Hansen RF, Resnick HS, Walker ME. Prevalence, case characteristics, and long-term psychological correlates of child rape among women: a national survey. *Child Maltreat.* 1999;4(3):187-200.

60. Widom CS. Posttraumatic stress disorder in abused and neglected children grown up. *Am J Psychiatry.* 1999;156(8):1223-1229.

61. Putnam FW. Ten-year research update review: child sexual abuse. *J Am Acad Child Adolesc Psychiatr.* 2003;42(3):269-278.

62. Hébert M, Cénat JM, Blais M, Lavoie F, Guerrier M. Child sexual abuse, bullying, cyberbullying, and mental health problems among high schools students: a moderated mediated model. *Depress Anxiety.* 2016;33(7):623-629.

63. Luster T, Small SA. Sexual abuse history and number of sex partners among female adolescents. *Fam Plann Perspect.* 1997;29(5):204-211.

64. Miller BA, Downs WR, Testa M. Interrelationships between victimization experiences and women's alcohol use. *J Stud Alcohol Suppl.* 1993;11:109-117.

65. Saunders BE, Berliner L, Hanson RF. *Child Physical and Sexual Abuse: Guidelines for Treatment.* Charleston, SC: National Crime Victims Research and Treatment Center; 2003.

66. Mohler-Kuo M, Landolt MA, Maier T, Meidert U, Schönbucher V, Schnyder U. Child sexual abuse revisited: a population-based cross-sectional study among Swiss adolescents. *J Adolesc Health.* 2014;54(3):304-311.

67. Sachs-Ericsson N, Kendall-Tackett KA, Sheffler J, Arce D, Rushing NC, Corsentino E. The influence of prior rape on the psychological and physical health function of older adults. *Aging Ment Health.* 2014;18(6):717-730.

68. Springer KW, Sheridan J, Kuo D, Carnes M. The long-term outcomes of childhood abuse: an overview and a call to action. *J Gen Intern Med.* 2003;18(10):864-870.

69. Kendall-Tackett KA. *Treating the Lifetime Health Effects of Childhood Victimization.* Kingston, NJ: Civic Research Institute, Inc.; 2003.

70. Juster RP, McEwen BS, Lupien SJ. Allostatic load biomarkers of chronic stress and impact on health and cognition. *Neurosci Biobehav Rev.* 2010;35(1):2-16.

71. McEwen BS, Wingfield JC. The concept of allostasis in biology and biomedicine. *Horm Behav.* 2003;43(1):2-15.

72. Kendall-Tackett K. Psychological trauma and physical health: a psychoneuroimmunology approach to etiology of negative health effects and possible interventions. *Psychol Trauma.* 2009;1(1):35-48.

73. O'Donovan A, Neylan TC, Metzler T, Cohen BE. Lifetime exposure to traumatic psychological stress is associated with elevated inflammation in the Heart and Soul Study. *Brain Behav Immun.* 2012;26(4):642-649.

74. Blanco L, Nydegger LA, Camarillo G, Trinidad DR, Schramm E, Ames SL. Neurological changes in brain structure and functions among individuals with a history of childhood sexual abuse: a review. *Neurosci Biobehav Rev.* 2015;57:63-69.

75. Nemeroff CB. Paradise lost: the neurobiological and clinical consequences of child abuse and neglect. *Neuron.* 2016;89(5):892-909.

76. Teicher MH, Samson JA. Annual research review: enduring neurobiological effects of childhood abuse and neglect. *J Child Psychol Psychiatry.* 2016;57(3):241-266.

77. Finkelhor D, Hotaling GT, Lewis IA, Smith C. Sexual abuse and its relationship to later sexual satisfaction, marital status, religion, and attitudes. *J Interpers Violence.* 1989;4(4):379-399.

78. Schönbucher V, Maier T, Mohler-Kuo M, Schnyder U, Landolt MA. Disclosure of child sexual abuse by adolescents: a qualitative in-depth study. *J Interpers Violence.* 2012;27(17):3486-3513.

79. Fontes LA. Sin vergüenza: addressing shame with Latino victims of child sexual abuse and their families. *J Child Sex Abus.* 2007;16(1):61-83.

80. Brown LK, Kessel SM, Lourie KJ, Ford HH, Lipsitt LP. Influence of sexual abuse on HIV-related attitudes and behaviors in adolescent psychiatric inpatients. *J Am Acad Child Adolesc Psychiatry.* 1997;36(3):316-322.

81. Carey MP, Carey KB, Kalichman SC. Risk for human immunodeficiency virus (HIV) infection among persons with severe mental illnesses. *Clin Psychol Rev.* 1997;17(3):271-291.

82. Al-Fayez GA, Ohaeri JU, Gado OM. Prevalence of physical, psychological, and sexual abuse among a nationwide sample of Arab high school students: association with family characteristics, anxiety, depression, self-esteem, and quality of life. *Soc Psychiatry Psychiatr Epidemiol.* 2012;47(1):53-66.

83. Jehu D. *Beyond Sexual Abuse: Therapy with Women Who Were Childhood Victims.* Oxford, UK: John Wiley & Sons; 1988.

84. Jehu D, Gazan M, Klassen C. Common therapeutic targets among women who were sexually abused in childhood. *J Soc Work Hum Sex.* 1985;3(2-3):25-45.

85. Ready CB, Hayes AM, Yasinski CW, et al. Overgeneralized beliefs, accommodation, and treatment outcome in youth receiving trauma-focused cognitive behavioral therapy for childhood trauma. *Behav Ther.* 2015;46(5):671-688.

86. Brown LK, Danovsky MB, Lourie KJ, DiClemente RJ, Ponton LE. Adolescents with psychiatric disorders and the risk of HIV. *J Am Acad Child Adolesc Psychiatry.* 1997;36(11):1609-1617.

87. De Bellis MD, Keshavan MS, Clark DB, et al. Developmental traumatology: part II: brain development. *Biol Psychiatry.* 1999;45(10):1271-1284.

88. Catanzaro SJ. Mood regulation and suicidal behavior. In: Joiner TE, Rudd MD, eds. *Suicide Science: Expanding the Boundaries*. Berlin, Germany: Springer Science & Business Media; 2000:81-103.

89. Eisenberg N, Cumberland A, Spinrad TL, et al. The relations of regulation and emotionality to children's externalizing and internalizing problem behavior. *Child Dev.* 2001;72(4):1112-1134.

90. Cohen JA, Mannarino AP. Addressing attributions in treating abused children. *Child Maltreat.* 2002;7(1):82-86.

91. Feiring C, Taska L, Lewis M. A process model for understanding adaptation to sexual abuse: the role of shame in defining stigmatization. *Child Abuse Negl.* 1996;20(8):767-782.

92. Nooner KB, Linares LO, Batinjane J, Kramer RA, Silva R, Cloitre M. Factors related to posttraumatic stress disorder in adolescence. *Trauma Violence Abuse.* 2012;13(3):153-166.

93. Beitchman JH, Zucker KJ, Hood JE, daCosta GA, Akman D. A review of the short-term effects of child sexual abuse. *Child Abuse Negl.* 1991;15(4):537-556.

94. Brand EF, King CA, Olson E, Ghaziuddin N, Naylor M. Depressed adolescents with a history of sexual abuse: diagnostic comorbidity and suicidality. *J Am Acad Child Adolesc Psychiatry.* 1996;35(1):34-41.

95. Hotte JP, Rafman S. The specific effects of incest on prepubertal girls from dysfunctional families. *Child Abuse Negl.* 1992;16(2):273-283.

96. Maniglio R. Child sexual abuse in the etiology of depression: a systematic review of reviews. *Depress Anxiety.* 2010;27(7):631-642.

97. Nagy S, Adcock AG, Nagy MC. A comparison of risky health behaviors of sexually active, sexually abused, and abstaining adolescents. *Pediatrics.* 1994;93(4):570-575.

98. Friedrich WN, Fisher JL, Dittner CA, et al. Child sexual behavior inventory: normative, psychiatric, and sexual abuse comparisons. *Child Maltreat.* 2001;6(1):37-49.

99. McClellan J, McCurry C, Ronnei M, Adams J, Eisner A, Storck M. Age of onset of sexual abuse: relationship to sexually inappropriate behaviors. *J Am Acad Child Adolesc Psychiatry.* 1996;35(10):1375-1383.

100. Paolucci EO, Genuis ML, Violato C. A meta-analysis of the published research on the effects of child sexual abuse. *J Psychol.* 2001;135(1):17-36.

101. Brodsky BS, Oquendo M, Ellis SP, Haas GL, Malone KM, Mann JJ. The relationship of childhood abuse to impulsivity and suicidal behavior in adults with major depression. *Am J Psychiatry.* 2001;158(11):1871-1877.

102. Cohen JA, Deblinger E, Mannarino AP, Steer RA. A multisite, randomized controlled trial for children with sexual abuse-related PTSD symptoms. *J Am Acad Child Adolesc Psychiatry.* 2004;43(4):393-402.

103. Finkelhor D, Kendall-Tackett K. A developmental perspective on the childhood impact of crime, abuse, and violent victimization. In: Cicchetti D, Toth S, eds. *Developmental Perspectives on Trauma: Theory, Research, and Intervention.* Rochester, NY: University of Rochester Press; 1997:1-32.

104. Rosenfeld S, Lewis D. The hidden effect of childhood sexual abuse on adolescent and young adult HIV prevention: rethinking AIDS education, program development, and policy. *AIDS Public Policy J.* 1993;8(4):181-186.

105. Debowska A, Willmott D, Boduszek D, Jones AD. What do we know about child abuse and neglect patterns of co-occurrence? A systematic review of profiling studies and recommendations for future research. *Child Abuse Negl.* 2017;70:100-111.

106. Donenberg GR, Schwartz RM, Emerson E, Wilson HW, Bryant FB, Coleman G. Applying a cognitive-behavioral model of HIV risk to youths in psychiatric care. *AIDS Educ Prev.* 2005;17(3):200-216.

107. Hussey DL, Singer M. Psychological distress, problem behaviors, and family functioning of sexually abused adolescent inpatients. *J Am Acad Child Adolesc Psychiatry.* 1993;32(5):954-961.

108. Rotheram-Borus MJ, Mahler KA, Koopman C, Langabeer K. Sexual abuse history and associated multiple risk behavior in adolescent runaways. *Am J Orthopsychiatry.* 1996;66(3):390-400.

109. Walsh K, Resnick HS, Danielson CK, McCauley JL, Saunders BE, Kilpatrick DG. Patterns of drug and alcohol use associated with lifetime sexual revictimization and current posttraumatic stress disorder among three national samples of adolescent, college, and household-residing women. *Addict Behav.* 2014;39(3):684-689.

110. Messman-Moore TL, Long PJ. The role of childhood sexual abuse sequelae in the sexual revictimization of women: an empirical review and theoretical reformulation. *Clin Psychol Rev.* 2003;23(4):537-571.

111. Feinauer LL, Callahan EH, Hilton HG. Positive intimate relationships decrease depression in sexually abused women. *Am J Fam Ther.* 1996;24(2):99-106.

112. Ormhaug SM, Jensen TK, Wentzel-Larsen T, Shirk SR. The therapeutic alliance in treatment of traumatized youths: relation to outcome in a randomized clinical trial. *J Consult Clin Psychol.* 2014;82(1):52-64.

113. Wang PS, Lane M, Olfson M, Pincus HA, Wells KB, Kessler RC. Twelve-month use of mental health services in the United States: results from the National Comorbidity Survey Replication. *Arch Gen Psychiatry.* 2005;62(6):629-640.

114. Burns BJ, Costello EJ, Angold A, et al. Children's mental health service use across service sectors. *Health Aff (Millwood).* 1995;14(3):147-159.

115. McKay MM, McCadam K, Gonzales JJ. Addressing the barriers to mental health services for inner city children and their caretakers. *Community Ment Health J.* 1996;32(4):353-361.

116. McKay MM, Stoewe J, McCadam K, Gonzales J. Increasing access to child mental health services for urban children and their caregivers. *Health Soc Work.* 1998;23(1):9-15.

117. Ringel JS, Sturm R. National estimates of mental health utilization and expenditures for children in 1998. *J Behav Health Serv Res.* 2001;28(3):319-333.

118. Lane WG, Dubowitz H, Harrington D. Child sexual abuse evaluations: adherence to recommendations. *J Child Sex Abuse.* 2002;11(4):17-34.

119. Lippert T, Favre T, Alexander C, Cross TP. Families who begin versus decline therapy for children who are sexually abused. *Child Abuse Negl.* 2008;32(9):859-868.

120. Gould MS, Shaffer D, Kaplan D. The characteristics of dropouts from a child psychiatry clinic. *J Am Acad Child Psychiatry.* 1985;24(3):316-328.

121. Wierzbicki M, Pekarik G. A meta-analysis of outpatient therapy dropout. *Prof Psychol Res Pr.* 1993;24(2):190-195.

122. McPherson P, Scribano P, Stevens J. Barriers to successful treatment completion in child sexual abuse survivors. *J Interpers Violence.* 2012;27(1):23-39.

123. Kazdin AE, Mazurick JL, Bass D. Risk for attrition in treatment of antisocial children and families. *J Clin Child Psychol.* 1993;22(1):2-16.

124. Koverola C, Murtaugh CA, Connors KM, Reeves G, Papas MA. Children exposed to intra-familial violence: predictors of attrition and retention in treatment. *J Aggress Maltreat Trauma.* 2007;14(4):19-42.

125. Kazdin AE, Wassell G. Predictors of barriers to treatment and therapeutic change in outpatient therapy for antisocial children and their families. *Ment Health Serv Res.* 2000;2(1):27-40.

126. Fong HF, Bennett CE, Mondestin V, Scribano PV, Mollen C, Wood JN. Caregiver perceptions about mental health services after child sexual abuse. *Child Abuse Negl.* 2016;51:284-294.

127. Lane WG, Dubowitz H, Harrington D. Child sexual abuse evaluations: adherence to recommendations. *J Child Sex Abus.* 2002;11(4):17-34.

128. Nock MK, Kazdin AE. Parent expectancies for child therapy: assessment and relation to participation in treatment. *J Child Fam Stud.* 2001;10(2):155-180.

129. Garcia JA, Weisz JR. When youth mental health care stops: therapeutic relationship problems and other reasons for ending youth outpatient treatment. *J Consult Clin Psychol.* 2002;70(2):439-443.

130. Frank JD, Frank JB. *Persuasion & Healing: A Comparative Study of Psychotherapy.* Baltimore, MD: Johns Hopkins University Press; 1991.

131. Garfield SL. Research on client variables in psychotherapy. In: Bergin AE, Garfield SL, eds. *Handbook of Psychotherapy and Behavior Change.* 4th ed. New York, NY: Wiley; 1994:190-228.

132. McKay MM, Pennington J, Lynn CJ, McCadam K. Understanding urban child mental health service use: two studies of child, family, and environmental correlates. *J Behav Health Serv Res.* 2001;28(4):475-483.

133. Rushton A. A scoping and scanning review of research on the adoption of children placed from public care. *Clin Child Psychol Psychiatry.* 2004;9(1):89-106.

134. Shivack N, Sullivan CW. Use of telephone prompts at an inner-city patient clinic. *Hosp Community Psychiatry.* 1989;40(8):851-853.

135. Szapocznik J, Perez-Vidal A, Brickman AL, et al. Engaging adolescent drug abusers and their families in treatment: a strategic structural systems approach. *J Consult Clin Psychol.*1988;56(4):552-557.

136. Shaw M, De Jong M. Child abuse and neglect: a major public health issue and the role of child and adolescent mental health services. *Psychiatrist.* 2012;36(9):321-325.

137. Bartlett JD, Barto B, Griffin JL, Fraser JG, Hodgdon H, Bodian R. Trauma-informed care in the Massachusetts Child Trauma Project. *Child Maltreat.* 2016;21(2):101-112.

138. Chambless DL, Hollon SD. Defining empirically supported therapies. *J Consult Clin Psychol.* 1998;66(1):7-18.

139. Chorpita BF, Yim LM, Donkervoet JC, et al. Toward large-scale implementation of empirically supported treatments for children: a review and observations by the Hawaii Empirical Basis to Services Task Force. *Clin Psychol (New York).* 2006;9(2):165-190.

140. Weisz JR, Hawley KM, Pilkonis PA, Woody SR, Follette WC. Stressing the (other) three Rs in the search for empirically supported treatments: review procedures, research quality, relevance to practice and the public interest. *Clin Psychol (New York).* 2000:7(3):243-258.

141. Cohen JA, Mannarino AP, Deblinger E. *Treating Trauma and Traumatic Grief in Children and Adolescents.* New York, NY: Guilford Press; 2006.

142. Kazdin AE. Bridging the enormous gaps of theory with therapy research and practice. *J Clin Child Psychol.* 2001;30(1):59-66.

143. Weisz JR, Donenberg GR, Han SS, Wiess B. Bridging the gap between laboratory and clinic in child and adolescent psychotherapy. *J Consult Clin Psychol.* 1995;63(5):688-701.

144. Aarons GA. Mental health provider attitudes toward adoption of evidence-based practice: the Evidence-Based Practice Attitude Scale (EBPAS). *Ment Health Serv Res.* 2004;6(2):61-74.

145. Durlak JA, DuPre EP. Implementation matters: a review of research on the influence of implementation on program outcomes and the factors affecting implementation. *Am J Community Psychol.* 2008;41(3-4):327-350.

146. McHugo GJ, Drake RE, Whitley R, et al. Fidelity outcomes in the National Implementing Evidence-Based Practices Project. *Psychiatr Serv.* 2007;58(10):1279-1284.

147. Deblinger E, Heflin AH. *Treating Sexual Abused Children and Their Nonoffending Parents: A Cognitive Behavioral Approach.* Thousand Oaks, CA: Sage Publications; 1996.

148. Wolfe DA, McMahon RJ, Peters RD. *Child Abuse: New Directions in Prevention and Treatment Across the Lifespan.* Thousand Oaks, CA: Sage Publications; 1997.

149. Bolton FG, Bolton SR. *Working with Violent Families: A Guide for Clinical and Legal Practitioners.* Thousand Oaks, CA: Sage Publications; 1987.

150. Gil E. *Systemic Treatment of Families Who Abuse.* San Francisco, CA: Jossey-Bass; 1995.

151. Karp CL, Butler TL, Bergstrom SC. *Treatment Strategies for Abused Children: From Victim to Survivor.* Thousand Oaks, CA: Sage Publications; 1997.

152. Maddock JW, Larson NR. *Incestuous Families: An Ecological Approach to Understanding and Treatment.* New York, NY: W.W. Norton; 1995.

153. Berliner L, Saunders BE. Treating fear and anxiety in sexually abused children: results of a controlled 2-year follow-up study. *Child Maltreat.* 1996;1(4):294-309.

154. Cohen JA, Berliner L, March JS. Treatment of children and adolescents. In: Foa EB, Keane TM, Friedman MJ, Cohen JA, eds. *Effective Treatments for PTSD: Practice Guidelines from the International Society for Traumatic Stress Studies.* New York, NY: Guilford Press; 2000.

155. Cohen JA, Mannarino AP. A treatment outcome study for sexually abused preschool children: initial findings [published correction appears in *J Am Acad Child Adolesc Psychiatry.* 1996;35(6):835.]. *J Am Acad Child Adolesc Psychiatry.* 1996;35(1):42-50.

156. Cohen JA, Mannarino AP. Interventions for sexually abused children: initial treatment outcome findings. *Child Maltreat.* 1998;3(1):17-26.

157. Deblinger E, Lippman J, Steer RA. Sexually abused children suffering from post-traumatic stress symptoms: initial treatment outcome findings. *Child Maltreat.* 1996;1(4):310-321.

158. Deblinger E, Mannarino AP, Cohen JA, Steer RA. A follow-up study of a multisite, randomized controlled trial for children with sexual abuse-related PTSD symptoms. *J Am Acad Child Adolesc Psychiatry.* 2006;45(12):1474-1484.

159. Murray LK, Skavenski S, Kane JC, et al. Effectiveness of trauma-focused cognitive behavioral therapy among trauma-affected children in Lusaka, Zambia: a randomized clinical trial. *JAMA Pediatr.* 2015;169(8):761-769.

160. Cohen JA, Deblinger E, Mannarino AP. Trauma-focused cognitive-behavioral therapy for sexually abused children. *Psychiatr Times.* 2004;21(10):109-121.

161. Deblinger E, Stauffer LB, Steer RA. Comparative efficacies of supportive and cognitive behavioral group therapies for young children who have been sexually abused and their nonoffending mothers. *Child Maltreat.* 2001;6(4):332-343.

162. King NJ, Tonge BJ, Mullen P, et al. Treating sexually abused children with posttraumatic stress symptoms: a randomized clinical trial. *J Am Acad Child Adolesc Psychiatry.* 2000;39(11):1347-1355.

163. Kazdin AE, Weisz JR. Identifying and developing empirically supported child and adolescent treatments. *J Consult Clin Psychol.* 1998;66(1):19-36.

164. Gillies D, Taylor F, Gray C, O'Brien L, D'Abrew N. Psychological therapies for the treatment of post-traumatic stress disorder in children and adolescents: review. *Evid Based Child Health.* 2013;8(3):1004-1116.

165. Silverman WK, Ortiz CD, Viswesvaran C, et al. Evidence-based psychosocial treatments for children and adolescents exposed to traumatic events. *J Clin Child Adolesc Psychol.* 37(1):156-183.

166. Chambless DL, Ollendick TH. Empirically supported psychological interventions: controversies and evidence. *Annu Rev Psychol.* 2001;52:685-716.

167. Hodgdon HB, Kinniburgh K, Gabowitz D, Blaustein ME, Spinazzola J. Development and implementation of trauma-informed programming in youth residential treatment centers using the ARC framework. *J Fam Violence.* 2013;28(7):679-692.

168. Van Horn P, Lieberman AF. Using dyadic therapies to treat traumatized young children. In Brom D, Pat-Horenczyk R, Ford JD, eds. *Treating Traumatized Children: Risk, Resilience and Recovery.* New York, NY: Routledge; 2008:210-219.

169. Allen B, Timmer SG, Urquiza AJ. Parent-child interaction therapy for sexual concerns of maltreated children: a preliminary investigation. *Child Abuse Negl.* 2016;56:80-88.

170. Slade MK, Warne RT. A meta-analysis of the effectiveness of trauma-focused cognitive-behavioral therapy and play therapy for child victims of abuse. *J Young Investig.* 2016;30(6):36-43.

171. Carpentier MY, Silovsky JF, Chaffin, M. Randomized trial of treatment for children with sexual behavior problems: ten-year follow-up. *J Consult Clin Psychol.* 2006;74(3):482-488.

172. Wolpe J. Basic principles and practices of behavior therapy of neuroses. *Am J Psychiatry.* 1969;125(9):1242-1247.

173. Beck AT. *Cognitive Therapy and the Emotional Disorders.* Oxford, England: International Universities Press; 1979.

174. Foa EB, Rothbaum BO, Riggs DS, Murdock TB. Treatment of posttraumatic stress disorder in rape victims: a comparison between cognitive-behavioral procedures and counseling. *J Consult Clin Psychol.* 1991;59(5):715-723.

175. Keane TM, Fairbanks JA, Caddell JM, Zimering RT. Implosive (flooding) therapy reduces symptoms of PTSD in Vietnam combat veterans. *Behav Ther.* 1989;20(2):245-260.

176. Weisz JR, Hawley KM, Doss AJ. Empirically tested psychotherapies for youth internalizing and externalizing problems and disorders. *Child Adolesc Psychiatr Clin N Am.* 2004;13(4):729-815, v-vi.

177. Kazdin AE, Weisz JR. *Evidence-Based Psychotherapies for Children and Adolescents.* New York, NY: Guilford Press; 2003.

178. Ollendick TH, King NJ. Empirically supported treatments for children and adolescents. In: Kendall PC, ed. *Child and Adolescent Therapy: Cognitive-Behavioral Procedures.* 2nd ed. New York, NY: Guilford Press; 2000:386-425.

179. Grasso DJ, Joselow B, Marquez Y, Webb C. Trauma-focused cognitive behavioral therapy of a child with posttraumatic stress disorder. *Psychotherapy (Chic).* 2011;48(2):188-197.

180. Schoenwald SK, Hoagwood K. Effectiveness, transportability, and dissemination of interventions: what matters when? *Psychiatr Serv.* 2001;52(9):1190-1197.

181. Henggeler SW, Bourduin CM, Schoenwald SK, Rowland MD, Cunningham PB. *Multisystemic Therapy for Antisocial Behavior in Children and Adolescents.* 2nd ed. New York, NY: Guilford Press; 2009.

182. Kraemer HC, Wilson GT, Fairburn CG, Agras WS. Mediators and moderators of treatment effects in randomized clinical trials. *Arch Gen Psychiatry.* 2002;59(10):877-883.

183. Torrey WC, Drake RE, Dixon L, et al. Implementing evidence-based practices for persons with severe mental illnesses. *Psychiatr Serv.* 2001;52(1):45-50.

184. Saunders BE, Berliner L, Hanson RF. *Child Physical and Sexual Abuse: Guidelines for Treatment (Revised Report: April 26, 2004).* Charleston, SC: National Crime Victims Research and Treatment Center, US Department of Justice; 2004.

185. Hensler D, Wilson C, Sadler BL; Kaufman Foundation. Closing the quality chasm in child abuse treatment: identifying and disseminating best practices: the findings of the Kauffman Best Practices Project to Help Children Heal from Child Abuse. University of Washington Web site. https://depts.washington.edu/hcsats/PDF/kauffmanfinal.pdf. Published March, 2004. Accessed January 29, 2019.

186. Cohen JA, Mannarino AP. Factors that mediate treatment outcome of sexually abused preschool children. *J Am Acad Child Adolesc Psychiatry.* 1996;35(10):1402-1410.

187. Cohen JA, Mannarino AP, Knudsen K. Treating sexually abused children: 1 year follow-up of a randomized controlled trial. *Child Abuse Negl.* 2005;29(2):135-145.

188. King NJ, Tonge BJ, Mullen P, et al. Treating sexually abused children with posttraumatic stress symptoms: a randomized clinical trial. *J Am Acad Child Adolesc Psychiatry.* 2000;39(11):1347-1355.

189. Cohen JA, Mannarino AP, Kliethermes M, Murray LA. Trauma-focused CBT for youth with complex trauma. *Child Abuse Negl.* 2012;36(6):528-541.

190. Kane JC, Murray LK, Cohen J, et al. Moderators of treatment response to trauma-focused cognitive behavioral therapy among youth in Zambia. *J Child Psychol Psychiatry.* 2016;57(10):1194-1202.

191. O'Callaghan P, McMullen J, Shannon C, Rafferty H, Black A. A randomized controlled trial of trauma-focused cognitive behavioral therapy for sexually exploited, war-affected Congolese girls. *J Am Acad Child Adolesc Psychiatry.* 2013;52(4):359-369.

192. Cohen JA, Mannarino AP, Perel JM, Staron V. A pilot randomized controlled trial of combined trauma-focused CBT and sertraline for childhood PTSD symptoms. *J Am Acad Child Adolesc Psychiatry.* 2007;46(7):811-819.

193. The National Child Traumatic Stress Network. Home page. The National Child Traumatic Stress Network Wed site. https://www.nctsn.org/. Accessed January 29, 2019.

194. Medical University of South Carolina. Home page. Medical University of South Carolina Wed site. https://tfcbt2.musc.edu/. Accessed January 29, 2019.

195. CATS Consortium. Implementing CBT for traumatized children and adolescents after September 11: lessons learned from the Child and Adolescent Trauma Treatments and Services (CATS) Project. *J Clin Child Adolesc Psychol.* 2007;36(4):581-592.

196. de Arellano MA, Danielson CK. Culturally-Modified Trauma-Focused Treatment (CM-TFT). Unpublished Manuscript; Charleston, SC: Medical University of South Carolina; 2005.

197. Northern Virginia Family Service. Multicultural center. Northern Virginia Family Service Web site. https://www.nvfs.org/about-nvfs/locations/multicultural-center/. Accessed January 29, 2019.

198. Hébert M, Daignault IV. Challenges in treatment of sexually abused preschoolers: a pilot study of TF-CBT in Quebec. *Sexologies.* 2015;24(1):e21-e27.

199. Madigan S, Vaillancourt K, McKibbon A, Benoit D. Trauma and traumatic loss in pregnant adolescents: the impact of trauma-focused cognitive behavior therapy on maternal unresolved states of mind and posttraumatic stress disorder. *Attach Hum Dev.* 2015;17(2):175-198.

200. Dalgleish T, Goodall B, Chadwick I, et al. Trauma-focused cognitive behaviour therapy versus treatment as usual for posttraumatic stress disorder (PTSD) in young children aged 3 to 8 years: study protocol for a randomised controlled trial. *Trials.* 2015;16(1):116.

201. Jensen TK, Holt T, Ormhaug SM, et al. A randomized effectiveness study comparing trauma-focused cognitive behavioral therapy with therapy as usual for youth. *J Clin Child Adolesc Psychol.* 2014;43(3):356-369.

202. Goldbeck L, Muche R, Sachser C, Tutus D, Rosner R. Effectiveness of trauma-focused cognitive behavioral therapy for children and adolescents: a randomized controlled trial in eight German mental health clinics. *Psychother Psychosom.* 2016;85(3):159-170.

203. Cohen JA, Mannarino AP, Iyengar S. Community treatment of posttraumatic stress disorder for children exposed to intimate partner violence: a randomized controlled trial. *Arch Pediatr Adolesc Med.* 2011;165(1):16-21.

204. Nixon RDV, Sterk J, Pearce A, Weber N. A randomized trial of cognitive behavior therapy and cognitive therapy for children with posttraumatic stress disorder following single-incident trauma: predictors and outcome at 1-year follow-up. *Psychol Trauma.* 2017;9(4):471-478.

205. Nixson RD, Sterk J, Pearce A. A randomized trial of cognitive behavior therapy and cognitive therapy for children with posttraumatic stress disorder following single-incident trauma. *J Abnorm Child Psychol.* 2012;40(3):327-337.

206. Scheeringa MS, Weems CF, Cohen JA, Amaya-Jackson L, Guthrie D. Trauma-focused cognitive-behavioral therapy for posttraumatic stress disorder in three through six year-old children: a randomized clinical trial. *J Child Psychol Psychiatry.* 2011;52(8):853-860.

207. Dorsey S, Pullmann MD, Berliner L, Koschmann E, McKay M, Deblinger E. Engaging foster parents in treatment: a randomized trial of supplementing trauma-focused cognitive behavioral therapy with evidence-based engagement strategies. *Child Abuse Negl.* 2014;38(9):1508-1520.

208. Salloum A, Wang W, Robst J, et al. Stepped care versus standard trauma-focused cognitive behavioral therapy for young children. *J Child Psychol Psychiatry.* 2016;57(5):614-622.

209. Konanur S, Muller RT, Cinamon JS, Thornback K, Zorzella KP. Effectiveness of trauma-focused cognitive behavioral therapy in a community-based program. *Child Abuse Negl.* 2015;50:159-170.

210. Diehle J, Opmeer BC, Boer F, Mannarino AP, Lindauer RJ. Trauma-focused cognitive behavioral therapy or eye movement desensitization and reprocessing: what works in children with posttraumatic stress symptoms? A randomized controlled trial. *Eur Child Adolesc Psychiatry.* 2015;24(2):227-236.

211. Chemtob CM, Tolin DF, van der Kolk BA, Pitman RK. Eye movement desensitization and reprocessing. In: Foa EB, Keane TM, Friedman MJ, Cohen JA, eds. *Effective Treatments for PTSD: Practice Guidelines from the International Society for Traumatic Stress Studies.* New York, NY: Guilford Press; 2000.

212. National Institute for Health and Clinical Excellence. Post-traumatic stress disorder. National Institute for Health and Clinical Excellence Web site. https://www.nice.org.uk/guidance/ng116. Published December 2018. Accessed February 5, 2019.

213. de Arellano MA, Danielson CK. Culturally-modified trauma-focused therapy for treatment of Hispanic child trauma victims. Workshop at: the Annual San Diego Conference on Child and Family Maltreatment; January 2006; San Diego, CA.

214. Kolko DJ, Cohen JA, Mannarino AP, Baumann BL, Knudsen K. Community treatment of child sexual abuse: a survey of practitioners in the National Child Traumatic Stress Network. *Adm Policy Ment Health.* 2009;36(1):37-49.

215. Riggs DS, Cahill SP, Foa EB. Prolonged exposure treatment of posttraumatic stress disorder. In: Follette VM, Ruzek JI, eds. *Cognitive-Behavioral Therapies for Trauma.* New York, NY: Guilford Press; 2006:65-95.

Chapter 21

The Path to Prevention

Carol Plummer, PhD
Vincent J. Palusci, MD, MS, FAAP

Introduction

As an adverse childhood experience, child sexual abuse has been associated with a number of poor long-term health and behavioral outcomes.[1] The costs of sexual abuse are great in human terms (psychological, physical, developmental), but they also have an economic price tag. Although the US Department of Justice[2] has previously estimated costs for child sexual abuse in the United States, to understand the recent financial impact, it is helpful to look at the increased costs for child abuse and neglect overall. These now range from $71 billion to $124 billion depending on which direct and indirect costs are included.[3-5] It appears that child sexual abuse reports comprise 5% to 10% of all child maltreatment reports in the United States, and data from the US National Child Abuse and Neglect Data System for 2015 indicate that there were an estimated 60 000 sexually abused children that year among 794 000 children who were victims of maltreatment.[6] The costs from these cases are likely to be sizable. It is difficult to precisely estimate the total costs for sexual abuse and assault for children younger than age 18 years, but the total direct cost for all child abuse and neglect was estimated at more than $33 billion in 2007, with an additional $70 billion in indirect costs.[2] This is thought to be an underestimate because these numbers only reflect children meeting criteria for child protective services (CPS) substantiation or indication. More recent estimates put the total economic cost of child maltreatment at $2 trillion.[7]

Health care professionals have unique reasons for wanting to prevent child sexual abuse—to prevent physical and emotional pain in their patients, to spare future health problems, and because it is congruent with the goals of their profession regarding health and safety promotion. However, the details of why, how, when, and where health care professionals can promote prevention may seem murky or ill defined, especially because violence against children remains one of the least documented crimes.[8] This chapter clarifies these issues by providing both the rationale for prevention and some concrete ideas about how prevention can become a part of not only what health care professionals support in the community, but also what they do in the day-to-day care of their patients.

The Problem of Child Sexual Abuse and the Importance of Prevention

In the past several decades, our awareness of child sexual abuse and its connection to other social and health problems has skyrocketed. Self-report surveys conclude that at least 1 in 5 girls and 1 in 10 boys in the United States are sexually abused before the age of 18 years.[8,9] Incidence rates show that as many as one in 1000 children are sexually abused in the United States every year, but these rates are considered low because most sexual abuse never gets reported to authorities.[10] In fact, a large part of the problem is our being unable to identify when or where sexual abuse has occurred because there is often cover-up by the shamed child victims, denial by alleged offenders, and, at least initially, disbelief by caregivers. Statistics clearly show that a majority of offenders are known to or are even relatives of the child sexual abuse victims, further contributing to the secrecy and underreporting.[11]

In addition, more facts about the old problem of sexually exploited runaway youth highlight the newer problems of cyberstalking and using the Internet to facilitate child sexual exploitation. The sexual abuse of children through sex tourism and commercial sexual exploitation, nationally and internationally, as well as production of and use of child pornography, is also being publicized.[12] Abuse at childcare centers and by religious leaders, sports coaches, and nationwide perpetrator rings are also regular news items.[13] It is becoming clearer that sexual abuse and exploitation are strongly linked, and it is increasingly evident that both occur worldwide.[13] Although the façade of sexual abuse may change from place to place and over time, the vastness of its reach and the depth of its outcomes are undeniably great.

Although no one symptom can "rule out" or "rule in" sexual abuse, with the possible exception of pregnancy or certain sexually transmitted infections, symptoms and behaviors have been identified that should raise concerns for additional inquiry. The sexual abuse of children has long been linked to a variety of mental health and behavioral problems. Relationship difficulties, depression, suicidal tendencies, and eating disorders are related to a history of child sexual abuse.[14-16] In fact, juvenile delinquency and future criminal behavior have also been strongly linked to a history of childhood abuse.[17] Some children are more resilient than others after sexual abuse experiences, and not all are immediately symptomatic, yet a significant number report emotional reactions or distress.[18,19] Several variables, such as relationship to the perpetrator, age, duration, prior victimization, and use of force are also sometimes predictive of reactions the child may have to the abusive experience. In addition, some children may only exhibit short-term effects and others may show only long-term effects of the sexual abuse.

Many health care professionals are still unaware of increasing evidence that child sexual abuse predicts not only emotional and mental health problems but also future physical health ailments. A large retrospective study linked child sexual abuse with diabetes, heart disease, somatization, drug abuse, and other psychosomatic illnesses.[20] The distress resulting from adverse childhood experiences such as child sexual abuse often results in physical health problems that have long-term effects on those victimized as children. Although a former US surgeon general has declared child sexual abuse "a serious public health challenge," a unified plan to address this problem and prevent sexual abuse has not yet been prioritized in this country.[21] This lack of a well-defined prevention plan continues to contribute to weak public involvement in prevention, resulting in the perpetuation of the problem.

Defining Prevention

Prevention of child sexual abuse is, of course, recommended by all those who are familiar with the problems associated with sexual abuse and its sequelae. Because intervention with and treatment for sexual abuse are both difficult and expensive, efforts aimed at preventing abuse are promoted by agencies, government officials, and individual practitioners. Unfortunately, beyond a blanket endorsement of the concept of prevention, there are many different ideas about what the term actually means and what activities are considered *prevention*. Definitions for prevention may vary, but 3 categories of prevention are generally noted: primary, secondary, and tertiary. The most commonly used definitions of the levels of prevention categorize them in the following way:

1. ***Primary***: Efforts aimed at the general population for the purpose of keeping abuse from happening.
2. ***Secondary***: Efforts aimed at a particularly high-risk group to keep abuse from happening to them given that the risk to this group is elevated.
3. ***Tertiary***: Efforts aimed at preventing abuse from happening again to those who have already been victimized. This level of prevention may include treatment of the patient and offender for the original abuse.

The Centers for Disease Control and Prevention (CDC) has relabeled these levels of prevention in a new way to emphasize that abuse operates in a context and requires an entire spectrum of necessary prevention strategies over time.[22] These efforts are explicitly based on Bronfenbrenner's ecological model, which promotes intervening at the individual, relationship, community, and societal levels.[23] Approaches inferred from these new labels emphasize a shift away from risk reduction as the predominant prevention approach and toward promotion of positive social changes. Some argue that the prior definitions may limit prevention strategies by focusing primarily on the potential individual targets of abuse and how to intervene with them, rather than focusing on the environmental and societal context that supports and even condones abusive acts. These newer definitions of prevention focus on *when* the prevention effort occurs:

1. ***Primary***: This is taking action *before* abuse has occurred to prevent it from happening.
2. ***Secondary***: This level of prevention is intervening right *after* risk factors for abuse have occurred.
3. ***Tertiary***: Tertiary prevention is seen as that which takes the long view and *works over time to change conditions* in the environments that promote or support abusiveness.

Physicians and other health care professionals are invited to become more active in prevention efforts as part of this definitional shift. The National Sexual Violence Resource Center[24] has published information about how to involve a broader constituency in prevention through using the "Spectrum of Prevention." Prevention is explicitly seen not as the responsibility of any one agency, profession, or intervention, but as the responsibility of all to create a society less conducive to child sexual abuse. In this spectrum, individual skill development, community and provider education, coalition building, organizational change, and policy innovations are all components of the prevention solution.

Risk and Protective Factors

Through the use of an ecological model to examine child sexual abuse, both risk and protective factors can be examined on the individual, relationship and family, community, and broader societal levels. Prevention includes activities that diminish risk and bolster protective factors. Prevention, then, requires that those of us involved recognize not only what we are against, or what we want to avoid, but also what we are for and want to promote. Current efforts aimed at reducing child maltreatment, for example, emphasize "resiliency" as a deterrent to abuse.[25] Examining risk factors can inform us about which individuals might have the greatest vulnerabilities. Likewise, recognizing personal, family, or community strengths and supporting them is another approach to preventing negative life outcomes.

On an individual level, risks of child sexual abuse include being a female child and being younger than age 11 years.[26,27] More girls are reported as child sexual abuse victims, but most experts also believe there are a substantial number of male victims who are not reported because of societal double standards, pressure on boys and men to not express "weakness" or admit vulnerabilities, and increased embarrassment if the abuse is same-gender.[28] Although the mean age of children being sexually abused is generally reported to be between 9 and 11 years of age, other studies report that more than half of those sexually victimized are younger than age 7 years.[5,28-31] Undeniably, the vulnerability of younger or disabled children is heightened for several additional reasons other than offender age preference: difficulty in adults understanding communication of the very young or disabled child, difficulty for the child in verbalizing or otherwise communicating what has happened, heightened dependence on adults, and a higher likelihood of these children being tricked or successfully threatened.

Relationship dynamics and family characteristics may also influence the likelihood of abuse. Presence of a stepfather in the home, living with parents who have a conflictual relationship or substance abuse problems, and living apart from one's natural parents are all variables that increase risk of sexual abuse.[8] There is some evidence that low socioeconomic status may increase the possibility of sexual abuse, perhaps in part because of neediness, lack of supervision, or increased familial stress levels.[5] Studies of ethnicity and rural versus urban differences have been inconclusive. What is definitive is that sexual abuse exists in high numbers in all groups: racial, ethnic, socioeconomic, and religious.

On a community or even societal level, some factors may increase vulnerability to sexual abuse, such as having a weak friendship network, lack of employment opportunities, lack of institutional support from police and the judicial system, general tolerance of sexual assault within the community, settings that support sexual violence, weak community sanctions against sexual violence perpetrators, and being isolated from the broader community.[32] Other societal factors include poverty, societal norms that support sexual violence, societal practices that support male superiority and sexual entitlement, attitudes that maintain women's inferiority and sexual submissiveness, weak laws and policies related to gender equity, and high tolerance levels toward crime and other forms of violence.[32]

Perhaps in part because of different levels of supervision, freedom, self-reliance, and social roles of boys and girls, these community risks can be categorized with regard to gender. Boys are abused more often by nonrelatives compared with girls,[30] and girls are more likely to be sexually abused by family members,[33] but both are likely to know the perpetrator.[34] The Children's Bureau's Child Welfare Information Gateway[35] highlights that all efforts to support strengths in families and build resilience in children should also provide protective factors such as social supports, positive peer group, stable living situation, self-efficacy, and good school environment, among others.

It is clear that healing after abuse is enhanced by these factors, but it is less clear how preventative they may be to keeping sexual abuse from reoccurring. Palusci and Ilardi[36] identified a number of risk and protective factors associated with recurrence of child sexual abuse after a first confirmed report. A small but important number of second sexual abuse reports (4%) could be linked to first reports in 2010 using data for 2010-2015 from the National Child Abuse and Neglect Data System. Similar to first reports, girls; children with emotional and behavioral problems; and families with poverty, violence, substance abuse, and behavioral problems also have increased risk for recurrent sexual abuse. This worsens when additional maltreatment co-occurs with sexual abuse. Unfortunately, few if any of the services used by child protective services (eg, counseling, foster care placement, family preservation, domestic violence intervention, other referrals made by CPS) after the first sexual abuse report were significantly associated with reduction in the risk for sexual abuse recurrence.

Some Key Points to Understand About Sexual Abuse of Children

Before discussing details of prevention efforts, including the role of health care professionals in prevention, a few key points need to be stressed. This list highlights what is known about child sexual abuse and provides guidance in potential responses. These points help to frame the work by providing a common understanding of the dynamics of child sexual abuse that should guide prevention and intervention efforts.

Discovery of Child Sexual Abuse: More of a Process Than an Event

Not all children who have experienced sexual abuse will be clearly identified, or perhaps even identified at all, before coming for medical services. Although some cases of sexual abuse are immediately apparent because of the presence of sexually transmitted infections or acute physical injury, the vast majority of child sexual abuse is discovered through a child's own accidental or purposeful disclosure of abuse. Children often grapple with whether to tell, who to tell, and when to disclose so as to minimize negative outcomes to themselves or their families. These children may be faced with adults who are unprepared to respond appropriately because of lack of information, fear, or adults' own emotional reactions. Even when adults listen, they may respond in ways that upset the child or contribute to a retraction of the report or they may misinterpret the message, either exaggerating or minimizing the situation.[37,38]

One goal of prevention is to minimize harm after sexual abuse is discovered, and thereby reduce the risk of further victimization. When children are officially questioned, much effort is put into reducing the number of times an interview occurs and increasing the sensitivity in interviewing to help children tell their stories accurately and without retraumatization. However, at any point in the investigative process, a true disclosure can be changed by a child victim to stop removal from the home, foster care placement, court proceedings, and so on. It is important for health care professionals to recognize that they may need to provide care and intervention at the initial report or, for a variety of reasons, long after the first or most recent incident of abuse. In fact, health care professionals may not be informed until the abuse has resumed or been ongoing for a period of years. Awareness of this issue also means knowing the possibility of children being tricked or forced into behaviors or situations that are nearly unbelievable to us, including sexual activities with other children, animals, maternal caregivers, teachers, and religious leaders; child pornography; and being prostituted or trafficked (even by their own parents). Full disclosure of such events may only be revealed over months or years, or as adults.

Children React in a Wide Variety of Ways After Victimization

Some children victimized by sexual abuse will be primarily relieved once the sexual abuse has stopped. Others will experience ongoing posttraumatic stress disorder, some will not want to discuss it, and others will need to vent their experience and emotions. It is impossible to "diagnose" the accuracy of a child's report or predict any long-term medical or psychological needs based on the immediate presentation of symptoms, especially because many children are actually asymptomatic.[39] Although children may react favorably to specialized evaluation techniques such as videocolposcopy during a physical examination, such responses do not allow one to interpret the accuracy of their victimization history and need for long-term mental health treatment.[40]

Parents Are Central for Both Successful Prevention and Intervention

Parents are critical to healing after abuse, but they will react differently than their children will and differently than one another. Assessment of and attention to parents are critical components of successful intervention. Parents may need referrals for mental health treatment or crisis support. Health care professionals play a central role in informing parents regarding the necessity of and techniques for talking to their children, supervising behaviors, and selecting care providers in order to prevent the sexual abuse of their children.[41,42] Furthermore, if there are questions or abuse allegations, physicians and other health care professionals may be asked for or want to offer referral services for parents.

Some Children Are More Vulnerable to Child Sexual Abuse

Prevention is important for everyone before abuse ever occurs; it is even more important for those who have been previously abused or who have special needs. Children with physical disabilities, cognitive impairments, or developmental delays all have greatly elevated risk of being sexually abused.[43-47] For that reason, parents and caregivers of these children need to be especially informed of their unique vulnerability and need for safety. Studies have shown that children who have already experienced sexual abuse have increased risk of experiencing additional sexual abuse and of experiencing other types of interpersonal violence, both as children and later as adults.[27,48-51]

History of Child Sexual Abuse Prevention Efforts

Educational Efforts Targeting Children

Since the late 1970s, when efforts first were made to prevent child sexual abuse in the United States, educational methods have been the main approach. Programs were designed to help children understand what abuse is, to instruct them on ways to avoid potentially dangerous situations, and to inform them of what to do if grooming (ie, gradually acclimating a child to activities that will ultimately lead to sexual abuse) or actual abuse took place. This child-education component was initially mandated in 1979 by federal authorities at the National Center on Child Abuse and Neglect (NCCAN) when deciding to fund child sexual abuse prevention programs.[52] Approaches to preventing sexual abuse were designed differently from those aimed to address neglect or physical abuse. Sexual abuse had been shrouded in secrecy and silence for so long and in most cases only the offender and the child were aware of it. Offenders were perceived to have few incentives to report themselves and limited motivation to willingly stop the behavior. In addition, many children didn't even know what this behavior (sexual abuse) was and had no knowledge of where or how they could seek help or what to do if they were approached in a potentially dangerous situation. For these reasons, educating children was seen as a necessary first step.

Educational programs for children often focused on victimization prevention. Many aimed to alter children's level of knowledge, skills, and resources regarding potential sexual abuse. For example, factual information was given to make children more aware of abuse as well as to address attitudes that may have contributed to self-blame. Many programs addressed lies that may be told by perpetrators to confuse children or keep them quiet and isolated. These messages challenged ideas presented by some offenders (eg, "You shouldn't have worn that outfit"; "Your mother will be mad at you if you tell"; "This is how uncles always show love to their nieces"). Most programs addressed myths about sexual abuse (eg, offenders are mostly strangers, it is the victim's fault, sexual abuse only happens to girls or in "bad" neighborhoods). Programs also endorsed and emphasized communication with trusted adults. Some of this was to build support networks for consulting with trusted adults regarding all kinds of problems or confusion. Building communication was a strategy to help prevent abuse by involving adults when luring of the child had begun but had not yet led to abuse. Other programs focused solely on the need for children to report abuse and to keep telling until someone believed and helped them.

Other programs for children, albeit in smaller numbers, also focused on educating children about related topics. These included bullying prevention, respect for others, protecting your own child when you become a parent, and even "offender prevention." Offender prevention pertains to programs that actually try to alter behaviors and attitudes in those youth who may be considering sexually abusive acts. These programs may emphasize morals, laws, or social norms. Many of these programs were developed later in the 1980s and 1990s and were integrated into already existing child abuse prevention programming.

Child education programs developed quickly over the next decade, resulting in millions of children receiving a wide variety of programs—from weak to strong, comprehensive to one-shot deals, risk reduction to reporting directions, assertiveness training to avoidance oriented, antisex to discussing a "continuum" of touching experiences.[53] These early efforts showed promise and had the ability to reach children and did so with broad adult approval.[54,55] Unfortunately, the quality of programs was thought to vacillate from very useful to potentially harmful or confusing.[56,57]

Educational Efforts Targeting Adults

Several groups of adults were particularly targeted in the earliest years of sexual abuse prevention programming. These included parents, teachers, mental health professionals who treated children and victims, and the general public. A plethora of newspaper articles, books, movies, and talk shows about the sexual abuse of children saturated the public in the early to mid-1980s. Although awareness of the problem undoubtedly increased, these efforts may have helped create a backlash that challenged claims of the astronomical rates of abuse, the extent of damage to victims and families, and even the veracity of specific victim statements. An overreaction to concerns about sexual abuse has been termed "moral panic" by some writers[58] and may have resulted in overzealous pursuits of those perceived to be offenders in large childcare center cases or bizarre stories being publicized about ritual abuse, baby killing, and other unusual child sexual abuse claims.[59] Even nonsensationalized public awareness efforts had their weaknesses in the earliest years of our awareness of sexual abuse. For example, most programs were aimed at the generic public, meaning that they were primarily focused on images and approaches that would appeal to white, middle-class Americans. Few programs were in other languages, focused on messages to subcultures, or had a distinct audience in mind.

Programs for parents initially accompanied almost every child-oriented educational effort. This was partly because parents had never before heard of talking with children about sexual abuse and had grave concerns about what would be said and how it would be communicated. Educational programs for parents were not just about gaining entry to work with children, but often became that, even though prevention advocates also attempted to engage parents as partners in prevention. Once parents realized the programs appeared to be safety oriented, did not differ from their personal values, and had some developmental appropriateness (or claimed to), they gave consent for their children to attend programs. They also stopped coming to parent education meetings themselves, either expecting that the experts would do a great job or believing that they knew what they needed to know after the media blitz or from a prior meeting they had attended.

Concerns About Sexual Abuse Prevention Efforts

Prevention programs, and especially those geared toward children, are not without critics. Early criticism focused on the fear that children would make false allegations, "practice" sex, be traumatized by the topic, or be incapable of understanding concepts. As is the case in arguments against sex education, some felt that parents and not schools should educate their children about sexual abuse. Others countered that when incest was the problem, relying on parents alone meant that these children would be at great risk and would never get prevention messages from parents.

Most critics today do not advocate completely dismantling child education about child sexual abuse, but they do encourage expanding the emphasis to decrease placing the sole responsibility on the shoulders of children for their own protection. Although there is no empirical evidence that any program actually promotes children taking full responsibility to prevent sexual abuse, there is no doubt that some programs have underemphasized their parent education, public awareness, and advocacy efforts to focus on child education.

Numerous efforts were neglected while children, parents, certain professionals, and the public were given awareness information. These areas included a broader focus on community ownership of the problem, organizational responses, long-term changes in social norms, and rigorous efforts to see if offending behaviors could be stopped so there were fewer offenders, to name a few. However, even today, parents who educate their children about sexual abuse continue to disproportionately focus on strangers as potential offenders and provide limited information, particularly in terms of the nature of sexual abuse and the secrecy associated with it. Parents with no direct or indirect experience with child sexual abuse are least likely to talk with their children about the issue in general and, when they do, provide less information.[60]

Bolen[33] suggests that potential offenders should be targeted by providing school-based programs for youth that promote healthy relationship patterns rather than a "victim-based paradigm" because there is such a diversity of approaches taken by offenders. Unfortunately, though the idea of outreach to offenders is gaining in popularity and has promise, no solid empirical evidence exists yet to show whether this will produce change in the rates of sexual abuse or whether new or potential offenders are amenable to change. One study[61] found that nearly half of offenders had no bad feelings about sexually abusing children, suggesting the limited value for prevention programs directed at them. The authors of a systematic review noted that there are major weaknesses in the scientific evidence, particularly regarding adult men—the main category of sexual abusers of children. They suggested that better coordinated and funded high-quality studies including several countries are urgently needed and that, until conclusive evidence is available, realistic clinical strategies might involve reduction of specific risk factors for sex crimes, such as sexual preoccupation, in abusers at risk of reoffending.[62]

The sex offender registry, initially driven by concerns about missing and exploited children, has been considered a prevention strategy by some. Efforts to learn where offenders are, to monitor their movement, and to limit their access to children have been expanding over the past decade. Those in the child sexual abuse prevention movement, though initially strongly supportive of the idea, have often withdrawn support for this direction, deeming it a poor substitute for other prevention efforts. First, it reinforces the idea that most offenders are those "dangerous stranger pedophiles," ignoring the role of family members. Second, it may reduce other prevention efforts by diverting funds away from primary prevention programs and give parents a false sense of security that reduces their perception of the need for them to be involved in other prevention efforts. Third, it inequitably has penalized offenders who are young, poor, minority, and mentally challenged. For example, professionals recognize the dangers of labeling youth with sexual behavior problems as "offenders" and the unfortunate outcome of dating relationships resulting in persons placed on the registry when in peer consensual liaisons. Finally, many of these offenders are maltreated children who have grown up, and extremely punitive measures may make some people feel some release for their anger but not really solve the overall problem. In fact, leaving no room for offender rehabilitation and reentry into society exacerbates the long-term problem.

The biggest questions of how best to prevent sexual abuse, how to reduce rates over time, and eventually eliminate it remain unanswered. However, there are numerous signs that prior efforts have been useful and new methods such as a public health approach need to be further explored and researched.[63] Study after study has characterized the merits of past prevention efforts with regard to learning and skill acquisition for children and adults as a result of policy change, education, or media campaigns. Although some argue that sexual abuse has not decreased as a result of sexual abuse prevention efforts,[34] actual rates of sexual abuse do seem to be decreasing. One proposed explanation is that sexual abuse prevention efforts may be at least part of the reason.[64] Few studies have actually found that participation in a prevention program resulted in reduced rates of sexual abuse for participants, however, with only anecdotal reports on successes and actions taken to stay safe as evidence. Even if initial abuse rates were not changed, one study did find that college women (n = 825) who had participated in a child sexual abuse prevention program as children were significantly less likely to experience subsequent sexual abuse than those who had not completed such a program.[65]

Prevention Today: Trends and Future Directions

Set Standards and Use Best Practices

The variability in past prevention programming aimed toward children has resulted in many efforts to find more effective prevention programs. One current trend in child-focused sexual abuse education programs is toward "best practices" for ensuring quality. The National Children's Alliance has instituted a number of national initiatives to promote high-quality programming.[66] Another example is Prevent Child Abuse Iowa, which provides a list of prevention resources for their funded programs.[67]

Similarly, the New Jersey Task Force on Child Abuse and Neglect has created a booklet titled *Standards for Prevention Programs: Building Success through Family Support* based on research findings about effective programs.[68] Included in their list of factors used to evaluate programs are conceptual standards (ie, the content and approaches to imparting information to the target group), practice standards, and administrative standards. Recommendations for programs include being family centered, community based, culturally competent, and using a strengths-based approach. Other suggestions include being easily accessible, being linked to informal and formal supports, and having a long-range plan and ongoing evaluations. These efforts are promising and may help to build the highest quality into programs that currently vary greatly in their level of comprehensiveness. Evidence-based interventions will be useful, but standardizing programs across settings and cultures may not entirely work. At the same time that high standards must be set, there must remain room for creativity and the use of feedback from diverse community settings to respond to their unique needs and situations. Also, some programs may be hampered in their opportunity to be truly comprehensive, reach broader audiences, and use creative methods because of lack of funds, a problem that has been identified by many prevention program leaders.[69] Demands for quality will need to be combined with demands for adequate funding for prevention so that truly valuable programs can exist.

Meaningfully Involve Parents

As discussed earlier, parents have generally been included in sexual abuse education programs. The earliest child sexual abuse prevention programs included strong parent education components, but in subsequent years, parent attendance dwindled, shifting the focus even more to children.[70-72] Parents are in the best position to prevent sexual abuse because it can begin at a very young age (before children have contact with school), because parents know how to talk to their own children, because children are more likely to believe their parents, because parents know what their children need to know, and because children will understand from the conversation that parents are approachable.[73,74] Promising outcomes in parent education on sexual abuse include substantial parental support for in-school programs[71] and the finding that programs may increase the confidence of parents to talk with their children about sexual abuse.[75,76] At the same time, survey results have indicated that parents may mistakenly believe their own children are well supervised and able to avoid danger, and as such they do not want to frighten them unnecessarily.[73] Some results of parent education have been encouraging, yet new methods of engaging parents meaningfully with information they truly need must still be creatively developed. Reppucci et al[72] found that parents are enthusiastic about parent programs "but in different formats, at different times and in different environments than the current typical parent-teach organization one evening, one-time meeting."

Prevention advocates are currently developing programs that better meet parents' needs. These include a topical focus on Internet safety and common lures for teens at malls, areas of newer concern for parents and for which parents are offered information they truly believe they require. Programs may need to reach out to parents in different formats (eg, take-home DVDs or interactive Internet training programs), videos played in waiting rooms of doctor's offices, meetings held over lunch in employment settings, and the incorporation of sexual abuse prevention messages into general pamphlets about the health care of children. A medical program for educating parents during primary care pediatric visits has been recommended but not studied systematically across populations.[41]

Broaden the Targets of Prevention Messages

Awareness programs need to include professionals, the general public, and even offenders or potential offenders. A survey of 87 sexual abuse prevention programs found that one-fourth of these programs had included some adolescent offender prevention messages or approaches in their overall education.[69] One approach developed by Dr. Gene Abel teaches parents to watch for sexual behavior problems in their children so patterns of dysfunction can be identified and interrupted earlier.[62] This program uses data about current offenders—including how they developed without effective interventions—to prevent young people who are at some risk for developing sexual problems from doing so. In large part it engages parents to help prevent their own children from developing sexual problems by recognizing concerning signs early and by taking them to sex-specific therapists rather than fearfully retreating into denial and ignoring these concerns.

Bystanders also are being encouraged to be more proactive, rather than silently ignoring concerns that a professional colleague, relative, or neighbor is displaying concerning behavior toward children. A booklet by *Stop It Now* details an approach that can be taken to ask questions of, and show concern for, a friend, colleague, or loved one who may have interest in sexual contact with children, or who may have acted inappropriately toward them.[77] Approaching a potential offender may alert them to a friend's awareness and force reconsideration of certain preabusive or abusive behavior. However, care must also be taken that this is done advisedly; in some cases, discussing concerns with an offender may only make the abuse go deeper underground or may inappropriately reassure the concerned party that nothing is occurring. This method and others need to be undertaken with awareness of the dynamics of sexual abuse and the potential for harm as well as good coming from prevention innovations. One thing is certain: sexual abuse prevention will need to involve many types of people and many diverse approaches if we are to alter the family and community context where sexual abuse occurs.

Support Quality Education of Children

School-based educational programs that teach children what abuse is and how to avoid and report it have merit.[78,79] Those studies with the most compelling findings revealed the age of the child, number of sessions, participant involvement, and use of behavioral skills training to be significant moderator variables. Dozens of studies have reported that children can and do learn information, change attitudes, and even gain skills from quality prevention education that is child-focused.[78,80] Despite this, communities should be wary of relying on children to be solely or primarily responsible for their own safety and protection, a technique that has not been used in other forms of child maltreatment. All communities must do more than simply educate children about sexuality or abuse. Health care professionals are well aware that good sex education programs, including messages about positive sexuality and good choices, are sorely lacking. To provide quality sexual abuse prevention, it is necessary to have a model for healthy sexual development and behavior to provide to children and to their parents.

Create Diverse Approaches for Diverse Communities

Different forms of abuse in distinctive communities and cultures will require unique types of prevention strategies. For example, as abuse of children in schools is addressed, administrators may need to establish stronger policies on student-to-student sexual harassment, working to change norms on allowable on-campus behavior. Prevention for children with disabilities will require special techniques and sensitivities to address their unique needs and abilities.[81] Teachers may need to address attitudes of sexual entitlement, provide sex education, and demand training on how to respond when sexual abuse is suspected or disclosed. Recent high-profile cases in which teachers, both male and female, have sexually exploited young students have also expanded our awareness that schools need to do more to screen teachers, set appropriate student-teacher relationship standards, and train bystanders to take action when it appears a teacher colleague is acting inappropriately. Education of a whole range of groups, including health care professionals, is necessary to help in the prevention of child sexual abuse.

Some groups are effectively addressing child sexual abuse as a public health problem and are attempting to change the willingness of adults to report abuse based on public awareness efforts. For example, *Stop It Now* found that there was an increased willingness to report abuse after they conducted a multiyear public education campaign on the importance of reporting.[77] Another program, Stewards of Children, which offers both in-person and Web-based formats for childcare professionals, was found to affect knowledge, attitudes, and preventive behaviors, and no differences were found between training modalities (ie, in-person versus Web-based).[82]

Some communities have chosen to focus on offender prevention. Efforts such as billboards and telephone hotlines aimed at current offenders, education programs for parents of children with sexual behavior problems that could lead to offending, and socialization skills training for youth are being evaluated. Hotlines have been used by friends or family of suspected offenders, and they encourage concerned adults to take appropriate action. Importantly, each of these approaches needs to be designed, evaluated, and updated based on specific local cultural values to maximize relevance and community endorsement and ownership.

One innovative community-based approach was developed by a group called Generation Five. In addition to providing community-specific consultation and capacity building to make programs emerge from theory and be relevant to the participants, Generation Five encourages taking a look at the long view as we try to change society to eradicate child sexual abuse. They anticipate it will take five generations to totally rid society of sexual abuse, and they prescribe tasks for each generation as we work for long-term outcomes. They promote "transformative justice" that does not focus on punitive responses to abuse but on communities addressing a wide range of problems that may ultimately result in children being victimized.[83]

Address the Internet and Media

The expanded use of the Internet by young people and by sexual offenders has placed children at additional risk of being lured into sexual contact. The World Wide Web is an invaluable teaching tool, but it can also enable exposure to unsavory topics or materials, as well as provide an avenue for luring children into sexually abusive situations. Although the public is broadly aware of this risk, school-based child education programs have only recently incorporated strong Internet-safety programs into their sexual abuse prevention curricula. Further, still fewer parents are monitoring their children's Internet use, and many do not believe that their own child is personally at risk of such exploitation. Although the risk of victimization may be low,[84] strong parent engagement and concrete training are necessary to minimize the risk to children in terms of Internet predators.

It is unlikely that prevention advocates or parents will force a discontinuation of children's use of the Internet because of these problems or because of the difficulties in monitoring its use. However, one promising approach targets children and youth with information on how to have "Netsmartz," with interactive Internet games, school programs, and print material that instructs them on safe practices, both online and in their broader lives.[85]

Organizational Interventions

Another type of prevention activity receiving attention is aimed at changing organizations to maximize safety for children. Nationally known speaker and consultant on the prevention of child sexual exploitation and sexual violence Cordelia Anderson[86] has highlighted the work of groups as diverse as the Boy Scouts of America, the National Alliance of Youth Sports, the Chicago Children's Museum, and the Greater Twin Cities Youth Symphonies, which have all done work to prevent child sexual abuse. Actions taken by these groups include developing organizational policies, installing security hardware, creating training mandates, instituting supervision and hiring requirements, making public statements about their commitment to child safety, and adopting proactive risk management plans. Even consideration of facility design to minimize one-on-one opportunities between unsavory adults and vulnerable children has resulted in cameras or mirrors in youth facilities or doors left off stalls where younger children may need assistance while toileting.

All organizations can develop policies and procedures that acknowledge that child sexual abuse occurs, in and outside of child-serving agencies. Youth-serving organizations have an implicit responsibility to their clientele. The CDC[87] and American Academy of Pediatrics[88] have made recommendations to prevent child sexual abuse in youth-serving and health care organizations. Doctors' offices, clinics, hospitals, community mental health centers, and other health care facilities that serve children could also enhance children's safety and decrease their own liability by taking similar actions. However, even organizations that do not solely or primarily focus on children can and should be involved in the same prevention process.

Involve Health Professionals in Prevention Efforts

There are several reasons that health professionals, particularly pediatricians, should be involved in prevention efforts. Most health professionals already understand and appreciate the linkages among prevention, intervention, and treatment, but it is equally critical that health care personnel embrace the importance of professionals having a role in prevention beyond merely treating and reporting suspicious injuries. Ray Helfer, a physician who spearheaded the creation of the Children's Trust Funds to promote prevention, suggested decades ago that health professionals should be an important part of a multifaceted approach with concurrent maneuvers to prevent violence.[89] The approaches listed include community commitment, mass media messages, training for new parents, early childhood development programs for all preschoolers, interpersonal skills programs for all school-aged children, and adult education programs for those caring for children.

Health care professionals are sometimes reluctant to intervene in potential cases of abuse. There are several reasons for this: lack of knowledge, fear of offending the patient (or caregiver), time pressures, potential discomfort for the patient when asked questions, fear of loss of control of the provider-patient relationship, and attitudes about accountability. Pediatricians, for example, do not always report suspected abuse or neglect.[90] Hamberger and Patel[91] have found these hesitancies in cases of domestic violence, and many of the same factors are relevant in cases of child sexual abuse. It is vital for health care professionals to be knowledgeable regarding current issues of sexually abused patients, and examining barriers to optimal service provision is important for every health care professional. If the child is treated medically, the physician's lack of knowledge about abuse may impede discussion with the child regarding sexual abuse and therefore, subsequent intervention. Often this interaction replicates the child's experience of family denial or minimization.[92] For example, touch is often experienced as invasive, intrusive, and noxious. Persistent revictimization themes may emerge during medical treatment. The patient may even feel that the medical experience triggers associations with childhood abuse. In addition, because of a patient's difficulty with trust or inability to remember, abuse issues may only be revealed to the provider over time.

Health professionals have unique relationships with families and special opportunities to intervene to prevent child sexual abuse. Dubowitz[93] has suggested that it is important for physicians to be able to ask sensitive questions, gather information, and use astute observation and careful assessment skills if they are to be successful in these endeavors. Palusci and Haney[94] provide a number of effective practices for comprehensive screening. Keys to effectiveness are: professional comfort with hearing sensitive issues, an ability to teach children about sensitive issues, familiarity with normal genital anatomy and routine child and parent concerns, an ability to diagnose and treat suspected maltreatment, and knowledge of the child welfare system.

Physicians specializing in forensic examinations and emergency department physicians charged with evaluating alleged abuse should be attuned to the need for thorough assessments. Physical examinations should include discussions with the patient and his or her family as part of the process. Physicians, nurse practitioners, and nurses can also assist in communicating messages that may prevent additional abuse.[74] Anticipatory guidance should be provided by health care professionals to parents and families about a variety of topics during childhood. However, pediatricians also report that they need additional training and support to make anticipatory guidance regarding abuse prevention more effective.[95] These messages can be in the form of pamphlets, video education, or interpersonal discussions that communicate safety information to victims, parents, and caregivers. Prevention messages may be critical if no medical evidence is found, if a child victim changes his or her story, or if action by child protective services or prosecutors is not possible because of the lack of medical evidence.

Lack of medical evidence,[96] victim recantation,[97,98] and general lack of evidence for legal action[9,99] are, in fact, very common. Health care professionals need to communicate to families that medical evidence is often not present (depending on the type of abuse), that coming in for help was the right thing to do, and that resources are available if other concerns arise.[31] Given that maternal support is important for a child's recovery and that maternal adjustment is predictive of the child's adjustment, attention to the needs of the maternal caregiver is critical.[100,101] Mothers need to not only believe that health care providers care about the child victim but that their needs and feelings as a nonoffending parent are also of interest. Professional support of mothers during early discovery and disclosure has been shown to have a positive relationship to maternal emotional stability.[56] Thus, supporting a mother with empathy and patience during this crisis may be one of the best ways to support the child victim. The mother, particularly in cases of incest, will need to be understood before she can take guidance or challenges, and her strength will determine the ability of a child or children to remain in a home. In cases in which nonoffending fathers are actively involved after the sexual abuse, it is likely that support for them is equally important, but few studies have examined the role of fathers in child adjustment after sexual abuse.[102]

Screening for family and community violence should be included in routine health visits, even though some pediatricians need skills to better identify and manage injuries caused by such violence.[103] Collecting information about possible abuse experiences on intake forms is another way to learn about and create opportunities to address certain problems. Some physicians may be skeptical that patients would reveal information about a history of sexual abuse on health forms, though patients are more forthcoming if asked than if never asked.[104] In addition, by mentioning "unmentionable" topics, those providing health care show that they are aware of these issues and probably are knowledgeable about how to be helpful. The American Academy of Pediatrics has developed a violence prevention program called *Connected Kids: Safe, Strong, Secure* that includes a guide for office clinicians, provides 21 parent or patient information brochures and supporting training materials, and encourages implementing a strengths-based approach for clinicians to provide anticipatory guidance in order to help parents raise resilient children.[105]

Ten Steps Health Care Professionals Can Take to Prevent Child Sexual Abuse

In addition to the prevention opportunities in the health care setting, health care professionals can also involve themselves in communitywide efforts to change the societal conditions that promote or allow sexual abuse of children. These and other steps[106] provide avenues for the prevention of abuse that broaden collaboration and enlarge health care professionals' role in the prevention of sexual abuse.

1. ***Child education:*** Health care professionals can endorse and support quality, comprehensive child-focused education on child sexual abuse using their professional status to reassure parents and communities.[107] They can also serve on an advisory board for a local child abuse prevention agency, thereby assisting in networking alliances between prevention programs and the treatment field. Physicians and nurses can play a key role in promoting both healthy sexuality and sexual abuse education.

2. ***Parent involvement:*** Health care professionals can provide parents with ideas of how to speak with their own children about sexuality and sexual abuse, providing materials or consultation. They can promote issues of Internet safety, supervision, selecting safe babysitters, and choosing a quality childcare program. Posters in waiting rooms, take-home brochures, and lists of Web addresses readily available for referrals for parents' use can be used to further provide outreach. Additional resources on child abuse prevention programs that exist in and around the community and referrals of parents to area agencies for additional information or assistance can also be vital prevention interventions.

3. ***Community awareness:*** Health care professionals can offer to provide radio or TV public service announcements to build awareness of child sexual abuse as a public health issue and an issue that is related to physical health. Health care professionals need to promote awareness of the links between childhood trauma and future health problems, and they have the credibility to do so. They can participate in Child Abuse Prevention Month, promoting activities from their practices and in their offices; they can also donate money to the Children's Trust Fund in their state.

4. ***Bystander involvement:*** In personal or professional capacities, health care professionals should be willing to become involved when they are concerned about a child's safety and should seek supervision or consultation when necessary. Despite great demands on their time, health care professionals must be willing to make appropriate referrals to child protective services based on reasonable suspicions, rather than waiting to report abuse when they are certain. Child protective services investigates suspicions and has the authority, expertise, and responsibility for that job.

5. ***Early sexual behavior problem identification:*** Caregivers often consult with medical authorities about sexual or social behavior problems with their children, who may be exhibiting sexually reactive symptoms of being abused or early sexual deviancy. Behavioral problems are often nonspecific, but physicians can guide parents to seek additional assistance rather than ignoring these problems, while guarding against parental overreaction to self-exploration or age-appropriate sexual curiosity.[31,108] Consider having materials and referral sources on hand for sexual behavior problems. Even parents who won't verbally address their concerns may pick up a pamphlet.

6. ***Offender prevention:*** Support efforts to reach out to those with problematic sexual feelings or desires and make certain that referrals are made to therapists knowledgeable about the assessment and treatment of sexual deviance. Be alert to early signs of sexual problems in youth so that patterns of deviant behavior do not become established through lack of responsiveness.

7. ***Policy and organizational prevention efforts:*** Health care professionals should be willing to make changes in policy, hiring, supervision, and training in their own offices or organizations to put proven risk-reducing procedures in place. This can include establishing clinical practice guidelines to address these issues in the office, hospital, and clinic. For example, new initiatives might include routine staff trainings conducted for updates on family violence issues, and intake protocols for patients that ask about past or present traumatic events.

8. ***Improved clinical care and education:*** Pediatricians should recognize risk factors for violence when providing clinic care and be able to diagnose and treat violence-related problems at all stages of child development. Pediatricians need to identify, for example, issues with mental illness, substance abuse, and stress in family constellations, as well as inappropriate supervision; family violence and exposure to media violence; access to firearms; and gang involvement and other signs of poor self-esteem, school failure, and depression.[105] Pediatricians should also support early bonding and attachment, and educate parents on normal age-appropriate behaviors for children of all ages. Pediatricians can educate parents about parenting skills, limit setting, and protective factors to be nurtured in children to help prevent a variety of injuries. Consistent discipline practices and body safety techniques should be emphasized. Pediatricians can also provide information about what constitutes safe, appropriate dating and relationships, as well as information on safe sex practices. During adolescence, this can mean supporting parents to foster independence in teens and teaching children about adult roles and responsibilities. During an examination, health care professionals can teach children about sexuality and preventing victimization. Statements such as "I can examine you because I am a doctor and your parent is here" are helpful in reducing anxiety and providing key information. Also, with so many parents anxious about the possibility of abuse, encouraging open communication in families is important. Parents should be encouraged to tell their children to let them know if something bothers them.

9. ***Treatment and referral:*** Pediatricians need to know what they can handle through office counseling and when they need to refer families for help. They must also be cognizant of the resources available in their community to address these risks. This will require knowledge of the child welfare, emergency shelter, and substance abuse treatment systems and how to make referrals to appropriate therapists and mental health professionals. Health care professionals need to understand when to make reports, the reporting laws, and how the reporting process works for sexual abuse in their jurisdiction. When parents learn that their child has been sexually abused, it is essential for the health care professional to communicate to nonabusive parents that they are likely to feel distress and that counseling for their own reactions, in addition to treatment for their victimized child, is normative and advisable, at least short term.[109] Care must be taken not to communicate blame toward parents who are not the abusers, leaving clinical interventions to those who provide counseling. At the same time, health care professionals need to make a commitment to reporting suspected abuse and following up when necessary to promote children's safety.

10. ***Advocacy:*** Pediatricians should use their given status in the community to advocate for the needs of individual families and for the broader needs of children in society. This may include working on public policy and can best be achieved by working in conjunction with nonmedical organizations that address the needs of children in different arenas. Pediatricians can also work with medical schools and pediatric training programs to provide opportunities for students to learn these techniques and to assist in research evaluating the effectiveness and implementation of child abuse prevention programs.

Conclusion

It is an exciting time for those working to prevent child sexual abuse. We understand the immediate and long-term human and financial costs associated with child sexual abuse and have begun to estimate the lifelong savings that can accrue if it can be prevented.[74] There is a wealth of information on what programs are doing and where they are making a difference. At the same time, with decades of experience, it is now apparent that gaps exist in prevention efforts. A level of awareness has been reached so that stronger efforts can proceed to prevent child sexual abuse by addressing individual, family, community, and societal level changes. Programs must involve the cultures and communities they serve and be geared toward a specific message to specific populations. Although child-focused programs have grown and provide some protection, involvement of a much wider range of targets and approaches is necessary. In particular, quality programs that involve key adults, including parents and health care professionals, need support and financial backing. Involving the public, bystanders, organizations, offenders, social change advocates, the media, teachers, policymakers, and health care professionals will be important to ongoing and expanded success of child sexual abuse prevention efforts. Pediatricians and others caring for children have a special position in relation to society and the family and have a multitude of steps they can take to reduce and prevent child sexual abuse.

References

1. Felitti VJ, Anda RF, Nordenberg D, et al. Relationship of childhood abuse and household dysfunction to many of the leading causes of death in adults: the Adverse Childhood Experiences (ACE) study. *Am J Prev Med.* 1998;14(4):245-258.

2. Miller TR, Cohen MA, Wiersema B; US Department of Justice. Victim costs and consequences: a new look. https://www.ncjrs.gov/pdffiles/victcost.pdf. Published January 1996. Accessed January 22, 2019.

3. Pereznieto P, Montes A, Routier S, Langston L. The costs and economic impact of violence against children. Child Fund International Web site. https://www.childfund.org/uploadedFiles/public_site/media/ODI%20Report%20%20The%20cost%20and%20economic%20impact%20of%20violence%20against%20children.pdf. Published September 2014. Accessed January 22, 2019.

4. Reed SF. Total estimated cost of child abuse and neglect in the United States: statistical evidence. Purdue University Wed site. https://www.purdue.edu/hhs/hdfs/fii/wp-content/uploads/2015/06/s_nmfis02c02.pdf. Accessed January 22, 2019.

5. Fang X, Brown DS, Florence CS, Mercy JA. The economic burden of child maltreatment in the United States and implications for prevention. *Child Abuse Negl.* 2012;36(2):156-165.

6. US Department of Health and Human Services, Administration for Children and Families. Child maltreatment 2015. https://www.acf.hhs.gov/sites/default/files/cb/cm2015.pdf. Accessed January 22, 2019.

7. Peterson C, Curtis C, Klevens J. The economics burden of child maltreatment in the United States, 2015. *Child Abuse Negl.* 2018;86:178-183.

8. Finkelhor D. Current information on the scope and nature of child sexual abuse. *Future Child.* 1994;4(2):31-53.

9. World Health Organization. Gender and health in disasters. World Health Organization Web site. https://www.who.int/gender/other_health/genderdisasters.pdf. Published July 2002. Accessed January 22, 2019.

10. Barnett OW, Miller-Perrin CL, Perrin RD. *Family Violence Across the Lifespan: An Introduction.* Thousand Oaks, CA: Sage Publications; 1997.

11. Greenbaum J, Crawford-Jakubiak JE; Committee on Child Abuse and Neglect. Child sex trafficking and commercial sexual exploitation: health care needs of victims. *Pediatrics.* 2015;135(3)566-574.

12. Finkelhor D, Mitchell KJ, Wolak J. Online victimization: what youth tell us. In: Cooper SW, Estes RJ, Giardino AP, Kellogg ND, Vieth VI, eds. *Medical, Legal, and Social Science Aspects of Child Sexual Exploitation: A Comprehensive Review of Pornography, Prostitution, and Internet Crimes.* Vol 1. St. Louis, MO: STM Learning, Inc.; 2005:437-467.

13. Palusci VJ, Vandervort FE, Lewis JM. Does changing mandated reporting laws improve child maltreatment reporting in large U.S. counties? *Child Youth Serv Rev.* 2016;66:170-179.

14. Berliner L, Elliott DM. Sexual abuse of children. In: Myers JEB, Berliner L, Briere J, Hendrix CT, Jenny C, Reid TA, eds. *The APSAC Handbook on Child Maltreatment.* Thousand Oaks, CA: Sage Publications; 2002:55-78.

15. Tyler KA. Social and emotional outcomes of childhood sexual abuse: a review of recent research. *Aggress Violent Behav.* 2002;7(6):567-589.

16. Dube SR, Anda RF, Whitfield CL, et al. Long-term consequences of childhood sexual abuse by gender of victim. *Am J Prev Med.* 2005;28(5):430-438.

17. Goodkind S, Ng I, Sarri RC. The impact of sexual abuse in the lives of young women involved or at risk of involvement with the juvenile justice system. *Violence Against Women.* 2006;12(5):456-477.

18. Whiffen VE, MacIntosh HB. Mediators of the link between childhood sexual abuse and emotional distress: a critical review. *Trauma Violence Abuse.* 2005;6(1):24-39.

19. Feerick MM, Snow KL. The relationships between childhood sexual abuse, social anxiety, and symptoms of posttraumatic stress disorder in women. *J Fam Violence.* 2005;20(6):409-419.

20. Satcher D. The surgeon general's call to action to promote sexual health and responsible sexual behavior. https://www.ncbi.nlm.nih.gov/books/NBK44216/pdf/Bookshelf_NBK44216.pdf. Published July 9, 2001. Accessed January 22, 2019.

21. Grunbaum JA, Kann L, Kinchen S, et al. Youth risk behavior surveillance—United States, 2003 [published corrections appear in *MMWR Morb Mortal Wkly Rep.* 2004;53(24):536 and *MMWR Morb Mortal Wkly Rep.* 2005;54(24):608]. *MMWR Surveill Summ.* 2004;53(2):1-96.

22. Bronfenbrenner U. Toward an experimental ecology of human development. *Am Psychol.* 1977;32(7):513-531.

23. National Sexual Violence Resource Center. A national resource directory & handbook preventing child sexual abuse. National Sexual Violence Resource Center Web site. https://www.nsvrc.org/publications/nsvrc-publications/national-resource-directory-handbook-preventing-child-sexual-abuse. Updated September 2006. Accessed January 22, 2019.

24. American Academy of Pediatrics. The resilience project. American Academy of Pediatrics Web site. https://www.aap.org/en-us/advocacy-and-policy/aap-health-initiatives/resilience/Pages/Resilience-Project.aspx. Accessed January 22, 2019.

25. Snyder HN; US Department of Justice, Office of Justice Programs, Bureau of Justice Statistics. Sexual assault of young children as reported to law enforcement: victim, incident, and offender characteristics. https://www.bjs.gov/content/pub/pdf/saycrle.pdf. Published July 2000. Accessed January 22, 2019.

26. Mullen PE, Martin JL, Anderson JC, Romans SE, Herbison GP. Childhood sexual abuse and mental health in adult life. *Br J Psychiatry.* 1993;163:721-732.

27. Rew L, Esparza D. Barriers to disclosure among sexually abused male children: implications for nursing practice. *J Child Adolesc Psychiatr Ment Health Nurs.* 1990;3(4):120-127.

28. Gomes-Schwartz B, Horowitz JM, Cardarelli AP. *Child Sexual Abuse: The Initial Effects.* Newbury Park, CA: Sage Publications; 1990.

29. Anderson J, Martin J, Mullen P, Romans S, Herbison P. Prevalence of childhood sexual abuse experiences in a community sample of women. *J Am Acad Child Adolesc Psychiatry.* 1993;32(5):911-919.

30. Finkelhor D, Hotaling G, Lewis IA, Smith C. Sexual abuse in a national survey of adult men and women: prevalence, characteristics, and risk factors. *Child Abuse Negl.* 1990;14(1):19-28.

31. Palusci VJ, Cox EO, Cyrus TA, Heartwell SW, Vandervort FE, Pott ES. Medical assessment and legal outcome in child sexual abuse. *Arch Pediatr Adolesc Med.* 1999;153(4):388-392.

32. National Center for Disease Control and Prevention. Sexual violence in youth: findings from the 2012 National Intimate Partner and Sexual Violence Survey. https://www.cdc.gov/violenceprevention/pdf/2012FindingsonSVinYouth-508.pdf. Accessed January 22, 2019.

33. Romans SE, Martin JL, Anderson JC, O'Shea ML, Mullen PE. Factors that mediate between child sexual abuse and adult psychological outcome. *Psychol Med.* 1995;25(1):127-142.

34. Bolen RM. Child sexual abuse: prevention or promotion? *Soc Work.* 2003;48(2):174-185.

35. Child Welfare Information Gateway. Sexual abuse prevention programs. Child Welfare Information Gateway Web site. https://www.childwelfare.gov/topics/preventing/prevention-programs/sexualabuse/. Accessed August January 22, 2019.

36. Palusci VJ, Ilardi M. Risk factors and services to reduce child sexual abuse recurrence. *Child Maltreat.* In press.

37. Jensen TK, Gulbrandsen W, Mossige S, Reichelt S, Tjersland OA. Reporting possible sexual abuse: a qualitative study on children's perspectives and the context for disclosure. *Child Abuse Negl.* 2005;29(12):1395-1413.

38. Staller KM, Nelson-Gardell D. "A burden in your heart": lessons of disclosure from female preadolescent and adolescent survivors of sexual abuse. *Child Abuse Negl.* 2005;29(12):1415-1432.

39. Kelly P, Koh J, Thompson JM. Diagnostic findings in alleged sexual abuse: symptoms have no predictive value. *J Paediatr Child Health.* 2006;42(3):112-117.

40. Palusci VJ, Cyrus TA. Reaction to videocolposcopy in the assessment of child sexual abuse. *Child Abuse Negl.* 2001;25(11):1535-1546.

41. Finkel MA. An ounce of prevention or two...providing anticipatory guidance regarding personal space and privacy: a commentary. *Child Abuse Negl.* 2013;37(9):631-632.

42. Hanson RF, Adams CS. Childhood sexual abuse: identification, screening, and treatment recommendations in primary care settings. *Prim Care.* 2016;43(2):313-326.

43. Palusci VJ. Disability and the epidemiology of child abuse and neglect. In: Palusci VJ, Nazer D, Greydanus DE, Merrick J, eds. *Child Abuse: Children with Disabilities.* Hauppauge, NY: Nova Science Publishers; 2017:39-68.

44. Mandell DS, Walrath CM, Manteuffel B, Sgro G, Pinto-Martin JA. The prevalence and correlates of abuse among children with autism served in comprehensive community-based mental health settings. *Child Abuse Negl.* 2005;29(21):1359-1372.

45. Andrews AB, Veronen LJ. Sexual assault and people with disabilities. *J Soc Work Hum Sex.* 1993;8(2):137-159.

46. Nosek MA. Sexual abuse of women with physical disabilities. In: Krotoski DM, Nosek MA, Turk MA, eds. *Women with Physical Disabilities: Achieving and Maintaining Health and Well-Being.* Baltimore, MD: Paul H. Brookes Publishing; 1996:153-173.

47. Kelly L. Pornography and child sexual abuse. In: Itzin C, ed. *Pornography: Women, Violence and Civil Liberties: A Radical New View.* Oxford, England: Oxford University Press; 1993:113-123.

48. Briere J, Runtz M. Differential adult symptomatology associated with three types of child abuse histories. *Child Abuse Negl.* 1990;14(3):357-364.

49. Fergusson DM, Lynskey MT, Horwood LJ. Attentional difficulties in middle childhood and psychosocial outcomes in young adulthood. *J Child Psychol Psychiatry*. 1997;38(6):633-644.

50. Fleming J, Mullen P, Bammer G. A study of potential risk factors for sexual abuse in childhood. *Child Abuse Negl*. 1997;21(1):49-58.

51. Darkness to Light. Child sexual abuse statistics: the issue of child sexual abuse. Darkness to Light Web site. https://www.d2l.org/wp-content/uploads/2017/01/all_statistics_20150619.pdf. Accessed January 17, 2019

52. Plummer CA. The history of child sexual abuse prevention: a practitioner's perspective. *J Child Sex Abus*. 1998;7(4):77-95.

53. McCurdy K, Daro D. Child maltreatment: a national survey of reports and fatalities. *J Interpers Violence*. 1994;9(1):75-94.

54. Miller-Perrin CL, Wurtele SK. The child sexual abuse prevention movement: a critical analysis of primary and secondary approaches. *Clin Psychol Rev*. 1988;8(3):313-329.

55. Finkelhor D, Asdigian N, Dziuba-Leatherman J. The effectiveness of victimization prevention instruction: an evaluation of children's responses to actual threats and assaults. *Child Abuse Negl*. 1995;19(2):141-153.

56. Plummer CA. Child sexual abuse prevention is appropriate and successful. In: Gelles RJ, Loseke DR, Cavanaugh MM, eds. *Current Controversies in Family Violence*. Newbury Park, CA: Sage Publications; 2004:257-270.

57. Reppucci ND, Haugaard JJ, Antonishak J. Is there empirical evidence to support the effectiveness of child sexual abuse prevention programs? In: Gelles RJ, Loseke DR, Cavanaugh MM, eds. *Current Controversies in Family Violence*. Newbury Park, CA: Sage Publications; 2004;271-284.

58. Edwards SM, Lohman JSS. The impact of "moral panic" on professional behavior in cases of child sex abuse: an international perspective. *J Child Sex Abus*. 1994;3(1):103-126.

59. Schreiber N. Interviewing techniques in sexual abuse cases: a comparison of a daycare abuse case with normal abuse cases. *Swiss J Psychol*. 2000;59(3):196-206.

60. Deblinger E, Thakkar-Kolar RR, Berry EJ, Schroeder CM. Caregivers' efforts to educate their children about child sexual abuse: a replication study. *Child Maltreat*. 2010;15(1):91-100.

61. Elliot M, Browne K, Kilcoyne J. Child sexual abuse prevention: what offenders tell us. *Child Abuse Negl*. 1995;19(5):579-594.

62. Långström N, Enebrink P, Laurén EM, Lindblom J, Werkö S, Hanson RK. Preventing sexual abusers of children from reoffending: systematic review of medical and psychological interventions. *BMJ*. 2013;347:f4630.

63. Mian M, Collin-Vézina D. Adopting a public health approach to addressing child sexual abuse and exploitation. *Child Abuse Negl*. 2017;66:152-154.

64. Finkelhor D, Jones LM; US Department of Justice, Office of Justice Programs. Explanations for the decline in child sexual abuse cases. https://www.ncjrs.gov/pdffiles1/ojjdp/199298.pdf. Published January 2004. Accessed January 22, 2019.

65. Gibson L, Leitenberg H. Child sexual abuse prevention programs: do they decrease the occurrence of child sexual abuse? *Child Abuse Negl.* 2000;24(9):1115-1125.

66. National Children's Alliance. National initiatives. National Children's Alliance Web site. http://www.nationalchildrensalliance.org/national-initiatives/. Accessed January 23, 2019.

67. Prevent Child Abuse Iowa. Iowa child sexual abuse prevention and treatment resource. Prevent Child Abuse Iowa Web site. http://www.pcaiowa.org/prevention/sexual-abuse-prevention/. Accessed January 17, 2019.

68. New Jersey Task Force on Child Abuse and Neglect. New Jersey standards for prevention programs: building success through family support. State of New Jersey Web site. https://www.state.nj.us/dcf/news/reportsnewsletters/taskforce/Standards.for.Prevention.Programs.pdf. Accessed January 22, 2019.

69. Plummer CA. Prevention of child sexual abuse: a survey of 87 programs. *Violence Vict.* 2001;16(5):575-588.

70. Berrick JD. Parental involvement in child abuse prevention training: what do they learn? *Child Abuse Negl.* 1988;12(4):543-553.

71. Elrod JM, Rubin RH. Parental involvement in sexual abuse prevention education. *Child Abuse Negl.* 1993;17(4):527-538.

72. Reppucci ND, Jones LM, Cook SL. Involving parents in child sexual abuse prevention programs. *J Child Fam Stud.* 1994;3(2):137-142.

73. Finkelhor D. *Child Sexual Abuse: New Research and Theory.* New York, NY: The Free Press; 1984.

74. Wurtele SK. Comprehensiveness and collaboration: key ingredients of an effective public health approach to preventing child sexual abuse. *Sex Abuse.* 1999;11(4):323-325.

75. Wilson CG, Golub S. Sexual abuse prevention programs for preschool children: what do parents prefer? *Psychol Rep.* 1993;73(3 pt 1):812-814.

76. Abel GG, Harlow N. *The Stop Child Molestation Book: What Ordinary People Can Do in Their Everyday Lives to Save Three Million Children.* Bloomington, IN: Xlibris; 2001.

77. Stop It Now. Let's talk: speaking up to prevent child sexual abuse. Stop It Now! Web site. https://www.stopitnow.org/sites/default/files/documents/files/lets_talk.pdf. Accessed January 22, 2019.

78. Rispens J, Aleman A, Goudena PP. Prevention of child sexual victimization: a meta-analysis of school programs. *Child Abuse Negl.* 1997;21(10):975-987.

79. Finkelhor D, Strapko N. Sexual abuse prevention education: a review of evaluation studies. In: Willis DJ, Holden EW, Rosenberg M, eds. *Prevention of Child Maltreatment: Developmental and Ecological Perspectives.* New York, NY: Wiley & Sons; 1991:150-167.

80. MacMillan HL, MacMillan JH, Offord DR, Griffith L, MacMillan A. Primary prevention of child physical abuse and neglect: a critical review: part I. *J Child Psychol Psychiatry.* 1994;35(5):835-856.

81. Palusci VJ. Preventing maltreatment in children with disabilities. In: Palusci VJ, Nazer D, Greydanus DE, Merrick J, eds. *Child Abuse: Children with Disabilities.* Hauppauge, NY: Nova Science Publishers; 2017:235-267.

82. Rheingold AA, Zajac K, Chapman JE, et al. Child sexual abuse prevention training for childcare professionals: an independent multi-site randomized controlled trial of Stewards of Children. *Prev Sci.* 2015;16(3):374-385.

83. Generation Five. Transformative justice docs. Generation Five Web site. http://www.generationfive.org/resources/transformative-justice-documents/. Accessed January 23, 2019.

84. Finkelhor D, Turner HA, Shattuck A, Hamby SL. Prevalence of childhood exposure to violence, crime, and abuse: results from the National Survey of Children's Exposure to Violence. *JAMA Pediatr.* 2015;169(8):746-754.

85. National Center for Missing and Exploited Children. NetSmartz home page. NetSmartz Web site. https://www.netsmartz.org/Home. Accessed January 23, 2019.

86. Anderson C. Sexual abuse prevention with organizations. Paper presented at: Imagine: The National Conference on Sexual Abuse Prevention; August 10-12, 2005; Huntsville, AL.

87. Saul J, Audage NC; Centers for Disease Control and Prevention. Preventing child sexual abuse within youth-serving organizations: getting started on policies and procedures. https://www.cdc.gov/violenceprevention/pdf/preventingchildsexualabuse-a.pdf. Accessed January 22, 2019.

88. Committee on Practice and Ambulatory Medicine. Policy statement—use of chaperones during the physical examination of the pediatric patient. *Pediatrics.* 2011;127(5):991-993.

89. Helfer RE. A review of the literature on the prevention of child abuse and neglect. *Child Abuse Negl.* 1982;6(3):251-261.

90. Flaherty EG, Sege RD, Griffith J, et al. From suspicion of physical child abuse to reporting: primary care clinician decision-making. *Pediatrics.* 2008;122(3):611-619.

91. Hamberger L, Patel D. Why health care professionals are reluctant to intervene in cases of ongoing domestic abuse. In: Kendall-Tackett KA, ed. *Health Consequences of Abuse in the Family: A Clinical Guide for Evidence-Based Practice.* Washington, DC: American Psychological Association; 2004;63-80.

92. Trepper T, Barrett MJ. *Systemic Treatment of Incest: A Therapeutic Handbook.* New York, NY: Brunner/Mazel; 1989.

93. Dubowitz H. Preventing child neglect and physical abuse: a role for pediatricians. *Pediatr Rev.* 2002;23(6):191-196.

94. Palusci VJ, Haney ML. Strategies to prevent child maltreatment and integration into practice. *APSAC Advisor.* 2010;8-17.

95. Sege RD, Hatmaker-Flanigan E, De Vos E, Levin-Goodman R, Spivak H. Anticipatory guidance and violence prevention: results from family and pediatrician focus groups. *Pediatrics.* 2006;117(2):455-463.

96. Bays J, Chadwick D. Medical diagnosis of the sexually abused child. *Child Abuse Negl.* 1993;17(1):91-110.

97. Rieser M. Recantation in child sexual abuse cases. *Child Welfare.* 1991;70(6):611-621.

98. Sorenson T, Snow B. How children tell: the process of disclosure in child sexual abuse. *Child Welfare.* 1991;70(1):3-15.

99. Myers JEB. *The Backlash: Child Protection Under Fire.* Thousand Oaks, CA: Sage Publications; 1994.

100. Everson MD, Hunter WM, Runyon DK, Edelsohn GA, Coulter ML. Maternal support following disclosure of incest. *Am J Orthopsychiatry.* 1989;59(2):197-207.

101. Goodman R. A modified version of the Rutter Parent Questionnaire including extra items on children's strengths: a research note. *J Child Psychol Psychiatry.* 1994;35(8):1483-1494.

102. Dubowitz H, Black MM, Cox CE, et al. Father involvement and children's functioning at age 6 years: a multisite study. *Child Maltreat.* 2001;6(4):300-309.

103. Trowbridge MJ, Sege RD, Olson L, O'Connor K, Flaherty E, Spivak H. Intentional injury management and prevention in pediatric practice: results from 1998 and 2003 American Academy of Pediatrics Periodic Surveys. *Pediatrics.* 2005;116(4):996-1000.

104. Diaz A, Manigat M. The healthcare provider's role in the disclosure of sexual abuse: the medical interview as a gateway to disclosure. *Child Health Care.* 1999;28(2):141-149.

105. American Academy of Pediatrics. Connected kids: safe, strong, secure. American Academy of Pediatrics Web site. https://www.aap.org/en-us/advocacy-and-policy/aap-health-initiatives/Pages/Connected-Kids.aspx. Accessed January 22, 2019.

106. American Professional Society on the Abuse of Children. Practice guidelines: integrating prevention into the work of child maltreatment professionals. https://apsac.memberclicks.net/assets/documents/PracticeGuidelines/integrating%20prevention%20into%20the%20work%20of%20child%20maltreatment%20professionals%20.pdf. Accessed January 22, 2019.

107. Pulido ML, Dauber S, Tully BA, Hamilton P, Smith MJ, Freeman K. Knowledge gains following a child sexual abuse prevention program among urban students: a cluster-randomized evaluation. *Am J Public Health.* 2015;105(7):1344-1350.

108. Crisci G. Youth sexually abusing youth. Paper presented at: Imagine: The National Conference on Child Sexual Abuse Prevention; August 2006; Florence, AL.

109. Plummer CA. Non-abusive mothers of sexually abused children: the role of rumination in maternal outcomes. *J Child Sex Abus.* 2006;15(2):103-122.

Index

A

Note: Page numbers followed by 'f' and 't' refer to figures and tables respectively.

C

D

H

I

J

K

L

M

N

O

P

Q

R

S

T

U

V

W

Y

Z

www.ingramcontent.com/pod-product-compliance
Lightning Source LLC
LaVergne TN
LVHW060014210926
848481LV00013B/3707
9781936590742